KINESIOLOGY | THE SCIENCE OF MOVEMENT

KINESIOLOGY | THE SCIENCE OF MOVEMENT

JOHN PISCOPO, Ed. D., A.C.S.M.
State University of New York at Buffalo, New York

JAMES A. BALEY, Ph.D., F.A.C.S.M.
Jersey City State College, New Jersey

John Wiley & Sons
New York   Chichester   Brisbane   Toronto

Cover and Text Design
by Laura C. Ierardi
Anatomical Illustrations
by Steve Klose

Library of Congress Cataloging in Publication Data:

Piscopo, John, 1922-
 Kinesiology, the science of movement.

 Includes index.
 1. Kinesiology.   I. Baley, James A., joint
author.   II. Title.

QP303.P53   612'.76   80-21545
ISBN 0-471-03483-5

Printed in the United States of America

10 9 8 7 6 5 4 3 2 1

DEDICATION

To my wife Carolyn and daughters Carol, Nancy and Annette

J. Piscopo

To my wife Estelle and sons Jim, Tim, Gary, Scot and Brian

J. A. Baley

FOREWORD

In the last twenty years there has taken place a tremendous shifting of attitudes in the scientific community and the lay public toward the role of physical activity in basic education, human development, the maintenance of physical fitness and of health status, and the treatment of a multitude of disease conditions, most significant of which include patients with asthma, certain psychiatric disorders, and coronary heart disease. Despite the proliferation of knowledge about physical activity and its required regular performance throughout life, the emphasis of most investigators and writers has been directed toward issues of cardiorespiratory fitness and overall rehabilitation. The current textbook does a great deal to complement these important contributions through its skilled presentations of kinesiological topics, particularly as they relate to the prevention of injury among young athletes and extend to the aging process of the mature adult. Of all factors except the overt presence of disease, these two, more than any other single set of factors, prevent and inhibit more people from entering or maintaining a lifelong program of physical activity and fitness. If physical activity is important to a modern lifestyle, then those who promote it, supervise it, and participate in it must have a fundamental knowledge of how the body works and functions and of how to minimize and prevent injury. In addition, the modifications to physical activity required by the maturing process must be well understood.

In this textbook, Piscopo and Baley offer a comprehensive overview of kinesiology in which the traditional basic anatomical, mechanical and neuromuscular views are integrated into the more contemporary concepts of functional and applicative kinesiology.

The book should provide a fine foundation of the science of kinesiology, giving basic knowledge and understanding upon which students in the health science disciplines can successfully build.

John Naughton, M.D.
Dean
SUNY/Buffalo
School of Medicine
Past President, American College of
    Sports Medicine
Director, National Exercise and
    Heart Disease Project

PREFACE

This book is intended to serve as a text for undergraduate students in physical education and the allied health professions who are concerned with basic scientific information and understanding of human motion. The main thrust of the subject matter is the practical application of motion concepts to everyday motor tasks and sport skills.

The scope of this book differs from the traditional kinesiology text in which emphasis is limited to anatomical, neuromuscular, and mechanical aspects of motion involving children and youth. In view of the current and projected shifts in demographic data reflecting greater numbers of older persons in our society, we have included a comprehensive analysis of human aging and motor performance. A section dealing with exercise prescription presents a set of concise indications and contraindications for persons over age 50. Such topics as *aging* and body balance, agility, flexibility, physique, and body composition changes — all of which affect mobility and motor performance — will be of special concern to persons working with older people.

We have considered the study of kinesiology in its broad context. Topical areas have been included for students engaged in the study and analysis of movement, irrespective of their professional orientation. For example, students interested in *kinanthropometry* (relationship of size and shape of the body to motor performance) will find the topics on somatotype and its influence upon physical performance of interest.

The physical therapist and adapted physical education specialist will find the presentation on applied anatomy with illustrated drawings useful in analyzing, correcting, and preparing specific exercises and activities for individuals with limited physical and motor performance capabilities. We have discussed the structural, articular, and muscular aspects in considerable detail. We have also discussed the axial and appendicular skeleton, muscles, and ligaments including the upper and lower extremities, spinal column, thorax, and hip joint, giving particular attention to the knee articulation. These structures have been graphically drawn, showing relationships between anatomical shapes and forms and human movement.

Certain essential neuromuscular considerations basic to the study of human motion have been included in Part I. Students interested in the effects of neural, physiological, and motor learning parameters will find such topics as conditioned reflex, proprioception, reciprocal innervation and inhibition, motor unit, and kinesthesia presented with examples and illustrations of how these mechanisms control movement patterns.

Part II is devoted to the biomechanical elements of human movement. Descriptions and applications of mechanical principles emphasizing the effects of internal and external forces upon the body are examined. Such terms as vectors, scalars, kinematics, kinetics, statics, dynamics, laws of motion, friction, buoyancy, balance and equilibrium, and linear and angular motions are explored and explained. We have attempted to minimize the inclusion of complex equations and formulas. In certain sections, mathematical relationships serve as examples or clarify our discussion. Mechanical principles and concepts have been drawn from daily life skills, physical medicine, physical rehabilitation, sports medicine, and athletics.

Throughout this text, we have presented concepts at the beginning of each chapter followed by detailed descriptions and applications of our stated concept. The basic units are written in concise form. Each precept was selected and constructed in such a way as to encourage the reader to further pursue factual information about the concept initially stated. For example, the concept stated in Chapter 5 declares: "During rotary motion, the axis may lie either within the body or outside the body." The curious reader may wonder how this mechanical fact happens. The student soon discovers by reading the text that definitions, analysis, and interpretations are provided under "Motion Descriptions." The concept is then reinforced by examples that demonstrate the axis of rotation within and outside the body. Finally, summations are presented at the end of each chapter, which again reinforce learning by allowing the student to review and synthesize the initial concepts and details of the subject matter found between the concepts and summary.

Part III of this textbook deals with applied kinesiology. The material on gymnastics and aquatics is drawn, not only from pertinent research, but from our teaching and coaching background at several colleges and universities including the southern and eastern regions of the United States, particularly at Northwestern State University of Louisiana, The University of Southern Mississippi, Jersey City State College, and the State University of New York at Buffalo.

Chapter 11 contains kinesiological principles and a recommended skill analysis format for badminton, wrestling, cycling, baseball, and racquetball. In our individual and team sport analyses, we have attempted to emphasize how these principles are used in the execution of each athletic skill.

Common problems in posture and body mechanics are presented in Chapter 12. Persons who work with students manifesting body mechanics deficits will find the section on remedial exercises helpful in program development and instruction.

The application of kinesiological principles to injury prevention is discussed in Chapter 13. Students interested in coaching football, basketball, skiing, ice hockey, baseball, soccer, gymnastics and swimming will find valuable information and suggestions concerning the reduction of sport injuries.

A new procedure called *video-tape-laboratory* (VTL) is described with application of mechanical principles from selected sports. A VTL model is presented with specific instructions for developing a laboratory format that can be used in other physical activities.

The final chapter contains a review and digest of the material presented within the body of the book. It is hoped that this book, which is based upon our experiential background, experience and research will provide a sound foundation for all persons concerned with the analysis and study of movement.

John Piscopo
James A. Baley

ACKNOWLEDGMENTS

The assistance of many people was required in the preparation of this textbook.

This book could never have been written without the support, hardwork and patience of our wives. We are gratefully indebted to Carolyn and Estelle who spent countless hours typing multiple drafts and the final edition of the manuscript.

We especially thank the many students and colleagues who helped us in gathering materials for this book. An attempt to name each individual will surely result in the omission of a deserving person. However, certain names and organizations must be mentioned. We extend our sincere thanks and gratitude to our former and present students and colleagues who assisted us in securing photographs or participating as models. Appreciation is expressed to Glenn Sunby, Dick Criley, and Helen Weber for permission to use photos of various skills that illustrate the applications of kinesiologic principles.

We thank the following persons, organizations and institutions for allowing us to photograph their students and athletes; Don Wieder's Gym, East Brunswick, N.J.; Erie County Health Care Center for Children, E. J. Meyer Memorial Hospital, School #84, Board of Education, Buffalo, N.Y.; Niagara Community College and Niagara Wheatfield High School, Sanborn, N.Y.; Ken-Ton YMCA, Tonawanda, N.Y.; Al Stumpf of the School of Gymnastics, Buffalo, N.Y.; student athletes at Jersey City State College, N.J., Northwestern State University, Natchitoches, La., and State University of New York at Buffalo, N.Y. We wish to acknowledge the fine cooperation of publishers and authors for allowing us to use their illustrations.

We also appreciate the expertise and help of our photographers Marcia Garcia, Tom Jakabs, and Francis Grimmer and of Richard Macakanja and his staff of the Educational Communications Center, State University of New York at Buffalo for their splendid reproductions of drawings and photoprints. A special thanks is extended to Steve Klose and Dan Paterka for their professional excellence in drawing our anatomical illustrations.

Appreciation is expressed to Donald E. Nichols, Professor of Art, State University of New York at Buffalo for his assistance with the cover design and Paul Caputo, Assistant Librarian, Health Sciences Library, State University of New York at Buffalo for his help with the index. Finally, we especially thank the staff of the Health Sciences Library of the State University of New York at Buffalo for their help and cooperation in securing the data based materials and research references.

J. P.
J. A. B.

CONTENTS

PART 3 APPLIED ASPECTS OF KINESIOLOGY 315

9 ANALYSIS OF SELECTED TUMBLING AND GYMNASTIC SKILLS 316

10 ANALYSIS OF SELECTED AQUATIC SKILLS 365

1 INTRODUCTION: AN OVERVIEW

DEFINITIONS AND INTERPRETATIONS

Kinesiology has been an elusive term. Anatomists have identified and interpreted the word with roots in body structure and functioning of the muscular and joint articulation systems. Physiologists have often associated kinesiology with exercise, physiology, biochemistry; and the effect of body composition, space, and size upon movement. Mathematicians and engineers approached the study of movement through the investigation of mechanics and the application of physical laws to the biological functioning of the human organism. Medical personnel often identified kinesiology as an appendage or branch of physiology. Pedagogical kinesiologists are concerned with scientific principles about human movement that enhance the teaching process, and they relate to the behavioral sciences, as well as to the biological health fields. In recent years, the term *biomechanics* has been used interchangeably with kinesiology. Measurement and evaluation specialists and research-oriented personnel tend to adopt biomechanics as the central core of subject matter in kinesiology. It is obvious to the student that basic terms need definitions and clarification.

Kinesiology is the science of movement dealing with the interrelationship of anatomy, neuromuscular physiology, and mechanics.

Biomechanics is a branch of kinesiology that deals with the investigation and application of mechanics to the human organism. The elements of mechanics deal with the action of forces on bodies and with motion, comprised of kinetics, statics, and kinematics.

The authors view kinesiology as a study of the anatomical, neuromuscular-physiological, and mechanical phenomena that underlie human motor performance.

HISTORICAL PERSPECTIVE

Early Pioneers

Perhaps the foundations of kinesiology may be attributed to the great philosopher *Aristotle* (384–322 B.C.), who wrote:

> . . . *For that which jumps performs that movement by pressing both on its own upper part and on that which is beneath its feet. . . . Hence athletes jump farther if they have weights in their hands than if they have not, and runners run faster if they swing their arms, for in the extension of the arms there is a kind of leaning upon the hands and wrists.*[1]

The writings of Aristotle in ancient Greece provided a fundamental understanding of the mechanics of walking by applying logical analysis. For example, he deduced that man must be both biped and have the upper part of his body lighter, and the lower part heavier, in order to walk erect. From this basic logic arose the scientific phenomenon explaining the body's center of gravity, laws of gravity, and principles of leverage. Aristotle observed and studied animals walking, jumping, and flying. His conclusions about flexion and extension of jointed limbs, as animals bend and stretch, led to the present-day concept that rotary motion of bones around their axes creates translatory motion of the whole body.

Archimedes (287-212 B.C.) established the basis for densitometry (underwater weighing), whereby the volume of the body is determined from its displacement of water. His principles are continually used to determine body composition and the effects of fluid mechanics on swimming efficiency.

Claudius Galen (A.D. 131-201), a physician from ancient Rome, specialized in anatomy and physiology. Galen attended to Roman gladiators and, through his medical writings, was the first to describe such terms as *synarthrosis* and *amphiarthrosis* relevant to joint actions. Galen is credited with relating the discipline of anatomy to the science of movement.

Florentine Leonardo da Vinci (1452-1519) lived during the Renaissance. Da Vinci's talents embraced the fields of art and science. This scientist is popularly remembered by his famous painting of *Man in Square and Circle* (Figure 1.1), depicting two positions of the human male form structured within a square and circle mathematical model.

Da Vinci expounded such statements as, ". . . Nothing whatever can be moved by itself but its motion is affected through another; this is force, and an object offers as much resistance to the air as the air does to the object."[2] He offered examples that were later called by Newton the principle of inertia and the law of action and reaction. Da Vinci also

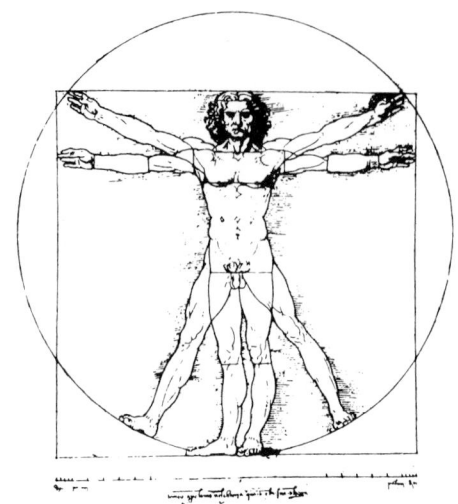

Figure 1.1 "Man in Square and Circle," by Leonardo da Vinci. From Asmussen, E., "Movement of Man and Study of Man in Motion: A Scanning Review of the Development of Biomechanics," in Paavo V. Komi (Ed.), **Biomechanics V-A**, University Park Press, Baltimore, Maryland, 1976, p. 39. Reprinted with permission.

contributed to the understanding of basic balance concepts involving the center of gravity in relation to its base of support in the human frame.

Although Galileo (1564-1643) is best known for his work in astronomy, his discoveries added to the body of knowledge surrounding balance and equilibrium, phenomena governing falling bodies, and laws of leverage. His demonstration that acceleration of a falling body is not proportional to its weight is a classic in the area of mechanics.[3]

Another Italian, Giovanni Alfonso Borelli (1608-1679), a pupil of Galileo, is credited with applying basic laws of mechanics and mathematical principles to muscular performance. Borelli's theories investigated the effect of lever action, air resistance, and water resistance upon various forms of locomotion, including walking, running, and swimming.

Sir Isaac Newton (1642-1727) of England presented the three basic laws of motion in his greatest work, *Principia Mathematica Philosophiae Naturalis*. He is also credited with the concept entailing parallelogram of forces. These basic mechanical precepts are presented not only in this text but in others on kinesiology, affirming the lasting value of Newton's contribution to the science of kinesiology.

Guillaume B. A. Duchenne (1806-1875) is considered the "father of medical electrophysiology." Duchenne applied electricity for the systematic determination of the dynamics of intact skeletal muscles. Duchenne applied an electrical stimulator to the skin as a substitute for a motor nerve and caused muscles to contract irrespective of the subject's control. His procedure became the basis of modern electrostimulation methods utilized in electromyography. Duchenne's book, *Physiologie des Mouvements*, is considered a classic text in the field of electrokinesiology.

Muybridge (1821-1904) and Marey (1830-1904) pioneered early moving picture photography. These researchers studied photographic techniques and recorded activities of man and animals. Muybridge used a number of cameras, equipped with quick-acting shutters, to take a series of instantaneous photographs of the gait of horses in 1878.[4] Marey followed Muybridge by developing a "chronophotography on a ribbon," which described various human and animal movements recording such motions as swimming fish, frogs; flying of birds; and walking, running, and swimming of man.[5] These men established photographic techniques as a bona fide modality in the analysis of motion.

The classic work of Barune and Fischer (1889) using frozen cadavers set the pattern for determining weights and center of mass of body segments. Their investigations provided initial methods in estimating the magnitude and location of gravitational forces acting on the human form.

Twentieth Century Notables

Many outstanding researchers and kinesiologists have contributed to today's sophisticated level of the science of human movement. Detailed enumeration of dedicated contributors is beyond the scope of this book; however, several individuals, in the view of the authors, have been preeminent. A brief sketch of these professional workers is presented.

A. V. Hill of England studied the efficiency of muscular work and contributed to the understanding of basic physiological changes that occur in work physiology and movement efficiency. T. K. Cureton of Springfield College and the University of Illinois has conducted hundreds of studies in track and field, swimming, and physical fitness. His work is continually cited by contemporary researchers and kinesiologists. Such names as Frances Hellebrandt of the University of Wisconsin and Arthur Steindler of State University of Iowa have had a profound effect upon advancing the scientific knowledge in body mechanics and medical kinesiology. Their work is frequently cited in this text. C. H. McCloy of Iowa left his mark as an expert in the analysis of sport activity.

Other notables, including Katherine Wells, formerly of Wellesley; Marion Broer of the University of Washington; John Cooper, Indiana University; James Hay, University of Iowa; Richard Nelson, Pennsylvania State University; Ruth Glassow, of the University of Wisconsin; Stanley Plagenhoef, University of Massachusetts; Kathryn Luttgens, Boston-Bouvé College of Northeastern University; Geofry Dyson, Winchester College of England; P. V. Karpovich of Springfield College; Marlene Adrian, Washington State University; Ernest Jokl of the University of Kentucky; Gladys Scott, State University of Iowa; J. V. Basmajian of Emory University; and John Bunn, formerly of Springfield College, have contributed valuable knowledge in their specialties within kinesiology, which has been a truly eclectic, interdisciplinary subject from the fields of anatomy, neuromuscular physiology, and physics. The subdiscipline of biomechanics is emerging as a new focus of attention in the analysis of movement. Annual international meetings and symposia held throughout the world have adopted the title *Biomechanics*; these gatherings include papers and reports of many specialists from the broad field of kinesiology such as muscle metabolism, electromyography, neuromuscular control, orthopedics, muscular strength and endurance, gait, anthropometrics, motion in sports, instrumentation, and motor learning. Each of these specialties has a common denominator: facilitation of a better scientific understanding of how man moves in work, play, and sport. The student is referred to a review of research by Atwater,[6] which deals with differences and trends surrounding the study of kinesiology.

FUNCTIONAL APPROACH TO THE STUDY OF KINESIOLOGY

What skills and competencies should a student of physical education or kinesiology be expected to exhibit? What are the basics in the study of kinesiology? Where should emphasis be placed regarding the quantitative skills in the analysis of movement? How important is applied anatomy in motion analysis? These queries are frequently asked by the practitioner and consumer of scientific information about human movement.

A recent national conference titled *Kinesiology: A National Conference on Teaching*, which was attended by many professional kinesiologists, discussed issues and problems and made several recommendations for development of vital competencies for movement analysts, particularly for those individuals involved in exercise programs and sports. The following are samples of general recommendations for *exit* competencies from basic courses:[7]

1. Understand the human body as a mover
2. Design a specific exercise regimen and give reasons for the exercises
3. Know how to describe movement
4. Develop a terminology to facilitate communication with others.

Implicit in the above concepts is a sound knowledge of anatomy. We feel that emphasis should be placed upon the musculoskeletal system of the human body. Anatomy provides the essential background for the comprehension of human kinetics. *Applied anatomy* and *neuromuscular physiology* together with the application of *mechanics* furnish the student with information that the authors view as essential for the understanding of both qualitative and quantitative kinesiology. This textbook accents the conceptualized approach as typified by enumerated concepts introducing each chapter. Although we recognize that quantitative information and skills are important, particularly for those students who aspire toward further study in the subdiscipline of biomechanics, mastery of qualitative concepts is a primary first step toward the development of quantitative skills and techniques.

The Kinesiology Academy of the National Association for Sport and Physical Education of the American Alliance for Health, Physical Education, Recreation, and Dance has recently published guidelines and standards for undergraduate kinesiology. In this possibly historic work, the Academy, after a nationwide polling of teachers of kinesiology, has set forth recommended content and minimal entrance and exit competencies, facilities, and equipment needed to conduct such a course.[8] In addition to course knowledge in anatomy, muscle function, neuromuscular considerations, and mechanical aspects, the Academy has listed important competencies that focus on the application of concepts. These concerns concentrate on the improvement of performance in motor skills, the evaluation of exercises for special purposes, and the evaluation of equipment used in athletics and exercise.

Specifically, a basic level of competence is recommended in the following categories:[9]

1. The student is able to observe and describe a movement technique accurately.

2. The student is able to determine the anatomical and mechanical factors basic to the performance of an observed movement.

3. The student is able to evaluate the suitability of a performer's technique with reference to the task at hand.

4. The student is able to identify those factors that limit performance and to establish a priority for change in those factors most likely to lead to improvement in performance.

The above guidelines have served the authors as a principal criterion in the writing of this text.

MOVEMENT AND HUMAN PERFORMANCE

Movement is a universal need of mankind. Human motion pervades the daily life of all living organisms. The efficient performance of physical activities and skills depends upon the application of basic principles of applied anatomy, neuromuscular physiology, and biomechanics. Kinesiology attempts to unite these scientific disciplines for a better understanding of human motor performance.

The physical education teacher strives to improve motor skills and the concomitant values surrounding physical activity. The coach endeavors to improve and refine techniques in the performance of athletes. The activity therapist and medically oriented professional are concerned with improvement in mobility and motor skills of individuals with structural and functional limitations. The athlete is primarily concerned about "how" to perform an athletic skill in an optimum manner. Persons conducting programs for older people are concerned with ways and means of maintaining mobility and locomotion.

The authors believe these specific goals can best be attained by exploring, examining, and analyzing movement precepts and laws found in the phenomena of man in motion and derived from the study of the science of *kinesiology*.

REFERENCES

1. Braun, Genevieve L., "Kinesiology: From Aristotle to the Twentieth Century," *Research Quarterly*, 12:163–173, May, 1941.
2. *Ibid*., p. 167.
3. Rasch, Philip J., and Burke, Roger K., *Kinesiology and Applied Anatomy*, 6th ed. Philadelphia: Lea and Febiger, 1978, p. 2.
4. Braun, *op. cit.*, p. 171.
5. *Ibid*.
6. Atwater, Anne E., "Kinesiology/Biomechanics: Perspectives and Trends," *Research Quarterly for Exercise and Sport*, 51:193–218, February, 1980.
7. Hay, James (Editor), "Kinesiology: A National Conference on Teaching." *Kinesiology Newsletter*. National Association of Sport and Physical Education—AAHPER, Summer, 1977, pp. 5, 6.
8. National Association for Sport and Physical Education. Kinesiology Academy, "Guidelines and Standards for Undergraduate Kinesiology," AAHPERD, March, 1979, pp. 1–6.
9. *Ibid*., p. 5.

PART 1

ANATOMICAL, NEURAL,
PHYSIOLOGICAL, AND
MOTOR LEARNING
ASPECTS OF MOVEMENT

2

STRUCTURAL, ARTICULAR, AND MUSCULAR CONCEPTS APPLIED TO HUMAN MOVEMENT

CONCEPTS

1. Bone, although composed largely of inorganic salts, grows, develops, repairs itself, and adapts to its environment.

2. Bones are shaped to perform their assigned function most effectively.

3. Ossification of bones begins before birth and procedes from the center of the future shaft of long bones toward the ends. The process is not fully completed until about age 20 when the bony epiphyses at the ends of long bones ossify.

4. Muscles are structured to best perform the specialized functions they are assigned. The arrangement of muscle fibers, line of pull, point of insertion, length of the tendon, length of the muscle, and muscle mass vary in different muscles according to their function.

5. Skeletal muscles are arranged in groups to oppose one another and to produce opposite actions such as flexion versus extention, inward rotation versus outward rotation, and abduction versus adduction.

6. Most muscles can produce more than one type of movement. The movement produced is dependent upon the involvement of other muscles. A muscle may act as an agonist, antagonist, stabilizer, or neutralizer.

7. Ligaments bind the adjacent bones together at all articulations. The size and position of each ligament is related to the stress placed upon the area it protects.

8. The shape of several long bones and the arrangement of adjacent bones in several areas of the body is such that they act as shock absorbers.

9. The shape of several long bones and the arrangement of adjacent bones in several areas of the body are such that they position the center of weight nearer the center of the base of support.

10. Joints, where ends of adjacent bones rub against one another frequently, possess a synovial membrane that secretes synovial fluid. They also possess bursae, which release a lubricating fluid.

11. Ball and socket joints of the hip and shoulder permit a large range of movement. Soft tissues are utilized to deepen the socket, thereby decreasing the probability of dislocation.

12. The thorax is designed to permit an increase in three diameters in order to make inhalation possible.

13. The shoulder mechanism (which includes the scapulae, humeral and clavicular bones, and the glenohumeral, acromioclavicular, and sternoclavicular joints) is designed principally for mobility.

14. The relationship between the radius and ulna facilitates pronation and supination of the hand.

15. The complex movements required of the hand are made possible by a large number of bones (27) and muscles.

16. The large condyles of the femur, and the way in which they articulate with the head of the tibia, together with the numerous powerful ligaments, menisci, and powerful muscles acting upon the knee joint, make it wonderfully adapted to perform its function.

17. The foot is designed for strength and flexibility to support great weight while serving as a shock absorber.

STRUCTURAL ASPECTS OF THE HUMAN SKELETON

The 206 bones and their more than 200 joints or articulations make it possible for the 656 skeletal muscles to move the body in the thousands of movement patterns of sports, dance, aquatics, and occupational chores. In addition to serving as levers, bones (1) give form and structure to the body, (2) protect internal organs, (3) produce red blood cells, and (4) store calcium and phosphorus. Like the steel girders of a building, they provide form and strength but, unlike steel girders, bones are dynamic, living, developing, and growing parts of the human organism.

No engineer has designed a framework for a machine that can compare with that of the human body. Although bone consists largely of inorganic material (inorganic salts that are complex compounds of calcium and phosphorus), it can grow, develop, and repair itself. It is adaptable to the environment. It will atrophy when not used and hypertrophy as a result of increased use. When a child is

struck by poliomyelitis and the innervation to one leg is lost, the affected leg will not grow at the same rate as the unaffected leg and the bones of the affected leg will be shorter and thinner than those of the other leg even though the virus has no direct effect upon bone, circulation, or muscular tissue. When a tooth is lost, the alveolar process that had supported the tooth will be absorbed. Babies who are habitually placed with the back of the head on a hard bed usually develop a flat occiput. These are all manifestations of the adaptations of bones to environmental forces.

The 206 bones of the skeleton are divided into the axial and appendicular sections. The axial section includes the 8 bones of the cranium, 14 of the face, 6 of the ear, the hyoid, the 26 of the vertebral column, 24 ribs, and the sternum. The Appendicular section includes 2 clavicles, 2 scapulae, 2 humerus bones, 2 radii, 2 ulnae, 16 carpals, 10 metacarpals, 28 phalanges of the fingers, 2 femurs, 2 patellas, 2 fibulas, 2 tibias, 16 tarsals, 10 metatarsals, and 28 phalanges of the toes.

The shape, size, thickness, strength, and weight of these bones and the manners in which they articulate with one another are wonderfully adapted to perform the specialized functions demanded of them. A great range and variety of movement is required in the shoulder joint to throw, to swing while hanging by the hands, and to manipulate many tools. The shoulder joint is so constructed as to make this possible. The knee joint, on the other hand, permits a large range in flexion, no extension beyond the straight line, very little rotation, and almost no abduction or adduction. In walking, running, and jumping, stability and flexion posteriorly are required while abduction, adduction, rotation, and hyperextension are not essential. The thumb has a tremendous range of motion making it possible to grasp and utilize a variety of tools. Some anatomists and anthropologists believe that the great range

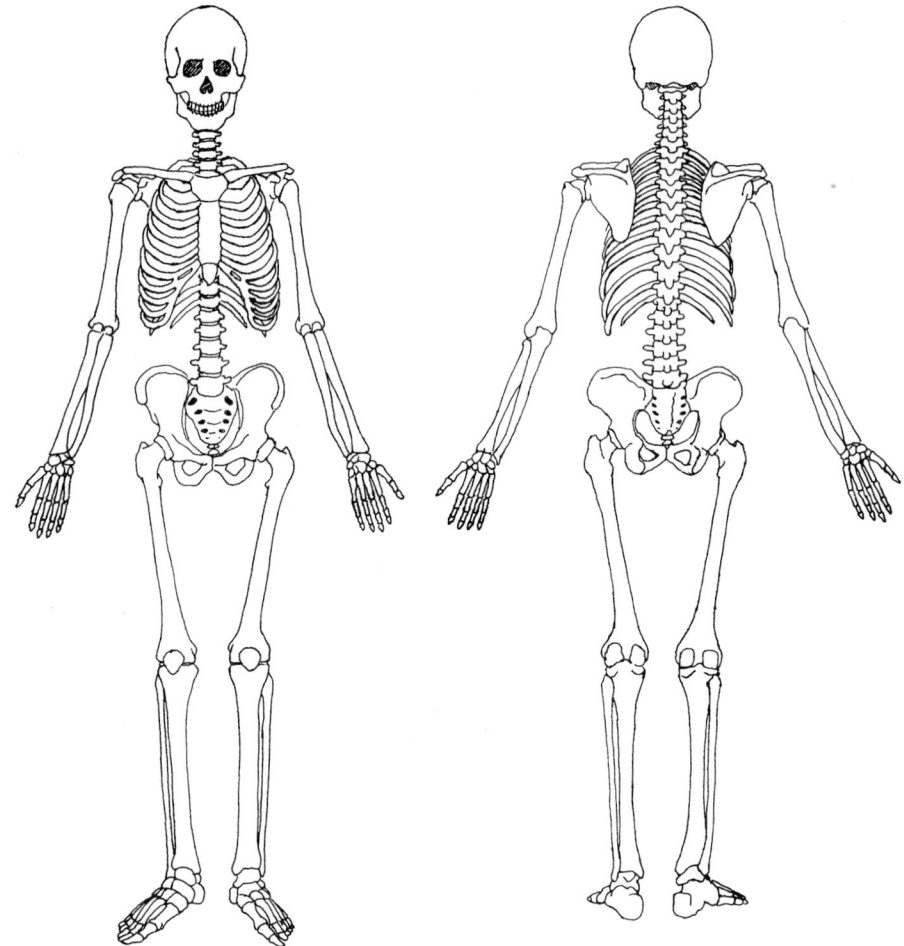

Figure 2.1   Front and rear views of skeletal system

of movement of man's thumb made possible the use of tools and thereby stimulated the development of his brain.

The skeleton provides pulleys (the sesamoid bones such as the patella, processes, trochanters, trochleas, and tubercles) over which muscle tendons pass before attaching to bones. These enable the muscles to secure better leverage to move the body parts. Articular surfaces are smooth and lubricated to minimize friction. The shape of the femur and the arrangement of the bones of the vertebral column and of the feet provide for efficient shock absorption. These shock absorb-

ers help to cushion the impact when a gymnast dismounts from the apparatus, when a broad jumper lands, and when a sprinter runs. Without these shock absorbers, the jar would be intolerable and might shatter bones or damage the brain. Tough but compressible, flexible, elastic cartilage is found between the articular surfaces of many bones to cushion impacts and jars. The vertebral column is so designed as to permit a great range of movement (flexion, extension, hyperextension, lateral flexion, and rotation), yet it can support tremendous weight. Weight lifters clean and jerk 500 pounds to arm's length overhead.

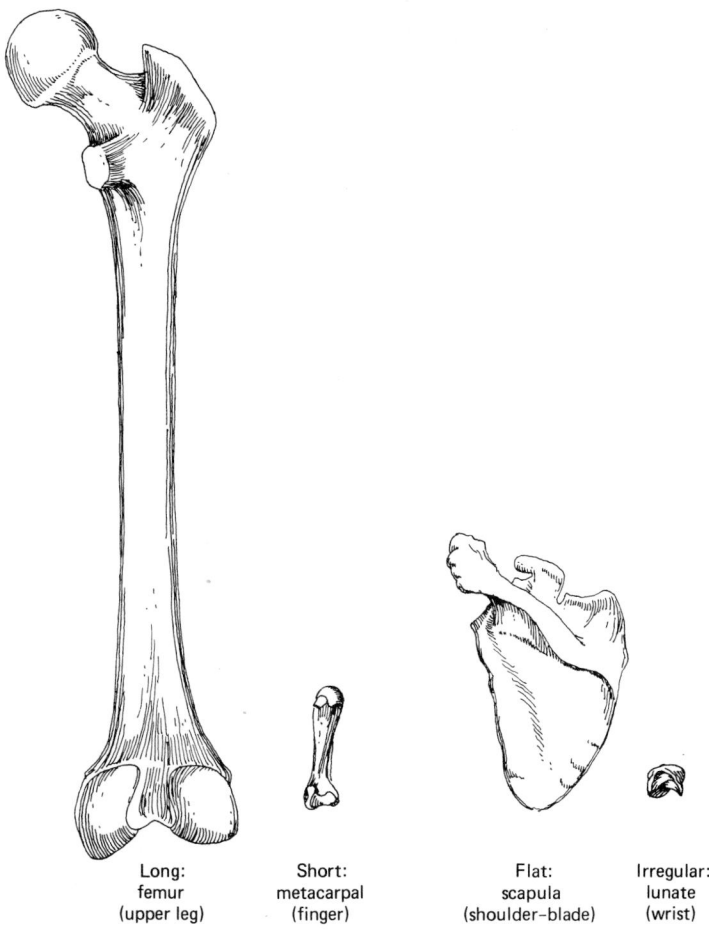

| Long:
femur
(upper leg) | Short:
metacarpal
(finger) | Flat:
scapula
(shoulder-blade) | Irregular:
lunate
(wrist) |

Figure 2.2 Shapes of bones

Understanders in balancing acts support four men on their shoulders.

Many more examples of the ingenious engineering of the human skeleton could be offered. Any student of the human body must stand in solemn wonder over the design and engineering of the human musculoskeletal system.

Form and Structure

There are many different sizes and shapes of bones (see Figure 2.2); however, they can be classified into 4 categories: *Long bones* have cylindrical shafts with broad, knobby ends

where tendons and fascia sheets attach. The shaft has thick walls called *compact bone* and a cavity through the center lengthwise known as the *medullary canal*. Both ends of these bones are specially shaped to form the kind of joint needed. The medullary canal is filled with *marrow*. The bones are designed to conserve weight and yet are sturdy enough to withstand great stress. Examples are the humerus, radius, ulna, femur, tibia, and fibula.

Short bones are small, chunky, solid bones. These bones are made up of a central spongy tissue with a thin hard surface. The carpals and tarsals are examples of these types of bones. *Flat bones* consist of a thin, hard surface enclosing spongy tissue. The principal function of flat bones, such as the sternum and the bones of the face and skull, is to protect vital organs. Although the scapulae and the pelvic bones are classified as flat bones and do provide protection for vital organs, they also facilitate movement. *Irregular bones* are those that do not fit into the other three categories. The 24 vertebrae, the sacrum, the coccyx, and bones of the ears are classified as irregular bones.

Composition and Structure of Bones.

Living bone consists of about 50 percent water and other fluids, and approximately 50 percent solids. About one-third of the solids are organic while two-thirds are inorganic. When all organic material and water are removed from bones, they crumble. When inorganic salts are removed from a long bone, which is fresh and moist, the bone can be tied into a knot. In adults, the proportions of fluid and organic material gradually decrease until the bones become quite brittle in elderly people and, consequently, are more easily fractured and heal more slowly.

The organic portion consists of cells, fibrous matrix, and ground substance. The fibrous matrix consists principally of fibrils of collagen, a protein substance. The ground substance consists mostly of mucopolysaccharides or protein-sugar compounds. This is a condensed tissue fluid, dispersed throughout the fibrous matrix. Inorganic salts, principally calcium phosphates, impregnate the organ matter. Blood vessels, lymph channels, and nerve branches permeate the bone tissue.

The structural basis of compact bone is the microscopic *Haversian system*. The *Haversian or central canals*, usually running the length of the bone, contain blood and lymph vessels and nerve fibers. Thin, cylindrical, concentric layers of bone tissue, called *lamellae*, are laid down around each Haversian canal. Between the layers of lamellae there are small cavities called *lacunae*. Tiny channels called *canaliculli* connect the lacunae with one another and with the Haversian canals. The canaliculi are filled with tissue fluid. Each lacunae contains an *osteocyte* or bone cell. This structure is illustrated in Figure 2.3.

Long bones consist of several parts. The tu-

Figure 2.3 Microscopic view of bone structure (Haversian system, lacunae, canaliculli, and Haversian canal)

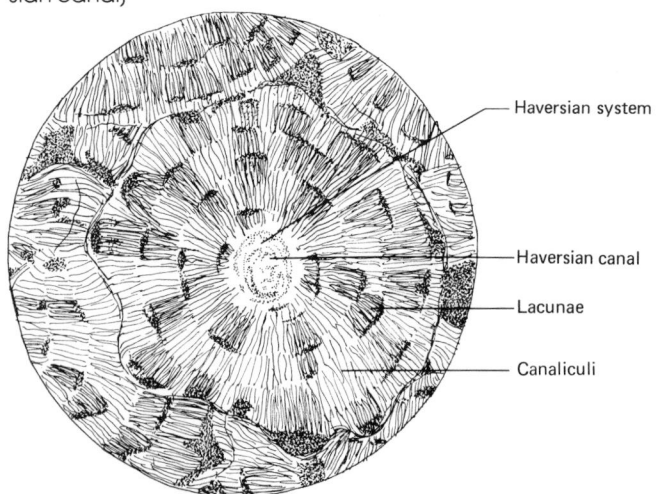

Haversian system

Haversian canal

Lacunae

Canaliculi

bular part is called the *shaft, body,* or *diaphysis*. Inside this part is the marrow-filled *medullary cavity*. Compact bone makes up the *ends* of the bone. On the ends are protrusions called *condyles, tubercles,* or *tuberosities*. Tendons and ligaments attach to these protrusions. Tendons passing over these protrusions are provided a more favorable angle of pull on the bone to which they are attached. If it were not for these protrusions, the line of pull of the muscles would be more nearly parallel to the long axis of the bone. The ends of adjacent bones are shaped to fit one another and to delimit or permit the kind of motion desired at the joint. The articular surface of the ends of long bones is covered with *hyaline cartilage*, which serves to improve the fit, decrease friction, absorb shocks, and prevent dislocations.

The surface of bones, except at articular surfaces, is covered by the *periosteum*. The periosteum attaches itself to the bone via tiny roots. Muscle tendons attach to the periosteum rather than to the bone. The periosteum is supplied with blood vessels and nerves. The pain of fractures, bone bruises, and shin splints arises principally from the periosteum. The *endosteum*, like the periosteum, is a connective tissue. It lines the medullary cavity and Haversian canals.

Ossification, or hardening of bone, occurs as a result of deposition of bone salts in the organic matrix of bones. The process begins well before birth near the center of the future shaft of long bones and progresses outward. The process is not fully completed until age 20 with ossification of the ends of long bones. This epiphyseal ossification progresses at various rates in different bones being totally completed by age 20. At *closure* the original cartilage is totally replaced by bone except for a thin *epiphyseal cartilage, epiphyseal plate,* or *epiphyseal disk*, which separates the shaft or diaphysis from the end or epiphysis. The newly formed bone *is called metaphysis*. *Closure* refers to bony union between the dia-

physes and epiphyses. The process of closure leaves an elevated ridge known as the *epiphyseal line* on the surface of the bone.

Injury to Bones

It is necessary that coaches and physical educators frequently appraise the ability of the bones of their students to withstand stresses imposed in contact sports, pyramid building, jumping, vaulting, and dismounting from apparatus. The thickness of bones at the wrist, ankle, and hips is one indication of the strength of bones. However, body size is not a reliable indication of the degree of maturity and strength of the bones. Although epiphyseal cartilage possess greater flexibility and compressibility than the bone that ultimately replaces it, the epiphyseal cartilage is highly susceptible to injury. Since closure of the epiphysis is not completed until age 20, many orthopedists caution against activities that may incur damage to the epiphysis.

In planning physical activity programs, it is important to know that the bones of males are more dense than those of females. It is also of interest to know that the bones of the Negroid skeleton are denser than those of the Caucasian skeleton.

STRUCTURE AND FUNCTIONS OF HUMAN ARTICULATIONS

Articulations or joints are points where two or more bones meet. Bones are usually, though not always, attached to one another at joints by connective tissue. The amount of movement permitted at various joints is highly variable, depending on the relationships between the needs for stability, protection of vital organs, and the type and range of movement required. All articulations of the body fall into one of three classifications, depending upon the amount of movement permitted (see Figure 2.4). These are as follows:

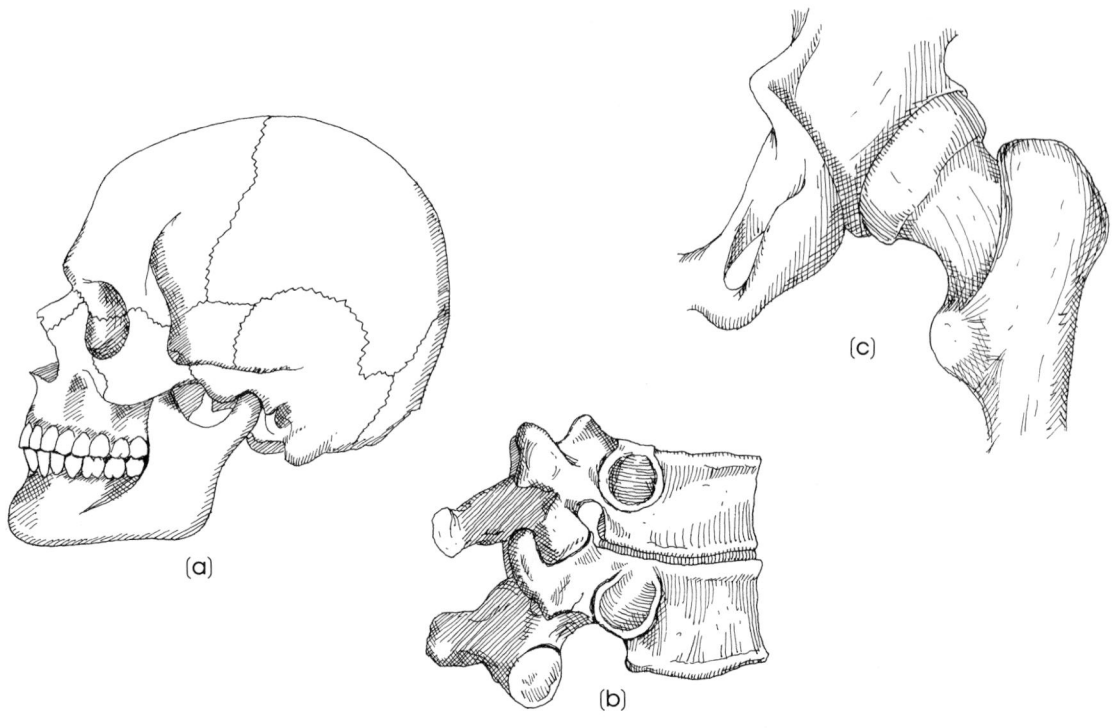

Three types of joints: A. Synarthrodial (bones of the skull)
B. Amphiarthrodial (thoracics of vertebral column)
C. Diarthrodial (hip–joint)

Figure 2.4 Three types of joints: (a) synarthrodial,
(b) amphiarthrodial, and (c) diarthrodial

1. **Diarthrodial**—freely movable. Examples: shoulder, hip, elbow, knee.

2. **Amphiarthrodial**—slightly movable. Examples: symphysis pubis and sacroiliac junctions.

3. **Synarthrodial**—immovable. Examples: sutures of the skull, coracoacromial union, midunion of the radius and ulna.

The *diarthrodial* joints are of greatest interest to people concerned with human movement. Characteristics of these joints are (1) an articular cavity, (2) the articulating surfaces covered with cartilage, usually hyaline, but occasionally fibrocartilage that makes the articular surfaces smooth, and (3) enclo-

sure of the joint in a ligamentous capsule, which is lined with a synovial membrane and secretes synovial fluid for joint lubrication.

Diarthrodial joints are classified into six structural types (see Figure 2.5) as follows:

1. **Gliding, arthrodial, or irregular.** The gliding surfaces are flat or slightly curved. Movement is nonaxial since the surfaces merely slide across one another. Examples are provided between the tarsals of the ankle or the carpals of the wrist.

2. **Condyloid, ovoid, or ellipsoidal.** In this type of joint, an oval-shaped head fits into a shallow cavity. Movements are biaxial since movement can be made in two planes, forward and backward, and from

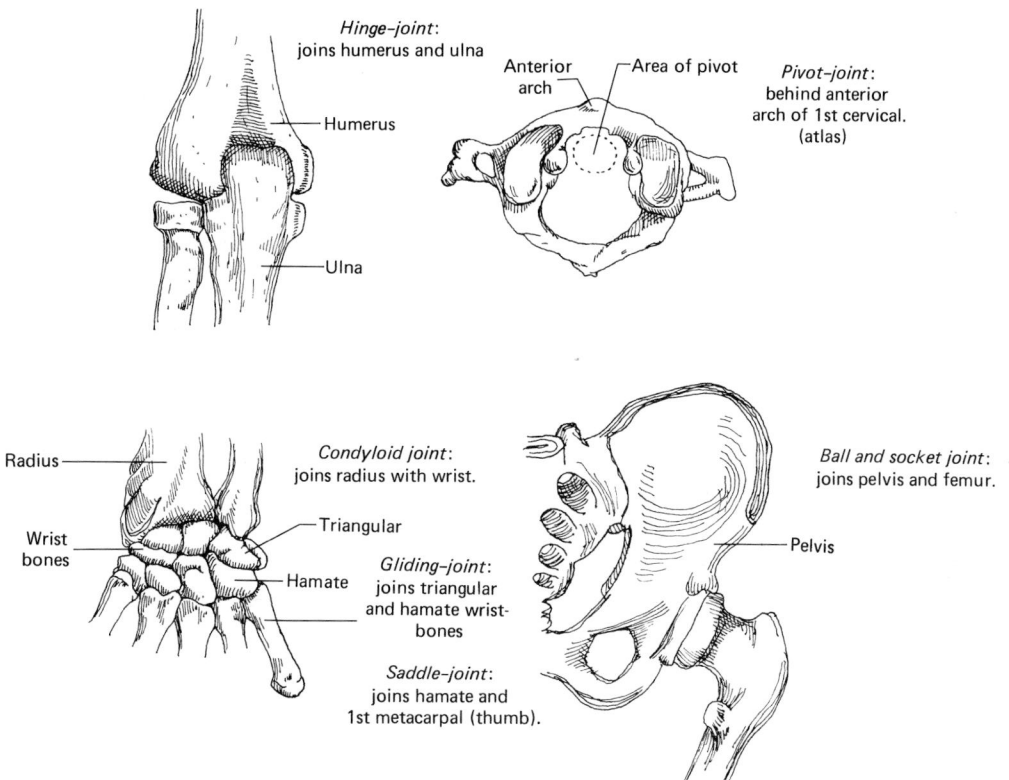

Hinge-joint:
joins humerus and ulna

Humerus

Ulna

Anterior arch

Area of pivot

Pivot-joint:
behind anterior
arch of 1st cervical.
(atlas)

Radius

Wrist bones

Condyloid joint:
joins radius with wrist.

Triangular

Hamate

Gliding-joint:
joins triangular
and hamate wrist-
bones

Saddle-joint:
joins hamate and
1st metacarpal (thumb).

Ball and socket joint:
joins pelvis and femur.

Pelvis

Figure 2.5 Illustrations of the six types of diarthrodial joints

side to side. Examples are the joints between the 2nd, 3rd, 4th, and 5th metacarpals and the proximal phalanx of the four fingers.

3. Saddle, sellar, or reciprocal (reception). These joints are similar to condyloid joints. The ends of the convex surface are tilted upward like a western saddle. Since these joints permit flexion, extension, abduction, adduction, and circumduction, they are biaxial. The carpometacarpal joint of the thumb is an example of this type of joint.

4. Hinge or ginglymus. A concave surface fits over a spool-like process to make possible a hinge-type movement. This joint is uniaxial since movement is permitted in only one plane. Examples are the elbow and the first and second joints of the phalanges.

5. Ball and socket, spheroidal, or enarthrodial. The ball-shaped end of one bone fits into a concave socket at the end of the other bone. These joints are triaxial, permitting movement about three axes. The variety and range of movement is greater than in any other joint. Examples are the shoulder and hip joints.

6. Pivot, trochoid, or screw. A ring-shaped bony structure rotates around a pivot-like process as between the atlas and the axis, or one long bone rolls around another near the end of both as between the radius and ulna. In the latter, a

CONCEPTS APPLIED TO HUMAN MOVEMENT | **15**

rounded surface (like the edge of a disk or a knob) on one bone fits into a concave notch on the other bone. Since the only motion permitted is rotation, this joint is uniaxial.

All joints without a separation or articular cavity are called *synarthrodial* joints. Since an articular cavity is absent, these joints do not have a capsule, synovial membrane, or synovial fluid. There is only one type of synarthrodial joint, the *fibrous* type. There are two types of amphiarthrodial joints: *ligamentous* and *cartilaginous*. In the cartilaginous type cartilage unites the bones. In the ligamentous type, the two bones may not touch one another but there is a ligamentous connection between the two. In the cartilaginous type, the bones are covered with hyaline cartilage, are separated by a disk of fibrocartilage, and are held together by ligaments. Motion is permitted only to the limits of compressibility of the disk. Examples are the bodies of the vertebrae, the symphysis pubis, and between the manubrium and the body of the sternum.

In the *fibrous* type of the synarthrodial class, the edges of bone are united by a thin layer of fibrous periosteum. No movement is permitted. Examples: sutures of the skull.

In the *ligamentous* type of the amphiarthrodial class, slight movement is permitted to the limits of the elasticity of one or more ligaments, which may be in the form of cords, bands, or sheets. The bones joined may be adjacent or separated. Examples are the coracoacromial joint, mid radioulnar joint, mid tibiofibular joint, and the interior tibiofibular joint.

Joint Functions

Joints make it possible for muscles to move bones. The greater the range and variety of movement in a joint, the less stability or resistance to displacement. Joint stability is dependent upon (1) ligaments, (2) muscle tension, (3) fascia, (4) atmospheric pressure, and (5) shape of the bone structure. *Ligaments* are strong, flexible, slightly elastic, fibrous tissues shaped like either straps or round cords; they attach the ends of bones to one another and serve to resist abnormal movements and movement beyond normal limits. *Tendons* of muscles pass over joints. A component of force of muscle pull is parallel to the long axis of the bone, thereby enhancing stability of the joint. The stronger the muscles whose tendons pass over a joint, the greater the joint's stability, and the less the probability of suffering a sprain or dislocation.

Steindler[1] showed that negative pressure exists in articular cavities; that is, pressure within the joint is less than atmospheric pressure. This serves to hold the bones together. Even when all the muscles and ligaments of the hip joint of a cadaver have been completely severed, the hip joint cannot be dislocated. However, when a hole is drilled through the acetabulum, the femoral head easily slips out of the socket. Bone structure is also an important determinant of the stability of a joint. The medial and lateral malleoli of the ankle add considerably to its stability. The deep socket at the hip joint gives it greater stability than does the shallow socket at the shoulder joint.

Range of motion in a joint is dependent upon (1) bone structure, (2) soft tissue near the joint, and (3) elasticity of muscles, tendons, and ligaments. The olecranon process of the ulna effectively limits hyperextension of the elbow joint when it strikes the epicondyle of the humerus. The ball and socket joint of the shoulder, on the other hand, with its shallow socket, permits a great variety and range of movements.

General Joint Movement Terms

When describing movements of the several body segments, and when analyzing sports movements to determine in which joints range of movement must be increased or which muscle groups need to be strengthened to improve performance, it is essential to use a commonly accepted or standardized language. The definitions of the terms for various movements that follow are standard. Physical educators and coaches should use these terms when describing techniques for execution of movement skills.

Flexion is movement of a segment of the body causing a decrease in the angle at the joint, such as bending the arm at the elbow or the leg at the knee. Flexion of the trunk or neck can be executed forward or sideward. Sideward bending is called *lateral flexion*. A body segment may also flex in the horizontal plane, as when the arm moves from a position in the frontal or lateral plane through the horizontal, or intransverse plane to the sagittal or anterior-posterior plane, as when executing a forehand or backhand drive in tennis. This is called *horizontal flexion* since the movement is in the horizontal plane. Flexion of the arm at the shoulder occurs when the extended arm is moved upward in the sagittal plane and the angle between the arm and the head and neck diminishes. The shoulder joint is fully flexed when the humerus is parallel to the long axis of the scapulae. When the arm is brought backward beyond a position parallel to the long axis of the scapulae it is said to be *hyperflexed*. *Dorsiflexion* (or to dorsal flex) occurs when the top of the foot is drawn toward the tibia. The opposite movement (pushing the foot downward) is called *plantar flexion*.

Extension is movement in the opposite direction to flexion. There is an increase in the angle at the joint, as in straightening the el-
bow or knee. *Horizontal extension* is the opposite movement to horizontal flexion; that is, the arm moves in the horizontal plane from the front toward the side of the body, as when moving the arm backward in the backswing for the forehand drive in tennis. *Hyperextension* is the extension of a body segment beyond its normal extended position, as in extending the leg at the hip backward beyond the line of the trunk. Hyperextension of the elbow is said to occur when the angle at the elbow exceeds 180 degrees. *Horizontal hyperextension* of the arm occurs when the arm is brought backward beyond the frontal or lateral plane of the body.

Abduction is movement of a segment away from the midline of the body, or, in the case of the fingers, away from the midline of the hand. Once initiated, abduction continues to be called abduction, even though, as in the case of the arm, after it has passed the first 90 degrees of its movement, it approaches the midline of the body. *Hyperabduction* refers to the movement of the upper arm after it has passed the vertical during abduction.

Adduction is the opposite of abduction — the return to anatomical position from an abducted position. Abduction and adduction cannot occur at the knee and elbow joints. Abduction at the wrist is called *radial flexion* while adduction is called *ulnar flexion*. *Hyperadduction* is adduction beyond the midline of the body. Obviously, this is impossible with the arms and legs because they strike the body. However, by combining slight flexion with hyperadduction, the upper arm can move across the front of the body and the thigh can move past the supporting leg. *Reduction of hyperadduction* refers to the return movement from hyperadduction.

Rotation is movement of a segment around its own longitudinal axis. *Rotation left or right* refers to rotation of the head and neck so that the anterior aspect turns to the left or right. *Outward or lateral rotation* refers to revolving of the thigh, the entire lower extremity, the upper arm, or the entire arm in such a way that the anterior side rotates outward. In *inward or medial rotation* the anterior aspect turns medially. *Supination* refers to outward turning of the forearm while *pronation* refers to turning inward of the forearm. *Reduction of outward rotation, reduction of supination, reduction of inward rotation,* and *reduction of pronation* refer to rotation of segments back to the mid or anatomic position. *Inversion* is bending of the foot so that the bottom of the foot is turned inward. *Eversion* is bending of the foot so that the bottom of the foot is turned outward.

Circumduction refers to a movement of a body segment in which the segment describes a cone with the apex at the joint and the base at the distal end of the segment. Circumduction is possible at the shoulder, hip, wrist, trunk, neck, ankle, the metacarpal-phalangeal, and the metatarsal-phalangeal joints.

Movements of the shoulder girdle require attention because of the unique construction and mobility of the scapulae, whose movements are not readily apparent. *Elevation* of the shoulder girdle occurs when the shoulder is lifted, as in shrugging the shoulders. *Depression* is the opposite of elevation. *Protraction* or *abduction* refers to the movement of the scapulae away from the midline of the body, as when broadening the shoulders. *Retraction or adduction* of the scapulae is the opposite movement to protraction. The scapulae can also be rotated to a degree. In *upward rotation* the lower tip of the scapulae moves away from the spinal column. In *downward rotation* the lower tip moves toward the spinal column.

To avoid confusion, it is recommended that when referring to joint action, terms such as *hip flexion* or *shoulder joint adduction* be used instead of "thigh flexion" or "arm adduction." The arms may be stabilized and the body may be pulled up toward the arms as in pulling up on the rings from a hang to a crucifix or the legs may be stabilized and the trunk pulled toward the thighs as in doing a sit-up.

MAJOR BODY ARTICULATIONS—STRUCTURE, FUNCTIONS, MUSCLES, AND LIGAMENTS

It has been pointed out that there are 206 bones and over 200 joints or articulations in the human skeleton. However, only 177 of the 206 bones engage in voluntary movement. It is these 177 bones with which the physical educator and coach are primarily concerned. The skeleton is divided into two major parts, the axial skeleton—which includes the skull, spinal column, sternum, and the ribs—and the appendicular skeleton—which includes the bones of the upper and lower extremities.

The structural forms of bones, particularly at their articulations with other bones, are amazingly adapted to perform the functions required at each specific joint. The bulbous ends of long bones increase the articular area, provide greater surface area for attachment of muscle tendons and ligaments, and improve the angle of insertion of muscle tendons. The *olecranon* process at the elbow not only prevents hyperextension of the elbow but also increases the length of the force arm. The posterior projection of the calcaneous provides a longer base for balance on the feet and also increases the length of the force arm of the *tendon of Achilles.* The *trochanter* on the proximal and lateral side of the femur provides a line of pull for the three gluteals and the outward rotators of the hip, which is more nearly at a right angle to the long axis of the femur. The *transverse processes* of the vertebrae increase the radius of rotation of the vertebrae to make the job of the muscles attaching to the vertebral column easier. *Sesamoid* bones, the *patella,* and soft tissues such as *bursae,* are located under tendons near their distal attachment to enable the tendon to insert into the bone nearer the vertical.

Muscles, too, are structured to perform best the specialized functions they are assigned. In running, the knee must be extended and the hip is flexed quickly. The large muscle mass, the short work arm, and the long resistance arm make it possible for this skill to be performed. The *gastrocnemius*, on the other hand, is required to exert substantial force over a short distance. Its many short muscle fibers and almost 90 degree angle of insertion enable this muscle to exert considerable pull upon the calcaneal bone, its distal attachment. Muscles are adapted to their specialized functions by means of the locus of the proximal and distal attachments, length and arrangements of their fibers, and number and size of their fibers.

Physical educators, coaches, teachers of dance and aquatics, and physical or exercise therapists can greatly enhance the probability that they will successfully achieve their objectives if a thorough knowledge and understanding of bones, articulations, ligaments, and muscles in the human body is acquired. Teachers will be less likely to ask students to attempt movements that may produce injury. They will know where range of movement has to be increased and which muscles strengthened to execute skills.

Movement of body segments occurs at articulations as a result of contraction of muscle tissue produced by chemical action initiated by nervous stimulation. In order to facilitate communication and description of specific body segments and of the entire body, it is necessary to identify *planes* in which movement takes place and *axes* around which the body or its segments may rotate. Additionally, it is necessary to define such words or concepts as: *center of gravity, line of gravity*, and the *fundamental and anatomic standing positions* from which movements are initiated.

These concepts are discussed more extensively in Chapter 8.

Fundamental Standing Position

In this position (see Figure 2.6) the person is standing with the feet slightly separated and parallel, arms at the sides, palms against the thighs. This position is generally utilized as the point of reference in describing all movements of the body's segments, except those of the forearm, hand, and fingers.

Anatomic Standing Position

This position (see Figure 2.6) is the same as the fundamental standing position except that the palms face forward with the elbows fully extended. This position is utilized as the point of reference for all movements of the forearm, hand, and fingers.

Planes and Axes of the Body

There are three cardinal planes (see Figure 2.7) and three axes of rotation (see Figure 2.8) perpendicular to these planes. Each plane is perpendicular to the other two. All three planes and all three axes intersect at the center of gravity. Each axis is perpendicular to the plane in which the motion occurs and perpendicular to the other two axes. The cardinal planes of the body are defined as follows:

1. The *cardinal sagittal, anteroposterior, or median* plane passes through the body from front to back dividing it vertically into two symmetrical halves, right and left.

2. The *cardinal coronal, frontal, or lateral* plane passes through the body vertically from side to side dividing it into two equal but not symmetrical halves, anterior and posterior.

3. The *cardinal transverse, horizontal, or transverse* plane passes through the body

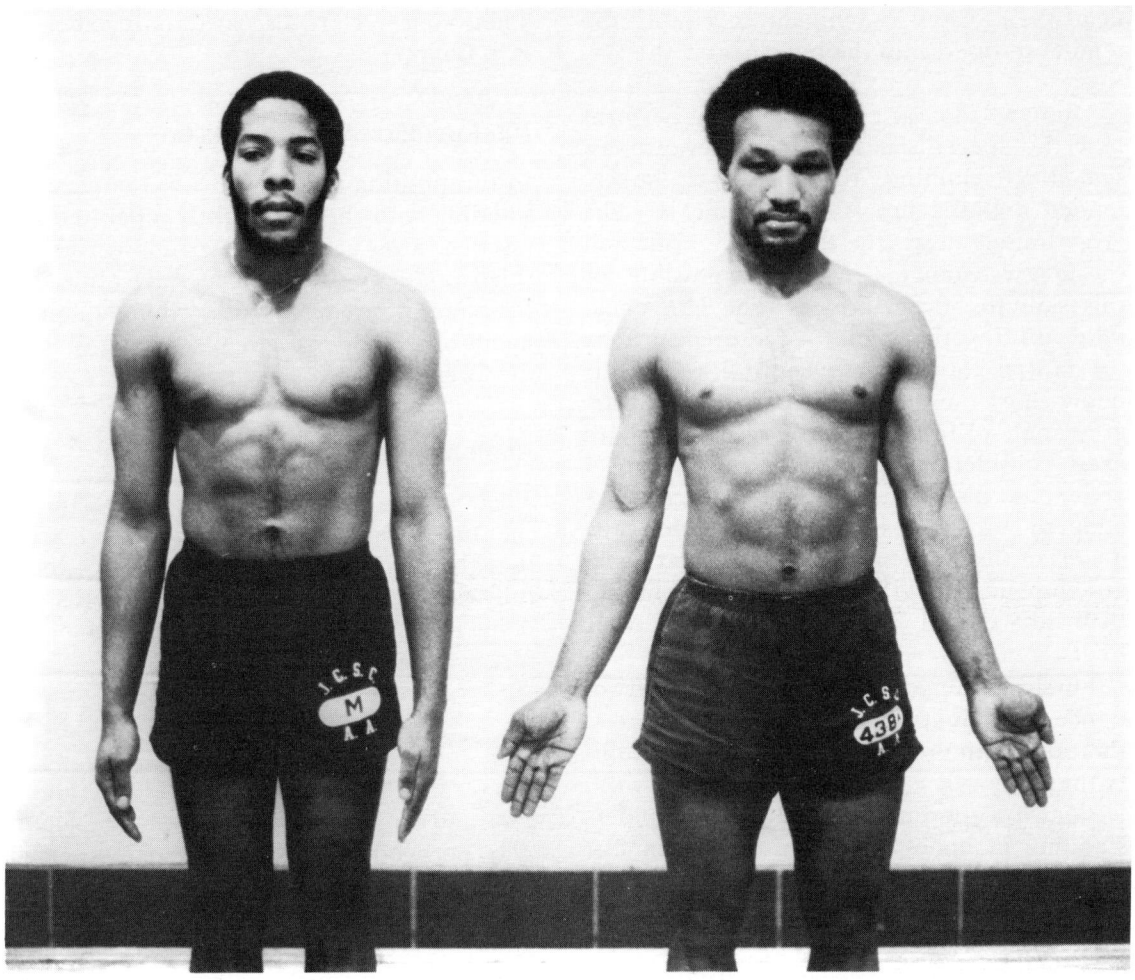

Figure 2.6 Fundamental and anatomic standing positions

horizontally from front to back dividing it into equal but not symmetrical upper and lower halves.

The line at which the cardinal anteroposterior and frontal planes intersect is the *gravitational line* or *line of weight* since it passes through the center of gravity and is perpendicular to the supporting surface. In balanced standing position, this line normally falls slightly less than two inches in front of the ankle joint. However, the student and

teacher of physical activities must keep in mind that the body is seldom in the anatomic or fundamental position. It has been found that even in "static standing" there is swaying and the line of gravity moves about. In static positions in sports where the athlete is prepared to move quickly at a signal such as in the sprinter's crouch, the offensive lineman's stance, and the body position of the tennis player waiting to return the service, the line of gravity is displaced forward, and the athlete is in a controlled off-balance position to

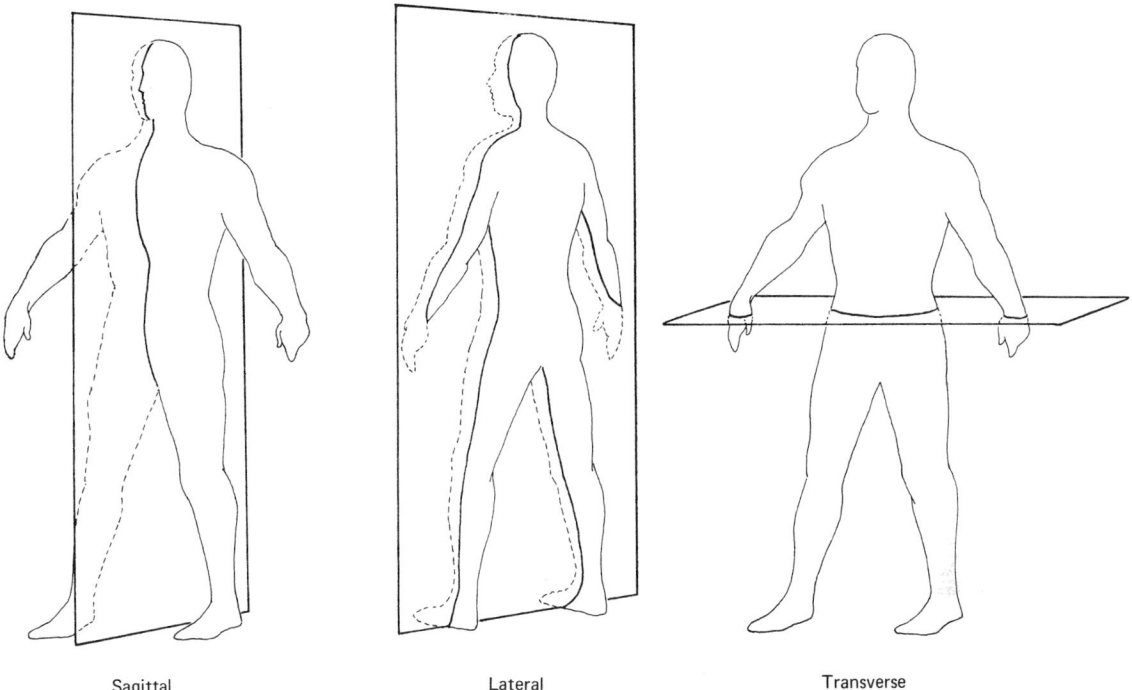

Sagittal   Lateral   Transverse

Figure 2.7 Three cardinal planes of the body

facilitate quick movement in the desired direction. In held static positions such as the one-hand balance or the scale in gymnastics, the line of gravity is constantly shifting and the performer is continually making corrections in body and segment positions through muscular contractions to maintain balance. When maintaining dynamic equilibrium, such as dribbling a basketball while evading other players, broken field running, skiing a slalom course, fancy skating, circling around the side horse, or performing on the parallel bars, the forces acting on the body are diverse, with constant changes in magnitude and direction. Considerations are the force and direction of a ball thrown to the player, potential impacts from other players, changing direction or speed of movement to avoid opponents or obstacles, momentum, and centrifugal and centripetal force. The fast moving player must accurately estimate the direction and magnitude of forces about to be thrust against his body. His compensatory movements and adjustments of his body positions must usually be initiated before the force is applied. Because these forces are irregular and unpredictable, the performer cannot depend exclusively upon developed skills but must focus attention on estimating the size and direction of these forces in order to initiate adjustment in body positions before actual impingement of the force.

Humans tend to move in manners that provide for the greatest conservation of energy. Sailors develop the habit of walking with their knees slightly flexed and their feet apart in order to widen the base of support laterally and lower the center of gravity as compensation for the rolling of the ship. Skaters, dancers, and gymnasts learn to block out sensations that cause vertigo or nystagmus when they repeat many fast spins. When changing

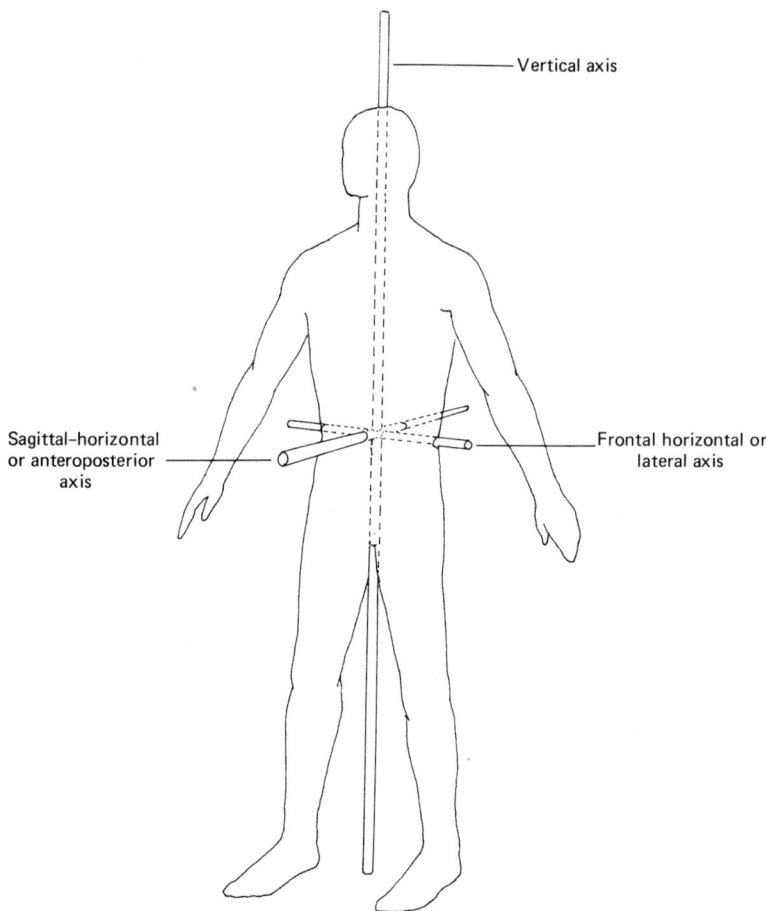

Vertical axis

Sagittal-horizontal or anteroposterior axis

Frontal horizontal or lateral axis

Figure 2.8 Three axes of the body (from Northrip, J. W., Logan, G. A., and McKinney, Wayne, C., **Introduction to Biomechanical Analysis of Sport**, 1977, William C. Brown Company, Publishers, Dubuque, Iowa)

direction, athletes displace their center of gravity laterally in order to utilize the force of gravity in executing the turn.

Following are definitions of the *axes* of the body:

1. The *frontal-horizontal* or *lateral* axis passes horizontally from one side to the other, lies in the transverse plane and lateral plane, and is perpendicular to the anteroposterior plane. In the fundamental standing position, the lateral axis lies in the lateral and horizontal plane and is perpendicular to the anteroposterior plane.

2. The *sagittal-horizontal* or *anteroposterior* axis passes horizontally from front to back, lies in the anteroposterior and the transverse planes, and is perpendicular to the lateral plane.

3. The *vertical* axis passes through the body vertically, lies in the anteroposterior and the lateral plane, and is perpendicular to the transverse plane.

When a movement is described as being one of the three planes, we mean that the movement is in a plane parallel to that plane. If we wish to indicate that the movement occurred in a plane that passed through the center of gravity, we would use the term *cardinal plane*. Similarly, movement about any of the three axes does not refer exclusively to movement around the cardinal axis. Flexing

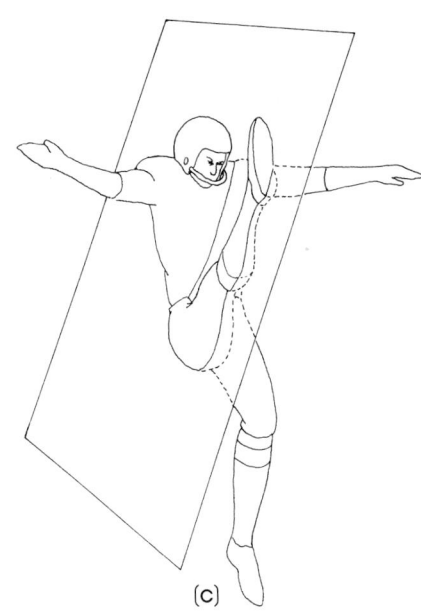

(c)

Figure 2.9c Diagonal plane—hip joint

the arm at the elbow with the arm next to the body is movement in the anteroposterior plane about the lateral axis even though the arm is lateral to the cardinal anteroposterior plane and the axis of the elbow joint is higher than the cardinal lateral axis.

Northrip, Logan, and McKinney[2] have pointed out the necessity for adding three new diagonal planes to the three cardinal planes in order that kinesiologists be able to accurately describe movements of the upper and lower limbs during ballistic actions. In movements such as pitching a ball, throwing a discus, or kicking a football, the limb moves in a plane diagonal to the longitudinal axis of the body. Further, the movement of the limb is around an axis perpendicular to this diagonal plane and, therefore, diagonal to the longitudinal axis of the body.

These authors have termed the three diagonal planes (1) the *high diagonal plane* involving the glenohumeral or shoulder articulation, (2) the *low diagonal plane* involving the same articulation, and (3) the *diagonal plane* involving the coxal or hip articulation (Figure 2.9a, b and c).

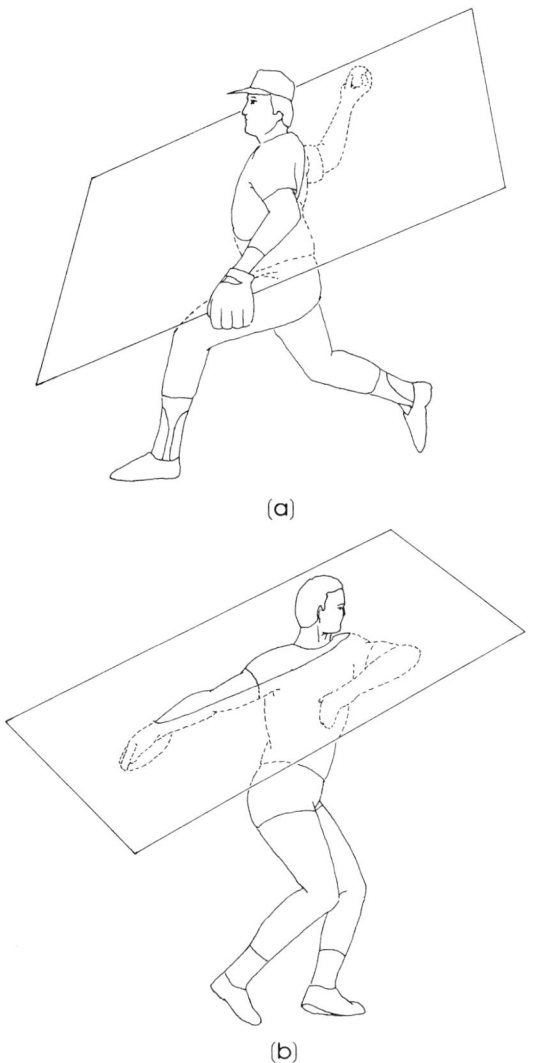

(a)

(b)

Figure 2.9a High diagonal plane—shoulder joint, (b) Low diagonal plane—shoulder joint

These authors indicate several reasons why limbs tend to move in planes diagonal to the longitudinal axis of the body during ballistic actions. First, major muscles acting on the humerus and femur, such as the pectoralis major and minor and the adductor longus and magnus, provide a diagonal line of pull. Second, when one limb is used to impart force to an object, the opposite limb must move in an opposite direction in order to maintain equilibrium. Third, when throwing, the glenohumeral joint is itself on the end of a lever arm (the breadth of the shoulders), which is rotating. As the vertebral column and thorax are rotated during the throw, the glenohumeral joint moves through an arc. If the humerus continues to move through a plane perpendicular to the axis of the shoulder, this plane will be diagonal to the longitudinal axis of the body due to rotation of the shoulder breadth axis. Fourth, the *crossed extensor reflex*, which causes simultaneous extension of the limbs opposite to those being flexed, is responsible for an "automatic relationship" in diagonal-type movements. (See Chapter 4.)

MUSCLES

Attachments

Muscles cause bones to move as a result of their ability to contract upon being stimulated. The proximal end of the muscle is attached to a heavier bone nearer the center of the body while the distal end of the muscle is attached to a lighter bone farther from the center of the body. Between the proximal and distal attachments, there are one or more joints or articulations. When the muscle contracts, movement of the bones about the joint occurs. The bone to which the proximal end of the muscle is attached is usually more stable while that to which the distal end is attached is usually the more movable. A muscle pulls equally on both ends. When the biceps contracts or shortens, the forearm is usually

brought upward toward the upper arm. However, if the forearm is stabilized, as when hanging from a horizontal bar when performing the chin-up, the upper arm is brought toward the forearm. The muscles that flex the hips may draw the trunk toward the thighs if the legs are held down or they may draw the legs toward the trunk if the trunk is stabilized.

Arrangement of Muscles

Voluntary muscles are arranged in groups that oppose each other. For example, muscles on the anterior aspect of the upper arm flex the elbow while those on the posterior aspect extend the elbow. The quadriceps femoris on the front of the thigh extends the knee while hamstring muscles on the back of the thigh flex the knee. Most muscles produce more than one type of movement upon contraction. As one of many examples, the latissimus dorsi functions in adduction, rotation, extension, and hyperextension of the humerus, depression of the shoulder girdle, and lateral flexion of the trunk.

When a muscle contracts, it will produce all the movements of which it is capable unless one or more other muscles contract to prevent undesired movements. Almost without exception, the desired movement is made possible by the contraction of many muscles. Muscles responsible for a specified movement are called *agonist*. Agonists may be further subdivided into prime and assistant movers. Muscles that directly oppose the action of another muscle or muscles are called *antagonists*. Muscles that insure that body parts move within the desired pathway are called *neutralizers*. For example, the right external oblique when contracting alone will flex the trunk to the right and rotate it to the left while the left external oblique will flex the trunk to the left and rotate it to the right. When they contract together they flex the trunk forward and neutralize one another's roles as lateral flexors and rotators of the trunk. Muscles that hold body parts steady in order to permit coordinated execution of the desired movement are called *stabilizers*. When the arm moves at the shoulder joint, the shoulder girdle must be held firm. When serving as stabilizers, muscles usually contract statically or isometrically, since their role is to hold the segment motionless. Obviously, a specific muscle may serve as an agonist in one movement, as an antagonist during another movement, as neutralizer in still another movement, and as a stabilizer in a fourth movement.

Multijoint Muscles

Multijoint muscles pass over and affect movement at more than one joint. The relatively short length of these muscles prohibits certain simultaneous movements at the joints over which they pass. For example, the hamstrings that both extend the hip joint and flex the knee joint cannot shorten enough to produce both complete hip extension and knee flexion at the same time. On the other hand, when the hip is flexed with the knees is in extension, the proximal end of the hamstring is drawn taut over the hip joint, causing it to assume the protective role of a ligament. This is called *ligamentous action*. At the distal end of the muscle there occurs an automatic shortening contraction that causes movement in the distal joint. This is called *tendon action*. The phenomenon is also observed in the rectus femoris when the hip is extended while the knee is flexed. The reader can observe the phenomenon by extending the fingers fully and then attempting to flex the wrist fully. It will be noted that as the wrist is flexed, the fingers will be less fully extended. This is because the multijoint muscles on the posterior side of the forearm cannot lengthen sufficiently and the multijoint muscles on the anterior side of the forearm cannot shorten sufficiently to permit both full extension of the fingers and full flexion of the wrist.

Agonistic and Antagonistic Interplay

The opposing actions of agonists and antagonists has been pointed out. In skillful execution of movement patterns, varying degrees of muscular force and speed of movement are required. When hitting a home run, maximal speed and force are required. When bunting, controlled movements are required. During controlled movements, voluntary resistance by antagonistic muscles is necessary. *Reciprocal inhibition* is the phenomenon that makes controlled movement possible. (See Chapter 4 for further discussion.)

Kinds of Muscle Action

Muscular contractions are of many types according to the task demanded. Contractions can vary in speed, force, and duration. In *maximum-force movements*, the agonist muscles contract at maximum speed and force. There are two types of maximum-force movements — *continuous force* and *ballistic*. In continuous-force movements, muscle tension is almost maximum throughout the range of the movement. Most weight training exercises are continuous-force movements as are some moves in gymnastics such as presses into handstands, pull up into a crucifix, and chinups. The muscles of football linemen pushing against one another are also undergoing continuous force contraction. A maximum-force movement of the *ballistic* type occurs when the body or one of its segments is moved quickly by a fast but short contraction of agonist muscles. After the initial burst of muscular activity, the muscle force is reduced and the action continues due to the momentum generated. The speed of movement gradually decreases due to the resistance of antagonist muscles, resistance in the joints, and external resistance such as the pull of gravity, the opposing momentum of a ball, or other forces. Near the end of ballistic movements, antagonistic muscles provide braking action through eccentric contraction. If the braking action is initiated too soon, the motion appears jerky and lacks fluidity, and maximum force will not be applied. If the braking action is initiated too late, the performer is likely to lose balance and/or not be in position for the next movement. There are many examples of ballistic movements in sports—swinging of clubs, rackets, or bats; throwing a punch, a ball, a discus, or a javelin; running, jumping, or dribbling a ball.

Slow-tension movements are used when speed and force are of secondary consideration to steadiness and accuracy. During slow-tension movements, the strength of contraction of the agonists and antagonists is almost equal in order to hold the body or its segments stabilized and steady. Examples are provided in aiming a gun, an arrow, or a dart; threading a needle; and movements in gymnastics such as holding a handstand, balancing on one foot, holding a V-sit with the hands touching the toes, and holding an L position or crucifix on the still rings.

Rapid-tension movements are those in which the direction of movement is quickly reversed, as in shaking a cocktail mixer, typing, or strumming a guitar. The maximal speed is determined by learning, the weight of the object being manipulated, and strength of the involved muscles.

When tension is developed within a muscle, it is said to be in contraction. While in contraction, a muscle may be shortening, lengthening, or maintaining its present length. When the tension developed in a muscle is greater than the resistance placed against it and the body part is moved, the muscle is in *concentric* contraction. In concentric contraction the muscle shortens and its proximal and distal attachments approach one another. *Concentric* means to move toward center. When the tension in a muscle is less than the resistance placed against it and the body part gives to the resistance, the muscle is in *eccentric* contraction. In eccentric contraction the muscle lengthens and its

proximal and distal attachments move away from one another. *Eccentric* means to move away from center. An *isotonic* contraction is one in which the tension within the muscle is uniform throughout the contraction. It is the custom to classify both concentric and eccentric contractions as of the isotonic type. A *static* contraction is one in which the tension developed within the muscle is exactly equal to the resistance applied and there is neither lengthening or shortening of the muscle. An *isometric* contraction is one in which the maximum tension that can be generated in the muscle is inadequate to overcome the resistance placed against it. As in the static contraction, there is neither shortening or lengthening of the muscle.

Examples from sports of concentric contractions are throwing, jumping, pole vaulting, executing a somersault, or striking a ball. Examples of eccentric contractions are catching a ball, absorbing the impact of landing by bending the knees and hips and allowing the feet to dorsi flex after a jump or somersault, or allowing the arms to extend slowly while lowering from a chin-up on the horizontal bar. Perhaps the easiest example to understand can be provided in an arm wrestling match between A and B. When A is pinning B's arm, A's muscles are undergoing concentric contraction while B's muscles are undergoing eccentric contraction. If neither is pinning the other, the muscles of both are undergoing an isometric contraction. The increase in size of muscle fibers and, consequently, in strength and power of the muscle is equal in exercise programs utilizing isometric exercises and those utilizing isotonic exercises when muscle tension developed is maximal or near maximal during every contraction. It has been found that the optimum number of repetitions in weight training, if the objective is to maximally increase strength and power, is 3 to 6 in 3 sets or series. The exercise should be done through the full range of movement. The optimum time to hold an isometric contraction is 6 seconds. Since in many movements (or attempted movements as in isometric exercises) different segments of a muscle serve as prime movers and different muscles serve as stabilizers and assistant movers at different points in the movement, an isometric exercise should be done at 2 or 3 different degrees of flexion, extension, abduction, adduction, or rotation of the involved joint. Isometric exercises offer the advantages of economy of time, cost, and storage space for equipment. Weight training exercises offer the advantages of "built-in" motivation (the amount being lifted and number of repetitions are known) and improved vascularization. Whenever a maximal contraction is made, air should be expired in a controlled manner by making an *s-s-s-s-s-s* or *f-f-f-f-f-f* sound This procedure will maintain a uniform intrathoracic pressure, which will circumvent the *Valsalva effect*. During a hard muscular contraction, the muscles of the thorax, abdomen, and spinal column come under hard contraction in order to stabilize the axial skeleton. As a consequence, intrathoracic pressure is elevated when the glottis is closed. This increased pressure may be great enough to slow the return flow of blood in the venae cavae with a resulting decrease in blood pressure. When the contraction has been completed and the pressure on the venae cavae is decreased, the damned up blood rushes into the heart and blood pressure is increased. Senile and hospitalized people with weak vascular walls have been known to suffer ruptured blood vessels as a result of performing an isometric contraction—straining at the stool, for example. One of the authors (Baley) has led thousands of people in hard isometric exercises and has known of no deleterious effects nor ever heard of any. However, the method of exhaling air during the contraction described earlier was always utilized.

Muscles that are required to sustain contractions, such as the postural muscles (the soleus and extensors of the hips and knees in particular), have larger amounts of *myoglobin* in the sarcoplasm, giving them a darker and redder appearance. The myoglobin probably stores oxygen, thus giving these muscles greater endurance. These are called *red fibers*. *Pale fibers* are better adapted to perform fast contractions. Wild geese and ducks, which demonstrate tremendous muscular endurance during their migratory flights, have been found to have red fibers in the muscles of the wings and breast. Domesticated fowl have pale fibers in the muscles of the breast and wings. However, when pale muscle fibers are transplanted to sites of red fibers, they become darker and redder.[3]

MICROSCOPIC STRUCTURE OF MUSCLE

The various muscles whose location and action we have just studied are groups of muscle bundles that join a tendon at either end. The muscle is covered by a fascia of fibrous connective tissue called *epimysium. Perimysium* covers each muscle bundle. The muscle bundle consists of thousands of *muscle fibers*. The individual muscle fibers are covered by *endomysium* (See Figure 2.10). The number of muscle fibers in every muscle is determined before birth. The thickness of each fiber increases as a result of strength conditioning programs. The greater the cross-sectional diameter, the greater the strength of the muscle. Cross-sectional diameter is measured at a right angle to the muscle fibers. As strength increases, the number of fibers remains constant but the individual fibers become thicker.

Muscle fibers are long cylindrical cells. The muscle fibers are thicker in some muscles than in others. Their thickness also varies within the same muscle. The length varies according to the length of different muscles. The polynucleated muscle cell is enclosed in the *sarcolemma*, a thin permeable membrane that adheres to the endomysium. The sarcolemma has remarkable electrical properties. Within the muscle cell is a protoplasm called *sarcoplasm*, which contains soluble proteins, glycogen, fat, phosphate compounds, and ions. Also suspended in this reddish viscous fluid are nuclei, mitochondria, phosphocreatine, and adenosine triphosphate (ATP).

Embedded in the sarcoplasm are *myofibrils*, which are responsible for the contractile power of muscles. The myofibrils run parallel to the long axis of the muscle fibers and attach to the sarcolemma at each end of the cell. Each muscle fiber contains many myofibrils. The electron microscope has revealed that each myofibril has alternating light and dark areas. The light areas are called *I bands* and the dark areas *A bands*. A dark line crosses the center of each I band. This is called the *Z line*. The A band receives its name from the fact that light waves passing through it are *anisotropic*, that is, after the light waves pass through the band, their velocity is not equal in all directions. The velocity of light waves after they have passed through the I bands, on the other hand, is equal in all directions and consequently the waves are called *isotropic*. The distance between one Z line and the next is called a *sarcomere*. The region in the center of the A band is called the *H zone*. In the center if the H zone is a darker area called the *M line*.

The I band is composed of thin protein fil-

Figure 2.10 Structure of a skeletal muscle and its fibers

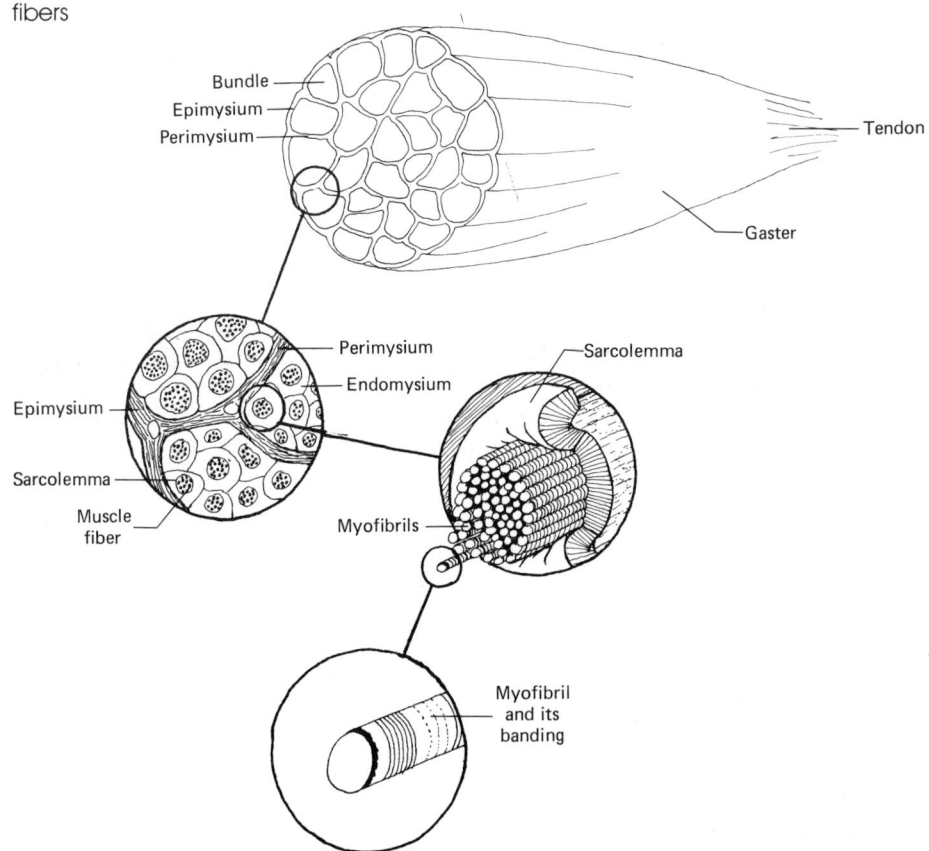

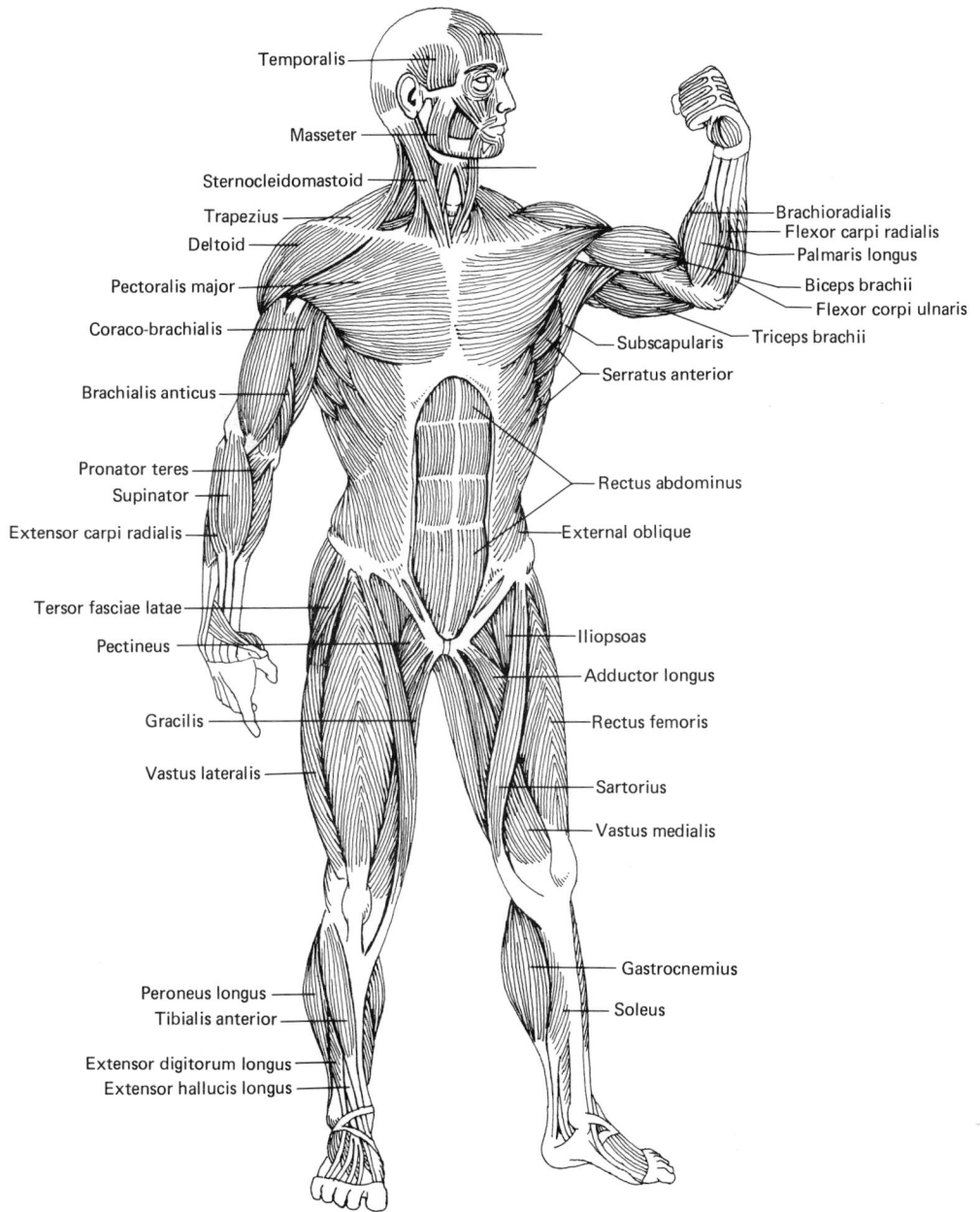

Figure 2.11 Superficial muscles—anterior side of body

aments called *actin filaments*. These actin filaments are anchored to the Z lines at one end of the sarcomere and extend partly into the region of the A band. The A band is also composed of protein filaments, but these are the thicker *myosin filaments*. The Z lines adhere to the sarcolemma, thereby helping to keep the actin filaments aligned and facili-

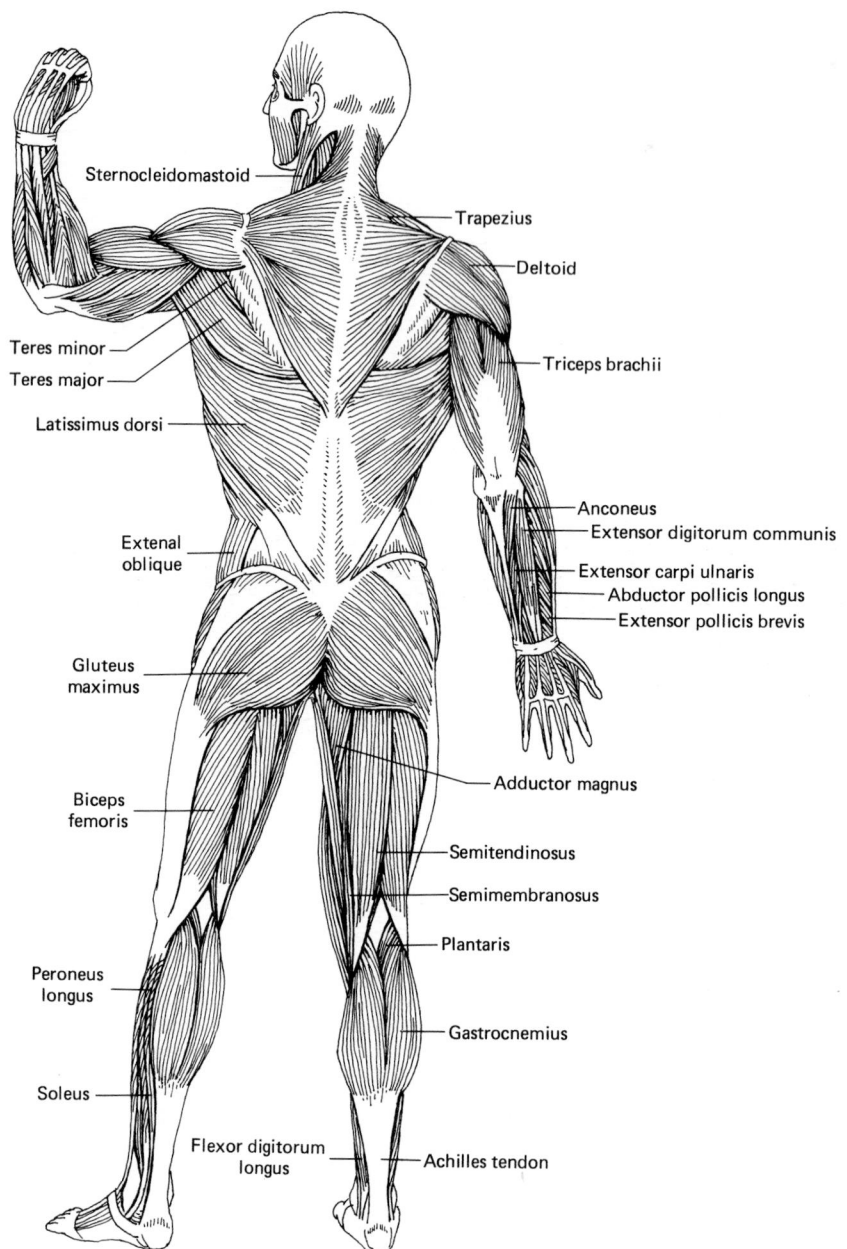

Sternocleidomastoid

Trapezius

Deltoid

Teres minor

Teres major

Triceps brachii

Latissimus dorsi

Anconeus

Extensor digitorum communis

Extensor carpi ulnaris

Abductor pollicis longus

Extensor pollicis brevis

Extenal
oblique

Gluteus
maximus

Adductor magnus

Biceps
femoris

Semitendinosus

Semimembranosus

Plantaris

Peroneus
longus

Gastrocnemius

Soleus

Flexor digitorum
longus

Achilles tendon

Figure 2.12 Superficial muscles—posterior side of body

tating the transmission of nervous impulses from the sarcolemma to the myofibrils. The actin filament actually contains two proteins in addition to actin—*tropomyosin* and *tropo-* *nin.* Each thin filament of the I band is shared by three thick filaments of the A band. The filaments of the two bands overlap slightly.

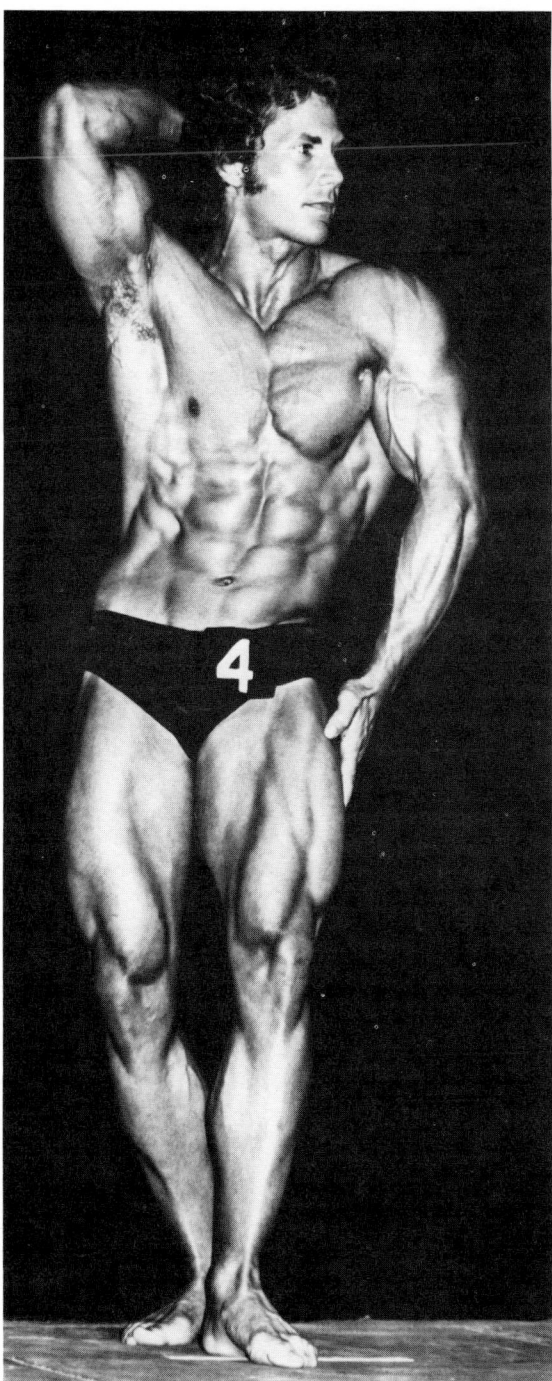

Figure 2.13 Mike Dayton, Teenage Mr. America. Photo by Bruce Klemens, Clifton, N.J.

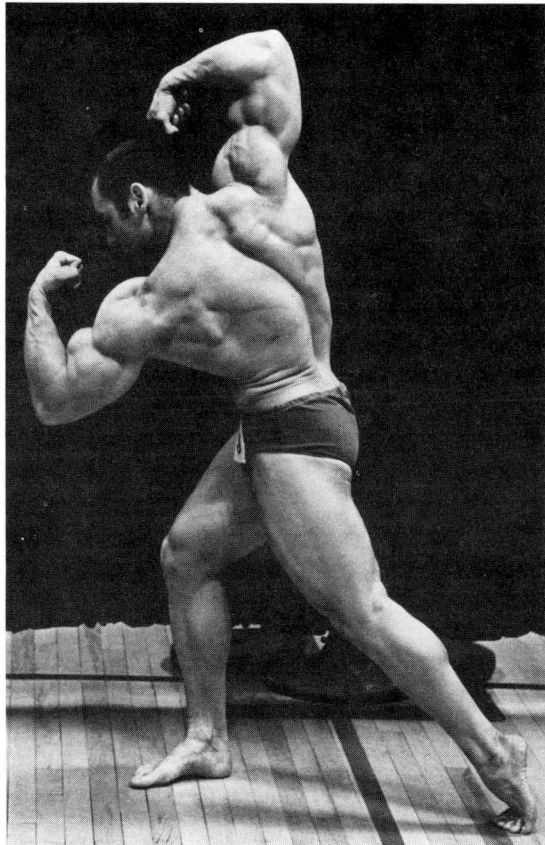

Figure 2.14 Bob Gallucci, Collegiate Mr. America. Photo by Bruce Klemens, Clifton, N.J.

Neither actin nor myosin can contract. However, in vitro, they can form a complex protein called actomyosin, which can contract. The myosin molecule has a "head" and a "tail." The enzymatic activity and its affinity for actin is located in the head. The heads project outward from the myosin filaments toward the actin filaments. These *cross bridges* are the only structural and mechanical connections between the actin and myosin filaments. During muscular contraction the actin filaments are pulled between the myosin filaments toward the Z line much like the bristles of two hairbrushes being pushed together. As the thin or actin filaments slide into the groups of thick or myosin filaments, the I band becomes narrower and, if contraction continues, disappears. As a consequence, the Z lines are drawn toward one another and the sarcomere shortens. The sum of the shortening of many sarcomeres constitutes muscular contraction.

MAJOR BODY ARTICULATIONS

The Pelvic Girdle

The responsibility of the pelvis is to transfer the weight of the upper body from the vertebral column to the legs and to provide protection to the urogenital organs and the large intestines. It is well suited to this job because of its shape and heavy bones. The pelvic girdle consists of two *innominate* bones and the *sacrum*. Each hip bone (*os innominatum*) is made up of three bones, the *ileum, ischium,* and *pubis*, which fuse into one bone at puberty (See Figure 2.15).

Ligaments of the Pelvis. The two hip bones are firmly bound to the sacrum by means of 6 ligaments—*anterior sacroiliac, posterior sacroiliac, interosseus, iliolumbar, sacrotuberous,* and *sacrospinous ligaments* (See Figure 2.16).

Movements Specific to the Pelvis. The pelvis is capable of four movements. These are as follows:

Increased inclination or forward tilt moves the pubis downward while the posterior aspect of the sacrum turns upward.

Decreased inclination or backward tilt moves the pubis forward-upward while the sacrum turns downward.

Rotation or lateral twist rotates the pelvis right or left around the vertical axis.

Lateral tilt elevates the iliac crest on one side while the other is lowered.

Movements of the pelvis are associated with and facilitate movements of the thighs and the spine. When the hip is flexed, as when

Figure 2.15 The male pelvis

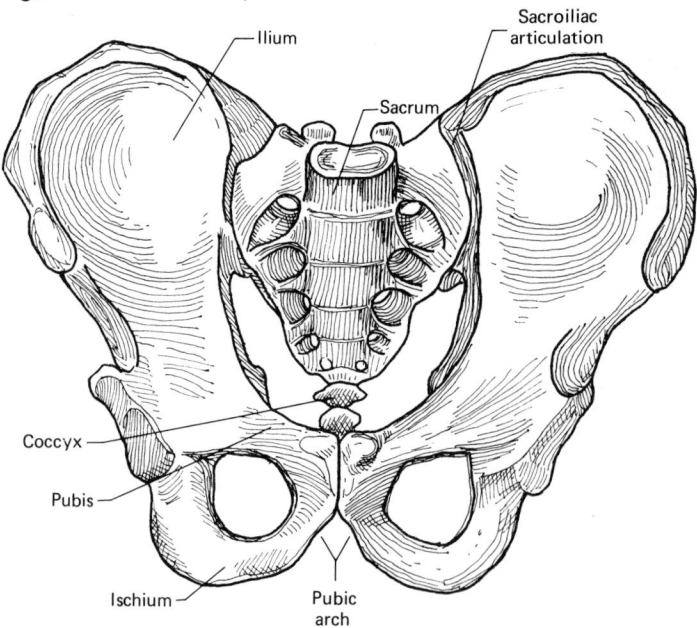

Ilium

Sacroiliac articulation

Sacrum

Coccyx

Pubis

Ischium

Pubic arch

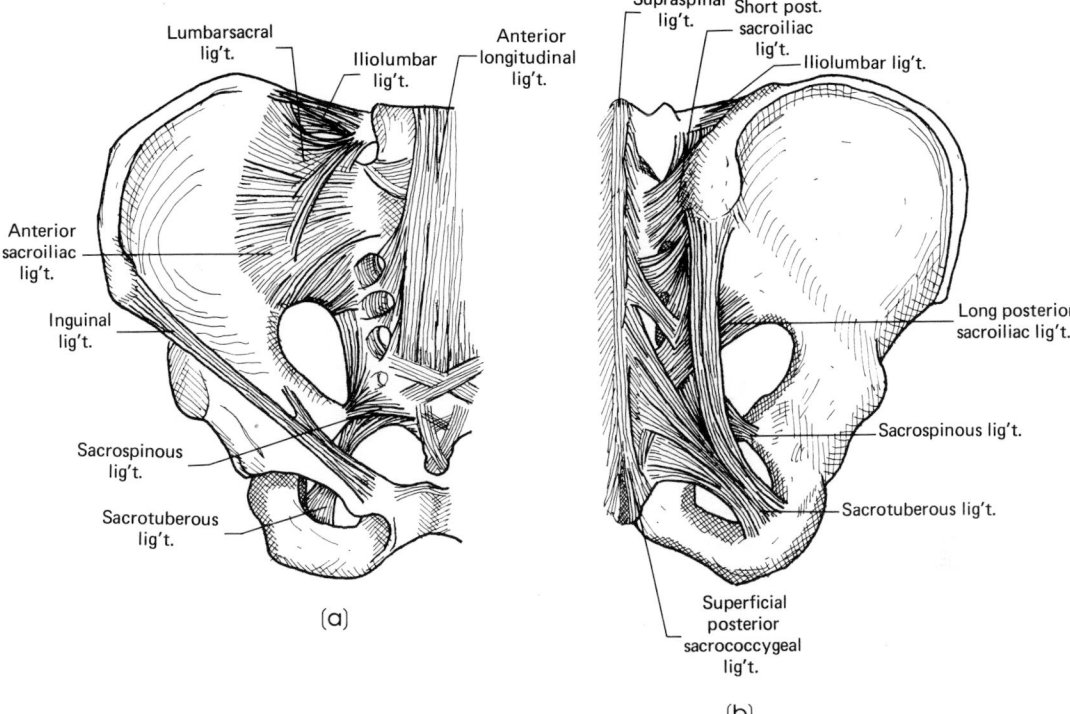

Figure 2.16 (a) anterior and (b) posterior views of pelvic ligaments

kicking a football, there is decreased inclination at the pelvis to increase the range of motion of the thigh. In this respect, the pelvis functions in the same manner as the shoulder girdle.

Muscles Attaching to the Pelvis. A large number of muscles attach to the pelvis. Following is a listing of these muscles according to their location:

Anterior Trunk
Rectus abdominis
External oblique
Internal oblique
Transversalis
Anterior Hip
Iliopsoas
Rectus femoris
Sartorius
Gluteus medius

Gluteus minimus
Tensor fascia latae
Anterior Knee
Rectus femoris
Medial Hip
Pectineus
Gracilis
Adductor magnus
Adductor longus
Adductor brevis

Posterior Hip
Gluteus maximus
Semitendinosus
Semimembranosus
Biceps femoris
Pyriformis
Quadratus femoris
Obturator internus
Obturator externus
Gimellus superior
Gimellus interior

Posterior Trunk
Erector spinae
Quadratus lumborum
Posterior Knee
Semitendinosus
Semimembranosus
Biceps femoris
Sartorius
Gracilis

The reader should note that two joint muscles that act upon both the hip and knee joints are listed under both groupings.

Vertebral Column

The superlative engineering of the vertebral column is manifested by its great stability, great range of movements, ability to support considerable weight, provision of attachments for many ligaments and muscles, transmission of gradually increasing weight to the pelvis, service as a shock absorber for jolts and jars, and provision of great protection to the delicate but important spinal cord.

The vertebral column is made up of 33 bones—7 cervical, 12 thoracic, and 5 lumbar vertebra, the sacrum, and the coccyx. The sacrum and the coccyx belong to both the pelvis and the vertebral column. The sacrum is formed of 5 fused vertebrae while 4 fused vertebrae form the coccyx. The coccyx is a vestegial tail bone.

The vertebral column has 4 curves when viewed from the side (see Figures 2.17 and 2.18). These curves serve as shock absorbers. They also move the weight of the thoracic cage and the pelvic girdle, which are anterior to the vertebral column, nearer the vertical line of gravity passing through the vertebral column. This is accomplished as a result of the concavity from the front of the thoracic and sacrococcygeal curves. The cervical and lumbar curves are convex from the front. The thoracic and sacrococcygeal curves exist before birth and consequently are called *primary curves*. Anterior concavity facilitates the fetal position. The cervical and lumbar curves are called secondary curves since they develop later. The cervical curve is formed as a result of the pull of muscles when the baby begins to lift its head. The lumbar curve develops as muscles develop that are attached to this area when the baby begins to walk. It will be noted that, beginning with the first cervical, the vertebrae become larger as they are called upon to carry an increasing amount of body weight.

All vertebrae have several common characteristics. These are: (1) the *body*, the largest portion and the part through which the weight is transmitted, (2) the vertebral *foramen*, the opening through which the spinal cord passes, (3) the *pedicles*, which connect

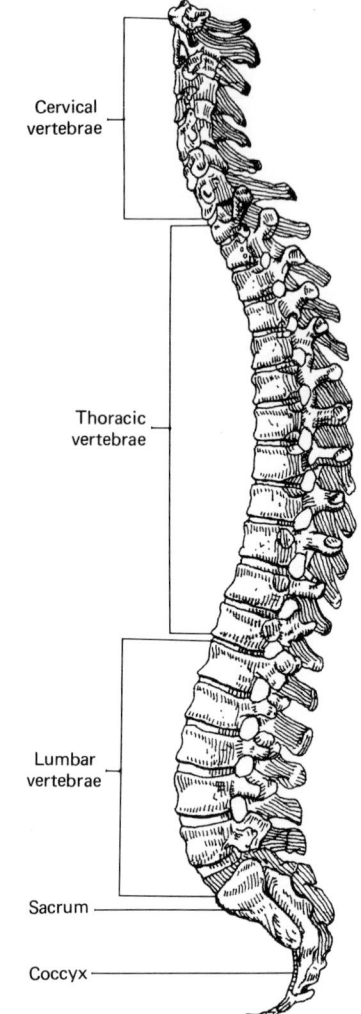

Cervical vertebrae

Thoracic vertebrae

Lumbar vertebrae

Sacrum

Coccyx

Figure 2.17 Vertebral column

the body to the posterior portion of the vertebrae, (4) *laminae*, the portion between the (5) *spinous process* and (6) the *transverse processes* on each side. Two articular processes on top and two on the bottom articulate with the adjacent vertebrae above and below. On the underside of each pedicle is an *intervertebral notch* through which nerves leaving the spinal cord pass. Thoracic vertebrae, in addition to the above features, have four articular facets where the ribs are attached.

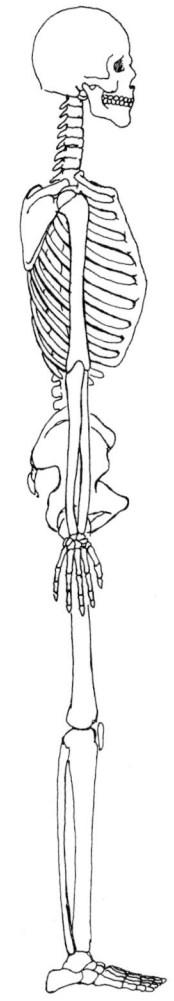

Figure 2.18 Side view of skeleton

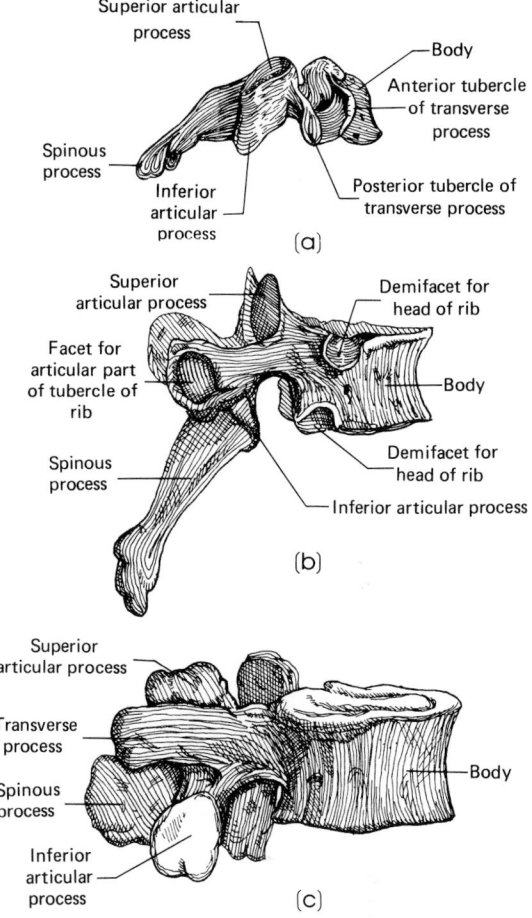

Figure 2.19 (a) Cervical, (b) thoracic, and (c) lumbar vertebrae

Figure 2.19 shows variations in the structure of vertebrae of three areas of the spine.

Between adjacent vertebrae are elastic disks of cartilage called *intervertebral disks*. In the center of the disk is a gelatinous material called the *nucleus pulposus*. The outer part of the disk is made up of a heavy and strong layer of fibrocartilage called the *anulus fibrosus*. When stress is placed on the disks, they are stretched rather than compressed. Excessive stress sometimes results in rupture of the nucleus pulposus. The protru-

sion of the nucleus pulposus may place pressure on the spinal cord or nerves emanating from it, thus causing radiating pains along the posterior side of the thigh. The disks are attached by thin cartilaginous plates to the vertebrae above and below, thereby contributing to the binding together of the vertebral column. The disks are the same diameter as the vertebral bodies except in the cervical area where they are not as wide laterally as the vertebral body. Altogether, the disks account for one-fourth of the length of the vertebral column.

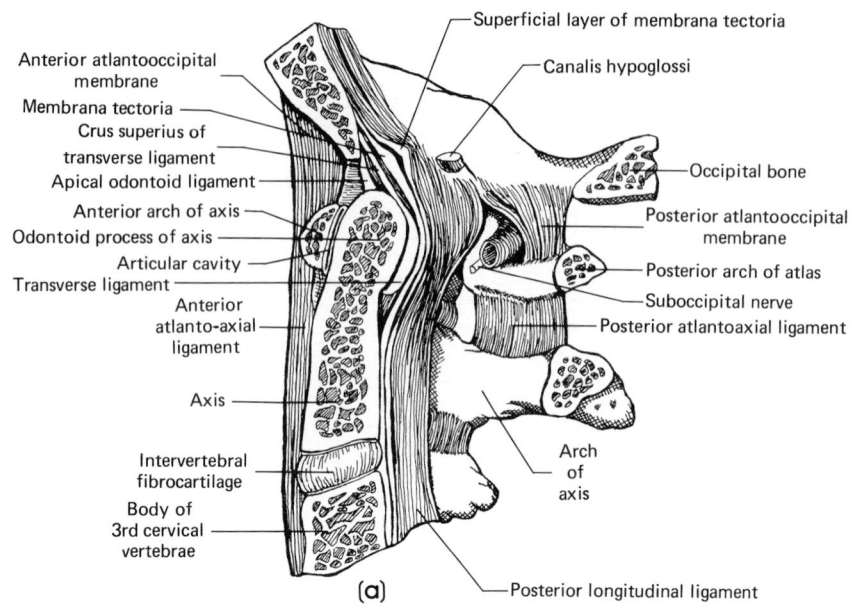

- Superficial layer of membrana tectoria

Anterior atlantooccipital membrane

Membrana tectoria

Crus superius of transverse ligament

Apical odontoid ligament

Anterior arch of axis

Odontoid process of axis

Articular cavity

Transverse ligament

Anterior atlanto-axial ligament

Axis

Intervertebral fibrocartilage

Body of 3rd cervical vertebrae

- Canalis hypoglossi

- Occipital bone

Posterior atlantooccipital membrane

Posterior arch of atlas

Suboccipital nerve

Posterior atlantoaxial ligament

Arch of axis

Posterior longitudinal ligament

(a)

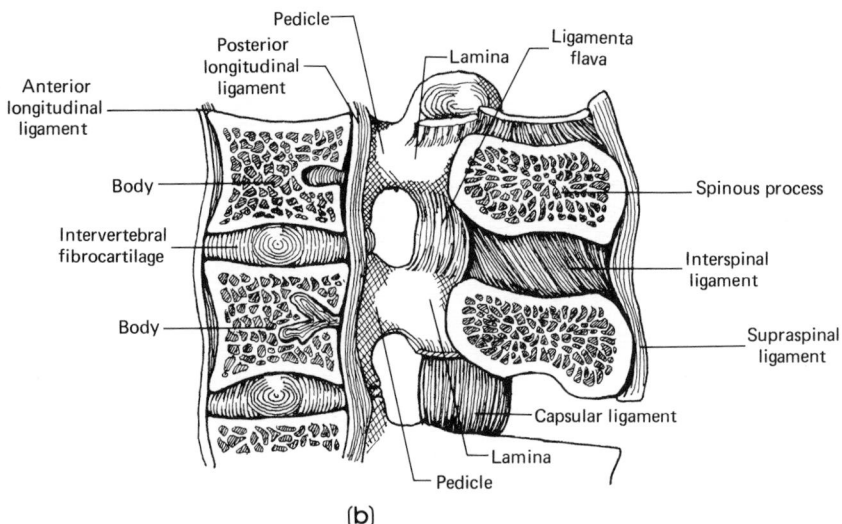

Pedicle

Posterior longitudinal ligament

Anterior longitudinal ligament

Body

Intervertebral fibrocartilage

Body

Lamina

Ligamenta flava

Spinous process

Interspinal ligament

Supraspinal ligament

Capsular ligament

Lamina

Pedicle

(b)

Ligaments of the Vertebral Column. The vertebrae are held together by several long ligaments that run the full length of the vertebral column. The *anterior longitudinal ligament* (see Figure 2.20*b*) is attached to the bodies of the vertebrae anterior to the pedi-cles and extends from the axis to the sacrum. The *posterior longitudinal ligament* (see Figure 2.20*c*) is attached to the posterior aspect of the vertebral bodies inside the vertebral foramen and extends the full length of the column. The *ligamentum flavum* (see Figure

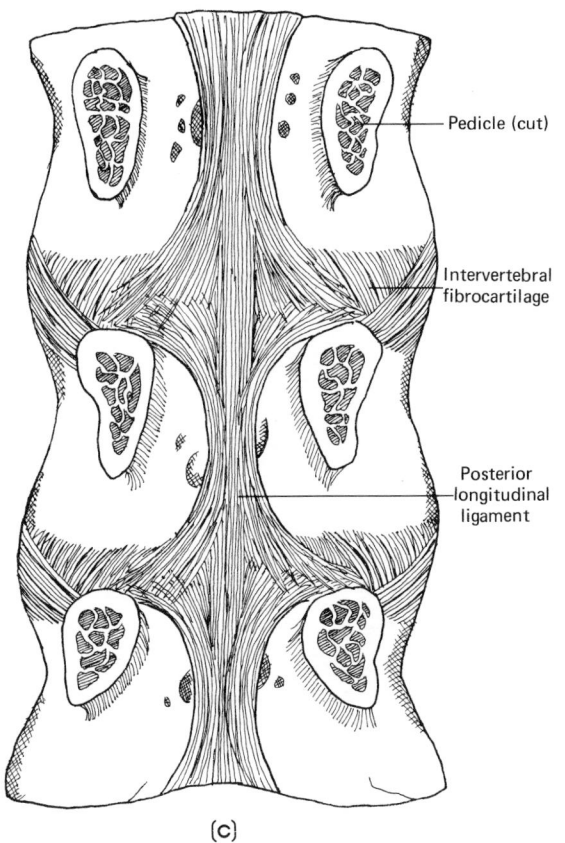

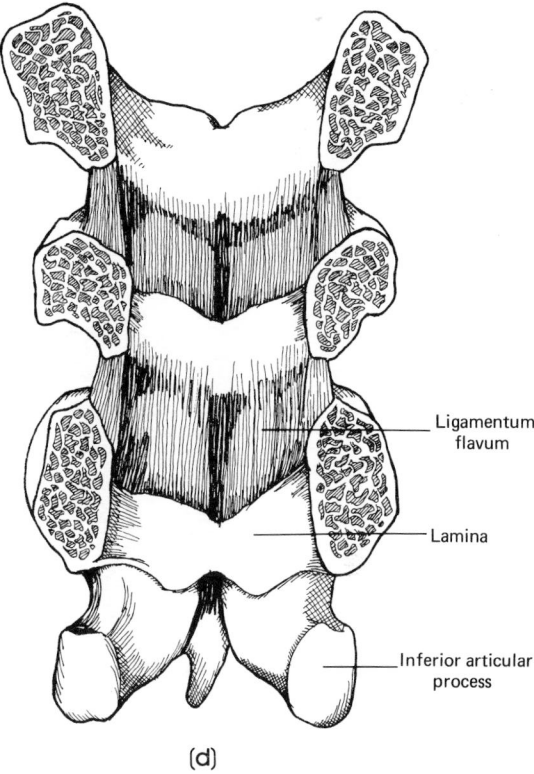

Pedicle (cut)

Intervertebral
fibrocartilage

Posterior
longitudinal
ligament

(c)

Ligamentum
flavum

Lamina

Inferior articular
process

(d)

Figure 2.20 Ligaments of the vertebral column (**a**) Medial (sagittal) section through the occipital bone and first three cervical vertebrae (**b**) Medial sagittal section of two lumbar vertebrae and their ligaments (**c**) Posterior longitudinal ligament of the vertebrae in the lumbar region (**d**) The ligamenta flava of the lumbar region, anterior aspect

2.20d) is also inside the vertebral foramen and connects the laminae to one another the full length of the column. The *supraspinous ligament* (see Figure 2.20*b*), a heavy cordlike ligament, is attached to the ends of the spinous processes. This ligament becomes the *ligamentum nuchae* in the cervical area where it assumes the characteristics of an extended membrane. Its uppermost attachment is on the occipital bone. Shorter ligaments appearing at each level are the *interspinous* and *intertransverse* ligaments. Ligaments of the oc-

cipital and first three corvical vertebrae are shown in Figure 2.20a.

Additional ligaments are located at the base of the skull. They connect the occipital bone to the axis and the atlas. The atlas and the axis, the two uppermost vertebrae, are uniquely formed. The *atlas* has two large concave articular surfaces that articulate with the occipital condyles of the skull. The atlas has no body, and its vertebral foramen accommodates the *odontoid process*, a peg-like projection from the axis, as well as the

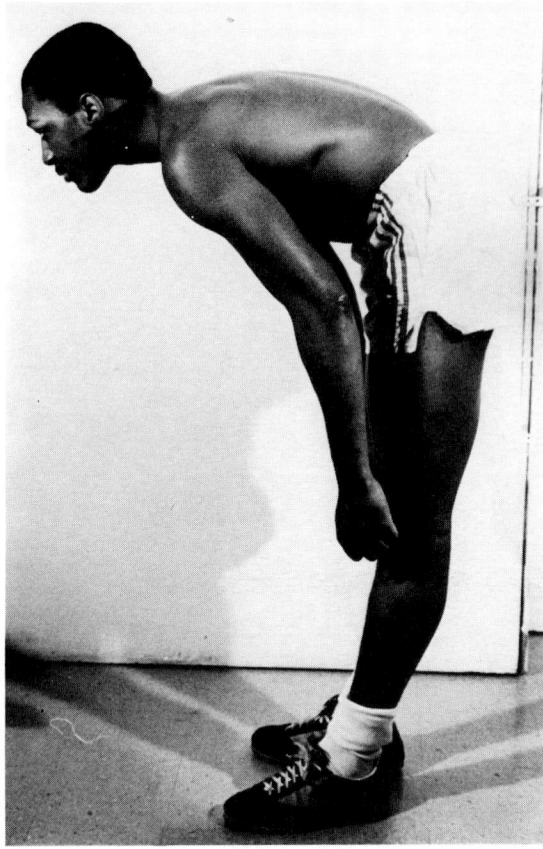

Figure 2.21a Flexion of the vertebral column combined with hip flexion

spinal cord. A very large ligament separates the ondontoid process and the spinal cord. This structure gives a considerable range of motion to the head.

Movements of the Vertebral Column. *Flexion* is a forward-downward movement of the trunk (Figure 2.21a). During the movement, the anterior portion of the vertebral disks are compressed and the articular processes slide on one another.

Extension is the return movement from flexion.

Hyperextension is a backward-downward movement of the trunk (Figure 2.21b). The greatest degree of hyperextension is possible

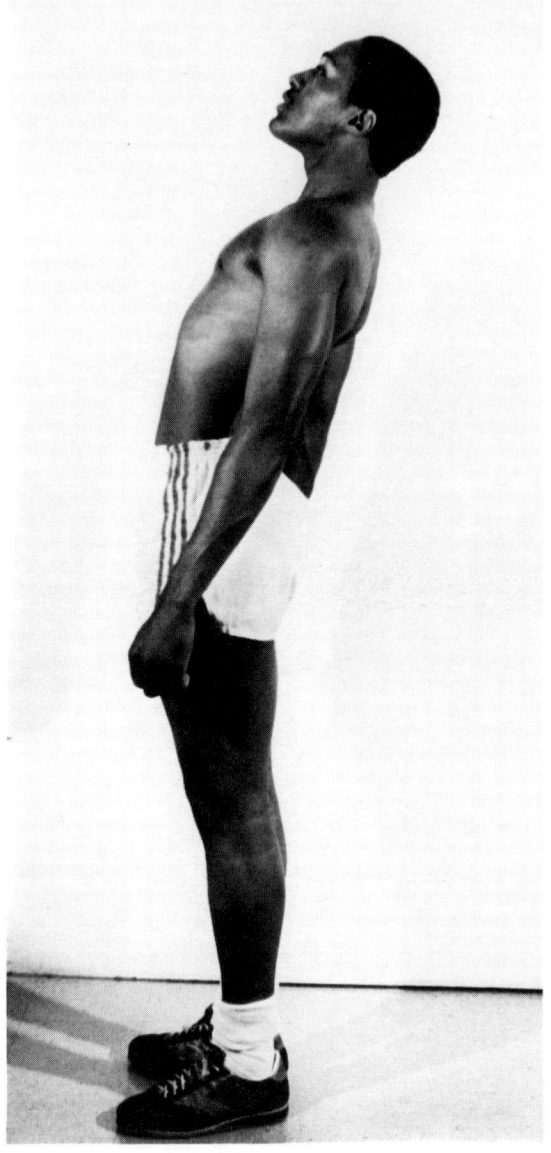

Figure 2.21b Hyperextension of the vertebral column

in the cervical and lumbar regions. Overlapping of the spinous processes in the thoracic region limits hyperextension.

Lateral flexion is sideward bending of the trunk (Figure 2.21c). Lateral flexion is limited in the thoracic region because of the ribs. Lateral flexion is always accompanied by tor-

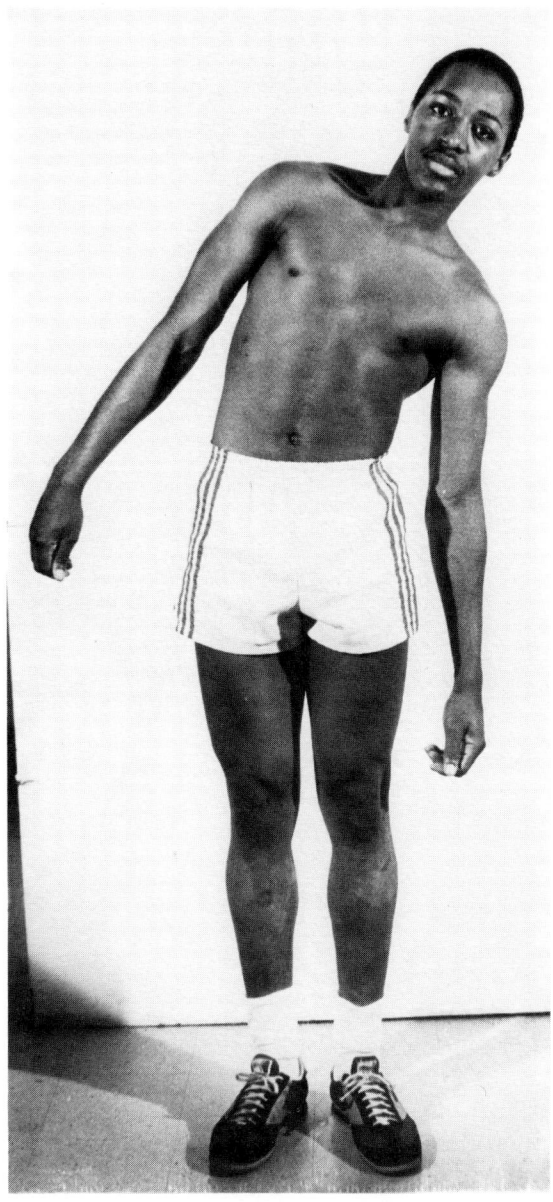

Figure 2.21c Lateral flexion of the vertebral column

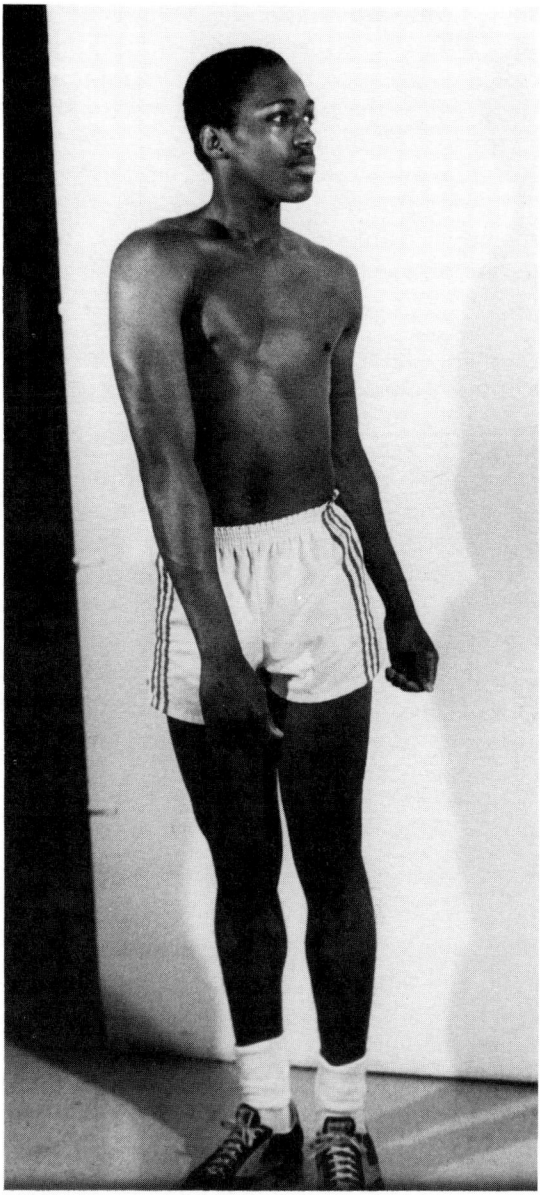

Figure 2.21d Rotation of the vertebral column to the left

sion or rotation of the vertebrae. During the lateral flexion in the standing and hyperextended positions, the vertebral bodies turn toward the direction of flexion. When lateral and forward flexion are combined, the torsion is reversed and the vertebral bodies turn in the direction opposite to the direction of lateral flexion.

Rotation is a rotatory movement of the vertebral column around the vertical axis (Figure 2.21d). The direction of rotation is indicated by the direction the front of the upper spine turns with relation to the lower. Therefore, rotation of the shoulders to the right is called rotation to the right, but rotation of the pelvis to the left while holding the shoulders still is also called rotation to the right. Rotation always involves some lateral flexion.

Circumduction is a circular movement of the upper trunk on the lower and is a combination of all the other movements except rotation.

Muscles Attaching to and Acting Upon the Vertebral Column: Exclusive Lateral Flexors.

Quadratus Lumborum (Figure 2.22)

Location: A flat sheet of fiber running vertically from the crest of the ilium and the transverse processes of the lower four lumbar vertebrae to the transverse processes of the upper two lumbar vertebrae and the lower border of the twelfth rib.

Action: Stabilization of the spine, stabilization of the ribs during inspiration, and lateral flexion of the trunk when only one of the pair contracts.

Flexors of the Vertebral Column

Rectus Abdominus (Figures 2.23 and 2.24)

Location: A slender muscle with parallel fibers divided horizontally by three tendinous areas and vertically into two sections by a tendinous strip approximately one inch wide called the *linea alba*. Runs from the crest of the pubis to the cartilages of the fifth, sixth, and seventh ribs.

Action: Spinal flexion, stabilization of the pelvis, and aiding in completion of the expiration by pulling downward on the ribs. When one rectus abdominus contracts alone, assists in lateral flexion.

External Obliques (Figure 2.25)

Location: Covers the front and side of the abdomen between the rectus abdominus and the latissimus dorsi with a sheet of parallel fibers running from the fifth through the

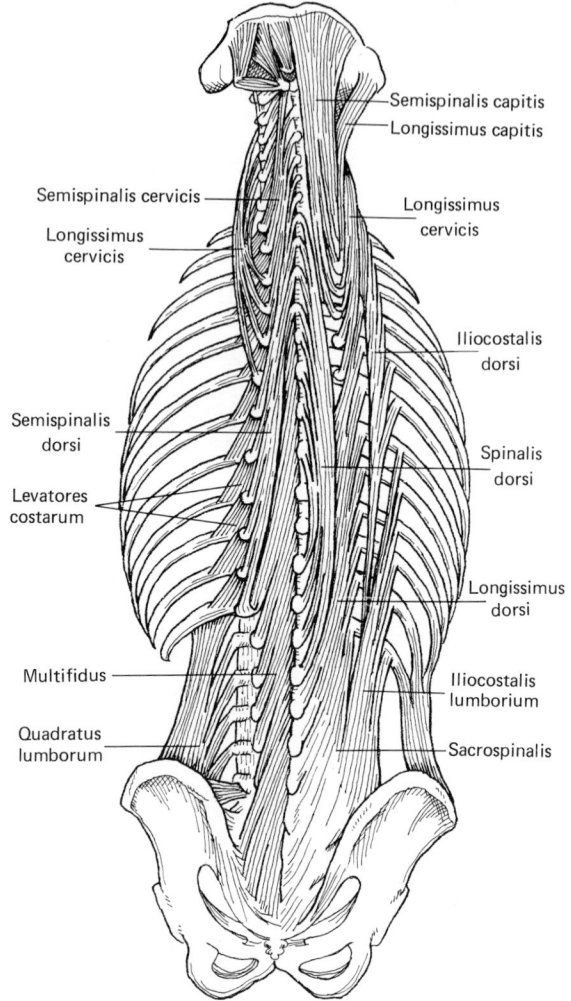

Figure 2.22 Deep muscles of back and neck

twelfth ribs to the crest of the ilium, the linea alba, the crest of the pubis, and the fascia of the thigh.

Action: Flexion of the vertebral column when the external obliques on both sides act together, and flexion, lateral flexion, and rotation to the opposite side if the muscles on one side act alone.

Internal Oblique (Figure 2.23)

Location: A flat muscle with fibers radiating from the lumbar fascia, the inguinal liga-

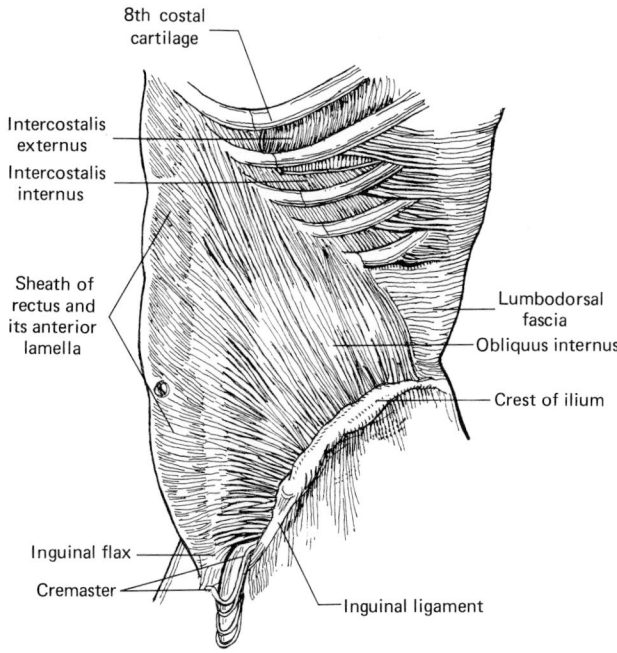

8th costal cartilage

Intercostalis externus

Intercostalis internus

Sheath of rectus and its anterior lamella

Inguinal flax

Cremaster

Lumbodorsal fascia

Obliquus internus

Crest of ilium

Inguinal ligament

Figure 2.23 Obliquus internus abdominis, intercostalis externus and internus, lumbodorsal fascia, inguinal flax, and inguinal ligament

Figure 2.24 Muscles of the abdominal area

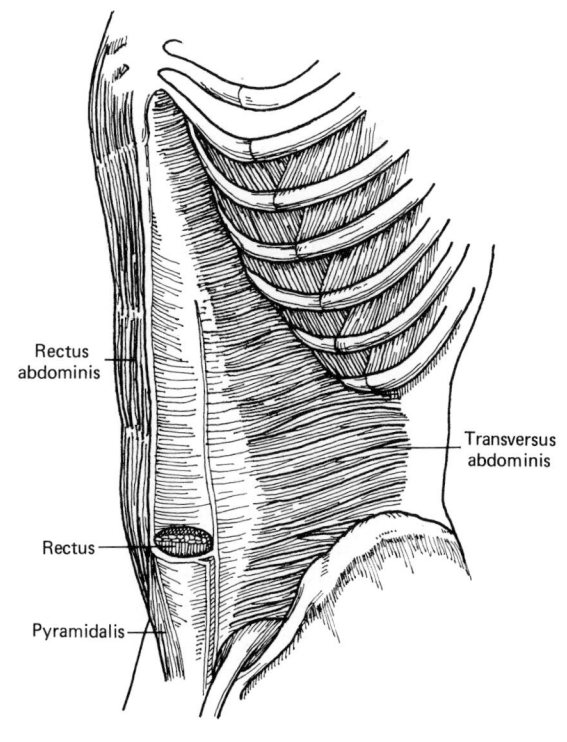

Rectus abdominis

Rectus

Pyramidalis

Transversus abdominis

ment, and the crest of the ilium to the cartilages of the eighth through tenth ribs and the linea alba. Its fibers are at right angles to those of the external oblique.

Action: Same as that of the external oblique, that is, flexion, lateral flexion, and rotation except that the internal oblique causes rotation to the same side.

Scaleni Anterior, Medius, and Posterior (Figure 2.26)

Location: Longitudinal fibers run from the transverse processes of the cervical vertebrae to the upper surface of the first and second ribs.

Action: Lateral flexion and assists in flexion of the cervical vertebrae. When the head is stabilized, may aid in respiration.

Sternocleidomastoid (Figure 2.27)

Location: A large superficial muscle in the

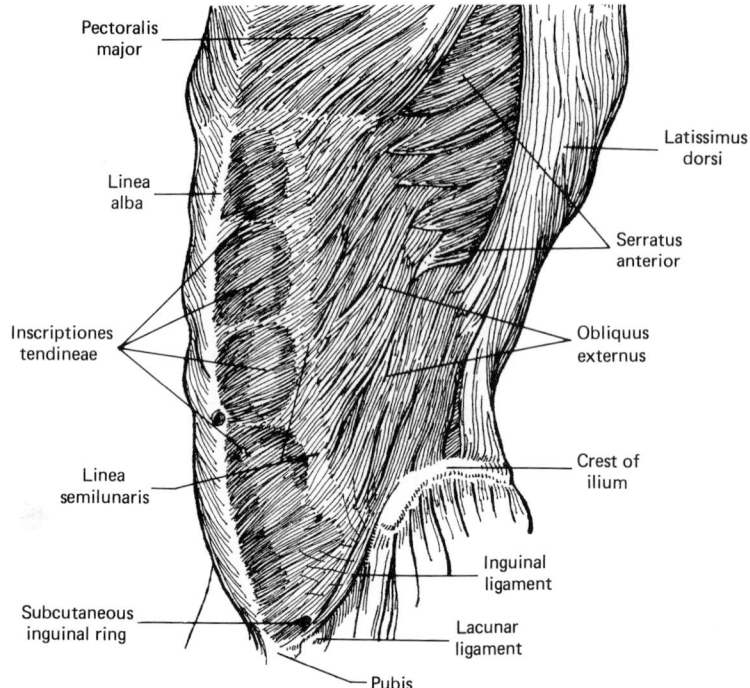

Labels on figure:
Pectoralis major
Linea alba
Inscriptiones tendineae
Linea semilunaris
Subcutaneous inguinal ring
Pubis
Latissimus dorsi
Serratus anterior
Obliquus externus
Crest of ilium
Inguinal ligament
Lacunar ligament

Figure 2.25 Pectoralis major, linea alba, inscriptiones tendinae, linea semilumaris, latissimus dorsi, serratus anterior, obliquus externus, and inguinal and lacunar ligaments

neck consisting of two groups of parallel fibers running from the sternum and the clavicle to the mastoid process of the skull.

Action: Flexion, lateral flexion, and rotation toward the opposite side, that is, the right sternocleidomastoid will rotate the head to the left.

Longus Colli

Location: Fibers run from the transverse processes of the third, fourth, and fifth cervical vertebrae, the anterior surface of the bodies of the first three thoracic and the last three cervical vertebrae to the anterior arch of the atlas, the anterior side of the bodies of the second, third, and fourth cervical vertebrae, and the transverse processes of the fifth and sixth cervical vertebrae.

Action: Assists in flexion and lateral flexion of the cervical region of the vertebral column.

Longus Capitis (Figure 2.26)

Location: Fibers run from the transverse processes of the third through the sixth cervical vertebrae to the occipital bone.

Action: Assists in flexion and lateral flexion of the head and cervical spine.

Rectus Capitis Anterior (Figure 2.22)

Location: From the lateral side of the atlas to the occipital bone.

Action: Assists in flexion of the head.

Rectus Capitis Lateralis (Figure 2.26)

Location: From the transverse processes of the atlas to the occipital bone.

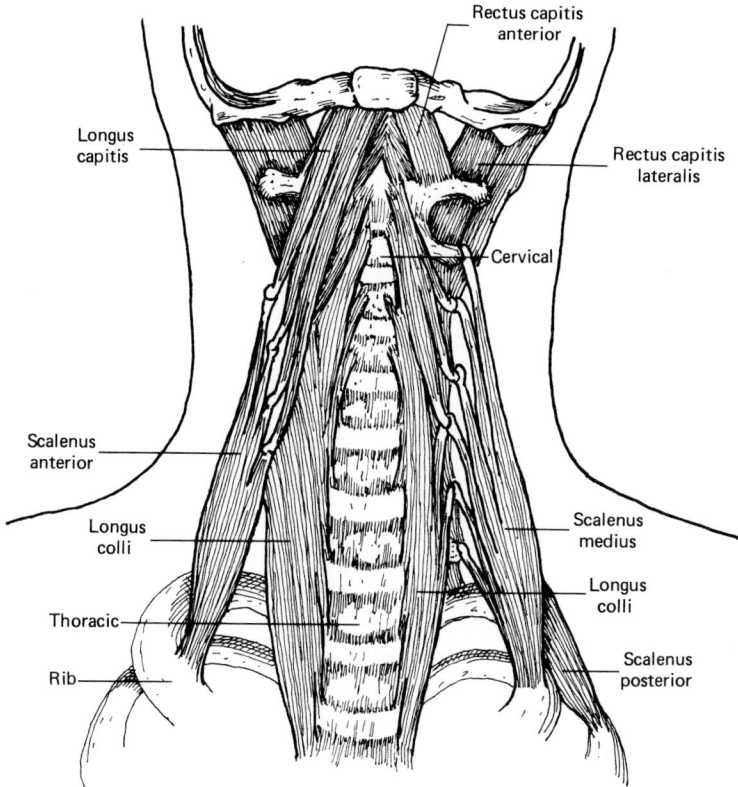

Figure 2.26 Anterior vertebral muscles of the cervical area

Action: Assists in lateral flexion of the head.

Extensors of the Vertebral Column.

Splenius Capitis and Cervicis

Location: The broad bands of parallel fibers angle outward and upward from the ligamentum nuchae, the spinous process of the seventh cervical, and spinous processes of the third to sixth thoracic vertebrae to the transverse processes of the upper two or three cervical vertebrae, the occipital bone, and the mastoid process of the temporal bone.

Action: Extension and hyperextension of the head and neck and support of the head in erect posture, when both sides act together.

Lateral flexion and rotation to the opposite side when one side contracts alone.

Intertransversarii

Location: From the transverse process of one vertebrae to that of the next, from the atlas to the first thoracic, and then from the tenth thoracic to the fifth lumbar—very small muscles.

Action: One side acting alone—lateral flexion of the vertebral column. Both sides acting together—extension and hyperextension of the spine.

Erector Spinae

Location: Begins as a large muscle in the lumbrosacral area but quickly divides into

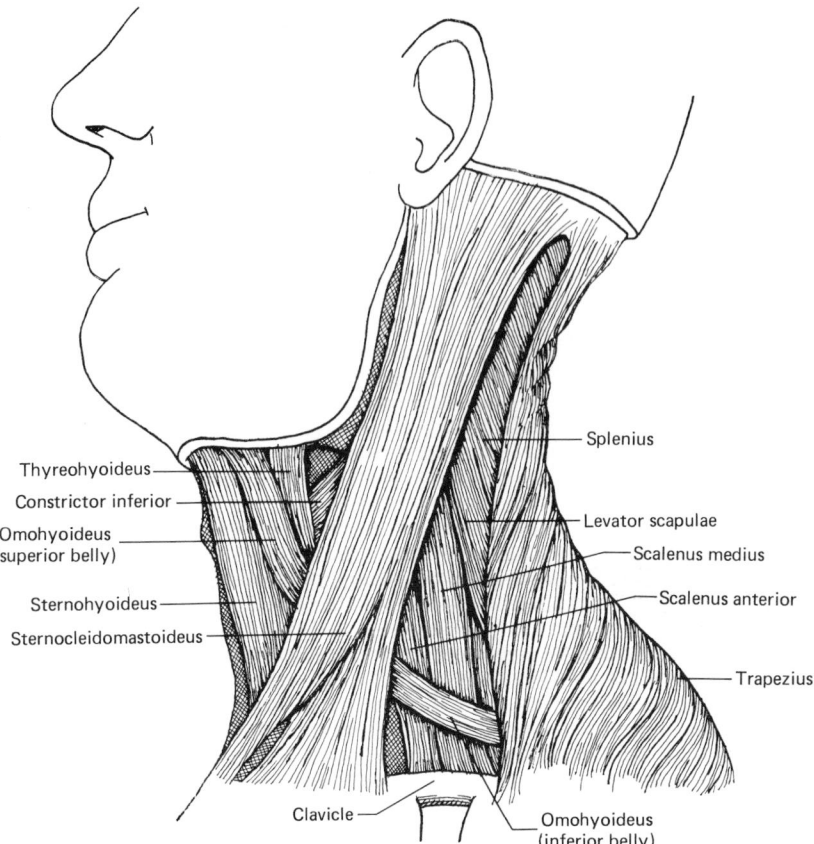

Figure 2.27 Muscle of the neck.

Thyreohyoideus
Constrictor inferior
Omohyoideus
(superior belly)
Sternohyoideus
Sternocleidomastoideus

Splenius
Levator scapulae
Scalenus medius
Scalenus anterior
Trapezius

Clavicle
Omohyoideus
(inferior belly)

three branches, the *iliocostal, longissimus,* and *spinalus* branches, which further subdivide. The iliocostalis branch divides into the *iliocostalis lumborum,* the *iliocostalis thoracis,* and the *iliocostalis cervicis.* The longissimus branch divides into the *longissimus thoracis,* the *longissimus cervicis,* and the *longissimus capitis.* The spinalis branch divides into the *spinalis thoracis* and *spinalis cervicis.* Slips of the several branches insert on the ribs, the transverse processes of the thoracic and cervical vertebrae, and the spinous processes of the cervical and thoracic vertebrae. The longissimus capitis inserts on the mastoid process of the skull.

Action: Extension and hyperextension of the head and vertebral column when both

sides contract. Lateral flexion when one side contracts alone. Rotation toward the side of the contracting pair in combination with other muscles.

Interspinales

Location: A deep posterior spinal muscle which joins the spinous processes of adjacent vertebrae from the axis to the second thoracic vertebrae and from the first lumbar to the sacrum.

Action: Extension and hyperextension of the vertebral column.

Rotatores Longi and Breves

Location: Small muscles from the transverse to the spinous processes of the first and second vertebrae.

Action: When both sides act together, extension and hyperextension of the vertebral column, and when one side acts alone, rotation toward the opposite side.

Multifidus

Location: Small deep posterior pairs of muscles running the full length of the vertebral column starting at the sacrum, the iliac crest, and the transverse processes of the lumbar and thoracic vertebrae and attaching to all the spinous processes except that of the atlas.

Action: Lateral flexion and rotation to the opposite side when one side acts alone and extension and hyperextension when both sides act together.

Semispinalis Thoracis

Location: From the transverse processes of the sixth to the tenth thoracic vertebrae to the spinous processes of the sixth and seventh cervical and the first through the fourth thoracic vertebrae.

Action: Lateral flexion and rotation to the opposite side if one side acts alone and extension and hyperextension when both sides act together.

Semispinalis Cervicis (Figure 2.22)

Location: From the tranverse processes of the first six thoracic vertebrae to the spinal processes of the axis down to that of the fifth cervical vertebrae.

Action: Lateral flexion and rotation to the opposite side when one side acts alone and extension and hyperextension when both sides act together.

Semispinalis Capitis (Figure 2.22)

Location: From the fourth, fifth, and sixth cervical vertebrae and the transverse processes of the seventh cervical and the first six thoracic vertebrae to the occipital bone.

Action: Lateral flexion of the head and cervical area when one side acts alone and extension and hyperextension of the head and neck when both sides contract.

Suboccipital Group

Location: These four muscles (*obliquus capitis superior* and *inferior* and the *rectus capitis posterior major* and *minor*) arise from the posterior surfaces of the axis and the atlas to insert on the occipital bone and the transverse processes of the atlas.

Action: Lateral flexion and rotation of the head to the same side when one side acts alone and extension and hyperextension of the head when both sides act together.

Psoas

Location: In the abdominal cavity behind the viscera. Arises from the bodies of the last thoracic and all the lumbar vertebrae and the transverse processes of all the lumbar vertebrae and inserts on the lesser trochanter of the femur.

Action: Primarily a hip flexor; however, in a supine position when the strength of the abdominals is inadequate, the psoas acts as a hyperextensor of the lumbar region during leg raising. Although the psoas is a very important muscle in sports involving running, jumping, kicking, and flexing of the hip, exercise programs which strengthen this muscle but inadequately develop the abdominal muscles are contraindicated for muscularly weak people or those with lordosis.

The Hip Joint

The hip joint (see Figure 2.28) has less freedom of movement than the shoulder joint, although the structure of both is quite similar. Both are ball and socket joints but that of the hip is much deeper. Nevertheless, a great range of movement can be developed in the hip joint as gymnasts and divers have demonstrated. The spherical head of the femur fits into the deep *acetabulum* formed at the junction of the ilium, ischium, and pubis of the

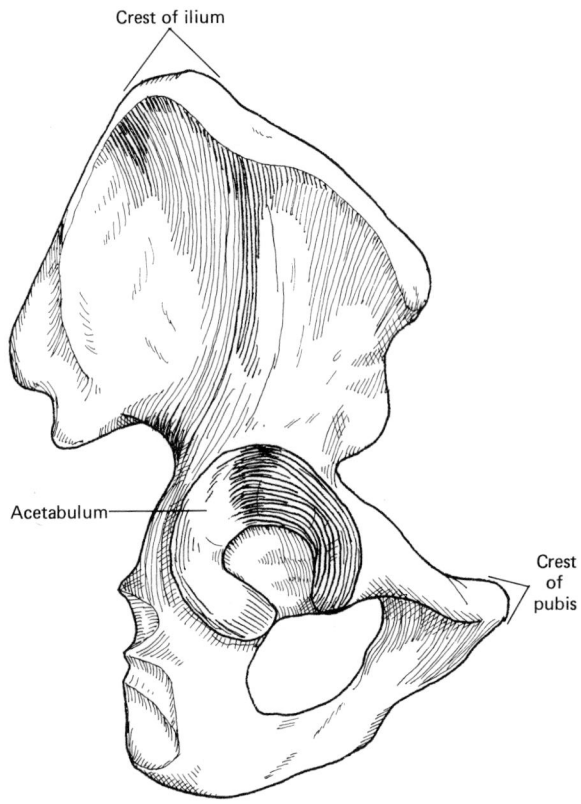

Crest of ilium

Acetabulum

Crest
of
pubis

Figure 2.28 Right hip bone showing acetabulum

pelvis. On the underside of the acetabulum is a notch or gap called the *acetabular notch*. *Hyaline cartilage*, which deepens the acetabulum since it is thicker at its periphery and thinner at its center, lines the acetabulum. The center of the hyaline cartilage is filled with fatty tissue covered by a *synovial membrane*. The *glenoid labrum*, a flat rum of fibrocartilage attached at its edge to the acetabulum, covers the hyaline cartilage. Like the hyaline cartilage, the glenoid labrum is thicker at its edges than it is at its center. This serves to hold the head of the femur more firmly. In order to absorb impacts of the femoral head against the acetabulum during running and jumping, the glenoid labrum is thicker above and behind. The head of the femur is also covered with hyaline cartilage,

which, just the opposite of that which lines the acetabulum, is thicker at the center and thinner at the edges. This serves to hold the head more firmly and to decrease the probability of a dislocation. There is a small pit near the center of the head called the *fovea capitis* to which is attached the *teres femoris*, a flat, narrow triangular ligament whose opposite end is attached to the *acetabular ligament*. It serves as a tight tether to decrease the probability of dislocation of the femoral head.

The neck of the femur serves to absorb shocks; however, in elderly people whose bones have become more brittle, it is a frequent site of fractures. When viewed from the side, the femur bows forward. This is another provision for the absorbtion of the stresses and strains imposed during running or jumping. When viewed from the front, the femur slants inward. This places the mechanical axis of the femur (Figure 2.29), the line connecting the centers of the two heads of the femur, in a more nearly vertical position. The wider the pelvis, the greater the slant. Since females have a relatively wider pelvis, the femur of females slants inward to a greater degree. This increases the difficulty of maintaining straight-forward thrust of the legs while running and introduces a rotatory component of force. Further, the angle between the neck and the shaft of the femur is more nearly a right angle in females. This angle is called the *angle of obliquity*.

Ligaments of the Hip Joint. The five powerful ligaments of the hip joint lend it considerable stability. The teres femoris and acetabular ligaments have already been mentioned. The *transverse acetabular ligament* is a strong flat band that passes across the acetabular notch to close the ring around the head of the femur. The *iliofemoral ligament* (Figure 2.30) is an extremely strong band in front of the capsule passing from that part of the rim of the acetabulum formed by the il-

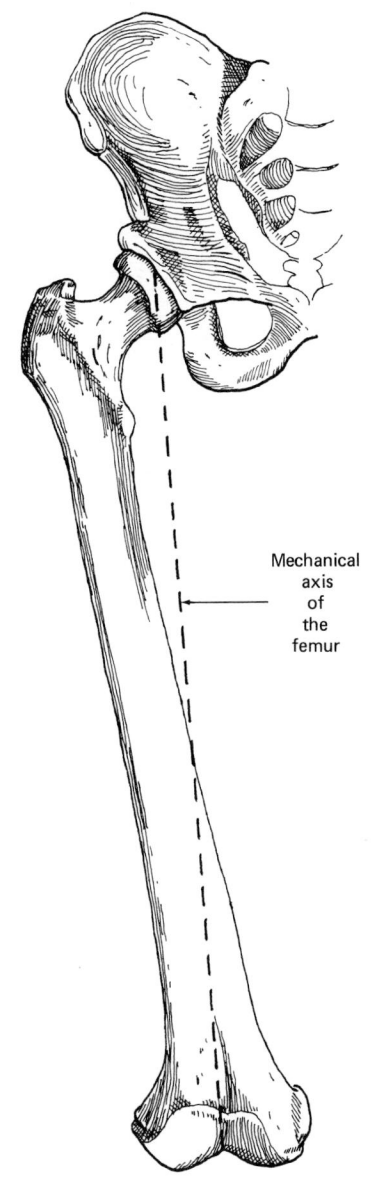

Figure 2.29 Mechanical axis of the femur

Mechanical
axis
of
the
femur

the capsule. It checks abduction, extension, and outward rotation. At the back of the capsule is the *ischiofemoral ligament*, which checks inward rotation and adduction when the hip is flexed.

Movements Specific to the Hip Joint. The hip joint permits the following movements:

Flexion is forward movement of the femur. When the knee is flexed, the thigh can be brought to the trunk. When the knee is extended the two joint hamstring muscles permit about 90 degrees of flexion. In extreme flexion, the pelvis contributes to the range of movement by tilting backward.

Extension is the reverse movement of flexion.

Hyperextension is backward motion of the femur beyond the line of the trunk. This movement is very limited due to tension in the iliofemoral ligaments and the psoas and iliacus muscles. Some gymnasts and dancers appear to have developed the ability to hyperextend the hip joint, but close observation will show that the femur is rotated outward, the pelvis is tilted forward (with some flexion at the hip joint of the supporting leg), and the lumbar region of the vertebral column is hyperextended.

Abduction is sideward movement of the femur away from the midline of the body. The range of movement is limited by tight antagonistic muscles rather than as a result of unique construction of the joint or ligaments. Hard stretching exercises and outward rotation of the femur make possible 90 degrees of abduction, as demonstrated in the side split.

Adduction is movement of the femur toward the midline of the body. It is limited by contact with the opposite thigh unless the moving leg is forward or rearward of the opposite leg. Adduction of the hip joint also takes place when the opposite hip is lowered (lateral tilt), as when flexing the trunk sideward.

Circumduction is movement of the femur

ium to the neck of the femur. It checks extension and both inward and outward rotation. The *pubofemoral ligament* passes from that part of the rim of the acetabulum formed by the pubis to the neck of the femur. It is a narrow band at the anterior and lower part of

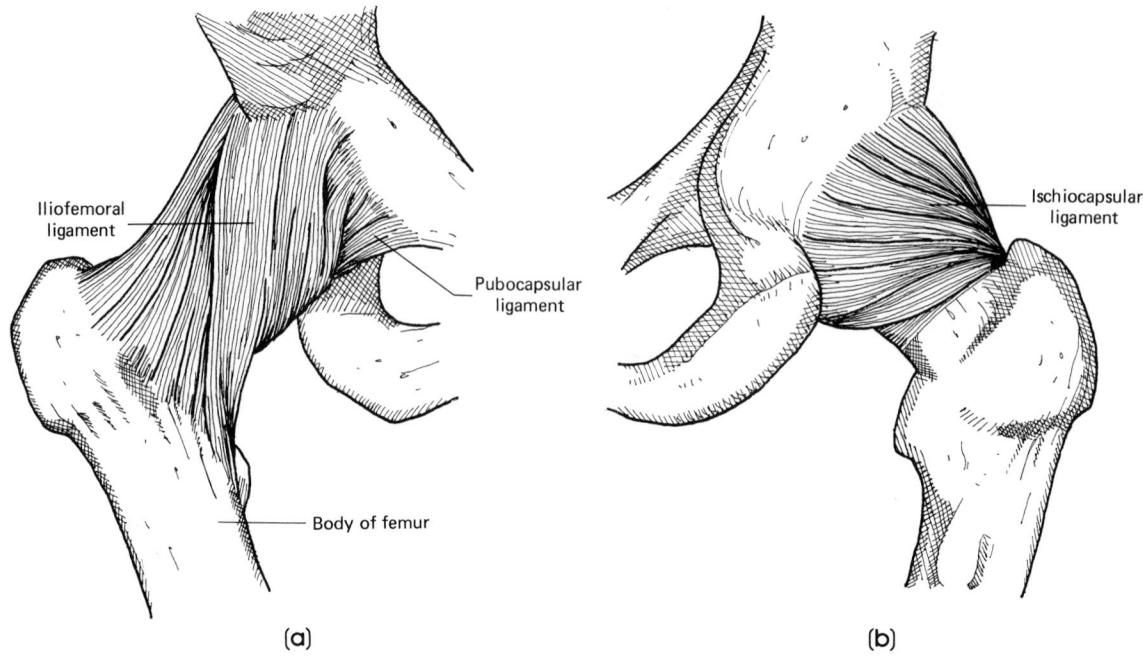

Iliofemoral
ligament

Pubocapsular
ligament

Body of femur

Ischiocapsular
ligament

(a)

(b)

Figure 2.30   Ligaments of the hip joint. (a) Anterior view, (b) posterior view

in a circle so that it describes a cone with its apex at the hip joint. Circumduction is a combination of all the preceding movements.

Rotation occurs around the central axis of the joint that passes through the hip and knee joints. Rotation is limited to 90 degrees because the neck of the femur strikes the side of the socket. *Inward rotation* occurs when the knee is turned inward while *outward rotation* occurs when the knee is turned outward.

Muscles of the Hip Joint.

The 16 muscles of the hip joint include 6 flexors, 4 extensors, 2 abductors, 4 adductors, and 6 outward rotators.

Flexors of the Hip

Psoas (Figure 2.31)

The proximal attachment of this muscle is on the last thoracic and all the lumbar vertebrae; consequently, it was described under

muscles attaching to the vertebral column. However, its principal function is that of flexing the hip. It is a powerful hip flexor, especially during the latter part of hip flexion where its angle of pull is considerably improved.

Iliacus (Figure 2.31)

Location: From the inner surfaces of the ilium and the sacrum over the front of the pelvis to the lesser trocanter via a tendon also arising from the psoas. Some authors classify these two muscles as one calling it the iliopsoas.

Action: Stabilization and flexion of the hip joint.

Sartorius (Figure 2.31)

Location: The spine of the ilium to the tuberosity of the tibia. This is the longest muscle in the body, curving around the medial

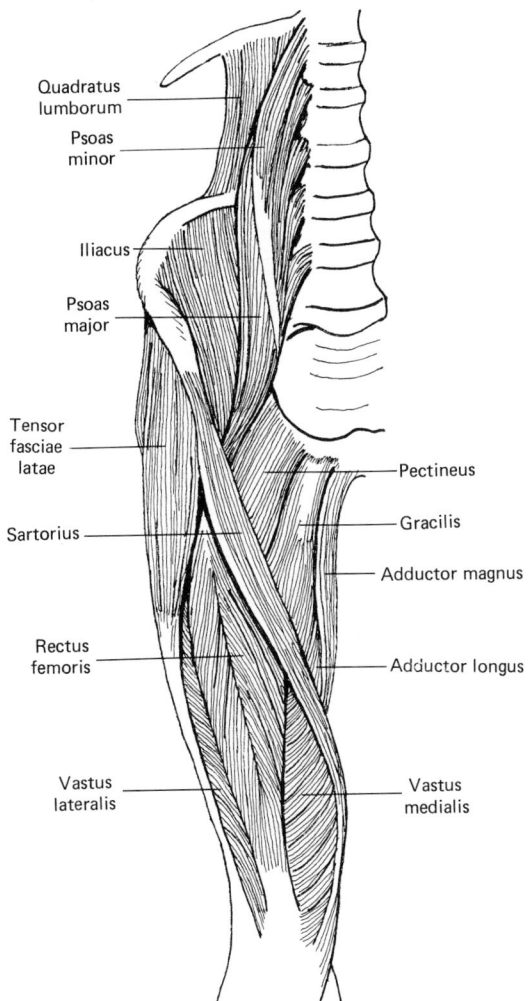

Figure 2.31 Muscles of the iliac and anterior femoral regions

side of the thigh, behind the medial condyle, and then to the tibia.

Action: Flexes, abducts, and outward rotates the thigh and inward rotates and flexes the lower leg.

Rectus Femoris (Figure 2.31)

Location: One head from the spine of the ilium and the second head from above the edge of the acetabulum via a common tendon to the patella.

Action: Hip flexion and abduction and knee extension. The construction of this muscle favors speed at the cost of force. Greater hip flexing force can be exerted when the knee is flexed. Called the "kicking muscle" because it moves the foot with great speed and power when it acts on both the hip and knee joints.

Pectineus (Figure 2.31)

Location: From the pubis to the lesser trochanter of the femur.

Action: Hip flexion and adduction and weak assistance during outward rotation.

Tensor Fasciae Latae (Figure 2.31)

Location: From the crest of the ilium to the iliotibial tract of the fascia lata of the thigh. This muscle does not insert on a bone.

Action: Flexes, abducts, and inward rotates the femur, and tenses the fascia latae.

Hip Extensors

Biceps Femoris (Figure 2.32)

Location: Long head from the tuberosity of the ischium and the short head from the linea aspera via a shared tendon to the lateral condyle of the tibia and head of the fibula.

Action: The long head extends the hip and assists in outward rotation and with the short head flexes and outward rotates the knee.

Semitendinosus (Figure 2.32)

Location: From the tuberosity of the ischium to the upper medial side of the tibia.

Action: Extension and inward rotation of the femur and flexion and inward rotation at the knee joint.

Gluteus Maximus (Figure 2.32)

Location: From the posterior crest of the ilium, the posterior surface of the sacrum, and the fascia in the lumbar area to the posterior side of the femur near the greater trochanter of the femur.

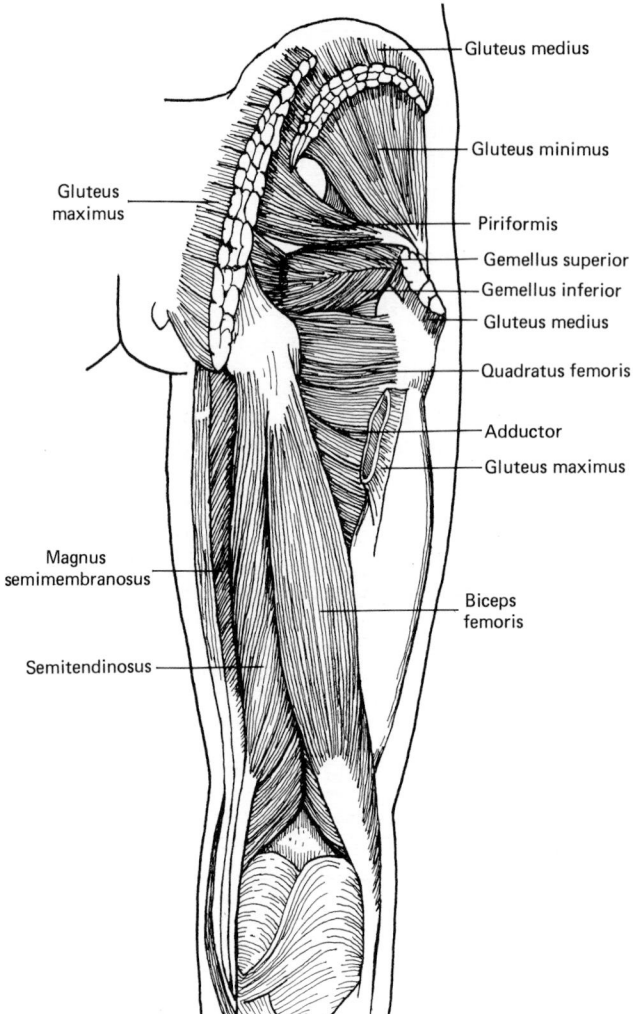

Labels on figure:
- Gluteus medius
- Gluteus minimus
- Piriformis
- Gemellus superior
- Gemellus inferior
- Gluteus medius
- Quadratus femoris
- Adductor
- Gluteus maximus
- Gluteus maximus
- Biceps femoris
- Magnus semimembranosus
- Semitendinosus

Figure 2.32 Gluteal and posterior femoral regions

Action: Powerful hip extension and outward rotation of the femur. The upper third, which lies above the center of rotation, abducts the femur while the lower two-thirds, which lies below the center of rotation, assists in adduction.

Hip Abductors

Gluteus Medius (Figure 2.32)

Location: From the medial side of the crest of the ilium to the lateral side of the greater trochanter of the femur.

Action: Powerful abduction of the hips. The anterior fibers flex and inward rotate the hip joint while the posterior fibers extend and outward rotate this joint.

Gluteus Minimus (Figure 2.32)

Location: From the outer surface of the ilium to the greater trochanter of the femur. It is beneath the gluteus medius.

Action: When the entire muscle contracts, it assists with abduction. When the anterior fibers contract alone, they produce inward rotation and flexion while contraction of the posterior fibers causes outward rotation and extension of the hip joint.

Hip Adductors

Adductor Longus (Figure 2.33)

Location: From the front of the pubis to the middle third of the thigh.

Action: Adducts and assists in hip flexion and outward rotation.

Adductor Brevis (Figure 2.33)

Location: from the pubis to the upper half of the linea aspera of the femur.

Action: Adducts and aids in flexing the hip joint in standing position but when the hip is already flexed, it extends and adducts the hip joint.

Adductor Magnus (Figures 2.31 and 2.33)

Location: From the pubis, tuberosity of the ischium and ramus to the linea aspera and medial condyle of the femur, as shown in Figures 2.31 and 2.33.

Action: Adduction of the hip joint when the entire muscle contracts, inward rotation and flexion when the upper fibers contract alone, and outward rotation and extension when the lower fibers contract alone.

Gracilis (Figure 2.31)

Location: From the symphysis pubis and the pubic arch to the medial side of the tibia below the condyle. This is a long slender muscle.

Action: Flexion when the knee is extended, adduction and inward rotation.

Outward Rotators

Location: The 6 outward rotators form a compact group behind the hip joint. Their horizontal fibers run from the posterior side of the pelvis to the greater trochanter of the femur. The 6 muscles are the *obturator externus, obturator internus, gemellus supe-*

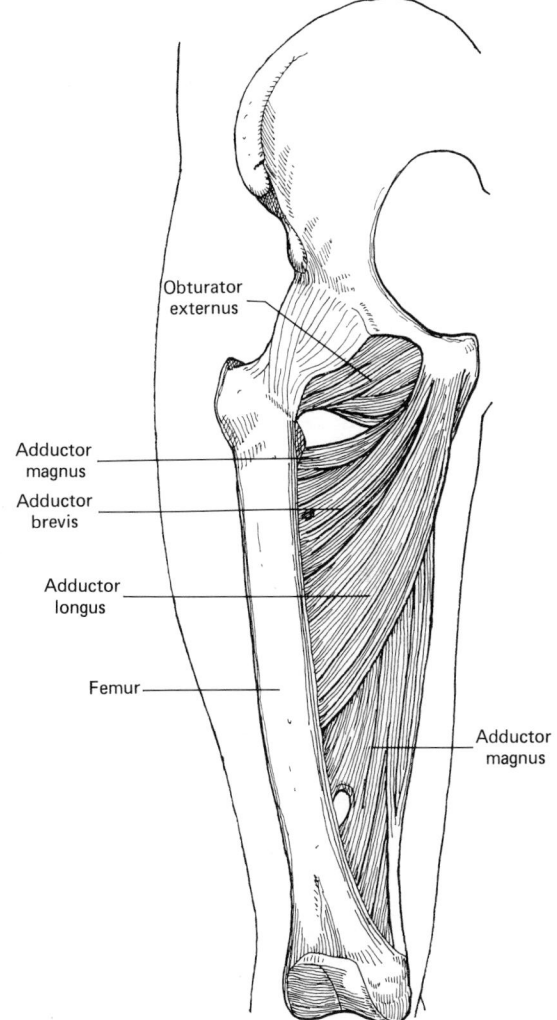

Figure 2.33 Deep muscles of the medial femoral region

rior, gemellus inferior, quadratus femorus, and piriformis.

Action: Hold the femoral head in the acetabulum, outward rotation, and abduction and adduction.

The Thorax

The thorax consists of the 12 ribs, the sternum, cartilage, ligaments, and muscles (see

Figure 2.34). The ribs have a long curving body. The point of greatest curvature is called the *angle*. The *head* of each rib articulates with the body of the thoracic vertebrae above (except for the first, tenth, eleventh, and twelfth rib). The tubercle of the first rib articulates with the transverse process of the first thoracic vertebra, the third with the third thoracic vertebra, etc. All of these are synovial joints with a ligamentous capsule.

The upper 7 ribs articulate directly with the sternum and are called *true ribs*, while the remaining 5 ribs, which do not articulate directly with the sternum, are called *false ribs*. The eighth, ninth, and tenth ribs attach to cartilage, which, in turn, attaches to cartilage of the rib above and thence to the sternum. The eleventh and twelfth ribs, called *floating ribs*, have no anterior attachment.

The sternum consists of the *manubrium, body,* and *xiphoid process*, which are joined by epiphyseal cartilages. The sternocostal articulations are: (1) *sternocostal* between the costal cartilages and the sternum, (2) the *costochondral* between each rib and its cartilage, (3) *interchondral* between costal cartilages, and (4) *intersternal* between the body and the manubrium and the body and the xiphoid process.

The angle formed between cartilages of the lowest ribs on one side of the sternum and those on the other side is called the *subcostal angle*. The subcostal angle is greater in people high in endomorphy than it is in those high in ectomorphy. The transverse diameter of the thorax is greater than the anterior-posterior diameter except in infants. Athletes and people high in mesomorphy generally possess a wide thorax, that is, one in which the transverse diameter is considerably greater than the anterior-posterior diameter.

Inspiration, regardless of how small, is dependent upon muscular contraction. Expiration at resting levels does not require muscular contraction. Forced expiration, which occurs during or after strenuous effort, does require the muscular contraction of the abdominal muscles and the depressors of the rib cage.

Movements Specific to the Thorax. Movement of the ribs is limited, because all, with the exception of the eleventh and twelfth ribs, are attached both anteriorly and posteriorly in order to offer greater protection to the heart and lungs. The thorax is designed in such a manner as to make possible increases in three diameters. Increase in these diameters augments the volume of the thoracic cavity and, because nature abhors a vacuum and the lungs expand with the chest, air rushes into the lungs when the respiratory muscles contract to expand the thorax. Increase in the *transverse diameter* occurs as a result of elevation of the ribs to a greater horizontal position and eversion of the lateral portion of the ribs. In *eversion* of the ribs, the lower edge of the central portion of the ribs turns upward and laterally, and the inner surface turns downward. The sternum is lifted upward and forward as the anterior ends of the ribs are elevated and, at the same time, the anterior ends of the lower ribs move laterally, increasing the subcostal angle and placing the diaphragm on a stretch to increase its power. The elevation of the ribs to a more horizontal position causes an increase in the *anteroposterior diameter* of the thorax as well as an increase in the transverse diameter discussed above. Increase in the *vertical diameter* is the result of contraction of the diaphragm and elevation of the upper two ribs. Extension of the thoracic vertebrae during forced inhalation makes possible further increase in the vertical diameter.

Respiratory Muscles

Diaphragm (Figure 2.35)

Location: This circular dome-shaped structure of both muscular and fibrous tissue separates the abdominal and thoracic cavities.

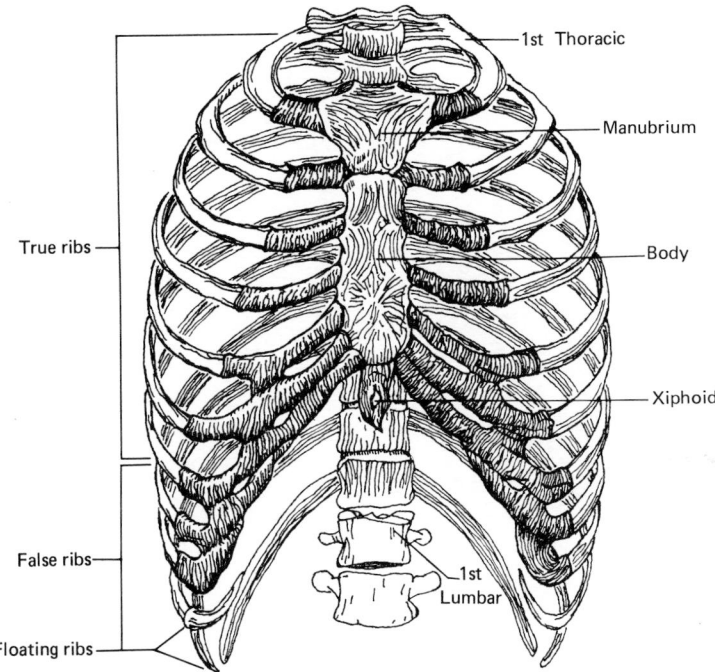

Figure 2.34 Thorax from the front

The muscular peripheral part attaches to the inner surfaces of the lower 2 to 6 ribs and their cartilages and the xiphoid process. All the fibers arch upward into the central tendon, which forms the top part of the dome.

Action: The diaphragm's function is inspiration. At rest, it may be the only muscle involved in inspiration. However, in people with a paralyzed diaphragm, respiration can proceed quite well. *Diaphragmatic breathing* with large excursions of this muscular partition produces a greater exchange of air than does *costal breathing* in which the ribs are elevated. Some females, perhaps for aesthetic reasons, limit the excursions of the diaphragm. By increasing the intraabdominal pressure as it moves downward, the diaphragm helps in defecation, vomiting, coughing, and other forms of expulsion.

Intercostals (Figure 2.36)

Location: As the name implies, the 11 pairs of external intercostals and the 11 pairs of internal intercostals run from the lower border of one rib to the upper border of the next lower rib. The fibers of the internal intercostals run at right angles to those of the external intercostals.

Action: Although studies have not completely resolved the uncertainty of the functions of these muscles, the weight of evidence seems to indicate that the external intercostals aid in inspiration while the internal intercostals aid in expiration. It is probable that the externals evert the ribs to expand the thorax while the internals invert the ribs.

Sternocleidomastoid (see Figure 2.27)

This muscle was described under the muscles of the vertebral column. However, it plays a role during forced inspiration provided that the cervical vertebrae are extended and held firm, enabling this muscle to elevate the sternum and clavicles.

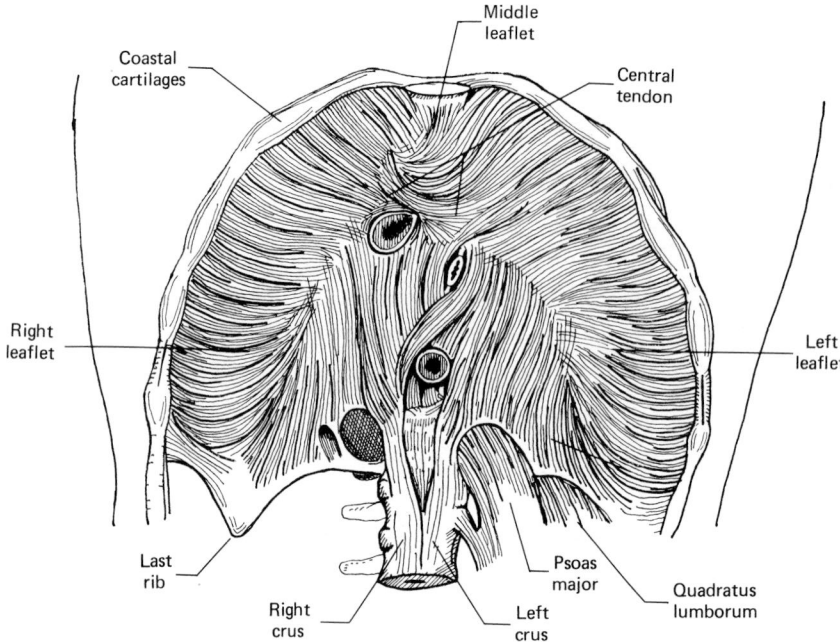

Figure 2.35   The diaphragm (under surface)

Labels on Figure 2.35:
- Middle leaflet
- Coastal cartilages
- Central tendon
- Right leaflet
- Left leaflet
- Last rib
- Right crus
- Left crus
- Psoas major
- Quadratus lumborum

Figure 2.36   Intercostals interni and externi

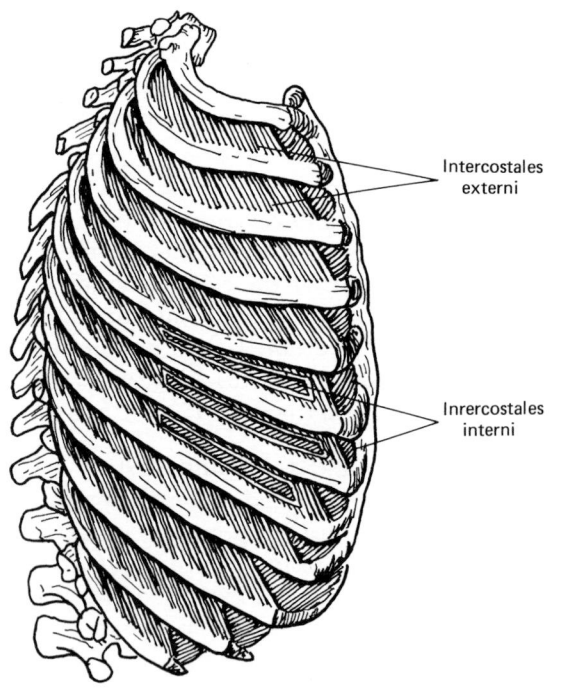

Labels on Figure 2.36:
- Intercostales externi
- Inrercostales interni

Scaleni (See Figure 2.26)

These three muscles were described under muscles of the vertebral column. However, they also play a role in respiration during both resting breathing and in forced inspiration by stabilizing the upper ribs to prevent the thorax from being pulled downward by the abdominal muscles.

Most of the following muscles are described in other sections of this chapter; however, they play various roles in respiration, which will be described.

Erector Spinae

Stabilize the vertebral column and pelvis against the pull of the abdominal muscles to prevent flexion of the spine and thereby facilitate preservation of greater vertical diameter of the thorax. This action forces the abdominal muscles to compress the abdominal viscera, aiding in expiration by enhancing the elastic recoil of the diaphragm.

Levatores Costarum

Assist in elevating the ribs during inspiration.

Pectoralis Major and Minor (see Figures 2.53 and 2.54)

Action: Elevate the sternum and the ribs when arms are held overhead and when hanging by the hands. Grasping an object overhead when winded and the practice of team mates assisting a fatigued athlete off the field with his arms over the shoulders of the two assisting team mates are sound practices since these positions keep the thorax high, the spine extended, and relieve the respiratory muscles of the weight of the arms and the shoulder girdle.

Quadratus Lumborum

Action: Enhances the effectiveness of the diaphragm by stabilizing the twelfth rib against the diaphragm's pull.

Serratus Posterior Superior

Action: Elevates the second through fifth ribs to aid in inspiration.

Transverse Abdominis

Action: A strong muscle of expiration and expulsion as in coughing, sneezing, or defecating as a result of its pressure against the abdominal viscera.

Transverse Thoracis (Figure 2.37)

Location: From the lower half of the inner surface of the sternum and costal cartilages to the lower borders of the costal cartilages of the second through the sixth ribs.

Action: Pulls downward to depress the costal cartilages to aid in expiration.

Lower Extremity—Knee, Ankle, and Foot

The ankle and knee are the most frequently injured joints during sports participation because they are subjected to greater stress than other joints in almost all sports. For this reason, coaches and physical educators should

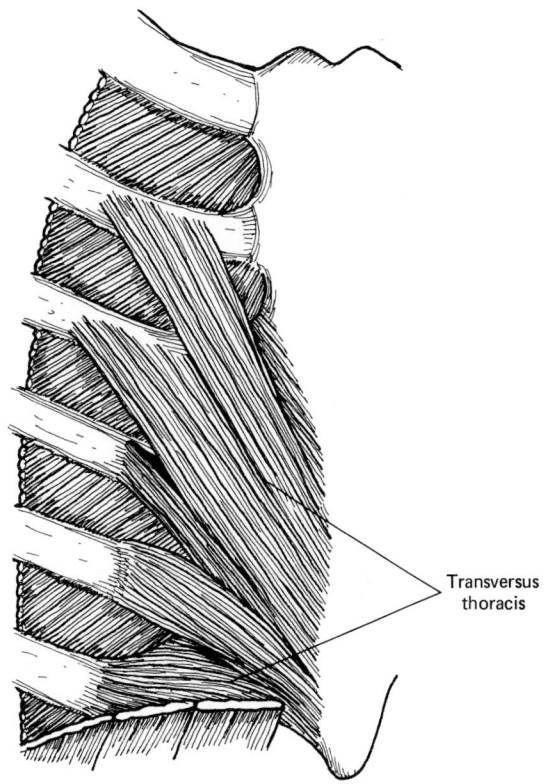

Transversus thoracis

Figure 2.37 *Posterior surface of sternum showing the transversus thoracis*

possess a thorough understanding of these joints. The joints of the lower extremity on each side of the body must support the entire weight of the body during walking and running. They must withstand the stresses of landing after jumping from a height, of sudden changes in direction of motion, and of uneven surfaces. They meet the requirements placed upon them with remarkable efficiency. To absorb stresses, the knee joint has massive condules. To prevent dislocation it has large strong ligaments and muscles. To facilitate running and jumping, its construction permits full flexion.

Knee Joint. Although the knee joint (Figure 2.38) is classed as a single hinge joint encased in a capsule, three articulations may be iden-

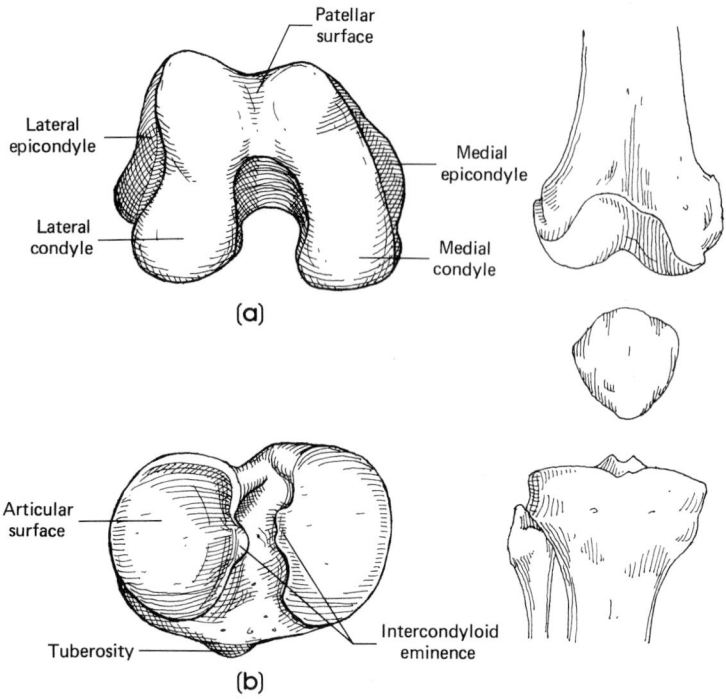

Figure 2.38 Bony structure of knee joint. (a) Articulation of femor, (b) articulation of tibia

tified. These are (1) between the medial condyles, (2) between the lateral condyles of the femur and tibia, and (3) between the patella and the femur. The femur angles inward from the pelvis in order to place the point of support more nearly under the center of weight. In order for this to be accomplished, and at the same time present a horizontal surface between the two condyles, the medial condyle projects further downward than the lateral condyle. This can be seen, however, only when the disarticulated femur is held vertically. The degree of inward slant of the femur is called the *angle of obliquity*. Although the medial condyle projects further downward, the lateral condyle is larger. Normally, the weight-bearing line passes slightly lateral to the center of each knee joint. In a condition known as *genu valgum* or knock-knees, the body weight passes laterally to the center of the knee. In *genu varum* or bow-legs, the body weight passes medially to the center of the knee. In both these conditions, a rotational force is exerted around the horizontal-frontal axis of the knee joint, which stresses the collateral ligaments and subjects the menisci to extra compression forces making the knee more prone to injury.

On the anterior side, the condyles are separated by the shallow depression of the patellar surface. Posteriorly, they are separated by the intercondylar fossa. The femoral condyles articulate with the slightly concave articular surfaces on the top of the tibia. Between the articular surfaces is a raised area called the *intercondyloid eminence*. Between the femoral condyles and the articular surfaces are the *medial* and *lateral menisci* or *semilunar cartilages (see Figure 2.41)*. This tough fibrocartilage absorbs the jars of walking, running and jumping, minimizes friction, and deepens the articular surface since the menisci are thicker at their periphery than they are at their center. Each meniscus is attached to both the anterior and the posterior intercondylar area of the tibia. The menisci are also attached to each other by the *transverse ligament*. Further, they are attached to the edges of the tibial condyles by the *coronary ligaments*. The inner borders are unattached. The lateral meniscus is further attached on its posterior side to the medial condyle of the femur by the posterior *meniscofemoral ligament*. The medial meniscus is attached to the *tibial collateral ligament*. Because of this attachment, the medial meniscus is more frequently damaged than the lateral. When the knee joint suffers a blow from the lateral side, or some other force causes the knee to be bent medially, particularly when the knee joint is in the extended position, the tibial collateral ligament is stretched and torn and may take the medial meniscus with it. In such injuries, the medial meniscus may also be crunched between the medial femoral condyle and the medial articular surface. A meniscus may be split, cracked, broken, or loosened by a tearing of its ligamentous attachments. These injuries are less likely to occur when the knee is flexed, at which time the ligaments are not as taut as when the knee is extended. For these reasons, players are advised to flex the knee and to shift the weight to the opposite foot when a blow from the lateral side is eminent.

The *patella* or *knee cap* is a large sesamoid bone. The tendon of the quadriceps femoris attaches to its upper borders while the *patellar ligament* attaches to its lower borders. The patellar ligament may be regarded as a continuation of the tendon of the quadriceps muscles. The *capsule* of the knee joint lies under the patella, folds around each condyle, but excludes the intercondyloid tubercles and the cruciate ligaments. The patella performs two functions: (1) it protects the knee joint and (2) it increases the angle of insertion of the patellar ligament. A number of bursae help to lubricate the knee joint. These include the *prepatellar, suprapatellar, infrapatellar* bursae and others. The head of the fibula articulates with the lateral condyle of the tibia forming the *proximal tibiofibular* joint.

Ligaments of the Knee Joint (Figures 2.39 and 2.40). The *patellar ligament* is a strong flat ligament that runs from the patella to the tuberosity of the tibia. The *tibial or medial collateral ligament* is a flat ligament that joins the medial epicondyles of the femur and the tibia. The medial meniscus is firmly attached to this ligament. The *fibular or lateral collateral ligament* is a rounded ligament that joins the lateral epicondyle of the femur to the lateral side of the head of the fibula. The *posterior or cruciate ligament* is a tough rounded ligament inside the knee joint runs from the back of the intercondylar area of the tibia upward and forward to the intercondylar fossa of the femur. The *anterior cruciate ligament* runs from the anterior intercondylar area of the tibia upward and backward to the intercondylar area of the femur. The posterior and anterior cruciate ligaments cross one another inside the knee joint. They prevent hyperextension, rotation when the knee is extended, and forward and backward sliding of the femur on the tibia. The *oblique popliteal ligament*, a broad, flat ligament, runs from the intercondyloid fossa and posterior aspect of the distal end of the femur to the posterior edge of the head of the tibia. The *transverse ligament* runs from the anterior edge of the lateral meniscus to the anterior edge of the medial meniscus. The *arcuate popliteal ligament* runs from the lateral condyle of the femur to the styloid process of the fibula. The *coronary ligaments* are parts of the capsule that connect the edges of both menisci with the head of the tibia. The *ligament of Wrisberg* runs from the posterior attachment of the lateral meniscus to the medial condyle of the femur (see Figure 2.41).

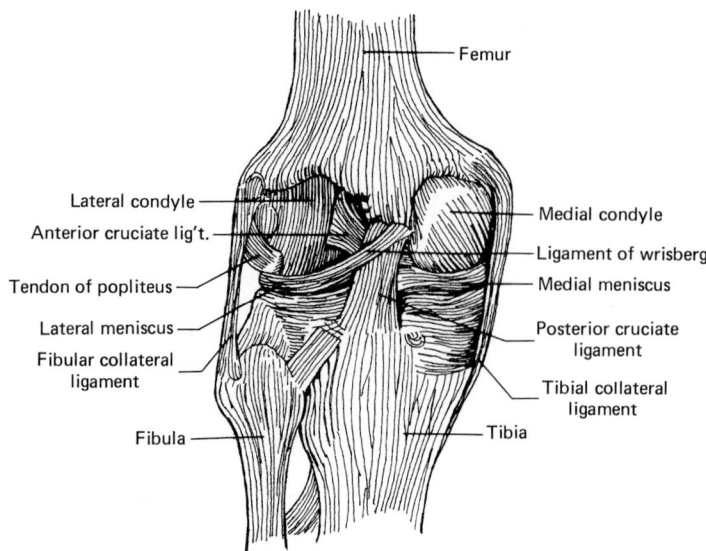

Figure 2.39 Interior ligaments of the left knee joint from behind

Figure 2.40 (a) Medial and (b) lateral aspects of the ligaments of knee joint

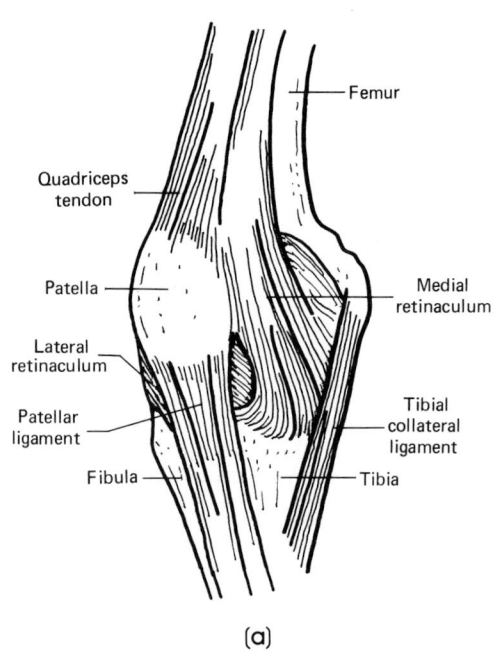

(a)

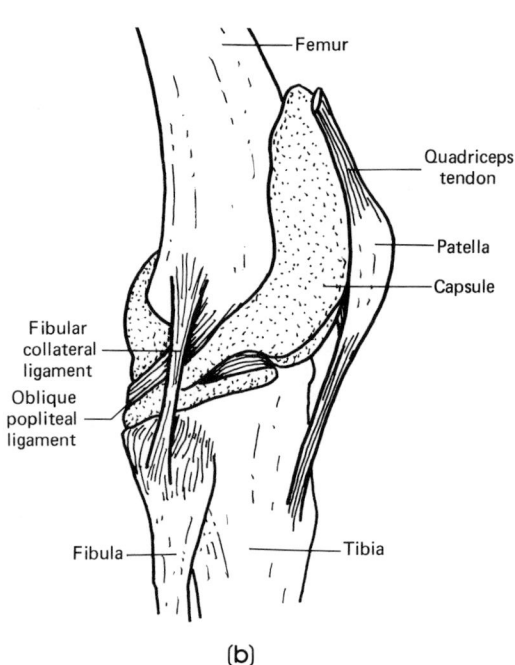

(b)

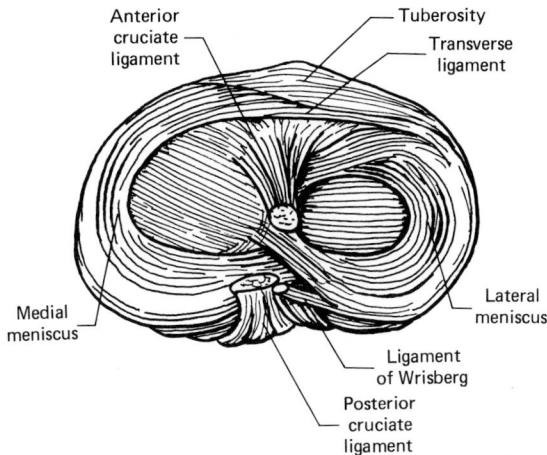

Anterior cruciate ligament
Tuberosity
Transverse ligament
Medial meniscus
Lateral meniscus
Ligament of Wrisberg
Posterior cruciate ligament

Figure 2.41 The menisci (semilunar cartilage) of the knee joint

Movements Specific to the Knee Joint.

Flexion is backward movement of the lower leg in the sagittal plane around the horizontal-frontal axis of the knee joint. This movement is not as simple, however, as those of other hinge joints. As the knee is flexed in a weight bearing position, the femoral condyles roll backward and glide forward in order that they maintain contact with the menisci. When the knee is extended, the femoral condyles roll forward and glide backward. Further, during the beginning of flexion and at the end of extension, there is slight inward rotation of the femur upon the tibia. This rotation is the result of the unequal size of the two femoral condyles, the lateral being broader and larger. Near the end of extension, after the lateral condyle has ceased its movement, the medial condyle continues to roll forward. During flexion or extension, in a non-weight-bearing position, it is the tibia that rotates on the femur rather than the femur on the tibia as in the weight-bearing position. During flexion, the anterior cruciate ligament becomes taut as it limits the backward movement of the femoral condyles. During extension the posterior cruciate ligament becomes taut as it limits the forward movement of the

femoral condyles on the tibia. It is because of these phenomena that the full squat with weights, the duck waddle, and similar exercises are contraindicated.

Extension is the return movement from flexion toward the straight line position of the femur and tibia.

Inward rotation is rotation around the long axis so that the lateral side moves forward while the medial side moves backward. Rotation at the knee joint is impossible when the knee is fully extended. However, when the knee is flexed to 90 degrees, varying amounts of rotation may be possible when the knee being rotated is not in a weight-bearing position.

Outward rotation is the opposite movement of inward rotation.

Muscles That Act on the Knee Joint.

Several muscles that act over the hip and knee joint have been discussed. These include the rectus femoris, gracilis, sartorius, semitendinosus, biceps femoris, and tensor fasciae latae.

Vastus Lateralis (see Figure 2.11)

Location: This muscle begins on the lateral surface of the femur below the greater trochanter and the upper half of the linea aspera and ends on the lateral and superior borders of the patella. It is a broad flat muscle on the lower and lateral side of the thigh.

Action: Extension of the knee.

Vastus Intermedius

Location: From the anterior and lateral side of the upper two-thirds of the body of the femur to the quadriceps femoris tendon. This muscle lies between the vastus lateralis and the vastus medialis and under the rectus femoris on the anterior aspect of the thigh.

Action: Extension of the knee.

Vastus Medialis

Location: On the medial aspect of the thigh originating from the linea aspera and

CONCEPTS APPLIED TO HUMAN MOVEMENT | **59**

the medial supracondylar line and inserting on the tendon of the quadriceps femoris.

Action: Knee extension, particularly the last few degrees.

Popliteus

Location: This thin flat triangular muscle is located behind the knee joint. It runs from the lateral side of the lateral condyle of the femur to the medial posterior side of the tibia.

Action: Flexion of the knee and rotation of the tibia.

Plantaris (Figure 2.42)

Location: This thin weak muscle on the back of the leg crosses both the knee and the ankle joints. It arises from the lateral supracondylar line of the femur and inserts on the posterior surface of the calcaneum.

Action: Provides weak assistance in flexion of the knee.

Gastrocnemius (Figure 2.42)

Location: This is a large, two-headed, superficial muscle on the back of the lower leg. One head arises from just above the posterior side of the lateral femoral condyle, and the other from the same area on the medial femoral condyle. About halfway down the leg, the fibers form the Achilles tendon, which inserts on the calcaneum.

Action: This muscle is a prime mover for plantar flexion at the ankle joint. It assists in knee flexion when plantar flexion occurs at the same time. It serves to stabilize the knee joint.

The Ankle and Foot. The 26 bones of the foot are wonderfully articulated and supported by ligaments and muscles to support the entire body weight, to absorb impacts, to facilitate propulsion, and to balance the body. These functions demand both strength and flexibility. Absorption of shock is provided for by the arrangement of bones in two arches—the *longitudinal* and the *transverse* or *metatarsal*. The longitudinal arch can be regarded as two arches running the length of the foot. The *medial longitudinal* arch is formed by the calcaneous, talus, navicular, the three cuneiforms, and the first, second, and third metatarsal bones. This arch is quite elastic. The *lateral longitudinal* arch is less elastic and consequently provides the stable base needed during standing. It is formed by the calcaneal, cuboid, and fourth and fifth metatarsal bones. The transverse or metatarsal arch is formed by the three cuneiform bones and the metatarsals. The bones are held in their arched position by ligaments, the plantar aponeurosis, and the extrinsic and intrinsic muscles of the foot. The height of the arch is not an indication of its strength, except where a low arch is associated with pronated feet.

The 26 bones of the foot include: (1) the 7 *tarsals* (*talus, calcaneus, navicular, cuboid,* and the first, second, and third *cuneiforms*); (2) 5 metatarsal bones, and (3) 14 phalanges. The most medial metatarsal is numbered first while the most lateral is numbered fifth. Each toe has 3 phalanges except the big toe, which has two.

The foot is joined to the lower leg at the articulation between the talus and the malleoli of the tibia and the fibula. The talus is held in its position by the *tibiofibular*, the *anterior* and *posterior lateral melleolar*, the three parts of the *medial* (*calcaneotibial, anterior talotibial,* and *tibionavicular), posterior talotibial* and *anterior* and *posterior talofibular* ligaments (see Figures 2.43 and 2.44).

The *subtalar* joint is located between the talus and the calcaneus. This joint is reinforced by the four *talocalcaneal* ligaments (*anterior, posterior, lateral,* and *medial talocalcaneal)* and the *plantar calcaneonavicular* or *spring* ligament. The broad, thick spring ligament, because of its elastic fibers, acts as a sling for the talus bone and helps to absorb impact.

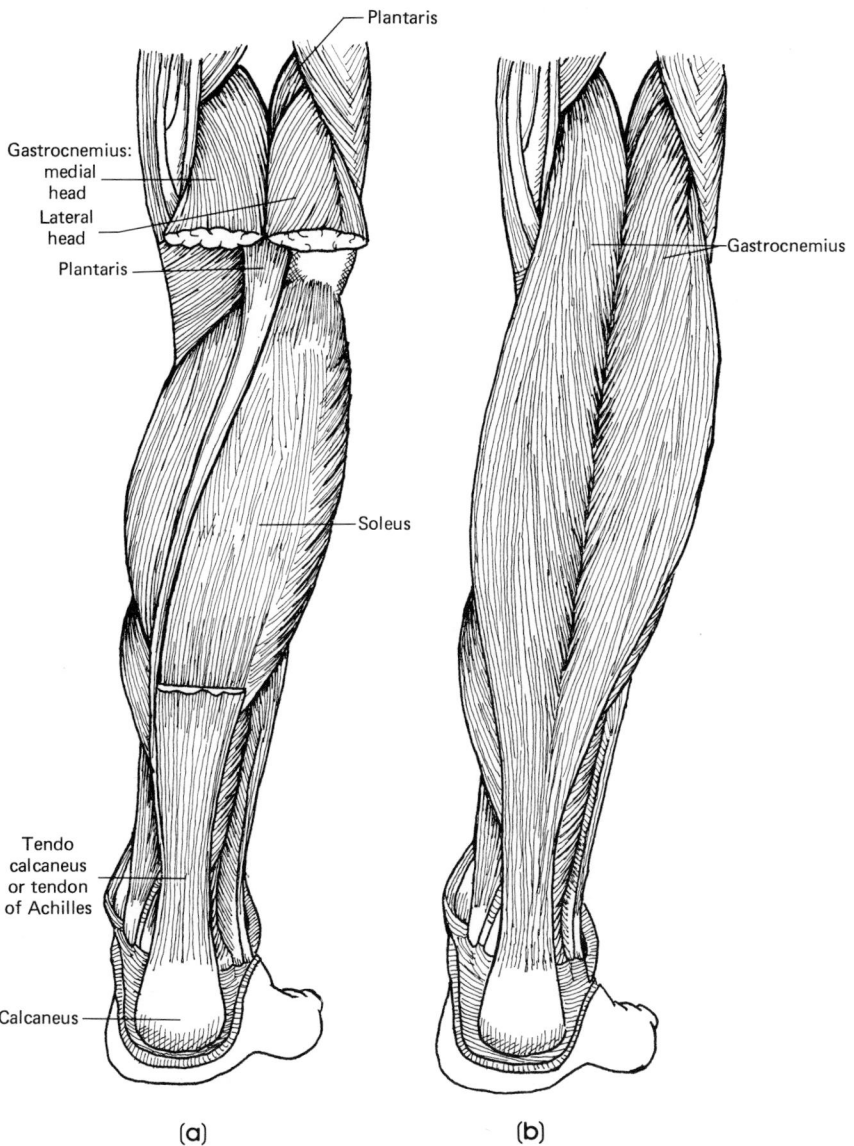

Figure 2.42 Muscles of the back of the leg. (a) Gastrocnemius cut away to reveal middle layer of muscles, (b) gastrocnemius intact

Articulations between the 7 tarsal bones are of the arthrodial type and permit gliding movements. The principle joint among these is the *talonavicular*. The articulations between the tarsals and the metatarsals are also arthrodial and permit only gliding motions.

The *intermetatarsal* joints are the articulations between the base of one metatarsal bone and its neighbor and between the head of one metatarsal bone and its neighbor. These joints facilitate flattening of the arches in weight-bearing position and return to the

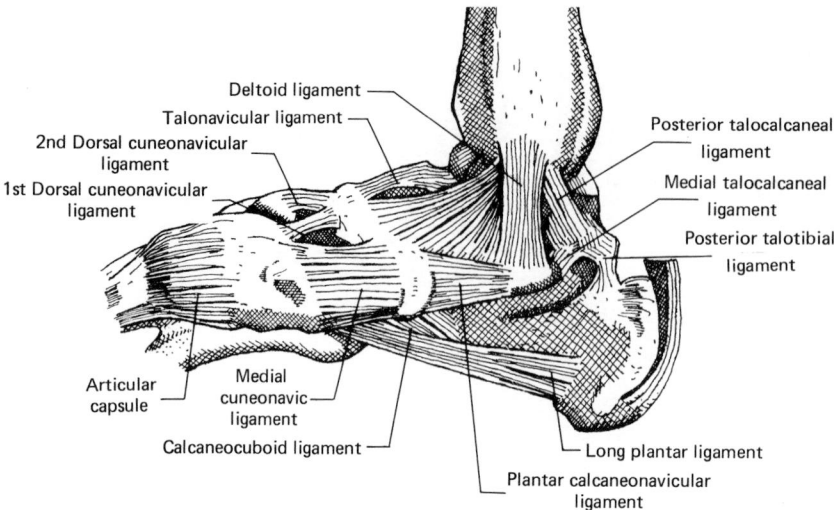

Figure 2.43 Ligaments of medial aspect of the foot

more highly arched position when the body weight is removed.

The metatarsophalangeal joints are the articulations between the distal end of the metatarsals and the proximal end of the first phalanx of each toe. Under the joint at the big toe are found two sesamoid bones. The metatarsophalangeal joints permit flexion, extension, and slight abduction and adduction.

Figure 2.44 Ligaments of the right ankle and tarsus, lateral aspect

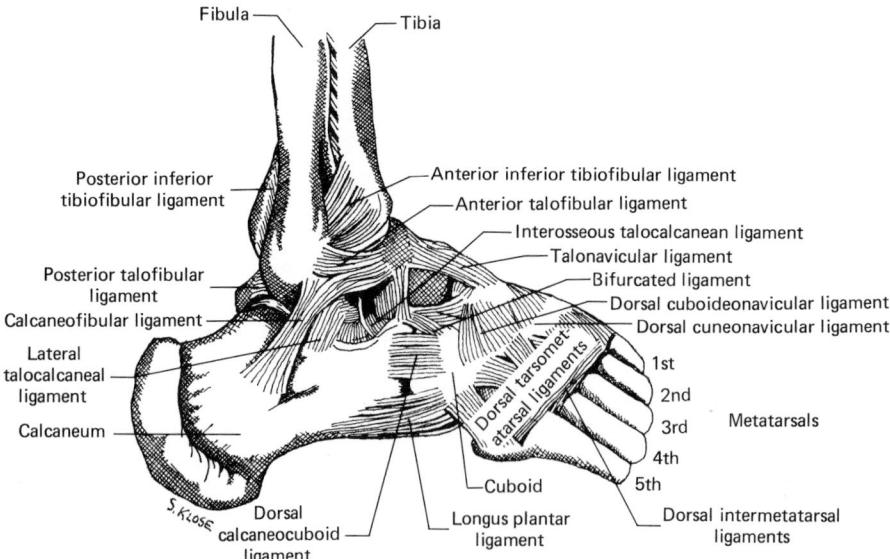

The hinge joints at the *interphalangeal* joints permit flexion and extension of the toes.

Movements Specific to the Foot.

Movements of the foot are the sum of movements at the ankle (articulations between the talus and the malleoli of the tibia and fibula), the subtalar joint, the 7 tarsal bones, and the intermetatarsal joints. These movements are as follows:

Dorsiflexion is movement of the foot toward the front of the leg.

Plantar flexion is movement of the foot away from the front of the leg as in pointing the toes.

Eversion is rotation of the foot around its long axis so that the bottom of the foot is turned outward. Eversion is usually accompanied by abduction or "toeing out." The combined movements are called *pronation*.

Inversion is rotation of the foot around its long axis so that the bottom or sole of the foot is turned inward. This movement is usually accompanied by adduction or "toeing in." The combined movements are called *supination*.

Muscles of the Ankle and Foot

Tibialis Anterior (Figure 2.45)

Location: This muscle is located on the lateral side of the tibia. It originates from the lateral condyle and upper two-thirds of the lateral surface of the body of the tibia and the adjoining interosseous membrane. It ends in a tendon that can be seen on the lower third of the anterior surface of the leg and that inserts on the medial and underside of the first cuneiform and the base of the first metatarsal.

Action: Dorsiflexion and supination of the foot.

Extensor Digitorum Longus (Figure 2.45)

Location: This penniform muscle is located on the lateral anterior side of the leg. It

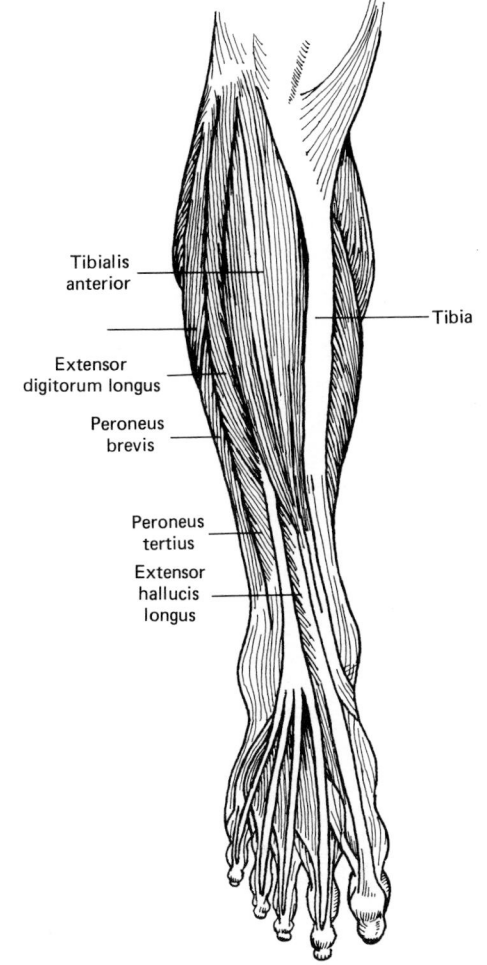

Figure 2.45 Muscles of the front of the leg

arises from the lateral condyle of the tibia, the upper three-fourths of the body of the fibula, and the adjacent interosseous membrane. It divides into four slips, which insert into the second and third phalanges of the four toes.

Action: Extension of the proximal phalanges of the four toes and dorsiflexion and pronation of the foot.

Extensor Hallucis Longus (Figure 2.45)

Location: This thin muscle runs from the anterior middle half of the fibula and the adjacent interosseous membrane to the base of the distal phalanx of the big toe.

Action: Extension of the proximal phalanx of the great toe and dorsal flexion and supination of the foot.

Peroneus Tertius (Figure 2.45)

Location: This muscle might be considered a part of the extensor digitorum longus. It arises from the lower third of the anterior side of the fibula and the adjacent interosseous membrane and inserts on the top of the base of the fifth metatarsal.

Action: Dorsiflexion and pronation of the foot.

Soleus

Location: This penniform muscle arises from the posterior surfaces of the tibia, fibula, and interosseous membrane and inserts, via the tendon of Achilles, into the calcaneous.

Action: Plantar flexion.

Peroneus Longus (Figure 2.46)

Location: This muscle arises from the head and upper two-thirds of the lateral surface of the body of the fibula and inserts into the lateral side of the base of the first metatarsal bone and the lateral side of the first cuneiform.

Action: Pronation and plantar flexion of the foot.

Peroneus Brevis (Figure 2.46)

Location: This muscle runs from the lower two-thirds of the lateral side of the fibula to the proximal end of the fifth metatarsal.

Action: In association with the peroneus longus, pronates and plantar flexes the foot.

Flexor Digitorum Longus (Figure 2.46)

Location: This muscle originates on the posterior surface of the shaft of the tibia and inserts on the proximal end of the distal phalanges of the four small toes.

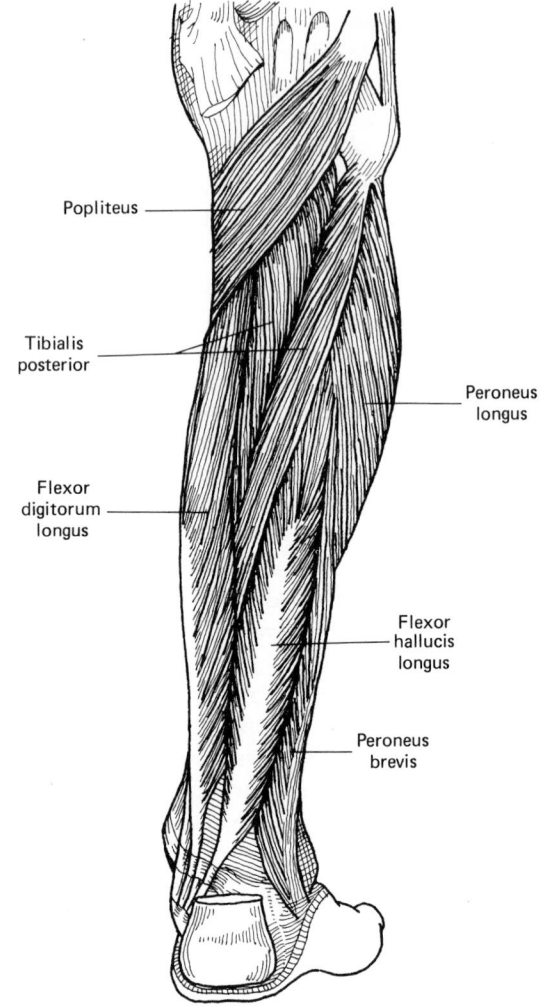

Figure 2.46 Deep muscles of the back of the leg

Action: A prime mover for flexion of the four small toes and an assistor in plantar flexion and supination of the foot.

Flexor Hallucis Longus (Figure 2.46)

Location: This muscle arises from the lower two-thirds of the posterior side of the shaft of the fibula and the adjacent interosseous membrane. After running down the lateral side of the leg, it inserts in the distal phalanx of the big toe.

Action: Flexion of the second phalanx of the big toe and assists in plantar flexion and supination of the foot.

Tibialis Posterior (Figure 2.46)

Location: This deepest posterior muscle arises from the interosseous membrane, the lateral posterior surface of the body of the tibia, and the upper two-thirds of the medial surface of the fibula. It inserts into the navicular bone and by fibrous slips into the calcaneus, the three cuneiforms, the cuboid, and the bases of the second, third, and fourth metatarsals.

Action: Supinates and assists in plantar flexion of the foot.

Intrinsic Muscles of the Foot. All but one (the extensor digitorum brevis) of the 11 intrinsic muscles are on the plantar surface. They are arranged in 4 layers. The muscles on the plantar surface are covered by fascia, which is divided into medial, central, and lateral portions. The very strong central portion, called the *plantar aponeurosis*, binds the calcaneous to the proximal phalanges of all five toes.

The first layer of intrinsic muscles of the foot include: (1) *abductor halluci,* (2) *flexor digitorum brevis,* and (3) *abductor digiti minimi.* The second layer includes: (1) *quadratus plantae* and (2) *lumbricales.* The third layer includes: (1) *flexor hallucis brevis,* (2) adductor hallucis, and (3) *flexor digiti minimi.* The fourth layer includes: (1) *dorsal interossei* and *plantar interossei.* The eleventh intrinsic muscle of the foot, as has been stated, the extensor digitorum brevis, is located on the dorsal side of the foot.

Shoulder Girdle and Upper Extremity

The scapula, clavicle, and arm function as a unit. This unit is sometimes termed the shoulder-arm mechanism. Understanding this arrangement requires recognition of the interdependence of the parts of this mechanism. To a lesser degree, the movement of any body part in daily activities and particularly in many sports skills is related to other body parts. Many muscles are involved in positioning body parts, serving as prime movers, antagonists, stabilizers, neutralizers, or assistors to maintain balance, stabilize body parts, and prevent undesired movements. However, because of the complexity of movements of the upper extremity, its great mobility, and the many skeletal parts involved, and because the arm and shoulder girdle articulate with the trunk only at the sternoclavicular joint, the authors believe it best to treat the arm and shoulder girdle as a unit.

The need for mobility of the shoulder-arm mechanism is greater than the need for stability. In the hip joint and lower extremity, the situation is reversed. The need for stability is greater than the need for mobility due principally to the amount of weight that must be supported by the hip joint. That the shoulder-arm mechanism is designed for mobility at the cost of stability will become increasingly apparent to the student as he studies its construction.

Two bones, the clavicle and the scapula (see Figure 2.47a and b), make up the shoulder girdle. When viewed from above, the clavicle shows a double curve with the curve at the *sternal end* being convex anteriorly and the curve at the *acromial end* being convex posteriorly. The three borders of the scapula, a flat triangular bone, are called the *medial, lateral,* and *superior borders.* Its three angles are called *superior, lateral,* and *inferior.* The surface next to the ribs is the *costal* surface and the posterior surface is the *dorsal* surface. On the dorsal surface is a bony projection called the *spine of the scapula,* which terminates in the flat *acromion process.* The junction of the spine and the acromion process is called the *acromial angle.* The area above the spine is the *supraspinous fossa* and the area below the spine is the *in-*

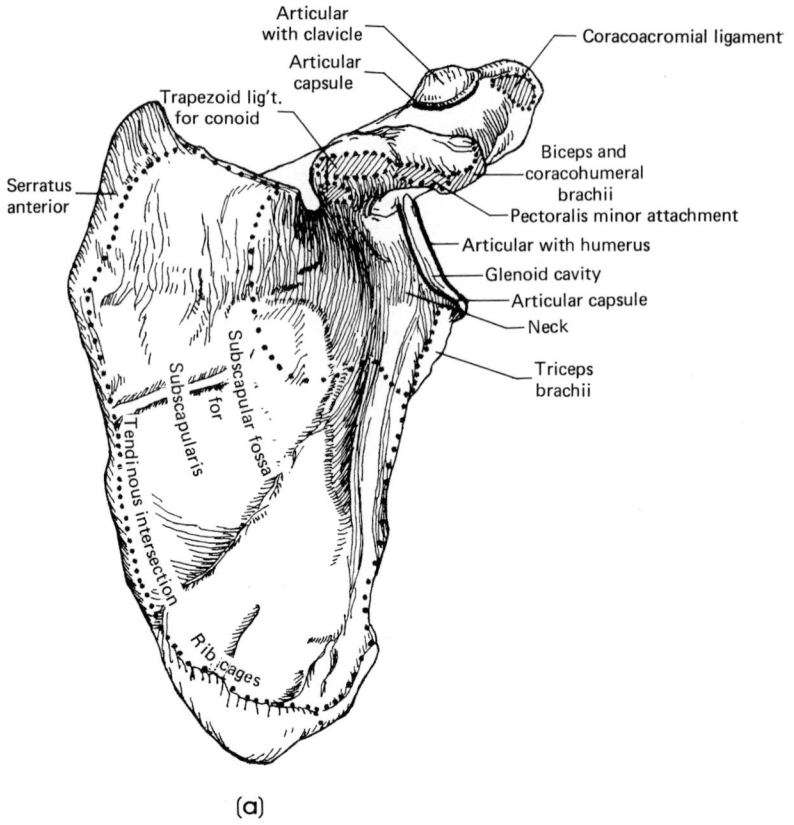

Articular
with clavicle

Articular
capsule

Coracoacromial ligament

Trapezoid lig't.
for conoid

Serratus
anterior

Biceps and
coracohumeral
brachii

Pectoralis minor attachment

Articular with humerus

Glenoid cavity

Articular capsule

Neck

Triceps
brachii

Subscapular fossa

for
Subscapularis

Tendinous intersection

Rib cages

(a)

Figure 2.47 Left scapula: (a) costal surface, (b) dorsal surface

fraspinous fossa. The *subscapular fossa* is on the costal surface. Medial to and slightly forward of the acromion process and above the glenoid cavity is the *coracoid process*. The acromion articulates with the clavicle, and the shallow *glenoid cavity* at the lateral angle articulates with the head of the humerus. The articulation of the head of the humerus and the glenoid fossa forms a diarthrodial ball and socket joint. The head of the humerus is covered with hyaline cartilage, which is thicker at the center of the head. The glenoid fossa is also lined with hyaline cartilage, which, however, is thicker at its circumference. These variations in thickness of the hyaline cartilage serve to decrease the probability that the head of the humerus will be

pulled out of its socket. The *glenoid labrum*, a flat rim of white fibrocartilage thicker at its periphery, also serves to deepen the glenoid fossa as well as to cushion it against impact of the head of the femur.

A loose *articular capsule* extending from the lip of the cavity to the neck of the humerus surrounds the joint. A *synovial membrane* lines the capsule. Friction between bones and between bone and tendons is minimized by several bursae as well as the *synovial fluid* secreted by the synovial membrane.

At the sternoclavicular joint, cartilage between the sternal end of the clavicle and the depression in the manubrium that receives it serves to absorb shocks received by the arm or shoulder. This cartilage also makes possible

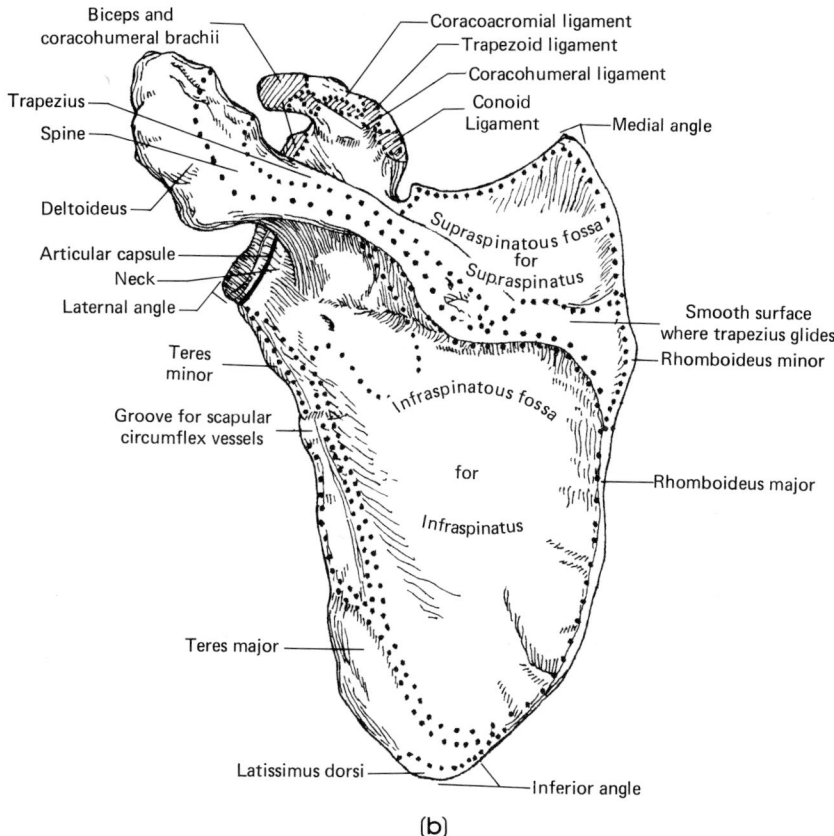

Biceps and
coracohumeral brachii

Coracoacromial ligament
Trapezoid ligament
Coracohumeral ligament
Conoid Ligament
Medial angle

Trapezius
Spine

Deltoideus

Articular capsule
Neck
Laternal angle

Teres minor

Groove for scapular
circumflex vessels

Supraspinatous fossa
for
Supraspinatus

Smooth surface
where trapezius glides
Rhomboideus minor

Infraspinatous fossa
for
Infraspinatus

Rhomboideus major

Teres major

Latissimus dorsi

Inferior angle

(b)

movements of the distal end of the clavicle up and down, forward and backward, and to a very limited extent in circumduction. Slight rotation of the clavicle is also permitted. All of these movements are utilized to place the glenoid fossa in a more favorable position for various movements of the arm.

The third joint of the shoulder-arm mechanism is the *acromioclavicular* joint. Acromioclavicular separation is a fairly common injury in sports. It occurs most often as a result of a fall on the tip of the shoulder.

Ligaments of the Shoulder-Arm Mechanism (Figure 2.48).
The ligaments that protect the shoulder joint are (1) the *coracohumeral* liga-

ment, (2) the three bands of the *glenohumeral* ligament, and (3) the *coracoacromial* ligament. Their names indicate their location. Up to 2 inches of separation is possible at this joint. The major portion of stability is provided by the muscles of the area.

The ligaments that protect the sternoclavicular joint are (1) the *intraclavicular* ligament (Figure 2.49), which joins the two clavicles, (2) the *anterior and posterior sternoclavicular* (Figure 2.49), and (3) the *costoclavicular* ligament (Figure 2.49), which runs from the underside of each clavicle to the rib below it.

The ligaments that protect the acromioclavicular joint are (1) the *acromioclavicular* ligament and (2) the *coracoclavicular* liga-

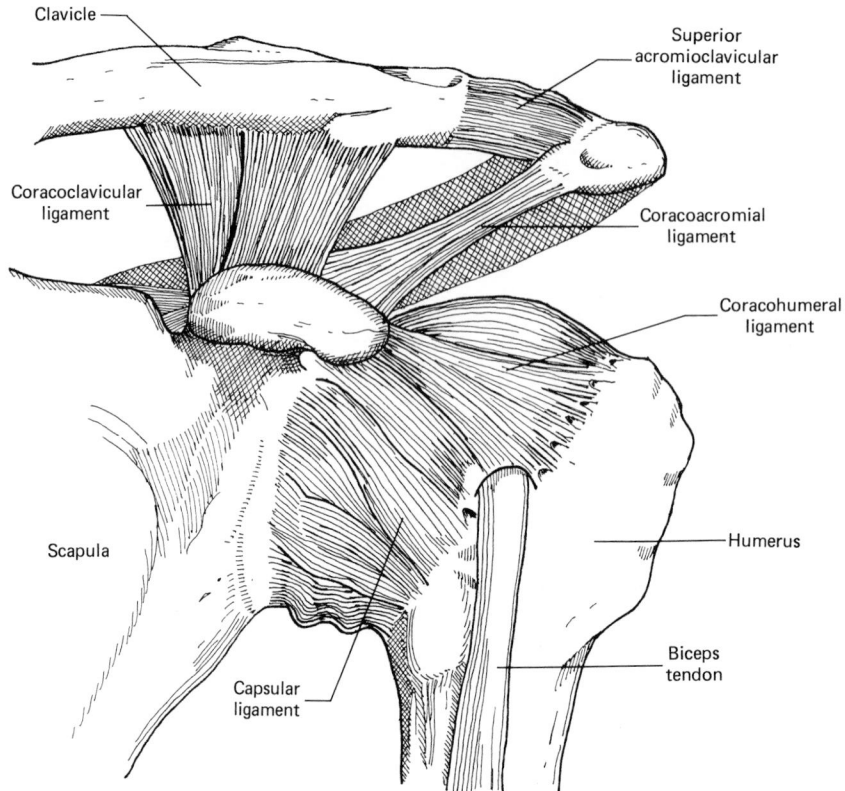

Figure 2.48 Ligaments of left shoulder joint and scapula

Figure 2.49 Ligaments of the sternoclavicular joint

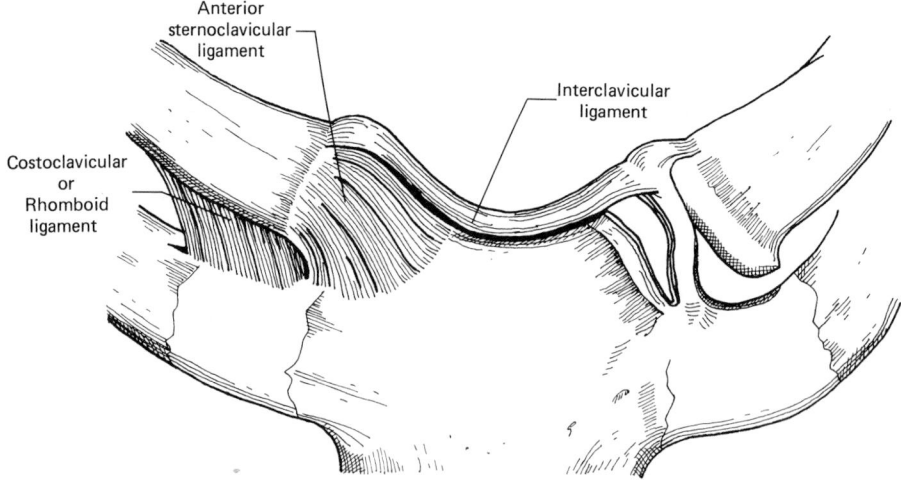

ment with its two parts, the *conoid* and the *trapezoid* ligaments.

Movements Specific to the Shoulder-Arm Mechanisms.

Following are the movements of the shoulder joint or the humerus at its articulation with the glenoid fossa:

Flexion is forward-upward movement in the sagittal or anteroposterior plane until the humerus reaches the frontal or lateral plane.

Hyperflexion is a continuation of flexion beyond the frontal plane (Figure 2.50).

Extension is movement of the humerus in a direction opposite to that of flexion until the humerus reaches the frontal plane.

Hyperextension is movement of the humerus downward-backward beyond the frontal plane (Figure 2.51).

Abduction is sideward-upward movement of the humerus in the frontal plane.

Adduction is the opposite movement of abduction.

Outward rotation is the turning of the humerus around its long axis so that the anterior side moves laterally.

Inward rotation is the opposite movement of outward rotation.

Horizontal flexion is a forward movement of the humerus in the horizontal plane from an abducted position.

Horizontal extension is a backward movement of the humerus in the horizontal plane from a horizontally flexed position.

Circumduction is a combination of movements in which the elbow describes a circle and the humerus a cone.

When the body is in other than an erect position, the above movements retain their terminology. Inward and outward rotation of the humerus should not be confused with pronation and supernation of the forearm.

Movements of the humerus are always in cooperation with movements of the scapula. The scapula positions itself so that its glenoid fossa will facilitate the desired movement of the humerus. All movements of the scapula involve motion in both the acromioclavicular and the sternoclavicular joints. Following are the *movements of the scapula:*

Abduction or protraction is movement of the vertebral border of the scapula away from the vertebral column. The vertebral border remains parallel to the vertebral column but there is a slight lateral tilt to the scapula as it moves around the rounded ribs.

Adduction or retraction is the opposite movement of abduction. The vertebral border moves toward the vertebral column.

Elevation is an upward movement of the scapula with no rotation. During this movement, the outer end of the clavicle moves upward.

Depression is the return movement from elevation. The scapula cannot be depressed below the normal resting position.

Upward rotation is a rotatory movement of the scapula in the frontal plane about an anteroposterior axis, which moves the genoid fossa upward to keep it under the upward moving humerus.

Downward rotation is the return movement of upward rotation. Downward rotation may continue until the glenoid fossa faces slightly downward.

Forward tilt is movement of the inferior angle of the scapula backward away from the thorax. This is rotation of the scapula around its frontal-horizontal axis in the anterior-posterior plane.

Backward tilt is a return movement of forward tilt.

Muscles of the Shoulder Mechanism

Deltoid (Figure 2.52)

Location: From the lateral third of the front of the clavicle, top of the acromion, and the spine of the scapula to the deltoid tuberosity of the humerus.

Action: The actions produced by this muscle's three parts must be considered separate-

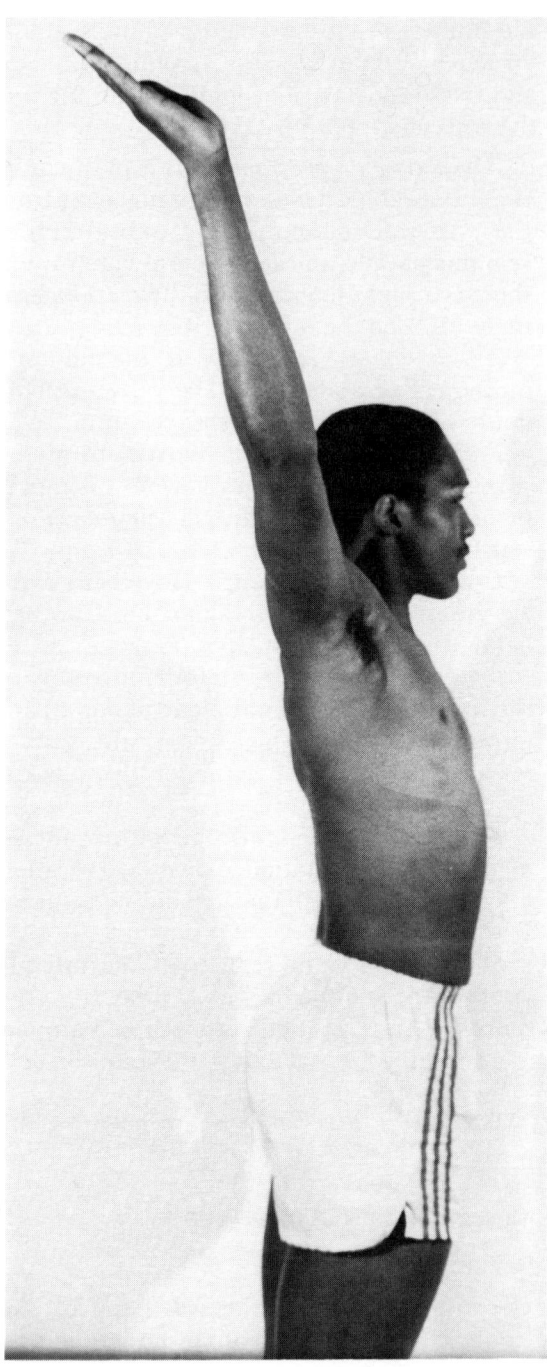

Figure 2.50 Hyperflexion of shoulder-arm mechanism

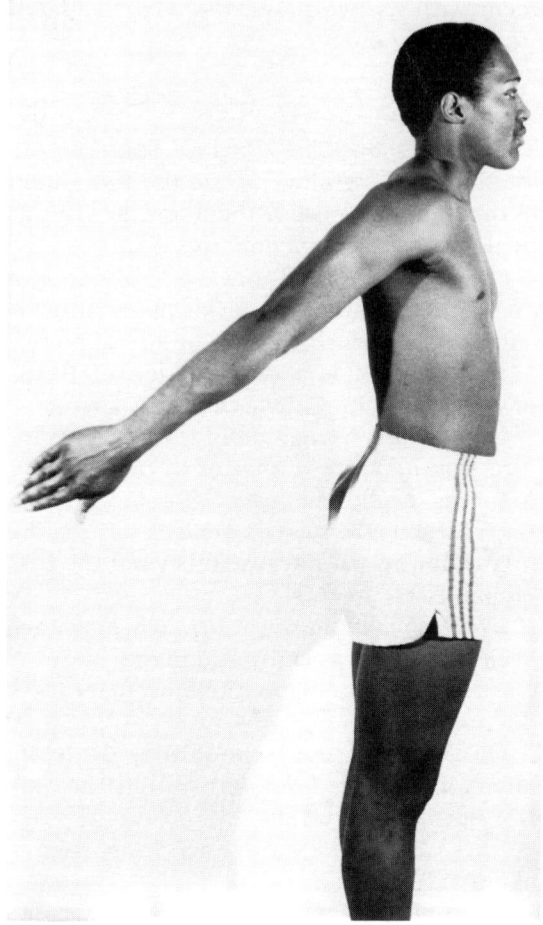

Figure 2.51 Hyperextension of shoulder-arm mechanism

ly. The *anterior portion* is a prime mover in flexion and horizontal flexion. It assists in inward rotation and abduction beyond 60 degrees. The anterior fibers of the *middle portion* serve as assistors in flexion and horizontal flexion while the posterior fibers assist in horizontal extension. The anterior and posterior fibers of the middle deltoid together are prime movers in abduction. The *posterior portion* is a prime mover in horizontal extension and assists in extension, adduction, and outward rotation. All three parts of the del-

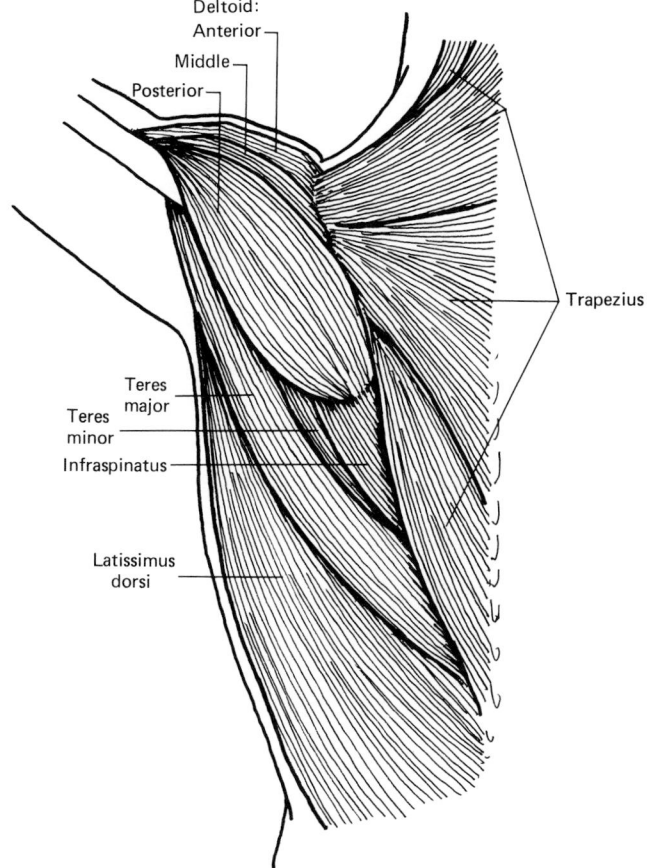

Deltoid:
Anterior
Middle
Posterior

Trapezius

Teres
major
Teres
minor
Infraspinatus

Latissimus
dorsi

Figure 2.52 Posterior superficial muscles that act
on the shoulder–arm mechanism

toid function in holding the head of the humerus against the glenoid fossa.

Pectoralis Major (Figures 2.53 and 2.54)

Location: This superficial fan-shaped muscle runs from the inner two-thirds of the clavicle, the front of the sternum, and the cartilages of the first six ribs to the bicipital
groove of the humerus. The fibers twist
through 180 degrees.

Action: The *clavicular portion* is a prime
mover in flexion, horizontal flexion, and inward rotation of the humerus. When the humerus is above the horizontal, this portion
abducts the humerus. The *sternal portion* is a
prime mover in extension and adduction.
This muscle is strongly involved in throwing,
punching, and pushing.

Trapezius (Figure 2.52)

Location: This large, superficial, triangular
muscle is divided into four portions in order
to facilitate descriptions of its functions. The
clavicular portion runs downward, laterally,
and forward from the skull and the cervical
region to insert on the lateral third of the

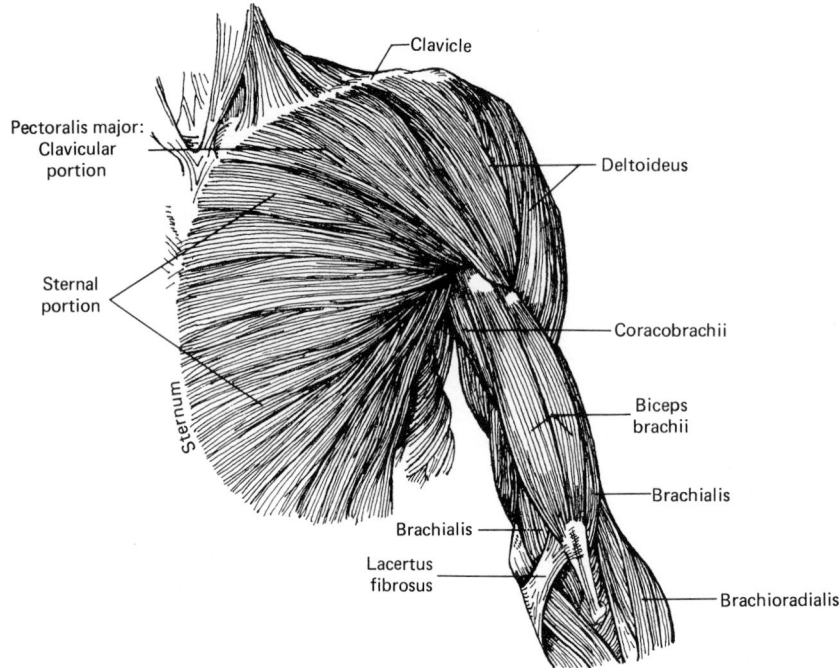

Figure 2.53 Superficial muscles of the chest and front of the arm.

Figure 2.54 Deep muscles of the chest and the front of the arm, with the boundaries of the axilla

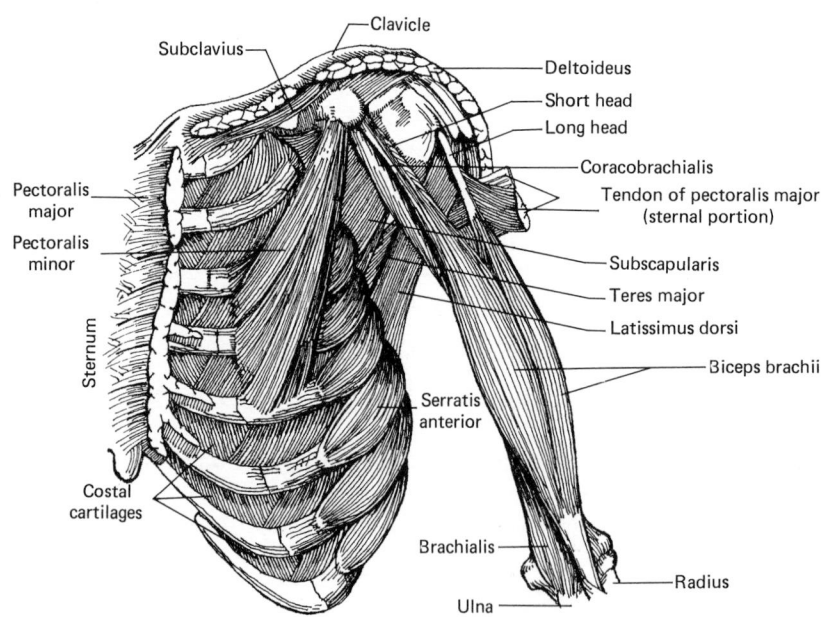

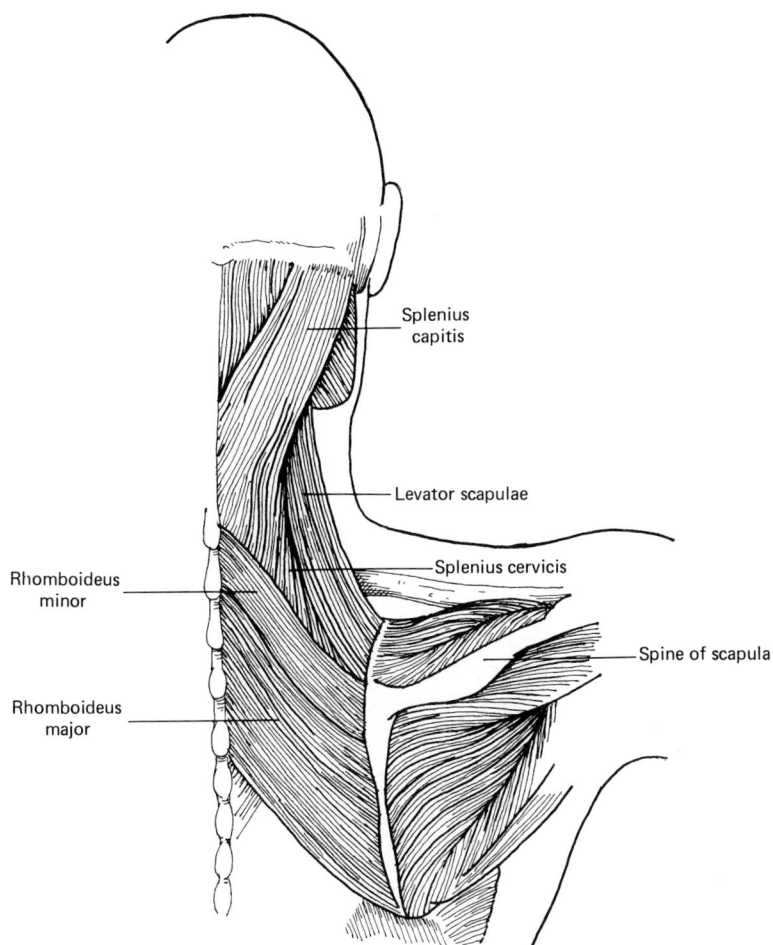

Figure 2.55 Posterior view of right shoulder showing the rhomboids and surrounding muscles that connect to vertebral column

Labels in figure:
- Splenius capitis
- Levator scapulae
- Splenius cervicis
- Spine of scapula
- Rhomboideus minor
- Rhomboideus major

clavicle. The *acromial portion* runs laterally and slightly downward from the lower cervical region to insert on the acromion process. The *horizontal portion* runs horizontally from the upper thoracic vertebrae to the spine of the scapulae. The *lower* portion runs upward and laterally from the lower thoracic vertebrae to insert on the medial side of the spine of the scapula.

Action: All four portions of this muscle support the shoulder girdle and the upper arm and move the scapula to position it for movements of the arm. The clavicular and acromial portions elevate the shoulder girdle and rotate the scapula upward. The horizontal portion adducts the scapula, rotates the scapula upward, and assists in elevation of the shoulder girdle. The lower portion rotates the scapula upward while the arm is being abducted. It also depresses the scapula.

Rhomboid Major (Figure 2.55)

Location: The parallel fibers of this flat muscle lie under the trapezius and run downward and laterally from the spines of the second, third, fourth, and fifth thoracic vertebrae to insert on the lower part of the vertebral border of the scapula.

Action: Serves to hold the vertebral border of the scapula against the ribs and to maintain proper distance between the vertebral column and the scapula when the arm is at rest. In cooperation with various other muscles, the rhomboids elevate, adduct, and rotate the scapula downward. The rhomboid major and minor must be considered as one muscle from the standpoint of function since they share the same nerve supply.

Rhomboid Minor (Figure 2.55)

Location: Next to and above the rhomboid major. The fibers run from the ligamentum nuchae and the spines of the seventh cervical and first thoracic vertebrae to insert on the vertebral border of the scapula just above the insertion of the rhomboid major.

Action: Same as that of the rhomboid major.

Levator Scapula

Location: The fibers run from the transverse processes of the upper four cervical vertebrae to the upper part of the vertebral border of scapula above the insertion of the rhomboid minor.

Action: Elevation and downward rotation of the scapula, support of the scapula while at rest, and lateral flexion of the neck when the scapula is stabilized.

Latissimus Dorsi (Figure 2.52)

Location: This is a very large superficial muscle that covers the lumbar and lower half of the thoracic regions. Its extensive medial attachment includes the iliac crest and the spines of all the lumbar and the lower six thoracic vertebrae. The fibers run upward and laterally to converge in their insertion at the bicipital groove on the humerus after curving around the medial side of the humerus. A few

slips of this muscle originate from the lower three or four ribs and the inferior angle of the scapula and join the others.

Action: It is a prime mover in adduction, extension, hyperextension, and medial rotation of the humerus. These movements are used in chinning, rope climbing, chopping wood, the crucifix on the rings, and many apparatus stunts. It also assists in depressing the shoulder girdle and in lateral flexion of the trunk.

Pectoralis Minor (Figure 2.54)

Location: This muscle is located under the pectoralis major. Its fibers arise from the anterior surfaces of the third, fourth, and fifth ribs and the fascia in the intercostal spaces between these ribs. They run upward and laterally to the corocoid process.

Action: Abduction and downward rotation of the scapula while moving the vertebral border away from the ribs. It also assists in forced inhalation when the scapula is stabilized.

Serratus Anterior (Figure 2.54)

Location: The fibers of this muscle run from the anterior surfaces of the upper eight or nine ribs, curve around the lateral side of the ribs, and pass backward between the ribs and the costal surface of the scapula to attach to the medial border of the scapula. The upper fibers are horizontal, the middle fibers slant slightly downward, and the lower fibers slant somewhat upward.

Action: The top bands abduct while the lower bands rotate the scapula upward. All the bands maintain the edge of the scapula near the ribs. When the scapula is stabilized, this muscle aids in respiration.

Subclavius (Figure 2.54)

Location: The fibers of this small, slender muscle run laterally and slightly upward from the first rib and its cartilage to attach to the middle third of the clavicle.

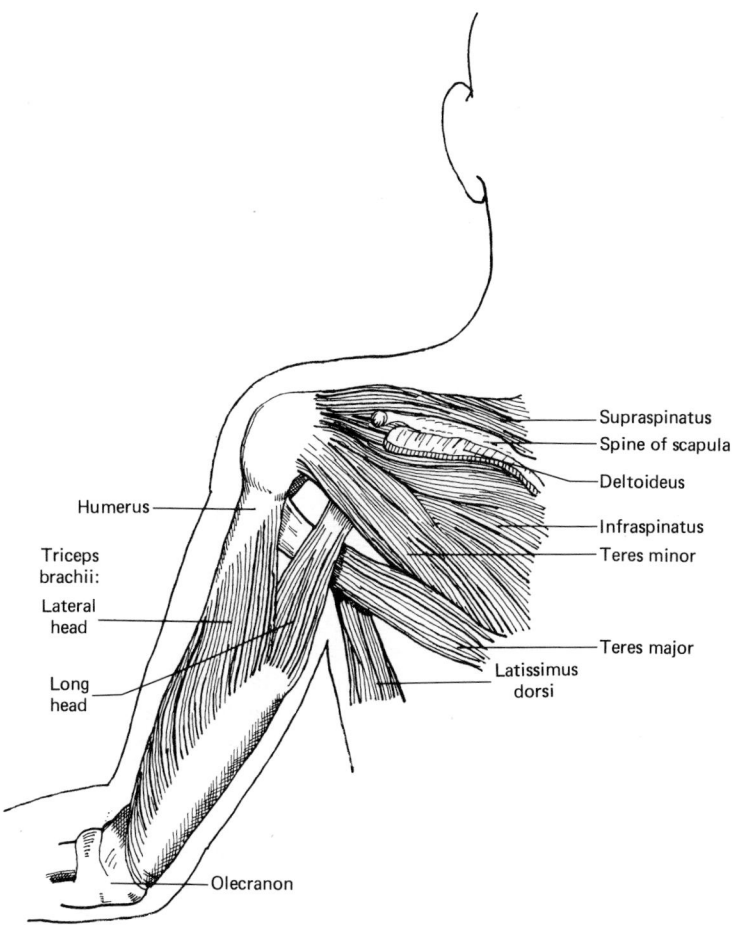

Figure 2.56 labels:
- Supraspinatus
- Spine of scapula
- Deltoideus
- Infraspinatus
- Teres minor
- Humerus
- Triceps brachii:
- Lateral head
- Teres major
- Latissimus dorsi
- Long head
- Olecranon

Figure 2.56 View of the left arm and shoulder from the rear showing muscles of scapula and triceps brachii

Action: The subclavius depresses the acromial end of the clavicle and pulls the clavicle toward the sternum.

Teres Major (Figure 2.56)

Location: The fibers of this muscle run from the lower third of the lateral posterior surface of the scapula upward and laterally and around the medial aspect of the humerus to attach via a flat tendon to the bicipital groove on the humerus.

Action: Adduction and inward rotation of the humerus.

Supraspinatus (Figure 2.56)

Location: This muscle lies against the scapula above the spine (supraspinous fossa) and under the trapezius. Its fibers originate on the medial two-thirds of the suprasinous fossa and run laterally and forward, passing under the acromion process to arch over the head of the humerus and insert on the greater tuberosity of the humerus.

Action: Abduction and elevation of the arm and stabilization of the head of the humerus against the glenoid fossa during all arm movements.

Infraspinatus (Figure 2.56)

Location: This muscle lies in and originates from the infraspinatus fossa. Its fibers converge in a tendon that attaches to the posterior part of the greater tuberosity of the humerus.

Action: Lateral rotation and horizontal abduction of the humerus. This muscle also holds the humeral head in the glenoid cavity whenever the arm is moved.

Teres Minor (Figure 2.56)

Location: The fibers run from the posterior (dorsal) surface of the lateral border of the scapula to the greater tuberosity of the humerus.

Action: Outward rotation and horizontal extension of the humerus and stabilization of the head of the humerus in the glenoid cavity.

Subscapularis (Figure 2.54)

Location: This muscle originates from almost the entire costal surface of the scapula. It inserts on the lesser tuberosity of the humerus.

Action: A prime mover for inward rotation of the humerus. It abducts and flexes the humerus in cooperation with the infraspinatus and the teres minor. It is also another of the muscles that stabilize the head of the humerus in the glenoid fossa.

Note

The last four muscles discussed—the supraspinatus, infraspinatus, teres minor, and subscapularis—form the *rotator cuff*. Their insertions on the neck of the humerus form almost three-quarters of a circle from the anterior aspect upward and to the posterior aspect. The muscles comprising the rotator cuff rotate the humerus but their most important assignment is that of holding the head of the humerus in the glenoid fossa.

Coracobrachialis (Figure 2.54)

Location: This slender muscle, located on the upper medial side of the humerus, connects the scapula with the humerus. It runs from the coracoid process to the anterior-medial surface of the humerus.

Action: This muscle is a prime mover for horizontal flexion and assistor in flexion. It holds the head of the humerus in the glenoid fossa when the arm hangs downward. It rotates the humerus inward from an outward rotated position.

Biceps Brachii (Figure 2.54)

Location: The short head shares a tendon with the coracobrachialis from the coracoid process, while the long head originates from the tubercle above the glenoid fossa and the glenoid labrum. The fibers of the long and short heads join just below the middle of the arm. The fibers of both heads form the distal tendon, which inserts on the tuberosity of the radius.

Action: This muscle is a prime flexor of the humerus. The long head stabilizes the shoulder joint and assists in abduction of the humerus. The short head assists in flexion, abduction, inward rotation, and horizontal flexion of the humerus. Both heads supinate the hand (by acting on the radioulnar joint) when the hand is in extreme pronation. In this action, the triceps contracts to prevent elbow flexion in order that the muscle's action for elbow flexion will be prevented while that for supination will be permitted to go on. The biceps is a prime mover in elbow flexion.

Triceps (Figure 2.56)

Location: This three-headed muscle is the only muscle on the posterior aspect of the arm. The long head arises from the tubercle below the glenoid fossa. The lateral head originates from the upper half of the posterior aspect of the humerus. The medial head originates from the lower two-thirds of the posterior side of the humerus. The fibers of the three heads join and then form a tendon that inserts on the olecranon process of the ulna.

Action: This muscle is, because of its favorable angle of pull, a powerful extensor of the forearm. The long head working alone assists in adduction, extension, and hyperextension of the humerus. It also pulls the head of the humerus into the glenoid cavity.

The Elbow and Radioulnar Joints

The elbow joint is classified as a hinge-type synovial joint. However, this joint is more complex than the usual simple hinge joint because the radius and ulna articulate with the humerus in different ways. A close examina-

Figure 2.57 Deep muscles of the right upper arm (anterior)

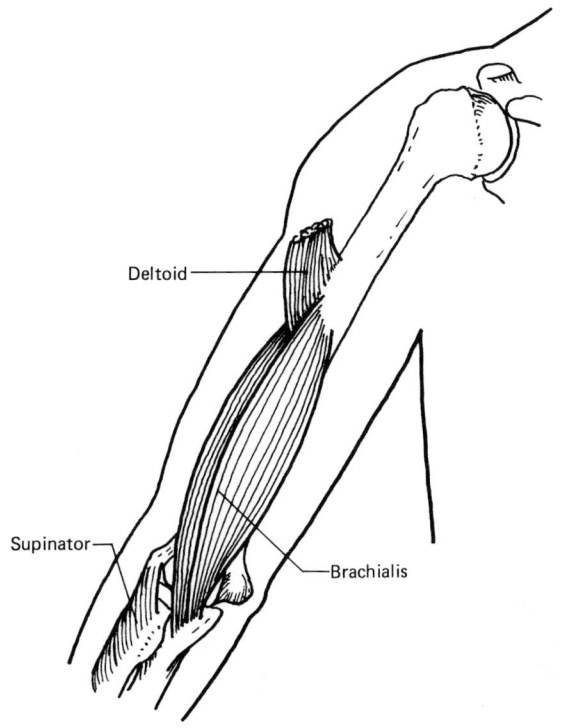

Deltoid

Supinator

Brachialis

tion of the shape and structure of the humeral, ulnar, and radial bones at this joint, as shown in Figures 2.58, 2.59, 2.60, will illustrate these differences. The *semilunar notch* of the ulna articulates with the back and underside of a spool-like process called the *trochlea* at the end of the humerus. The semilunar notch is given greater depth by the small *coronoid process* in front and the large *olecranon process* in the back. The olecranon process limits hyperextension of the elbow when it strikes the posterior side of the medial *epicondyle* of the humerus. This is a true hinge joint. The articulation between the head of the radius and the capitulum on the lateral side of the head of the humerus, on the other hand, is more like a ball and socket joint. Because the concave head of the ulna fits over the rounded capitulum, it would appear that abduction and adduction would be possible. However, these movements are prevented because the *anular ligament*, which encircles the head of the radius, binds it to the radial notch of the ulna. Since the ulna cannot be abducted or adducted, the radius is effectively prevented from engaging in these movements.

Elbow flexion and extension occur through a range of approximately 150 degrees.

A capsule and synovial membrane enclose the articulations between the radial head and the capitulum, the semilunar notch and the trochlea, and the radial head and radial notch of the ulna.

Rotation of the *radial head* in the *radial notch* at the proximal end and rotation of the *ulnar head* in the *ulnar notch* at the distal end make pronation and supination of the forearm possible. When inward and outward rotation of the arm at the shoulder joint is added to pronation and supination of the foeearm, the total range of movements is on the order of 270 degrees.

The distal radioulnar joint has a synovial cavity and capsule. The ligamentous *articu-*

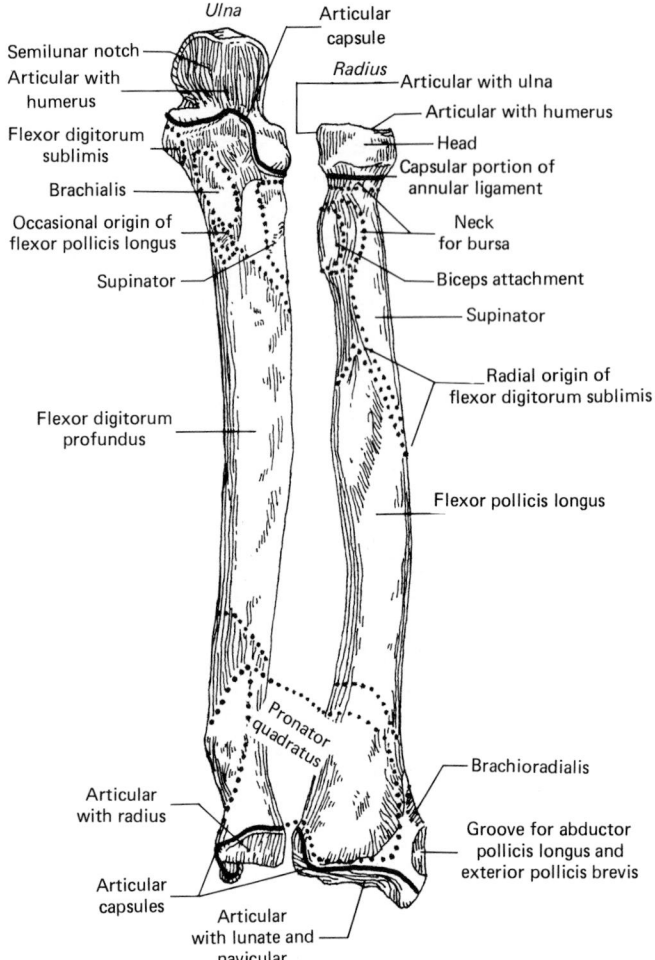

Labels on figure:

Ulna
Articular capsule
Semilunar notch
Articular with humerus
Flexor digitorum sublimis
Brachialis
Occasional origin of flexor pollicis longus
Supinator
Flexor digitorum profundus
Pronator quadratus
Articular with radius
Articular capsules
Articular with lunate and navicular

Radius
Articular with ulna
Articular with humerus
Head
Capsular portion of annular ligament
Neck for bursa
Biceps attachment
Supinator
Radial origin of flexor digitorum sublimis
Flexor pollicis longus
Brachioradialis
Groove for abductor pollicis longus and exterior pollicis brevis

Figure 2.58 Bones of the left forearm, anterior aspect

lar disk holds the head of the ulna against the ulnar notch of the radius and at the same time protects the head of the ulna from the proximal carpal bones.

Ligaments of the Elbow and the Radioulnar Joints. Ligaments at the elbow joint include: (1) *anterior*, (2) *posterior*, (3) *radial collateral*, and (4) *ulnar collateral*. There is one ligament at the proximal radioulnar joint. This is

the *anular ligament* (see Figure 2.61). Between the proximal and distal radioulnar joints are the *interosseus membrane* and the *oblique cord*. The proximal broader end of the ulna receives the weight of the body in arm support activities and the interosseus membrane transmits this force to the radius, which has its broader articulation at its distal end. In activities such as punching or catching a ball, in which the impact is received at the distal end of the radius, a portion of the impact is

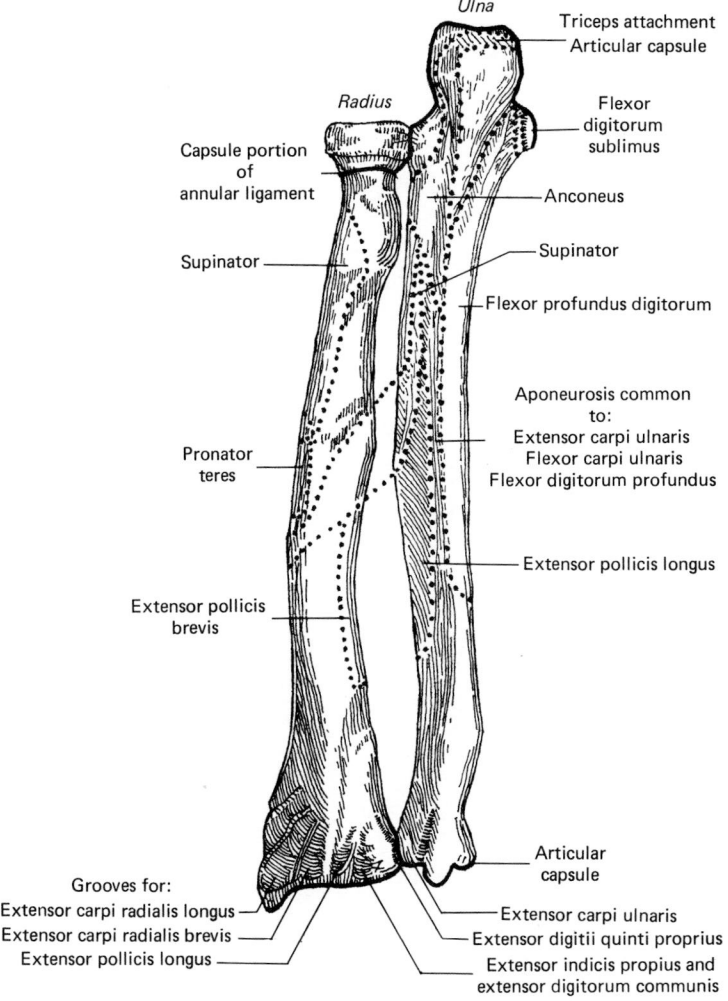

Labels on figure:

Ulna

Triceps attachment
Articular capsule

Radius

Flexor digitorum sublimus

Capsule portion of annular ligament

Anconeus

Supinator

Supinator

Flexor profundus digitorum

Aponeurosis common to:
Extensor carpi ulnaris
Flexor carpi ulnaris
Flexor digitorum profundus

Pronator teres

Extensor pollicis longus

Extensor pollicis brevis

Articular capsule

Grooves for:
Extensor carpi radialis longus
Extensor carpi radialis brevis
Extensor pollicis longus

Extensor carpi ulnaris
Extensor digitii quinti proprius
Extensor indicis propius and extensor digitorum communis

Figure 2.59 Bones of the left forearm, posterior aspect

transferred to the ulna by the interosseus membrane. This prevents the radius and ulna from sliding past one another when longitudinal forces are applied.

The distal radioulnar joint is protected by the *ligamentous articular disk*.

Movements of the Elbow and Radioulnar Joints. *Flexion* at the elbow joint decreases the angle between the upper arm and the forearm.

Extension at the elbow joint increases the angle between the upper arm and the forearm.

Hyperextension at the elbow joint moves the forearm beyond 180 degrees to the upper arm. Few males are able to hyperextend the elbow.

Pronation is rotation of the forearm around its longitudinal axis in which the palm turns medially.

Supination is rotation of the forearm

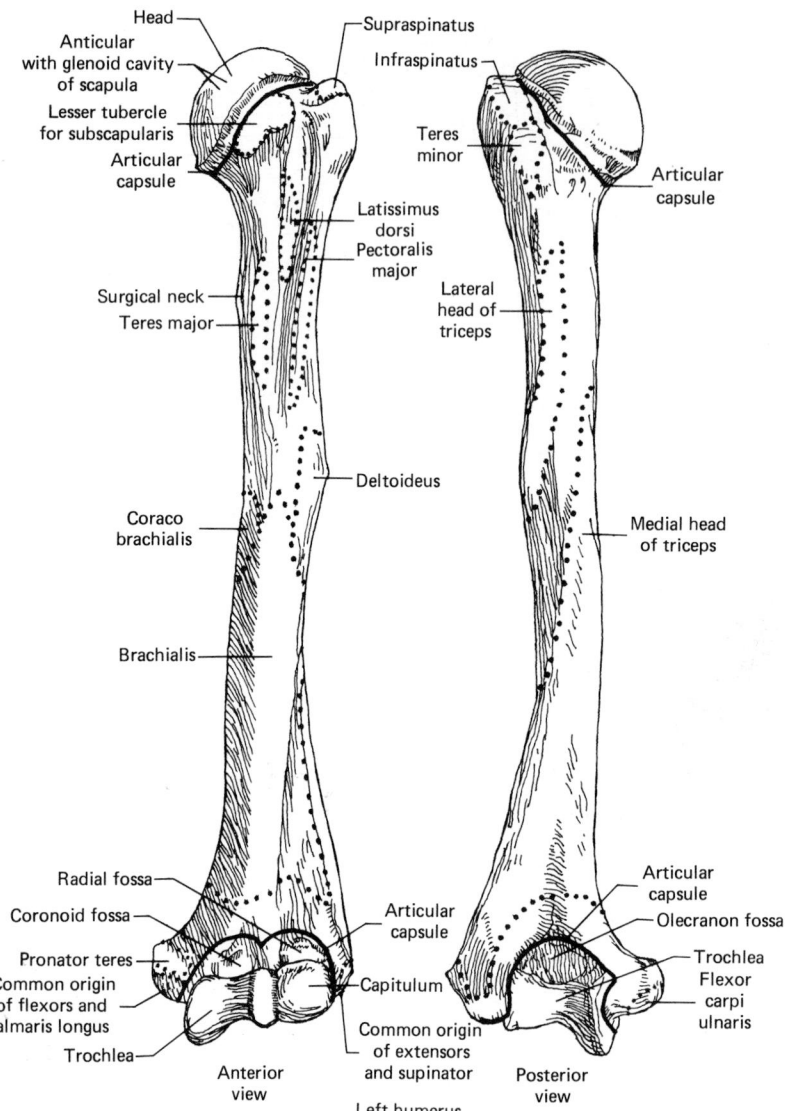

Figure 2.60 Humerus bone, anterior and posterior view

around its longitudinal axis in which the palm turns laterally.

Muscles of the Elbow Joint

Brachialis (Figure 2.62 and 2.57)

Location: This thin muscle is located between the biceps and the humerus. Its fibers run obliquely from the anterior surface of the lower half of the humerus to the tuberosity of the ulna and the front of the coronoid process.

Action: A powerful flexor of the elbow.

Brachioradialis (Figure 2.63)

Location: This muscle's origin is the supracondyloid ridge of the humerus and its insertion is the base of the styloid process on the

80 | ASPECTS OF MOVEMENT

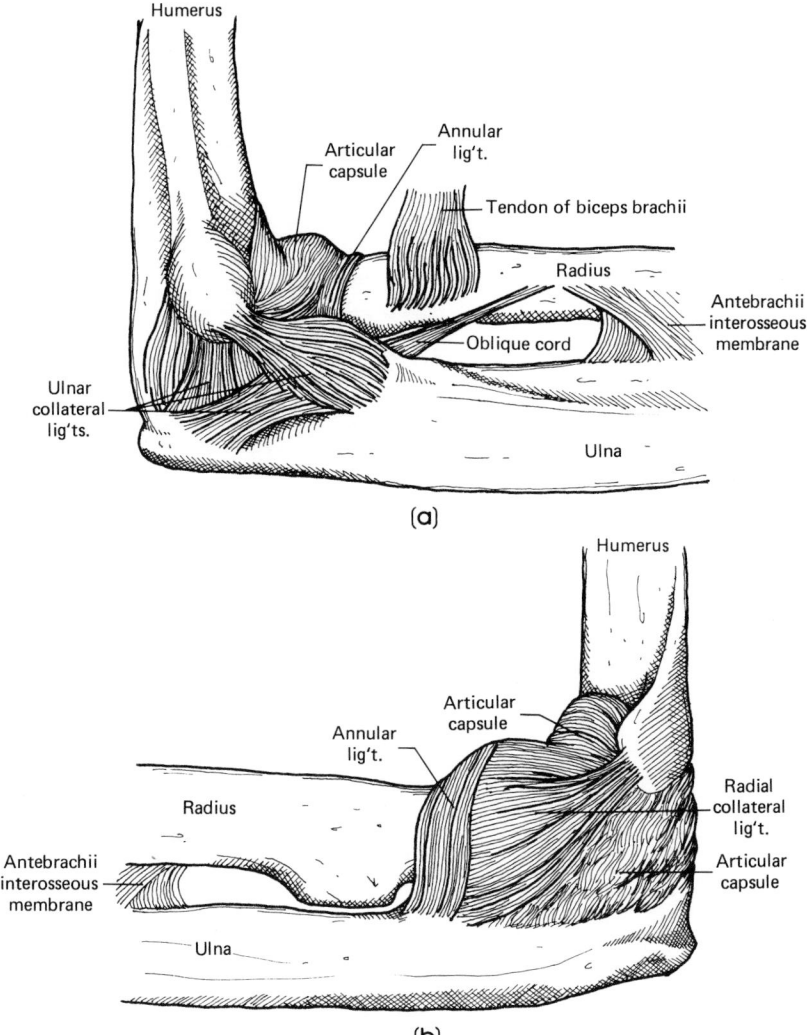

Humerus

Articular capsule

Annular lig't.

Tendon of biceps brachii

Radius

Antebrachii interosseous membrane

Oblique cord

Ulnar collateral lig'ts.

Ulna

(a)

Humerus

Articular capsule

Annular lig't.

Radius

Radial collateral lig't.

Articular capsule

Antebrachii interosseous membrane

Ulna

(b)

Figure 2.61 Lateral and medial aspects of elbow joint and ligaments. (a) Ligaments of left elbow joint, medial aspect; (b) lateral aspect of elbow joint

lateral surface of the radius. This superficial muscle accounts for the rounded curve on the forearm from the elbow to the wrist.

Action: A very effective flexor of the elbow.

Pronator Teres (Figure 2.63)

Location: This small, spindle-shaped mus-

cle has two heads, one from the medial epicondyle of the humerus and the other from the coronoid process of the ulna. The fibers run obliquely across the elbow to insert near the center of the radius.

Action: The pronator teres assists in pronating the forearm when speed of movement is desired or resistance is encountered.

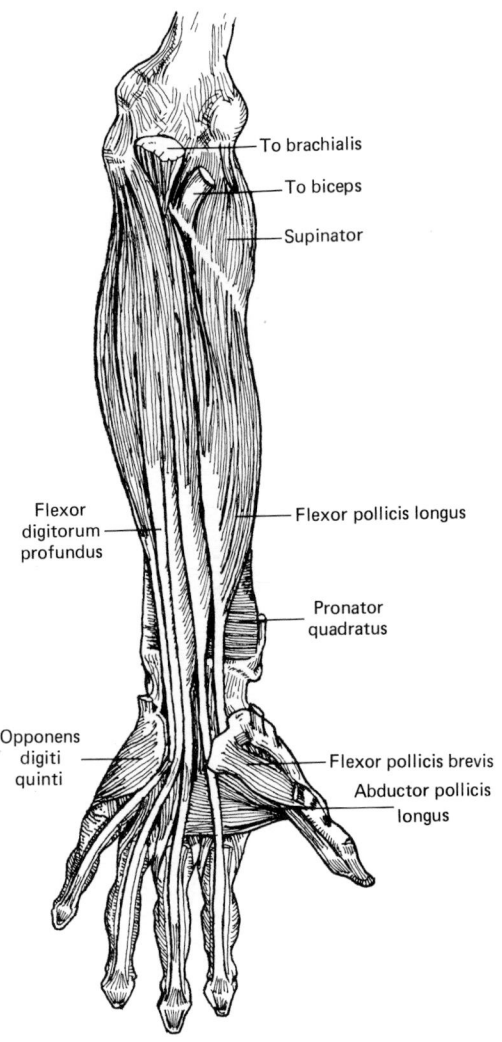

Figure 2.62 The front of the left forearm (deep muscles)

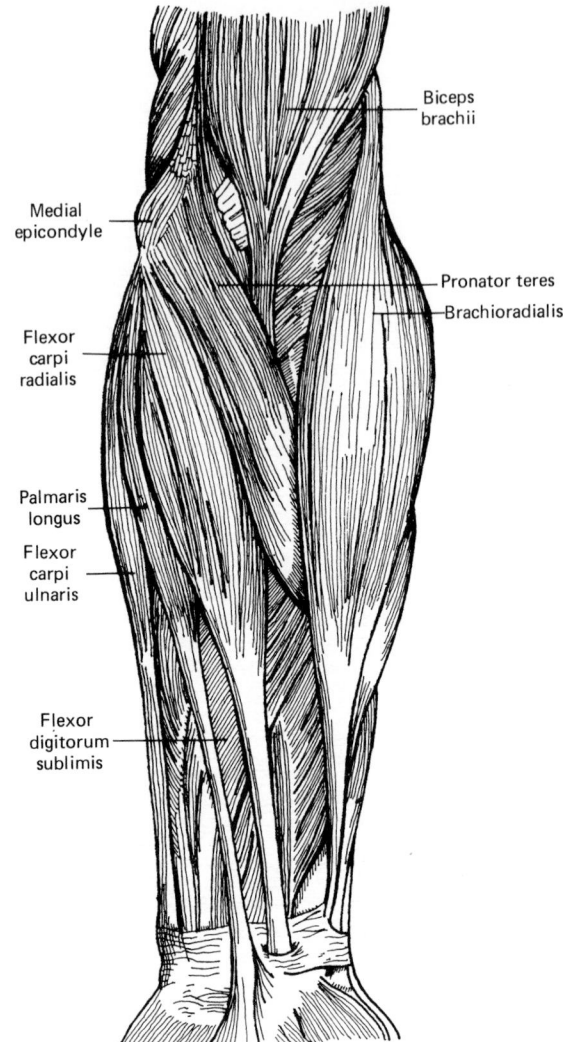

Figure 2.63 Front of the left forearm—superficial muscles

Flexor Carpi Radialis (Figure 2.63)

Location: Figure 2.63 shows this muscle on the anterior surface of the forearm; it originates at the medial epicondyle of the humerus and slants downward to insert on the palmar surface of the second metacarpal bone. A slip also runs to the base of the third metacarpal.

Action: The principal function of this mul-tijoint muscle is flexion and abduction of the wrist; however, it can assist in flexion of the elbow during strenuous movement.

Pronator Quadratus (Figure 2.62)

Location: This muscle is located on the anterior surface of the forearm near the wrist as shown in Figure 2.62. It attaches to the lower fourth of the anterior surface of the ulna and the lower fourth of the anterior surface of the radius.

Action: Pronation of the forearm.

Supinator (Figure 2.64)

Location: This muscle arises from the lateral epicondyle of the humerus and the supinator fossa of the ulna and attaches to the proximal third of the lateral surface of the radius.

Action: Supination of the forearm.

Palmaris Longus (Figure 2.63)

Location: This slender muscle is just medial to the flexor carpi radialis. It originates from the medial epicondyle of the humerus and inserts on the anular ligament of the *palmar aponeurosis.*

Action: Tightens palmar fascia and assists slightly in wrist flexion.

Flexor Digitorum Sublimis (Figure 2.63)

Location: The larger of the two heads of this muscle arises from the medial epicondyle, adjacent fascia, and the coronoid process as shown in Figure 2.63. The smaller radial head originates from the upper two-thirds of the front of the radius. At a point a little more than halfway down the forearm, four tendons are formed, each of which splits into 2 tendons at the base of the proximal phalanx to attach to each side of the middle phalanx of each of the four fingers.

Action: Flexion of the wrist and fingers. It also assists in elbow flexion when great power is required.

Flexor Carpi Ulnaris (Figure 2.63)

Location: This muscle is found on the medial side of the forearm. It originates from the medial epicondyle of the humerus, the medial aspect of the olecranon, and the upper two-thirds of the anterior aspect of the ulna. It inserts on the palmar surface of the pisiform and hamate bones and the fifth metacarpal.

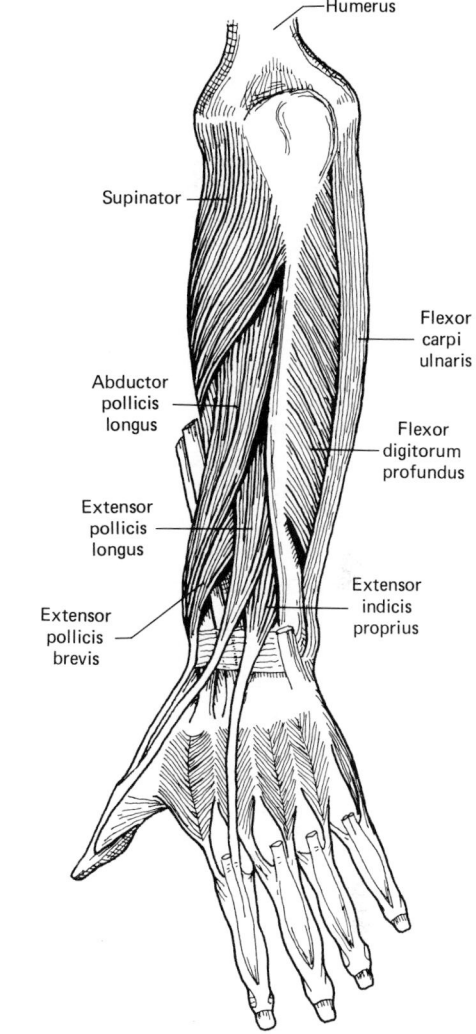

Figure 2.64 Posterior view of the deep muscles of the forearm

Extensor Carpi Radialis Longus

Location: This muscle, located on the radial or thumb side of the forearm, originates on the lateral supracondylar ridge of the humerus and inserts on the dorsal or posterior side of the second metacarpal.

Action: Extension and abduction of the wrist.

Extensor Carpi Radialis Brevis

Location: This muscle runs from the lateral epicondyle of the humerus to the posterior or dorsal side of the base of the third metacarpal.

Action: Extension and abduction of the wrist.

Extensor Digitorum

Location: This muscle is located in the center of the dorsal side of the forearm. It originates from the lateral epicondyle of the humerus. At its distal end, the muscle forms 4 tendons, each of which attaches to the dorsum of the proximal phalanx and then divides into 3 parts, the 2 collateral parts splitting and rejoining to attach to the back of the distal phalanx while the central slip inserts on the back of the base of the middle phalanx.

Action: Extension of the proximal phalanx and the wrist. Like all multijoint muscles, this muscle cannot fully extend both joints over which it operates at the same time. When the wrist is fully extended its contraction has little effect on the last two phalanges.

Extensor Digiti Minimi

Location: This long thin muscle is medial and parallel to the extensor digitorum. It originates from the tendon of the extensor digitorum and inserts into the dorsal expansions of the little finger.

Action: Extension of the proximal phalanx of the little finger, extension of the middle and distal phalanges of the little finger when the proximal phalanx is held in flexion, and extension of the wrist.

Extensor Carpi Ulnaris

Location: This muscle runs from the lateral epicondyle of the humerus and the middle half of the posterior border of the ulna to the medial side of the base of the fifth metacarpal.

Action: The principal function is that of adducting the hand. It is also a weak assistor in elbow flexion when the forearm is pronated and a weak assistor in extension of the elbow when the forearm is supinated. This paradox is explained by the muscle's relationship to the head of the radius in pronated and supinated positions.

Articulations of the Wrist and Hand

Great demands for finely coordinated movements of the wrist, hand, and fingers are demanded in many of mans' activities. Typing, playing a piano, arts and crafts, pitching a baseball, and sculpting are examples of a few of these complex activities. This creates a need for a complex structure. The 27 bones of the hand, as shown in Figure 2.65, include: (1) 8 carpal bones, (2) 5 metacarpal bones, and (3) 14 phalanges. These bones form over 20 joints and require 33 muscles to move them.

The irregularly shaped carpal bones in the wrist are arranged in 2 rows of 4 bones in each row. Those in the first row beginning on the thumb side are named as follows: *navicular, lunatum, triquetrum,* and *pisiform.* Those in the second row, beginning again from the thumb side, are named as follows: *multangulum major, multangulum minor, capitatum,* and *hamatum.* All of the carpal bones, with the exception of the pisiform, have six sides. The first row of carpal bones fit into the concavity formed by the ends of the radius and ulna between the styloid processes of the radius and ulna. The pisiform, however, does not articulate with the either the radius or the ulna. The second row of carpals articulates with the 5 metacarpals. The 8 carpals are so arranged that a shallow concavity exists on the volar, anterior, or palmar side, thereby providing a groove for tendons, nerves, and blood vessels to the hands and fingers.

The saddle joint between the multangulum major and the first metacarpal (thumb side) permits movement of the thumb in any

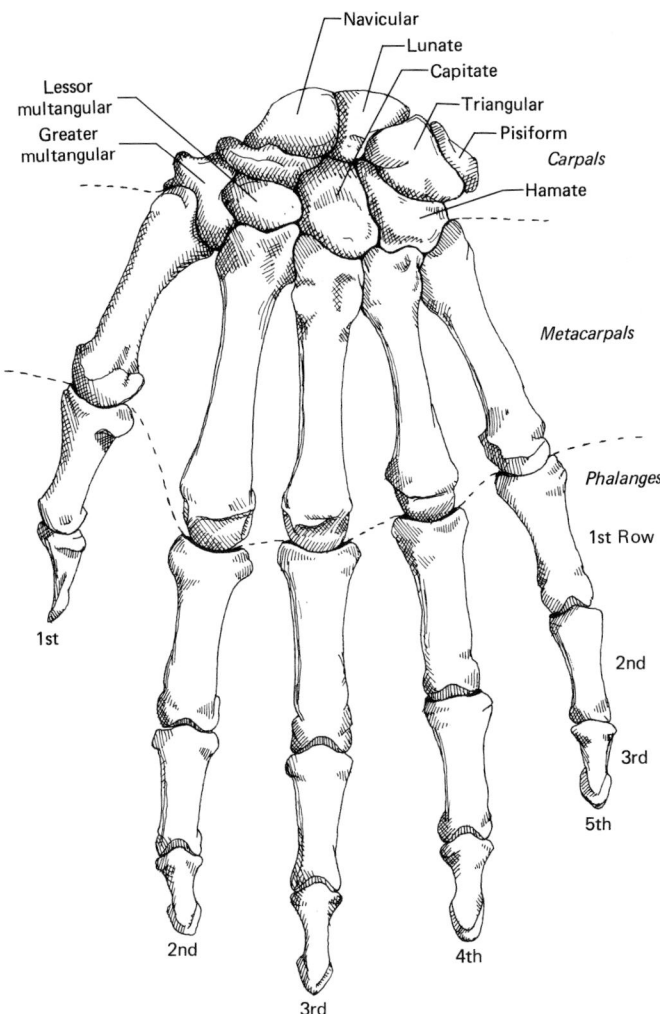

Navicular
Lunate
Capitate
Triangular
Pisiform
Carpals
Hamate
Lessor multangular
Greater multangular
Metacarpals
Phalanges
1st Row
1st
2nd
3rd
5th
2nd
4th
3rd

Figure 2.65 Bones of the left hand (dorsal surface)

plane. This range of movement, when coupled with flexion of the thumb, contributes greatly to the manipulative ability of the hands. The thumb is also turned on its axis so that flexion is somewhat toward the other phalanges rather than in the same plane. This is one of the major structural differences between man and the anthropoids. Many anthropologists believe that the ability of man to grasp and manipulate objects and to use them as tools was a basic cause for the development of his brain.

The major articulations in the wrist are (1) the *radiocarpal*, (2) the *intercarpal*, and (3) the *carpometacarpal*. Movement at the wrist is the sum of the gliding movements of the bones across one another. These joints are all classified as nonaxial diarthrodial joints.

Ligaments of the Wrist and Hand. The ligaments of the wrist include: (1) the *volar radiocarpal*, (2) *dorsal radiocarpal*, (3) *ulnar collateral*, and (4) *radial collateral*. These ligaments form a closed cover for this joint.

These ligaments are shown in Figures 2.66–2.68.

The ligaments of the carpometacarpal joints of the four fingers include: (1) the *dorsal* carpometacarpal, (2) *volar* carpometacarpal, and (3) *interosseus* carpometacarpal. These joints are enclosed by a capsule. The joints are further reinforced by the ligaments of the intermetacarpal articulations (the joints between the proximal ends of the metacarpal bones of the four fingers). These ligaments include: (1) the *dorsal basal*, (2) *volar basal*, (3) *interosseous basal*, and (4) *transverse metacarpal* ligaments.

In the *metacarpophalangeal* joints, the convex head of the metacarpal bones fit into a shallow depression on the proximal ends of the first phalanges. This ovoid joint is encased in a capsule and is reinforced by strong *collateral* ligaments. The *volar accessory* ligament deepens the fossa on the base of the phalanx.

The *interphalangeal* joints between adjacent phalanges of all five digits are all hinge joints. Strong *collateral* ligaments, an *accessory volar* ligament, and a capsule protect each joint (see Figure 2.66).

Movements Specific to the Wrist and Hand.

Movements at the wrist joint include the following:

Flexion of the hand moves the palm side toward the anterior aspect of the forearm in the sagittal plane.

Extension is the opposite movement of flexion.

Hyperextension is movement of the back of the hand toward the posterior side of the forearm. It is extension beyond the straight line position of the hand and forearm.

Radial flexion or abduction is sideward movement of the hand in the frontal plane. The hand moves toward the radial (thumb) side of the forearm. When the arms are in the anatomic position, the hand moves away from the midline of the body.

Ulnar flexion or adduction is a sideward movement of the hand toward the ulnar (little fingers) side in the frontal plane. It is the opposite movement to radial flexion or abduction.

Circumduction is a combination of all the preceding movements executed in sequence in either direction. The extended fingers describe a circle and the hand describes a cone (reciprocal reception).

Movements Specific to the Thumb and Metacarpophalangeal Joints (Figure 2.69).

Extension is sideward movement of the thumb away from the index finger.

Hyperflexion is movement of the thumb toward the ulnar side across the front of the palm.

Abduction is movement of the thumb away from and at right angles to the plane of the palm.

Adduction is the return movement from abduction.

Hyperadduction is continuation of adduction beyond the plane of the hand.

Circumduction is a sequential combination of all the above movements in either direction. The tip of the thumb describes a rough circle.

Opposition is the touching of the tip of the thumb to the tip of each of the four fingers. It is really a combination of abduction and hyperflexion.

Movements specific to the fingers at the metacarpophalangeal joints include the following:

Flexion is movement of the volar (front of the finger) toward the palm.

Extension is movement of finger away from the palm — the return from flexion.

Hyperextension is backward movement of the finger beyond the plane of the hand.

Radial flexion is sideward movement of the finger toward the thumb side.

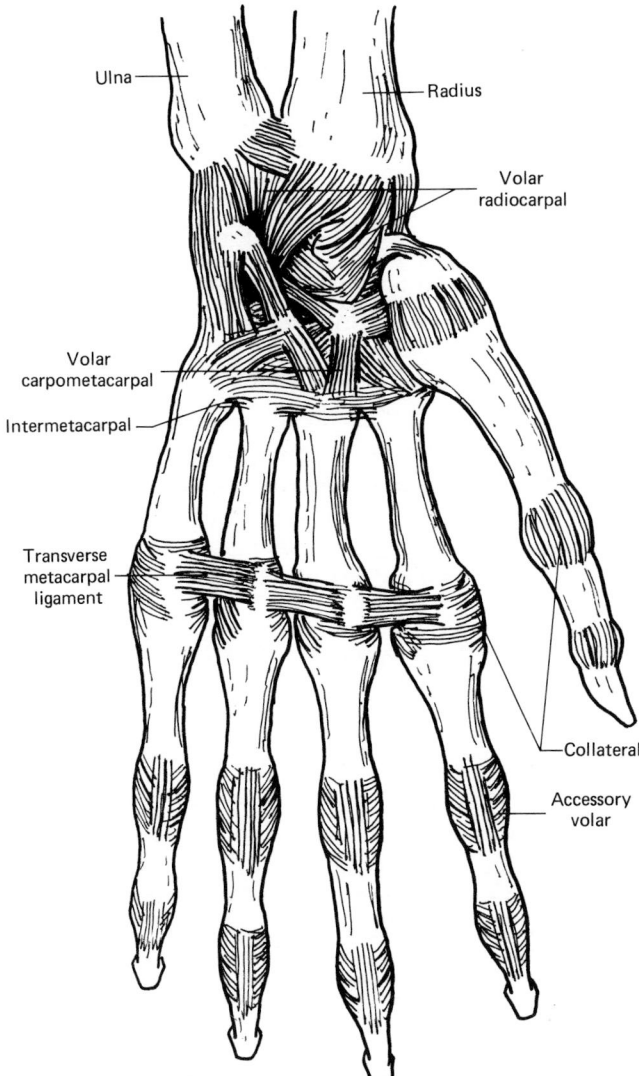

Figure 2.66 Anterior view of the ligaments of the left hand

Labels on figure:
Ulna
Radius
Volar radiocarpal
Volar carpometacarpal
Intermetacarpal
Transverse metacarpal ligament
Collateral
Accessory volar

Ulnar flexion is sideward movement of the finger toward the little finger side.

Circumduction is circular movement of the fingers in either direction.

Movements of the thumb at the metacarpophalangeal joint include the following:

Flexion is movement of the front of the thumb toward its base.

Extension is the return movement from flexion.

Hyperextension is continuation of extension beyond the straight line position of the first metacarpal and the phalanges of the thumb. Some people are unable to hyperextend the thumb.

The only movements possible at the inter-

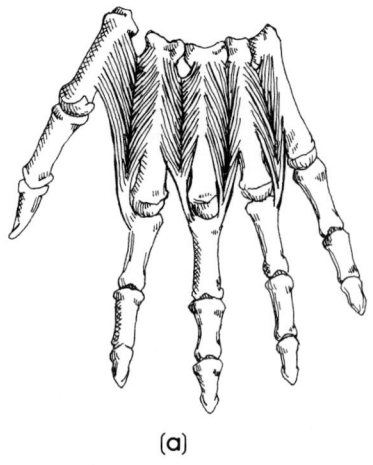

(a)

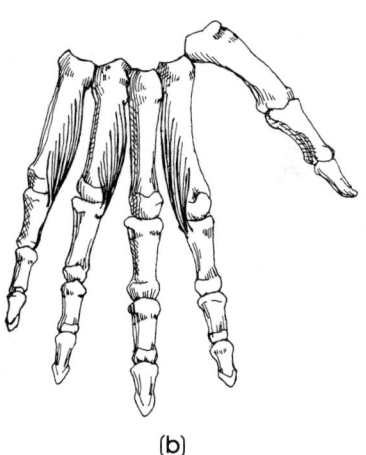

(b)

Figure 2.67 (a) Dorsal interossei of the right hand and (b) palmer interossei of the left hand

phalangeal joints are flexion and extension. Hyperextension is limited, if present.

Muscles of the Wrist and Hand. The location and function of muscles that act on the elbow or radioulnar joints, as well as the joints of the wrist and hand, have been described. The 6 muscles that originate in the forearm and act on the wrist and hand will be described. We will restrict ourselves to merely naming the intrinsic muscles of the hand.

Flexor Pollicis Longus (Figure 2.62)

Location: This muscle is located next to the radius and ulna on the anterior side. It runs from the middle three-quarters of the anterior aspect of the radius to the palmar surface of the base of the distal phalanx of the thumb.

Action: Flexion of the wrist and phalanges of the thumb and adduction of the thumb in cooperation with other muscles.

Flexor Digitorum Profundus (Figure 2.62)

Location: This deep, anterior, and medial muscle arises from the upper three-fourths of the medial and anterior aspects of the ulna and adjacent interosseus membrane and attaches to the palmar side of the proximal end of the distal phalanx of each of the four fingers.

Action: Flexion of the wrist and all three interphalangeal joints and adduction of the fingers.

Abductor Pollicis Longus (Figure 2.62)

Location: This deep posterior muscle arises from the lateral part of the posterior surface of the ulna, the adjacent interosseous membrane, and the middle third of the posterior surface of the radius. The muscle curves around to the lateral side of the forearm and inserts into the radial side of the base of the first metacarpal bone.

Action: Abduction of the hand and thumb, flexion of the wrist, and extension of the first metacarpal.

Extensor Pollicis Brevis (Figure 2.64)

Location: This muscle originates from the medial portion of the lower third of the posterior surface of the radius and the adjacent interosseous membrane. It inserts on the posterior side of the base of the first phalanx of the thumb.

Action: Extension of the proximal phalanx of the thumb; indirectly, extension of the first

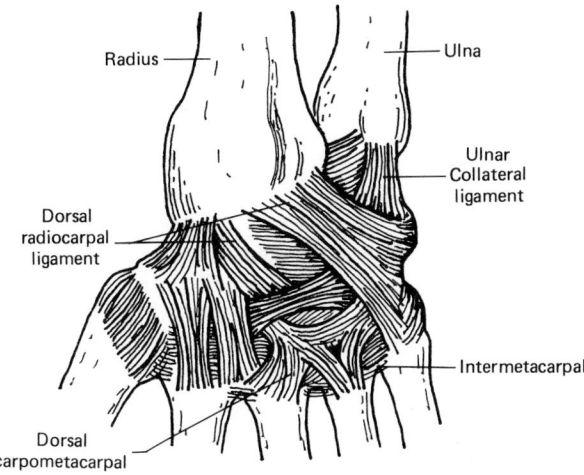

Radius

Ulna

Ulnar
Collateral
ligament

Dorsal
radiocarpal
ligament

Intermetacarpal

Dorsal
carpometacarpal

Posterior view of the ligaments
of the left wrist.

Figure 2.68   Posterior view of the ligaments of the
left wrist

metacarpal bone; and, in cooperation with
other muscles, abduction of the thumb.

Extensor Pollicis Longus (Figure 2.64)

Location: Arises from the lateral part of
the middle third of the posterior surface of
the ulna and adjacent interosseous membrane. It inserts on the posterior of the base
of the distal phalanx of the thumb.

Action: Extends the distal and proximal
phalanges of the thumb and the first metacarpal bone. It also adducts the thumb and
both extends and abducts the wrist.

Extensor Indicis

Location: Originates on the posterior surface of the ulna and adjacent interosseous
membrane. Its tendon joins the tendon of the
extensor digitorum, which inserts on the
posterior side of the index finger.

Action: Strong extension of the proximal
phalanx and weak extension of the middle
and distal phalanges of the index finger, adduction of the index finger, and extension of
the wrist.

Intrinsic muscles of the hand include the
following (Figure 2.70):

1. Abductor pollicis brevis
2. Opponens pollicis
3. Flexor pollicis brevis
4. Adductor pollicis
5. Flexor digiti Minimi
6. Opponens digiti minimi
7. Abductor digiti minimi
8. Palmaris brevis
9. Lumbricales
10. Palmar interossei
11. Dorsal interossei

SUMMARY

This chapter has been devoted to a review of
anatomic and structural considerations that
influence human movement. The structure
and function of bones, joints, ligaments, and
muscles have been reviewed. Forms of human
bones—long, flat, and irregular—have been

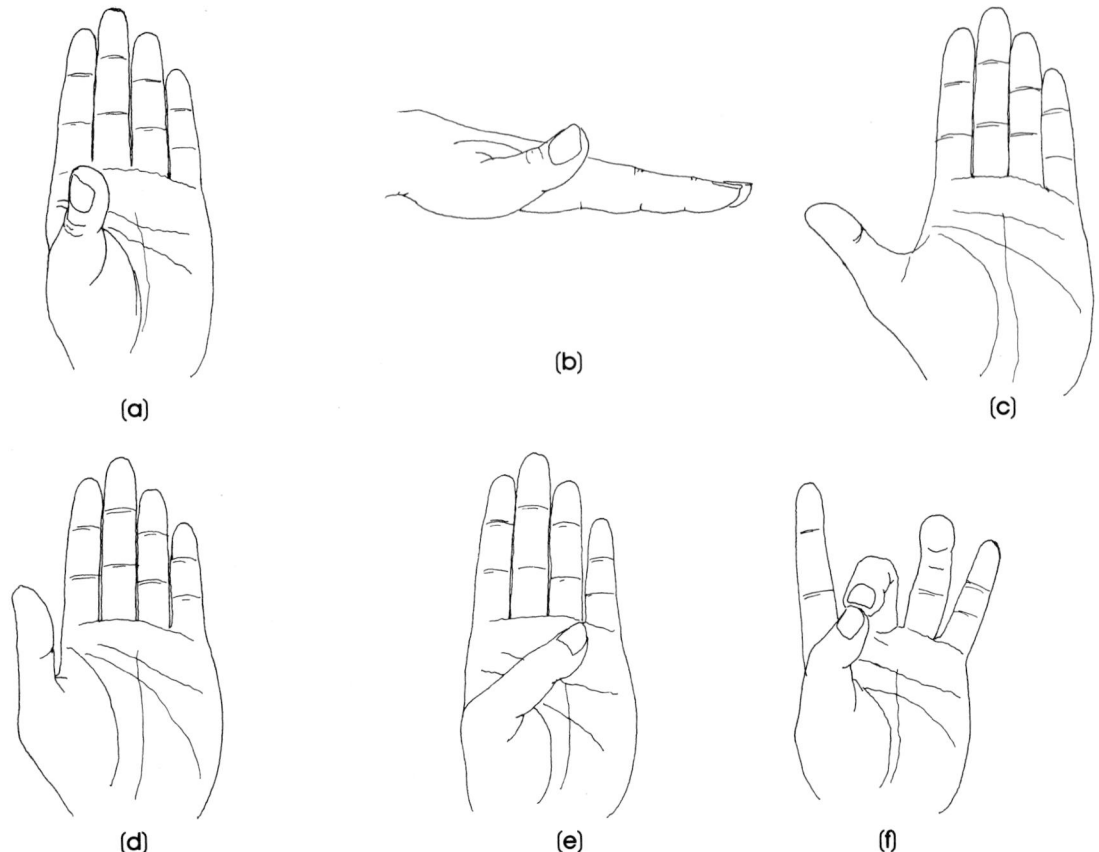

Figure 2.69 Movements of the thumb at the carpometacarpal joint. (a) Abduction, (b) hyperadduction, (c) extension, (d) flexion, (e) hyperflexion, (f) opposition

discussed. The composition of bones and their parts, such as the Haversian system, lamellae, canaliculli, osteocytes, diaphyses, condyles, tubercles, tuberosities, hyaline cartilage, periosteum, endosteum, epiphyseal cartilage, and metaphysis, have been studied. Ossification, closure, and injury to bone have been looked at from the point of view of physical educators, coaches, and others involved in human movement.

We have covered the three major types of articulations—diarthrodial, amphiarthrodial, and synarthrodial. We have also cov-

ered the 6 structural types of diarthrosis joints—gliding, condyloid, saddle, hinge, ball and socket, and pivot—and the 3 types of syarthrosis joints—cartilaginous, fibrous, and ligamentous. The characteristics of joints that give them stability and the characteristics that permit or limit the range of motion have been listed and explained.

Standard joint movement terms have been defined including those for the scapula, pelvis, vertebral column, hand, and foot as well as those for individual joints such as the shoulder, hip, knee, elbow, wrist, interphal-

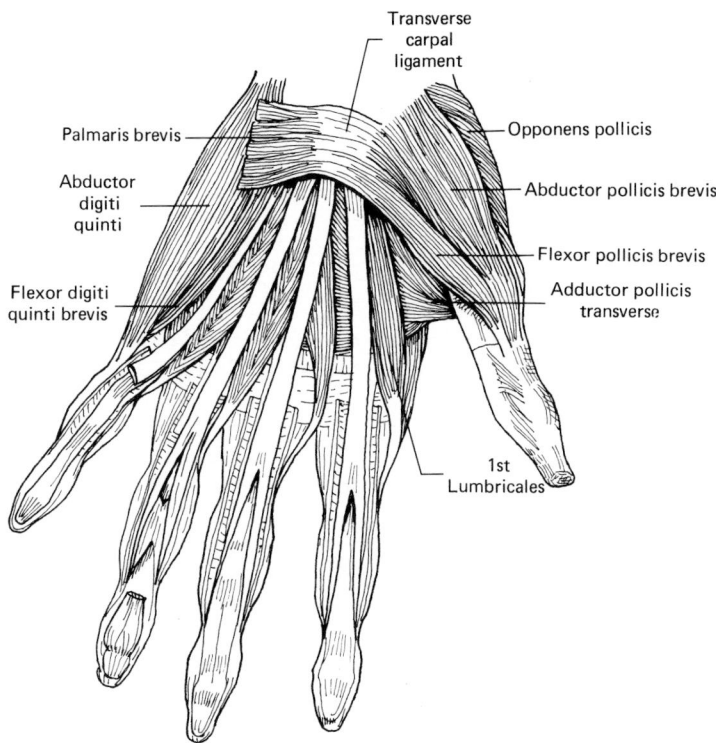

Transverse
carpal
ligament

Palmaris brevis

Abductor
digiti
quinti

Flexor digiti
quinti brevis

Opponens pollicis

Abductor pollicis brevis

Flexor pollicis brevis

Adductor pollicis
transverse

1st
Lumbricales

Figure 2.70 Muscles of the left hand, palmar surface

angeal, intercarpal, and intertarsal, and others. The range of movement in many of these body parts and joints has been presented.

Anatomic and fundamental standing positions, planes, and axes have been studied with respect to the influences upon human movement. The student who understands these concepts will be able to analyze sports movements more effectively and consequently be a more effective coach or physical educator.

Gross muscle structure and function were studied from the standpoint of origin, insertion, line of pull, action over two joints, and functions as an agonist, antagonist, neutralizer, or stabilizer. Ligamentous action, tendon action, reciprocal inhibition, maximum-force movements (continuous-force

and ballistic), slow-tension movements, rapid-tension movements, concentric contraction, eccentric contraction, isotonic contraction, static contraction, and isometric contraction have been defined and implications for the conduct of training programs have been specified. The advantages and disadvantages of weight training and isometric strength programs have been presented as have several suggestions for the conduct of such programs. The relationships between myohemoglobin, red fibers, pale fibers, and muscular endurance were explained.

The bony structure, movements, and ligaments protecting and muscles acting upon the body articulations were studied. This included function and location of ligaments and location, attachments, characteristics, and action of muscles. The following articulations were covered: pelvic girdle, vertebral column, hip joint, thorax, scapula, shoulder joint, elbow, radioulnar joints, wrist, carpometacarpal joints, metacarpophalangeal joints, interphalangeal joints, knee, ankle, tarsal joints, tarsometatarsal joints, intermetatarsal joints, and metatarsophalangeal joints. We have discussed the location (origin and insertion), structural characteristics, and function of 106 muscles. We have also cited 11 intrinsic muscles of the hand and the 11 intrinsic muscles of the foot. Physical educators and coaches can utilize this information in determining which muscles need to be strengthened and which tendons need to be stretched to perform specific skills with greater proficiency. They can also utilize this information to help determine which muscle has been injured after a trauma.

Finally, we have discussed the microscopic structure of muscle fibers and their parts—sarcolemma, endomysium, sarcoplasm, myofibrils, mitrochondria, I bands, A bands, Z line, sarcomere, H zone, M line, actin and myosin filaments, and cross bridges. The manner in which the myofibrils contract was also briefly discussed.

REFERENCES

1. Steindler, A., *Kinesiology of the Human Body* (3rd printing). Springfield, Ill.: Charles C. Thomas, 1970, pp. 60-61.
2. Northrip, John W., Logan, Gene A., and McKinney, Wayne C., *Biomechanical Analysis of Sport*. Dubuque, Iowa: William C. Brown, 1974, pp. 14-19.
3. Forsbert, A., Tesch, P., Sjodin, B., Thorstensson, A., and Karlsson, J., "Skeletal Muscle Fibers and Athletic Performance," *Biomechanics V-5* (edited by P. V. Komi). Baltimore: University Press, 1976, pp. 112-117.

3 ANTHROPOMETRICAL DIMENSIONS

CONCEPTS

1. Every person combines in varying degrees the qualities of three body types. The degree to which a person possesses the characteristics of each body type is rated on a seven-point scale.

2. Successful athletes in all sports rate average or above in mesomorphy. However, sports in which demands are made upon cardiovascular-respiratory or muscular endurance, or in which the body must be hurled through space, reward ectomorphy while sports in which a heavy object or an opponent (unlimited weight class) must be moved reward endomorphy or extreme mesomorphy.

3. Somatotype can be useful in counseling students for sports and in the selection of candidates for interscholastic teams.

4. Students rating at the extremes in ectomorphy or endomorphy should not be expected to perform as well in tests of motor fitness as medial types or those high in mesomorphy.

5. Body fat is classified into two types: (1) essential fat and (2) storage fat.

6. The most important factor accounting for the high incidence of obesity in Western societies is inactivity.

7. The caloric cost of identical amounts of activity is greater for the obese than it is for the lean person.

8. Fat cell number, rather than fat cell size, is the principal factor in obesity; consequently, obese people may have almost ten times the number of fat cells found in the person of average weight.

9. Evidence exists that exercise during the growing years will permanently delimit the number of fat cells.

10. Three methods for determination of somatotype are the Sheldon method, the Heath–Carter method, and Cureton's Simplified Physique Rating.

11. Although leanness/fatness may be assessed through either direct or indirect methods, the indirect methods, such as hydrostatic weighing or girth and skinfold measures, are most commonly used in physical education.

12. Most successful athletes have high body density because they have little storage fat.

13. Blacks have a higher crural index than Caucasians as well as higher body density, producing an advantage in jumping and running on the one hand, and a disadvantage in ability to float on the other.

14. The weight and center of gravity of various body segments has been computed and could be utilized by physical educators in computing moment of inertia and radius of gyration.

GENERAL CONSIDERATIONS

Anthropometry is the science of measuring the human body and its parts. The early Greek physician Hippocrates, before 400 B.C., recognized two extreme body types: *habitus apoplecticus*, the short thick type, and *habitus phthesicus*, the long thin type. In 1797 Halle classified human bodies into four types according to their dominant anatomic characteristics. These were abdominal, muscular, thoracic, and nervous. In 1828 Rostan recognized the same four basic types, which he renamed digestive, muscular, respiratory, and cerebral. In 1925 Kretschmer[1] suggested three types: pyknic (the round type), athletic, and leptosome or asthenic (linear type). The basic similarities of these various systems for classification of body type is rather obvious.

The system of body typing most widely used today is that developed by Sheldon and his associates.[2] Sheldon, like most of those preceding him, recognized three basic body types. However, he considerably refined and improved upon the systems used previously by recognizing that only a very small percentage of people can be characterized as belonging exclusively to one of the three basic types. Consequently, he developed a system for rating each person on the degree to which he possessed qualities of each of the three extreme body types. The degree is indicated via a seven-point scale, 1 indicating minimal possession of the qualities of the body type, 7 indicating maximal possession of the qualities, and 4 indicating an average amount. Each person is assigned three numbers, each number ranging from 1 to 7. Illustrations of several body types are presented in Figure 3.1.

ENDOMORPHY

The first component is called endomorphy, the second mesomorphy, and the third ectomorphy. The last part of the term (*morphy*) of the three types means body type. The prefix *endo* comes from the term *endoderm*, which refers to that part of the developing egg cell that becomes viscera. The endomorphic body type predominates in abdominal area.

Characteristics of Extreme Endomorphs

1. Large anterior-posterior diameter of body segments

2. Centralization of body mass

3. Body soft and round

4. Large trunk volume

5. Neck short and thick

6. Head large and round

7. Face wide and round

8. Chest broad and thick

9. Breasts often fat

10. Clavicles and scapulae well padded with fat

11. Costal angle wide

12. Vertebral column relatively straight

13. Upper arms and legs relatively short

14. Lower legs and forearms relatively short

15. Forearms, upper arms, and thighs taper to relatively small joints

16. Shoulders square and high

17. Hands and feet small

18. Muscles smooth with little or no definition

19. Buttocks heavy and fat with no dimpling

20. Abdomen large and full above navel and relatively long from xiphoid to pubis

21. Large anterior-posterior diameter through waist

MESOMORPHY

The second component is called mesomorphy. The prefix *meso* comes from the term *mesoderm*, which is the part of the develop-

ing egg cell that becomes muscle. The mesomorphic type predominates in muscle.

Characteristics of Extreme Mesomorphs

1. Muscles massive, prominent, and defined

2. Bones large and prominent

3. Body appears square and hard with
the mass distributed uniformly

4. Large transverse diameter of shoulders, forearms, and lower legs while anterior-posterior diameter is smaller than in
endomorphic types

5. Head square with thick and dense
bones

6. Face with prominent cheek bones and

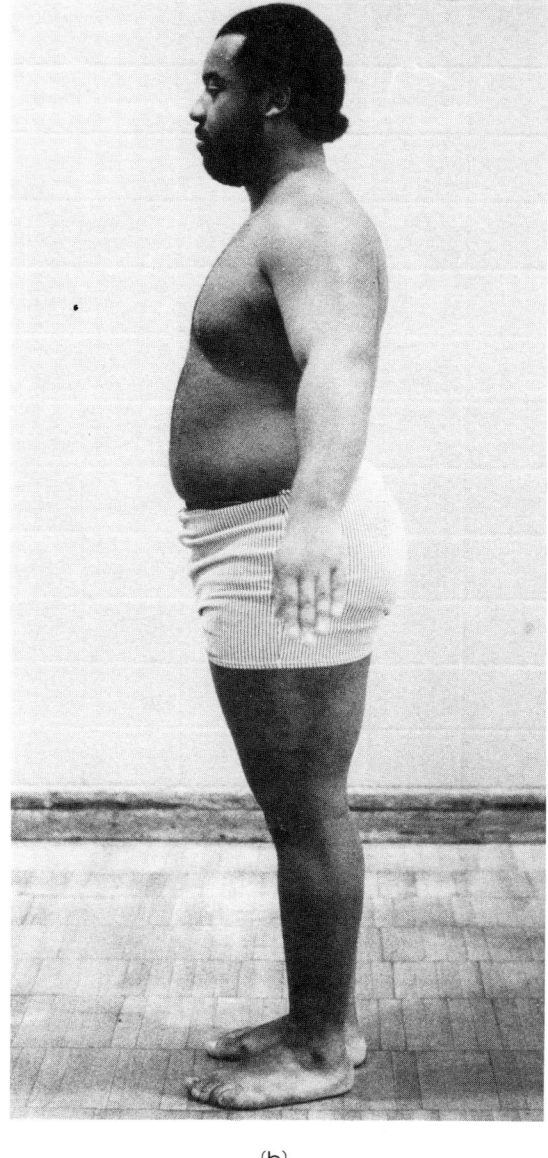

(b)

Figure 3.1 Mesomorphic Body Types (a) to (c) Endomorphic mesomorph 661

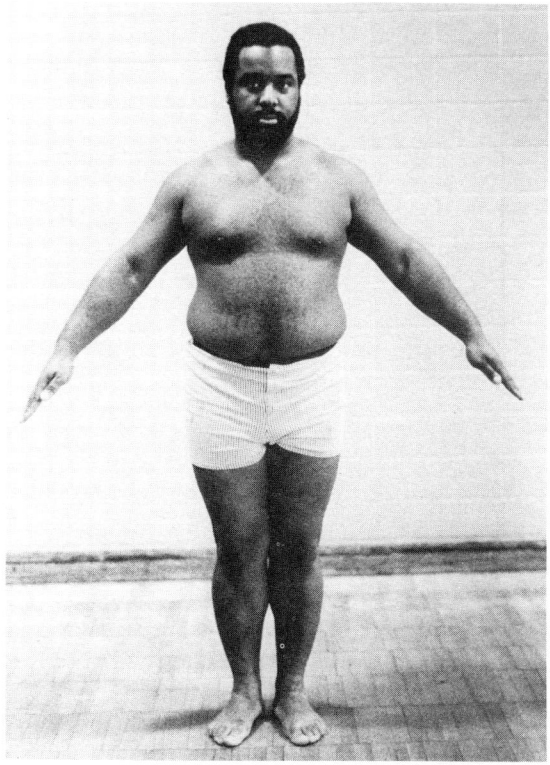

(a)

supraorbital ridges, square jaw, facial
mass greater than forehead

7. Neck long and strong with greater
transverse than anterior-posterior diameter

8. Thorax wide at apex, little curvature

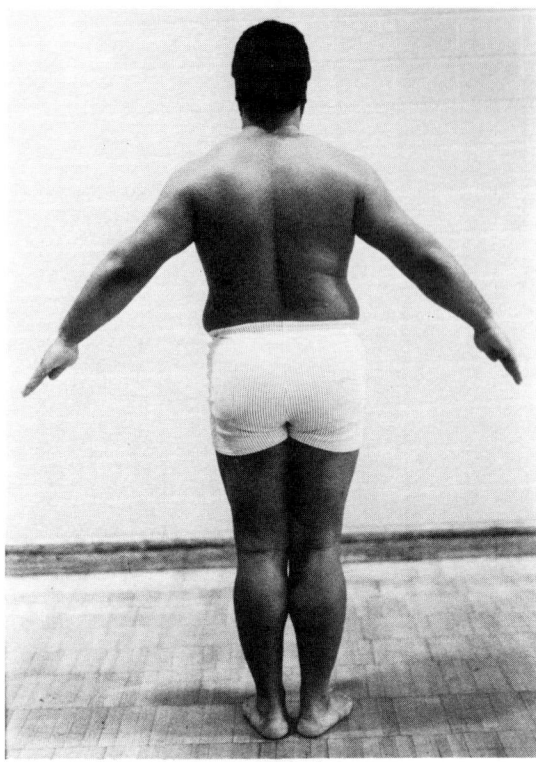

(c)

in thoracic spine, thoracic volume greater than abdominal volume

9. Thick ribs

10. Abdominal area well muscled and defined

11. Waist low and slender

12. Pelvic girdle broad and strong

13. Lumbar curve large

14. Shoulders broad with well-developed trapezius and deltoid muscles

15. Clavicles heavy and prominent

16. Upper arms and forearms well muscled and evenly proportioned

17. Wrists, hands, and fingers large

18. Buttocks well muscled with dimpling

19. Thighs and lower legs heavily muscled and uniformly proportioned

ECTOMORPHY

The third component is called ectomorphy. The prefix *ecto* comes from the term *ectoderm*, which is that part of the developing egg cell that becomes skin. The ectomorph has a large surface area relative to body volume, causing this type to lose body heat quickly. This is why, when swimming in cold water, the thin linear types of children shiver, show goose bumps and blue lips, and cry to leave, while the chubby endomorphs are quite comfortable.

Characteristics of Extreme Ectomorphs

1. Small anterior-posterior diameter

2. General impression of frailty, delicateness, linearity, leanness, and undernourishment

3. Bones small and thin

4. Long arms and legs relative to trunk

5. Face small with pointed chin and nose

6. Forehead large

7. Neck long and slender, forward head (poke neck) common

8. Lips delicate, thin, dry, and pale

9. Thorax narrow, thin, and longer than abdomen

10. Costal angle smaller than in endomorphs or mesomorphs

11. Ribs prominent

12. Scapulae protuberant

13. Clavicals prominent with deep clavicular hollows

14. Shoulders forward (kyphosis or round shouldered)

15. Abdomen short, hollow above navel and protuberant below navel with small anterior-posterior diameter at the navel

16. Arms and legs long and thin with little muscle

17. Hands and feet thin and long

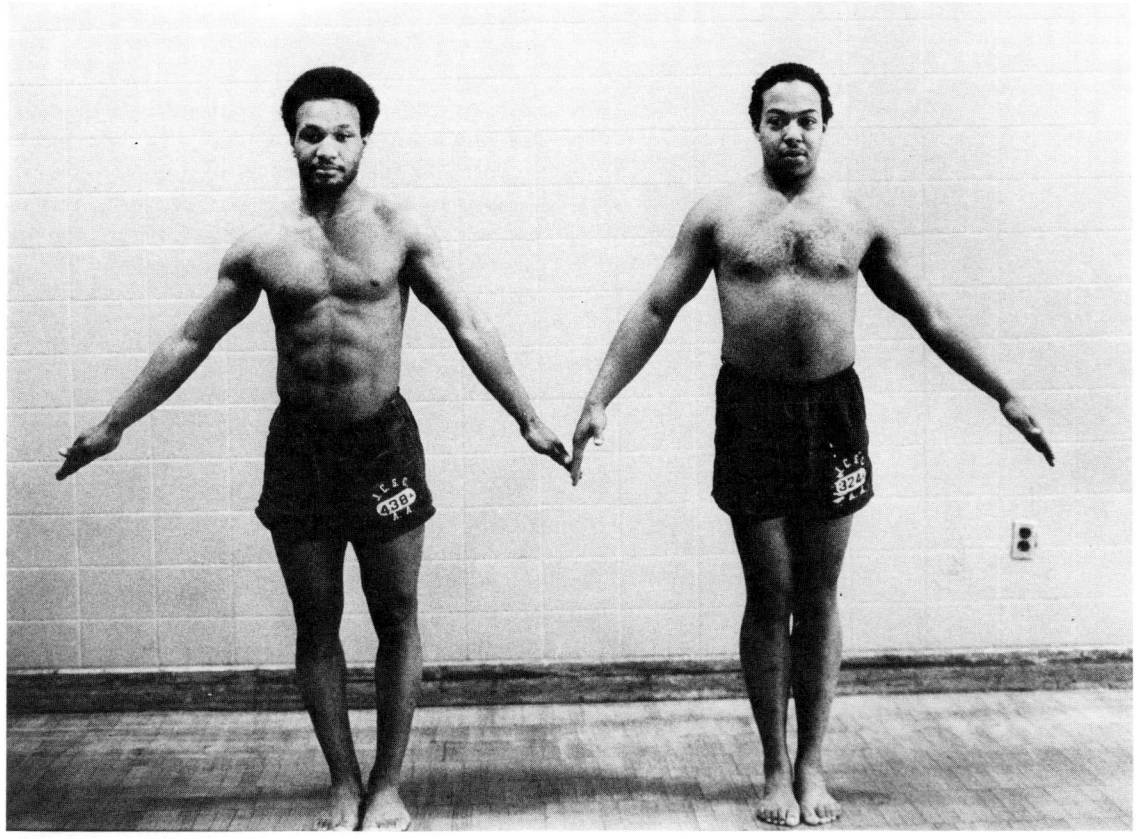

(d)

Figure 3.1d to 3.1f Man on left—mesomorph 463; man on right—endomorphic mesomorph 552

18. Forearms long compared to upper arms

19. Buttocks small, flat and thin

The extreme body types described above are rarely seen since most people combine, in varying degrees, qualities of all three body types. The seven-point scale for the three components implies that 343 different types exist. ($7 \times 7 \times 7 = 343$). Although, according to Sheldon, the three components are independent of one another, somatotypes of 111, 777, 272, 171, 515, etc., are never seen. Sheldon has described 76 somatotypes, of which 50 occur fairly frequently. It is obviously impossible for a person to rate high in both endomorphy and ectomorphy although some rate 5 or 6 in either ectomorphy or endomorphy and 6 or 7 in mesomorphy. In describing mixed somatotypes, compound terminology is used, the dominant component being the second term. Examples follow:

Ectomorphic-mesomorph— 145 to 254

Endomorphic-mesomorph— 542 to 551

Ectomorphic-endomorph— 415, 424, 523

Medial—434, 343, 543, 444

Ecto-medial— 135, 336

Endo-medial— 534, 532

Meso-medial— 252

ANTHROPOMETRICAL DIMENSIONS | **97**

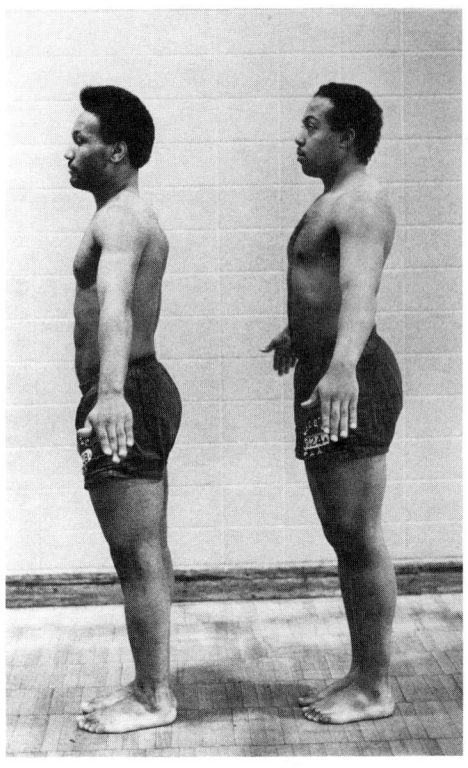

(e)

Study of Chart I will illustrate why it is impossible for a person to rate 5 or above in both endomorphy and ectomorphy as well as why it is unlikely that a person rating 7 in mesomorphy will rate 7 in either ectomorphy or endomorphy. Although Sheldon called the three characteristics components, which indicates that he regarded them as distinct, there does seem to be a relationship among the three.

SOMATOTYPE AND SKILL PERFORMANCE

Olympic champions in most sports are average or above in mesomorphy. The reason for this is because in almost all sports strength or muscular endurance is prerequisite to suc-

cess. The degree of mesomorphy predetermines the degree of strength that can be developed. In activities that require endurance, such as the marathon and mile run, ectomorphy assumes importance because the cardiovascular-respiratory system need not work as hard to transport oxygen and nutrients to the cells of thin people as it does in heavily muscled endomorphic-mesomorphs or mesomorphs. Ectomorphs have less tissue than endomorphs and mesomorphs. In sports where a heavy implement such as a shot or hammer or an opponent must be moved, endomorphy assumes greater importance because endomorphic mesomorphs possess greater bulk.

Sports could be ranked from those in which endurance plays the greatest role and body mass the least to those in which mass and power play the greatest role while endurance exerts the least. At one end would be the marathon run, and at the opposite end would be heavy weight lifting and wrestling competition and the guard or tackle position in football. The more important endurance, the greater advantage in ectomorphy. The more important mass, the greater the advantage in endomorphy. However, regardless of the event, successful athletes in all sports are average or above in mesomorphy. In endurance events against little resistance, however, a high degree of mesomorphy is a disadvantage because in these events strength and power are not needed and yet the heart has to work harder to pump blood.

Long third-class levers make possible greater speed due to their great range of motion. (See Chapter 7 for a more detailed explanation of human levers.) Athletes with long legs, and particularly those with long lower legs, have a mechanical advantage in jumping, running, vaulting, and hurdling.

In the 1972 Olympic Games, the flyweight weight lifting division (52 kg) was won with a total of 337.5 kg, while the heavyweight (110 kg) division was won with a total of 580.0 kg. The flyweight champion lifted 6.392 times

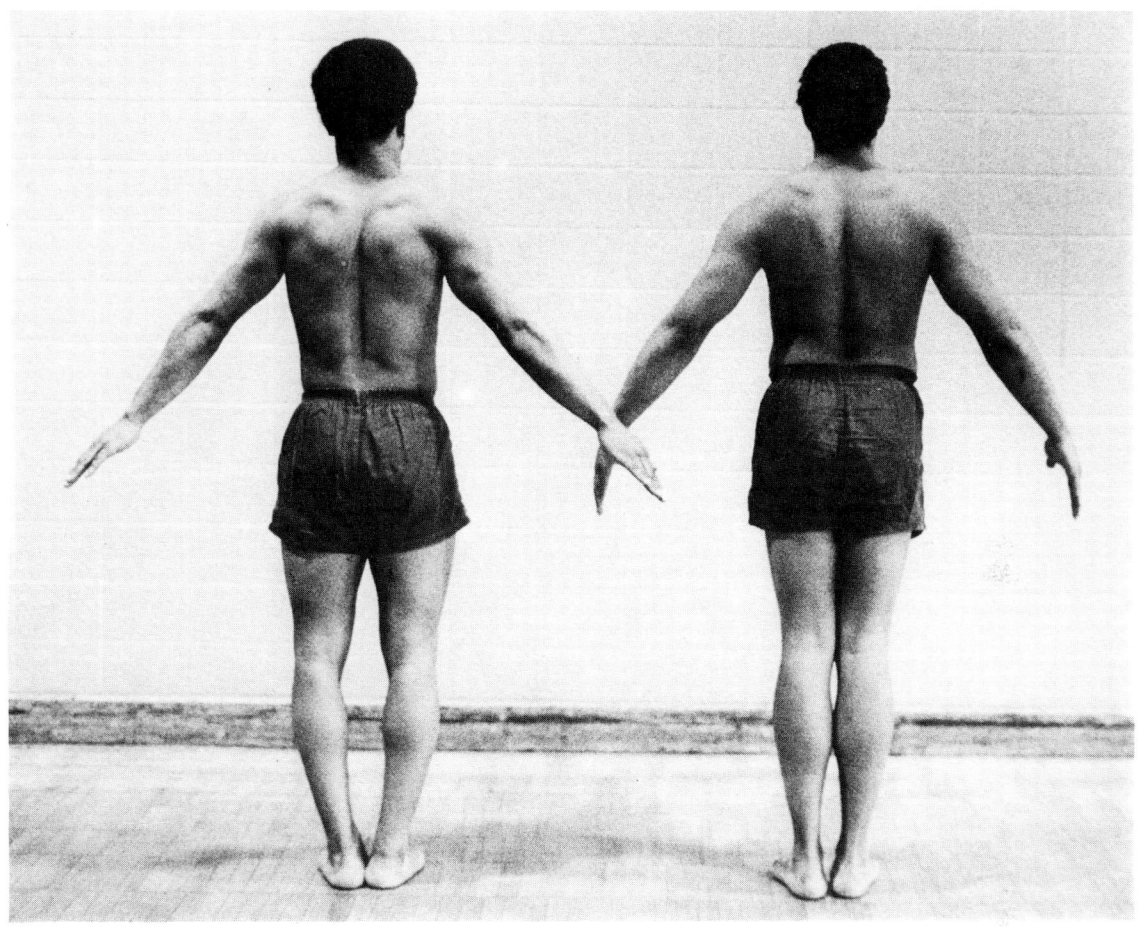

(f)

his body weight, while the heavyweight champion lifted 5.273 times his body weight. This difference is fairly consistent from one weight class to the next. The heavier the lifter, the less he can lift relative to his weight. This is because body weight increases as the cube of size, while force increases as the square, being roughly proportional to the cross-sectional diameter of the muscle. This explains why short, broad individuals excel in strength events and become efficient heavy laborers.

Total strength correlates less than 0.30 with age, height, or weight but correlates 0.61 with skeletal build. This suggests a positive relationship between somatotype and athletic events that demand strength and power. Football linemen, heavyweight wrestlers, hammer throwers, shot putters, and understanders in circus triples and four-man balancing acts are usually massive endomorphic-mesomorphs.

It was discovered some time ago that jumping animals have a high crural index (ratio of lower leg length × 100 to the length of the thigh).[3] A relatively long lower leg permits

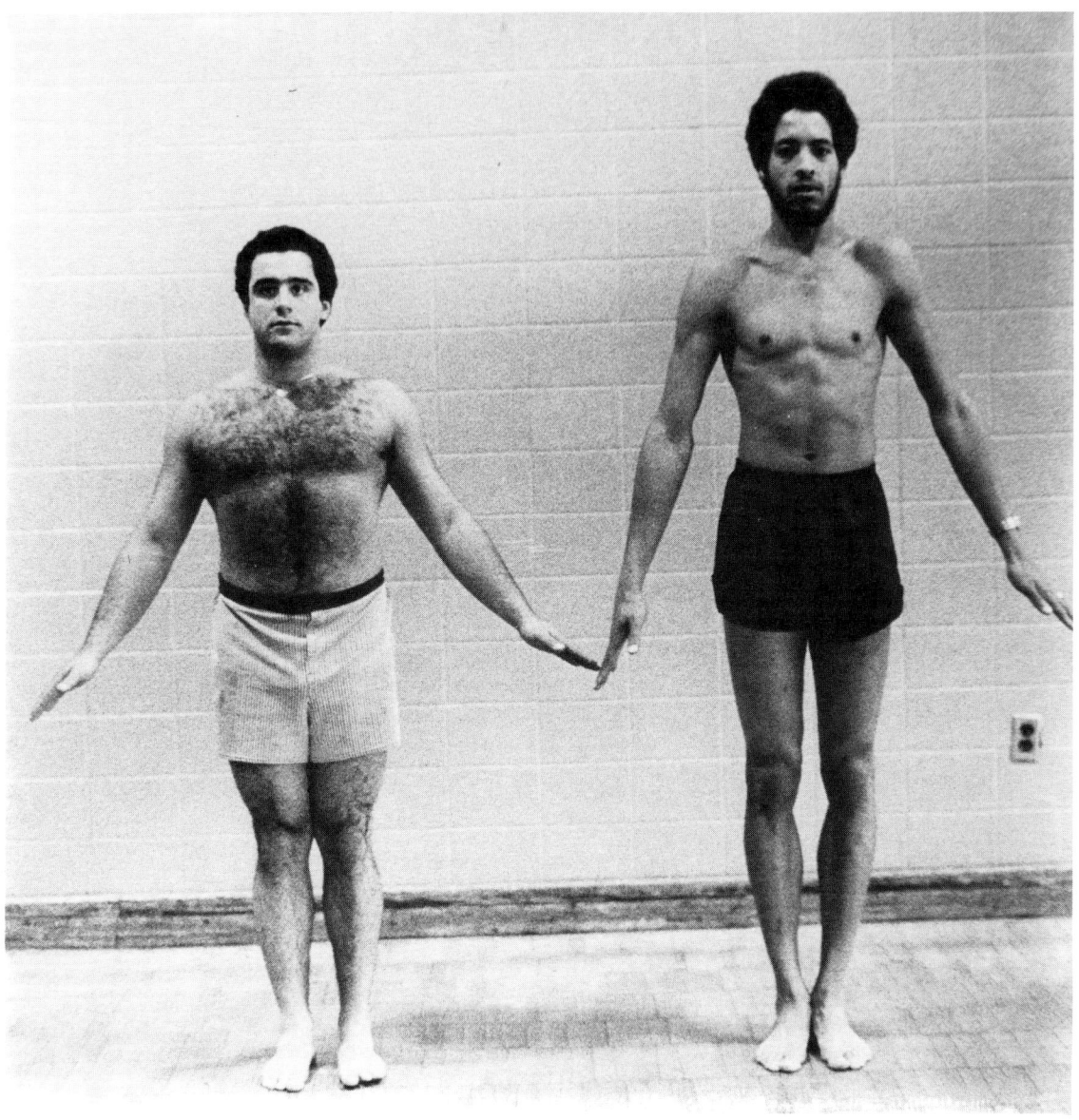

Figure 3.1g to 3.1i Man on left—endomorphic mesomorph 562; man on right—ectomorphic mesomorph 256

application of thrust against the supporting surface for a greater distance and for a greater period of time. This means that, all other factors being equal, people with a rela-

tively longer lower leg will be able to jump further than those with shorter lower legs.

The most common body type among football players is the endomorphic-mesomorphic

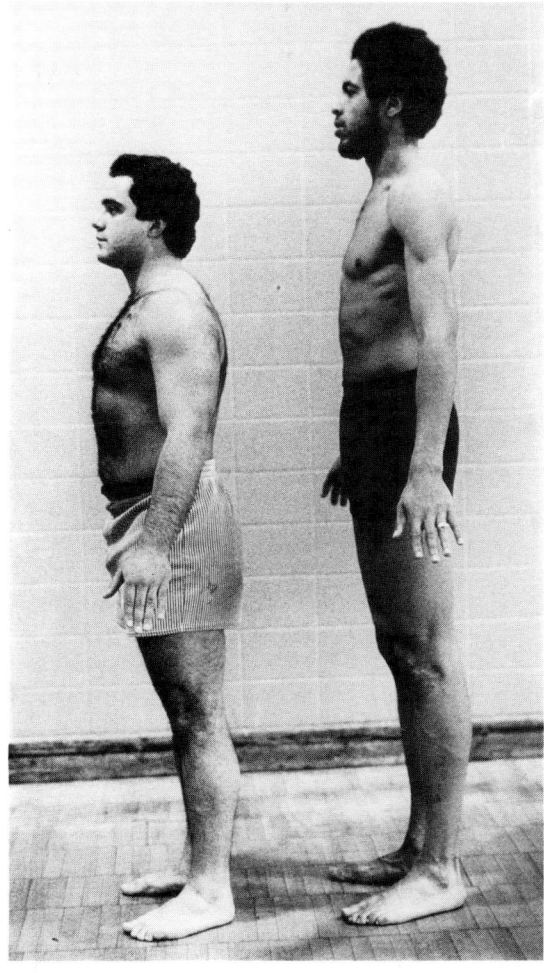

(h)

type. Backfield players are higher in ecto-morphy and lower in endomorphy than line-men.[4]

Students scoring highest in tests of strength rate highest in mesomorphy.[5,6] Static strength was found to be dependent on both meso-morphy and size in a study of extreme ecto-morphs and mesomorphs.[7]

The body type characteristics of champion male and female athletes in a number of

sports has been studied and reported upon.[8] These athletes were rated and analyzed, and their body type number was plotted on soma-tocharts. A total of 1039 male and female athletes was studied. The researcher found relatively clear-cut differences in the mean somatotype scores of champions in different sports as indicated by Table 3.1, taken from Carter's article.

He also found that when he plotted the so-matotype numbers of champion athletes in selected sports on a somatochart, they clus-tered in predictable areas of the somatochart. The somatochart is reproduced in Figure 3.2.

It should be noted that the level of meso-morphy is indicated by the vertical axis in-creasing as the top of the triangle is ap-proached. Endomorphy and ectomorphy are expressed along the two diagonal axes. The higher the level of endomorphy, the further to the left, and the higher the number for ectomorphy, the further to the right the indi-vidual's somatotype number is located. This is opposite to Cureton's somatotype chart, in which endomorphy increases toward the right while ectomorphy increases to the left.

The plotted somatocharts shown in Figures 3.3 and 3.4 indicate that somatotypes of champion athletes in specific sports are sim-ilar to one another and different from those of champion athletes in other sports.

The data on somatotypes of champion women athletes (see Table 3.2) is not nearly as complete as that for men, nor are the dif-ferences in somatotypes as striking. However, as increasing numbers of females compete in athletics, become more highly motivated, en-dure more rigorous training, and are provided better coaching and facilities, it is probable that differences in somatotype will assume in-creasing importance.

A total of 317 male physical education ma-jors from four countries were compared in terms of somatotype and body size.[9] The stu-dents were from universities in Brussels, Dun-edin, Prague, and San Diego. It was found

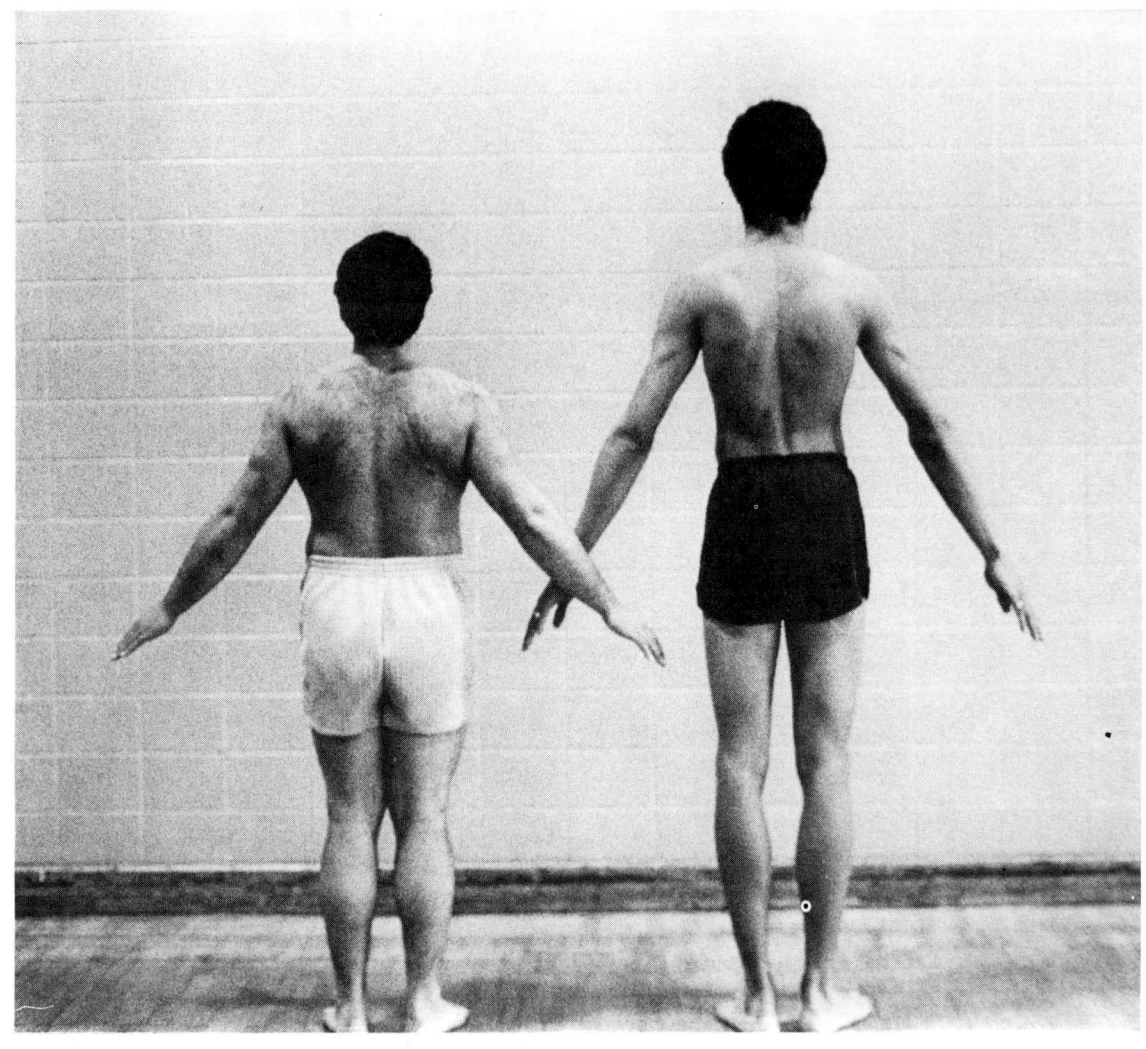

(i)

that the San Diego students were older, taller, heavier, and higher in endomorphy than the Prague or Brussels students. The Prague students were less endomorphic than the physical education majors from the other three countries. None of the four groups differed in mesomorphy, ectomorphy, or the height–weight ratio. The physical education majors from all four countries were high in mesomorphy. Students attracted to a career in physical education are those who enjoy and are successful in sports and other physical activities. These types are likely to be above average in mesomorphy.

The mean height (158.51 ± 5.04 cm) and weight (51.09 ± 7.08 kg) for college-age women gymnasts have been shown to be significantly less than values reported for all college-age women, while mean body density (1.064 ± .0101 gm/cc) is significantly higher.[10] Skeletal diameter, except for the wrist, elbow, and femur, of the women gym-

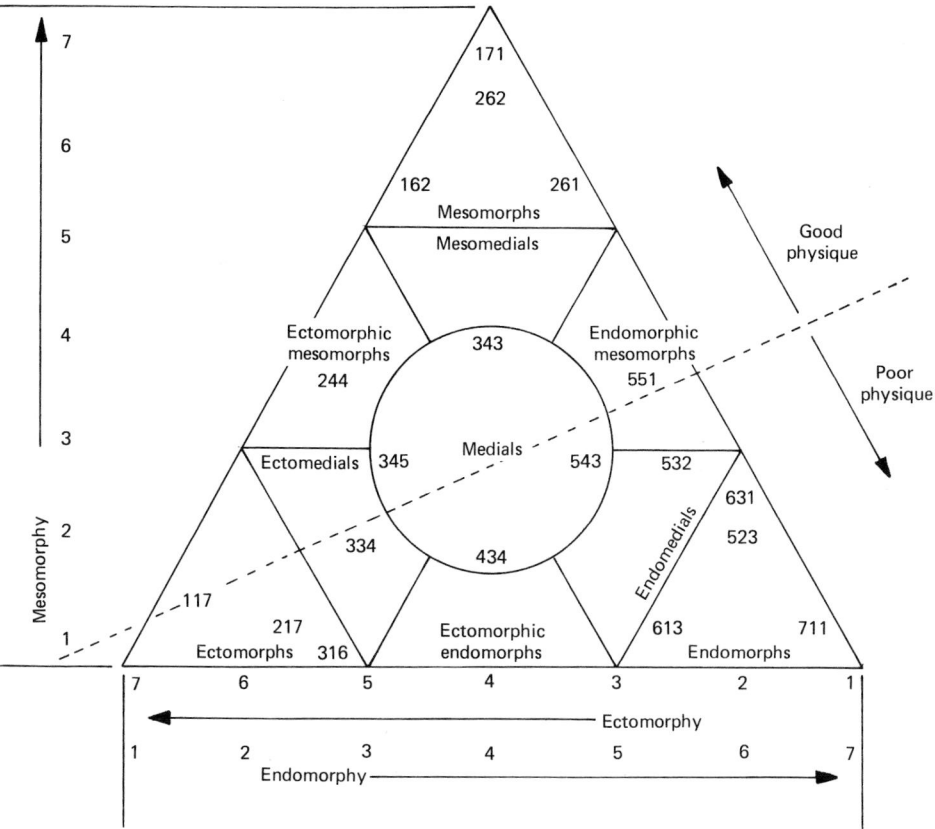

Chart 3.1 Relationship between body type numbers (with permission of T. K. Cureton)

nasts is smaller. Circumference measures are also smaller except for measures of the upper arm, forearm, neck, and thorax. This study shows that light-boned and strong women are attracted to and succeed in gymnastics.

Utilization of Somatotyping in Sports and Recreational Counseling

Although a need exists for additional research on the relationships between body type and performance in various athletic skills, the authors believe that the current evidence is sufficient to provide a base for counseling boys and girls into participation in those forms of athletics in which they will be most likely to succeed. Permitting a boy or girl

high in ectomorphy to pursue unrealistic goals in football, weight lifting, the field events, or wrestling may lead to frustration, a damaged self-concept, and injury. A short, extreme endomorph is unlikely to achieve a satisfying degree of excellence in basketball, distance running, jumping events, or pole vaulting.

Body type should also receive consideration (among many other factors) in recreational counseling for physical activity. People enjoy activities in which they are successful. Guidance should give some consideration to probable success in recreational activities recommended.

It has been well established that somatotype is a major determinant of the level of per-

Table 3.1 Mean Values for Selected Groups of Male Champion Athletes

Sample	N	Age (yr)	Ht. (cm)	Wt. (kg)	Endo- morphy	Meso- morphy	Ecto- morphy
San Diego State swimmers	24	19.9	179.3	74.9	2.4	5.4	2.6
Cureton's champion swimmers	21	21.4	183.4	79.6	2.9	5.4	2.7
English Channel swimmers	11	N.A.	171.5	86.4	4.1	5.1	2.0
San Diego State football players	35	21.3	184.4	94.4	4.2	6.3	1.4
U. of Iowa football players	20	19.9	182.1	86.1	3.2	6.2	1.6
"Oregon" football players	66	20.3	181.6	84.9	3.6	5.5	2.1
Cureton's track & field champions	19	24.2	179.6	72.6	2.5	5.2	3.1
1960 Olympic track & field throwers	14	23.6	189.2	100.3	2.8	6.7	1.4
San Diego State cross-country runners	17	20.2	179.3	65.7	1.8	3.9	4.0
Monte Vista H.S. cross-country runners	8	17.3	175.0	61.6	2.2	4.2	3.9
Olympic distance runners	34	25.9	176.5	63.2	1.5	4.6	3.6
Danish gymnasts	15	24.6	172.7	74.9	2.6	6.2	1.5
U. of Iowa gymnasts	10	22.3	176.5	71.8	2.0	5.8	2.6
U.S.S.R. gymnasts	5	N.A.	172.7	72.2	2.6	6.0	2.1
San Diego State basketball players	10	20.6	190.0	83.4	2.4	4.9	3.3
U. of Iowa basketball players	10	19.6	186.9	79.7	2.7	4.9	3.0
U.S.S.R. basketball players	8	N.A.	192.5	87.5	2.9	4.6	4.1
San Diego baseball players	151	19.7	179.3	78.2	3.8	5.0	2.7
U. of Iowa baseball players	10	20.3	180.3	80.7	3.8	5.2	2.2
British Empire Games wrestlers	33	27.0	173.2	77.2	2.1	6.2	1.6
U.S.S.R. wrestlers	34	N.A.	167.1	77.1	3.5	6.4	1.3
A.A.U. champion weight lifters	43	N.A.	N.A.	N.A.	2.9	6.5	1.2
British Empire Games weight lifters	29	26.2	167.9	73.1	1.8	7.6	0.9
U.S.S.R. weight lifters	54	N.A.	164.6	77.2	4.2	6.6	1.0
British Empire Games boxers	39	N.A.	171.5	65.8	3.0	5.1	2.8
San Diego State golfers	9	21.1	181.4	81.0	4.1	5.0	2.3
San Diego State rowers	21	20.2	183.6	79.8	2.7	5.1	2.6
N.Z. physical education majors	60	20.7	176.3	72.6	2.5	5.4	2.1
Finnish champion lumberjacks	40	33.0	173.7	73.1	2.0	5.5	3.0
U.S. college "nonathletes"	18	19.5	181.9	76.8	5.0	3.3	3.4

N.A. = not available.

Table 3.2 Mean Values for Selected Groups of Women Champion Athletes

Sample	N	Age (yr)	Ht. (cm)	Wt. (kg)	Endo- morphy	Meso- morphy	Ecto- morphy
U.S. professional golfers	26	27.8	167.6	62.4	4.1	4.0	2.7
San Diego amateur golfers	26	40.5	164.8	62.9	4.9	4.6	2.1
San Diego track and field	61	17.2	167.1	56.8	3.5	3.6	3.6
U.S.S.R. basketball players	10	N.A.	173.0	71.4	4.3	4.5	3.0
U.S.S.R. gymnasts	5	N.A.	157.0	53.9	3.8	5.2	1.6
N.Z. physical education majors	61	19.4	164.3	60.0	3.9	4.4	2.2

N.A. = not available.

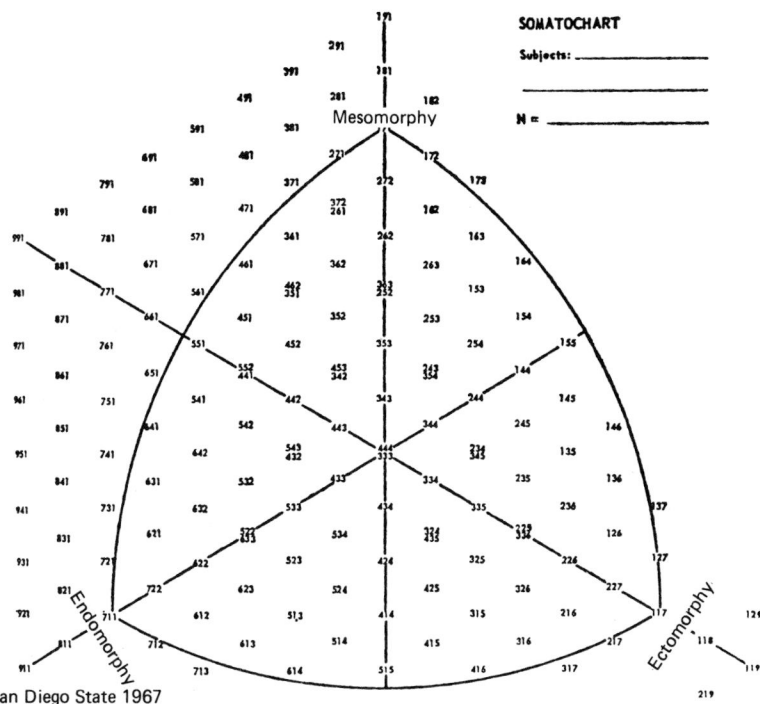

SOMATOCHART

Subjects: _____

_____

N = _____

Mesomorphy

Endomorphy

Ectomorphy

San Diego State 1967

Figure 3.2 Somatochart (from J. E. L. Carter, "The Somatotypes of Athletes—A Review," **Human Biology**, Vol. 42, Dec. 1970, pp. 535–569, with permission)

formance in measures of physical and motor fitness. Endomorphs and ectomorphs who are low in mesomorphy are unable to score well on these tests regardless of their efforts during the tests or as a result of conditioning activities previous to the tests. These types are simply unable to develop substantial amounts of strength, power, or agility. The endomorphs are also unable to develop endurance. These boys and girls will experience frustration, a damaged self-concept, and very likely decide to avoid participation in physical activities if the standard is one established for mesomorphs. Just as beginning or novice, intermediate, and advanced levels of competition, age group competition, separate competitive programs for males and females, weight categories and city, state, district, national, and international levels of competition have been

established, separate standards of excellence could be established in physical and motor fitness tests for the extremes in body type. This would serve to encourage those who need physical activity most to seek it out.

METHODS FOR DETERMINATION OF SOMATOTYPE

The Sheldon Somatotype

Sheldon's method for somatotyping requires that in photographing the subjects specific procedures be followed in both developing and printing the film. It is also necessary that a specific type of film be used. Three photographs are taken of the subject—front, side, and back views. Included in these pictures is a data board that shows the subject's age,

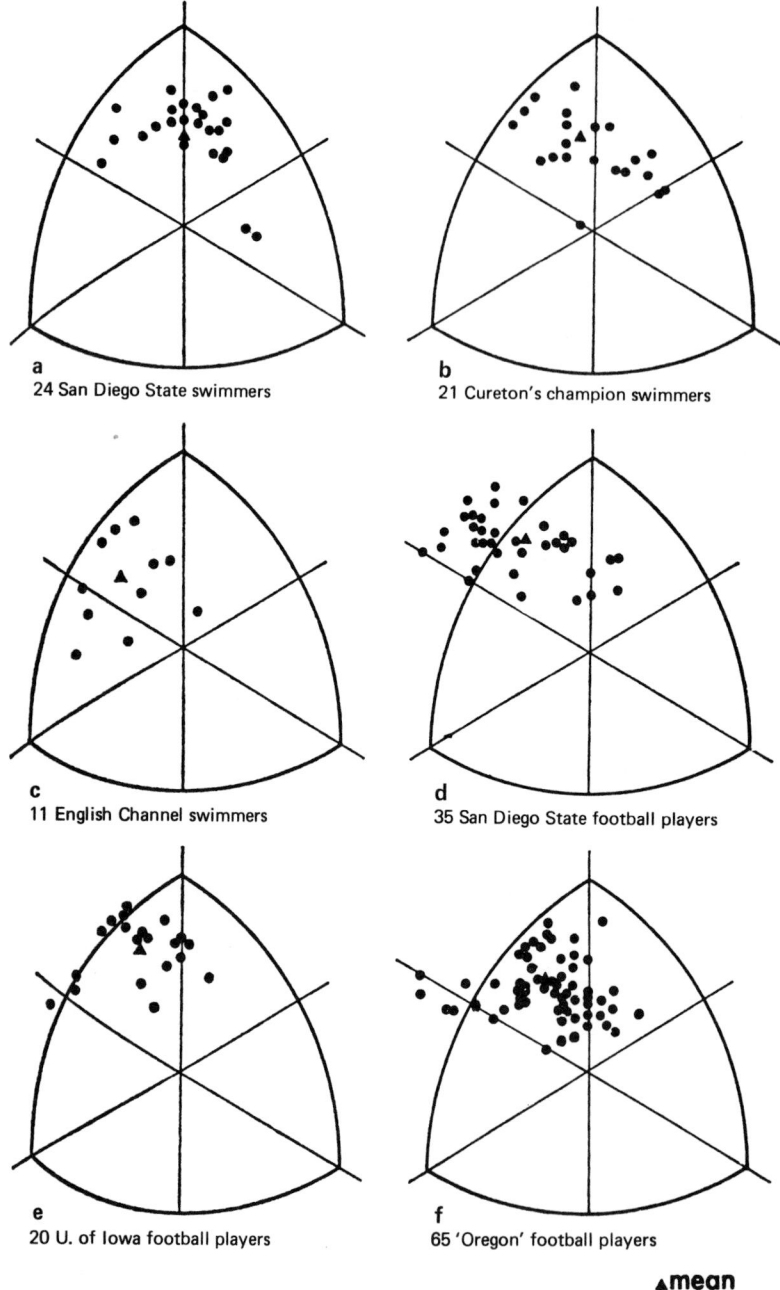

a
24 San Diego State swimmers

b
21 Cureton's champion swimmers

c
11 English Channel swimmers

d
35 San Diego State football players

e
20 U. of Iowa football players

f
65 'Oregon' football players

▲mean

Figure 3.3a Somatoplots of champion athletes—swimmers and football players (from J. E. L. Carter, "The Somatotypes of Athletes—A Review," **Human Biology**, Vol. 42, Dec. 1970, pp. 535–539, with permission)

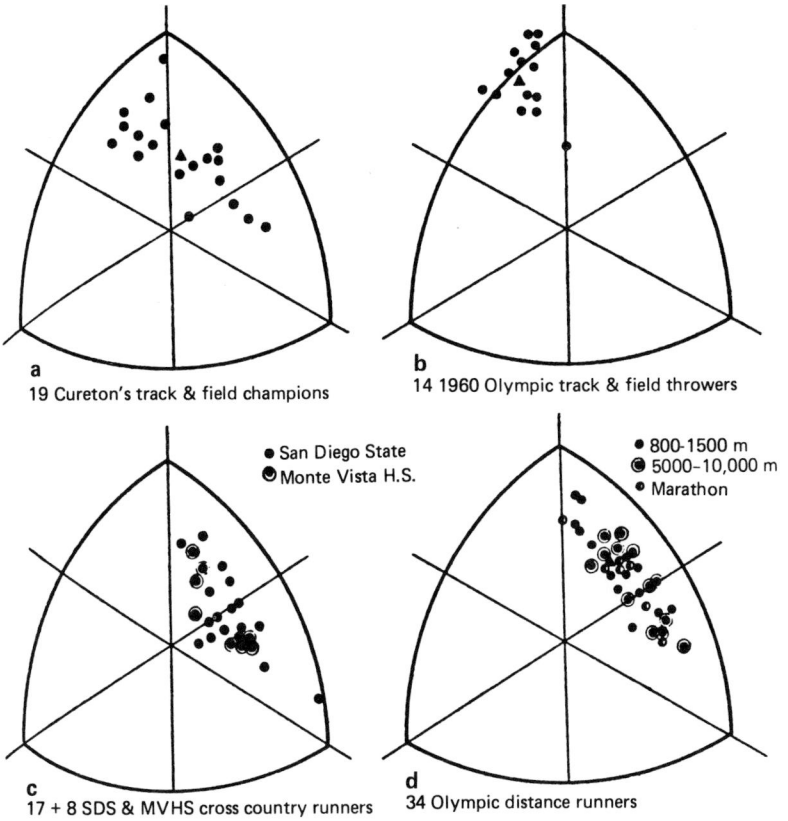

a
19 Cureton's track & field champions

b
14 1960 Olympic track & field throwers

• San Diego State
◑ Monte Vista H.S.

• 800-1500 m
◑ 5000-10,000 m
◔ Marathon

c
17 + 8 SDS & MVHS cross country runners

d
34 Olympic distance runners

Figure 3.3b Somatoplots of champion athletes— ▲ Mean
track and field, cross country and distance runners
(from J. E. L. Carter, **op. cit.**, with permission)

height, and weight. Next, the ponderal index is computed to aid in locating the somatotype. The ponderal index = height/-weight. Sheldon's *Atlas of Men*[11] presents an index for various combinations of height and weight to negate the necessity of doing this computation. Next, a table in this text is consulted to find the location of somatotypes for various intervals of ponderal index. The final somatotype assessment is made through anthroposcopy and inspection in the *Atlas*.

Heath-Carter Somatotype Rating Form

Heath and Carter[12] have presented a method for somatotyping that facilitates the process

for both men and women. Their procedure requires use of the Heath-Carter Somatotype Rating form, a copy of which is shown in Figure 3.5.

To obtain the rating for endomorphy, the skinfold measurements at the triceps, subscapular, and suprailiac areas are totaled. The closest value on the skinfold scale is then circled. The first component (endomorphy) for that column is also circled. In taking the skinfold measurements, a single fold of skin is pinched between the thumb and fingers, picking up all the fat but no muscle tissue. Skinfold calipers are used to measure the thickness of the skinfold in millimeters. See Chapter 14 for a more detailed treatment of skinfold measurement techniques.

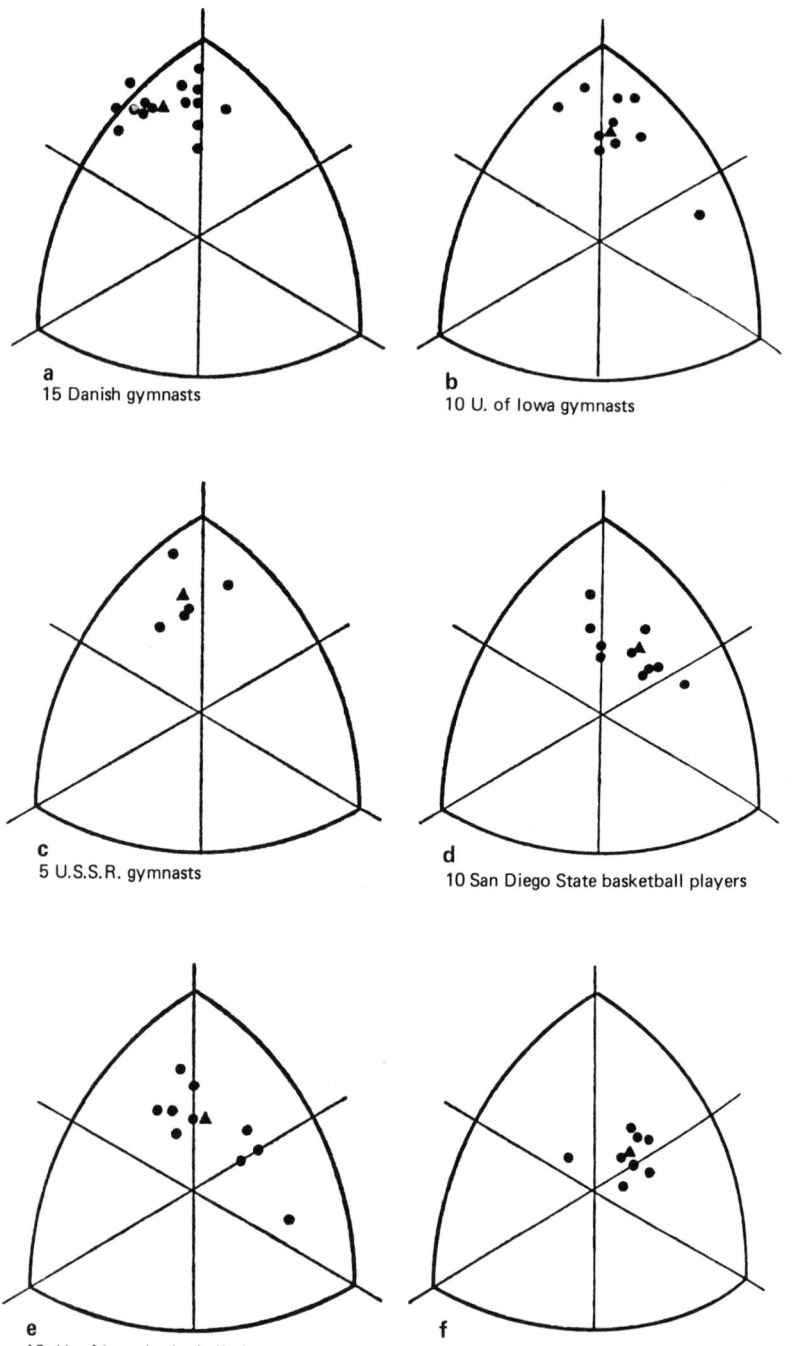

a
15 Danish gymnasts

b
10 U. of Iowa gymnasts

c
5 U.S.S.R. gymnasts

d
10 San Diego State basketball players

e
10. U. of Iowa basketball players

f
8 U.S.S.R. basketball players

Figure 3.3c Somatoplots of champion athletes—
gymnasts and basketball players (from J. E. L. Carter, **op. cit.**, with permission)

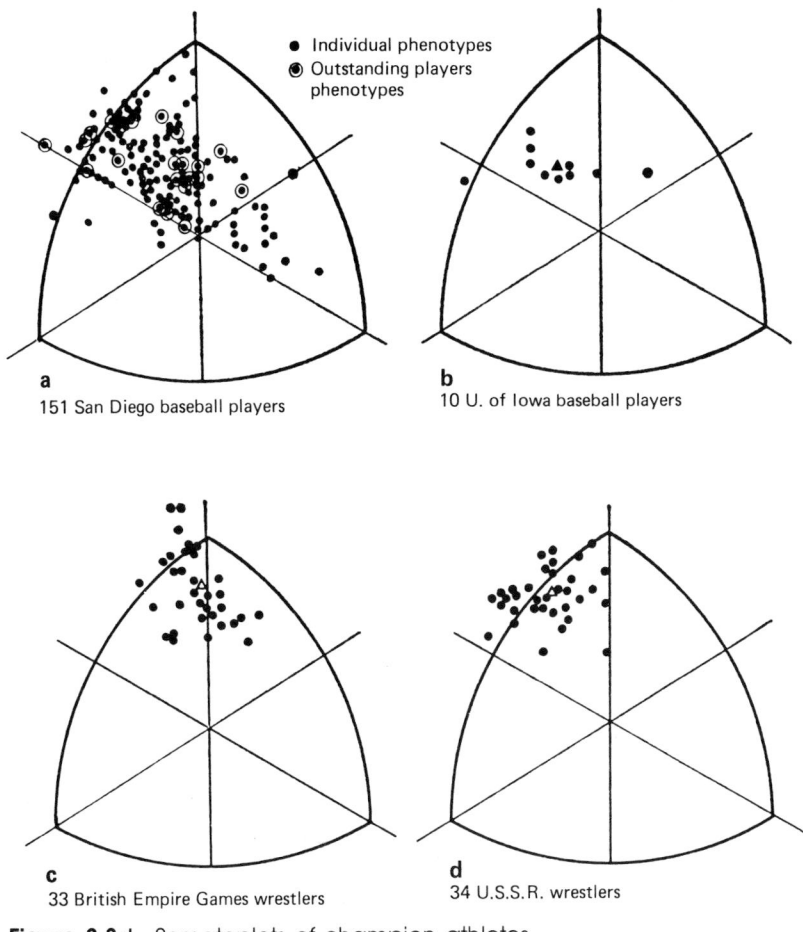

- ● Individual phenotypes
- ◉ Outstanding players phenotypes

a
151 San Diego baseball players

b
10 U. of Iowa baseball players

c
33 British Empire Games wrestlers

d
34 U.S.S.R. wrestlers

▲ Mean

Figure 3.3d Somatoplots of champion athletes— baseball players and wrestlers (from J. E. L. Carter, **op. cit.**, with permission)

Mesomorphy is computed on the Heath–Carter Somatotype Rating Form by first placing an arrow above the column containing the subject's height. Measurements of the width of the humerus at the elbow and the femur at the knee joint are made with calipers and recorded in centimeters. The closest figures in the appropriate row are circled. When uncertainty exists regarding whether to circle the next highest or the next lowest number, the one closer to the height column previously marked by an arrow is circled. Next, the triceps skinfold measure is subtracted from the biceps circumference (in

centimeters). After this, the calf skinfold measurement is subtracted from the circumference of the calf, again after converting all measures to centimeters. Next, these measures are circled in their proper rows. Circumference of both the biceps and the calf are measured at their greatest circumference.

Starting with the column furthest to the left containing a circled value, the number of columns each circled value deviates from this starting point is counted. The average of these deviations is computed by dividing the sum of the deviations of the four measures by four. The number of columns that the mean

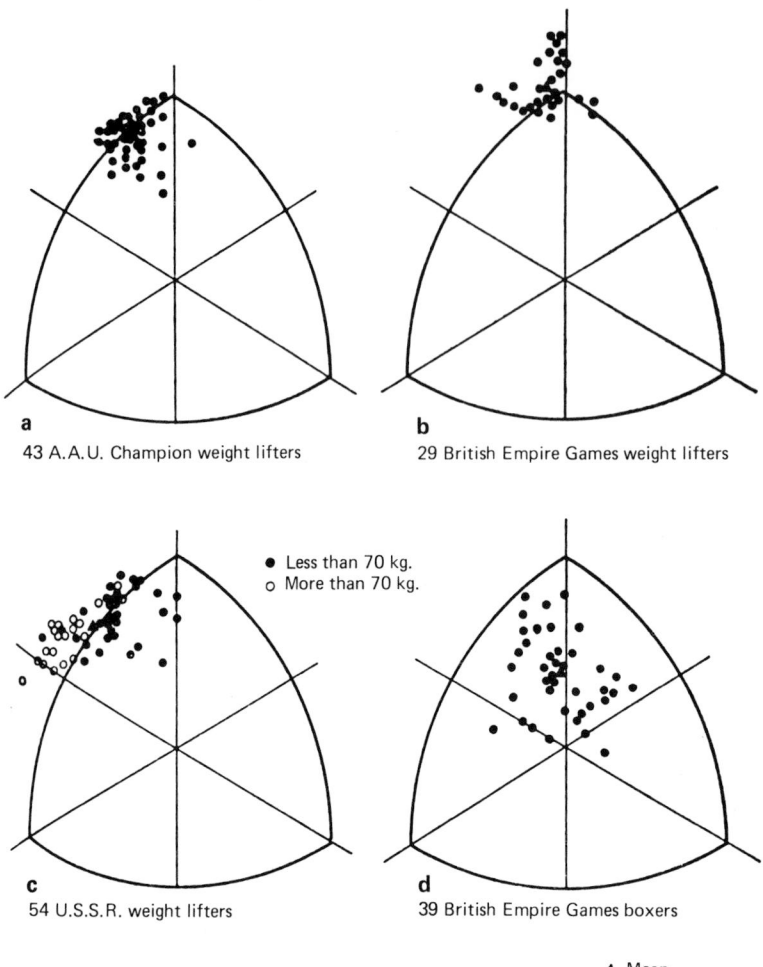

a
43 A.A.U. Champion weight lifters

b
29 British Empire Games weight lifters

• Less than 70 kg.
o More than 70 kg.

c
54 U.S.S.R. weight lifters

d
39 British Empire Games boxers

▲ Mean

Figure 3.3e Somatoplots of champion athletes—
weight lifters and boxers (from J. E. L. Carter, **op. cit.**,
with permission)

deviation is to the right of the original starting column is counted. An asterisk is placed
at this point. The number of columns that
the above point, identified by an asterisk, deviates from the height column, which had
been identified by an arrow, are counted.
This number is used to determine the second
component, mesomorphy. If the asterisk is to
the right of the arrow, count this number of
columns to the right of the column directly
above the 4 in the row identified as "second

component." If the asterisk is to the left of the
arrow, count this number of columns to the
left of the column directly above the 4 in the
row identified as "second component." Follow the column downward to the number in
the row marked "second component" to find
the somatotype number for mesomorphy.

The third component, ectomorphy, is obtained by dividing the cube root of the weight
into the height to secure the ponderal index.
The closest value is circled and the somato-

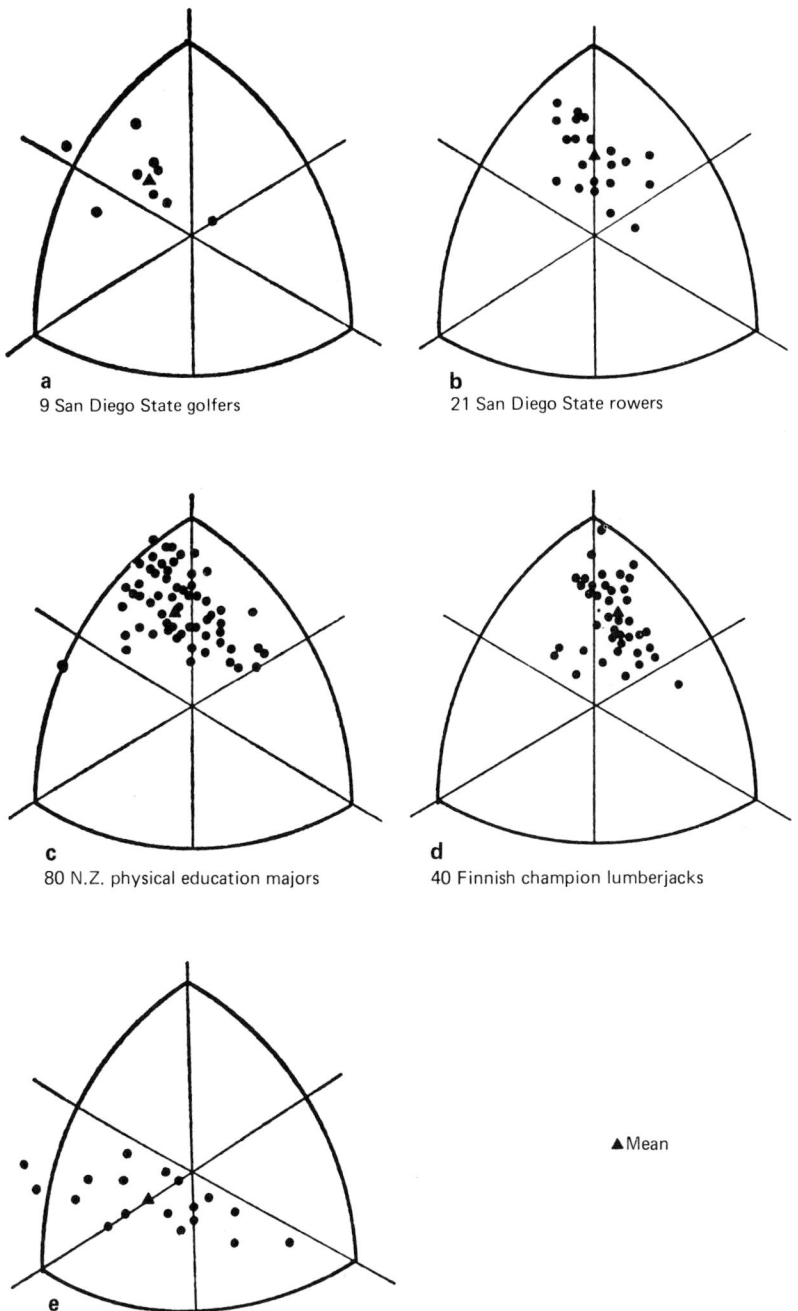

a
9 San Diego State golfers

b
21 San Diego State rowers

c
80 N.Z. physical education majors

d
40 Finnish champion lumberjacks

▲ Mean

e
18 U.S. college 'nonathletes'

Figure 3.3f Somatoplots of champion athletes—golfers, rowers, lumberjacks, physical education majors, and nonathletes (from J. E. L. Carter, **op. cit.**, with permission)

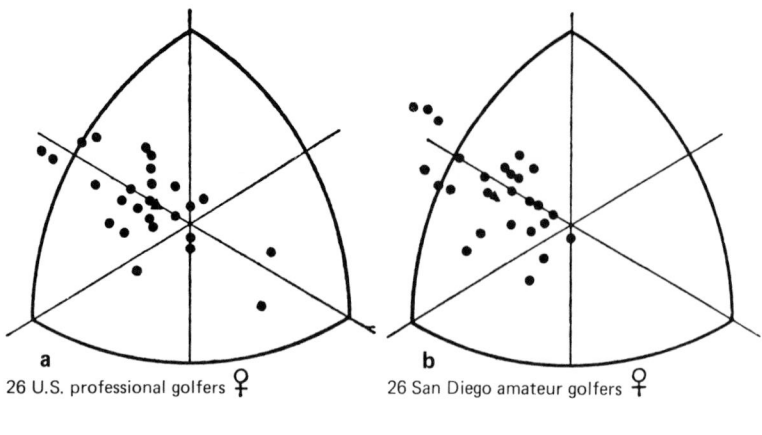

a
26 U.S. professional golfers ♀

b
26 San Diego amateur golfers ♀

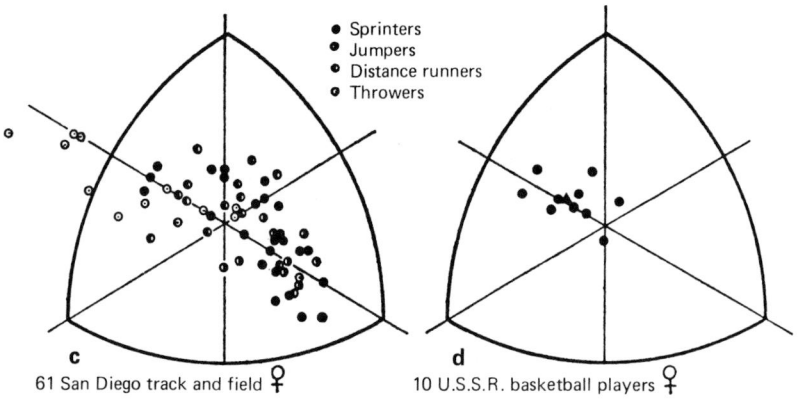

● Sprinters
● Jumpers
◔ Distance runners
◑ Throwers

c
61 San Diego track and field ♀

d
10 U.S.S.R. basketball players ♀

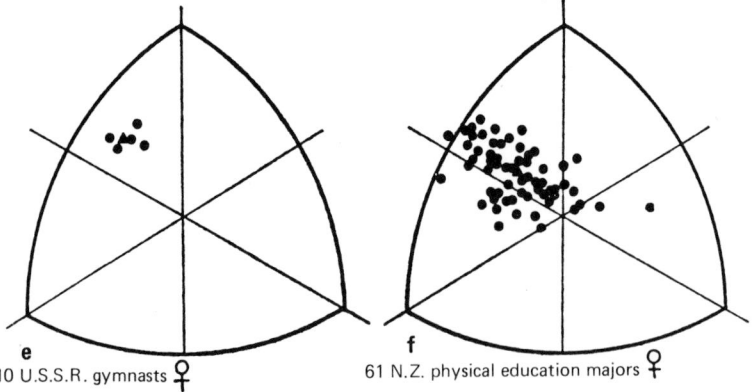

e
10 U.S.S.R. gymnasts ♀

f
61 N.Z. physical education majors ♀

Figure 3.3g Somatoplots of champion women athletes—golfers, track and field, basketball players, gymnasts, and physical education majors (from J. E. L. Carter, **op. cit.**, with permission)

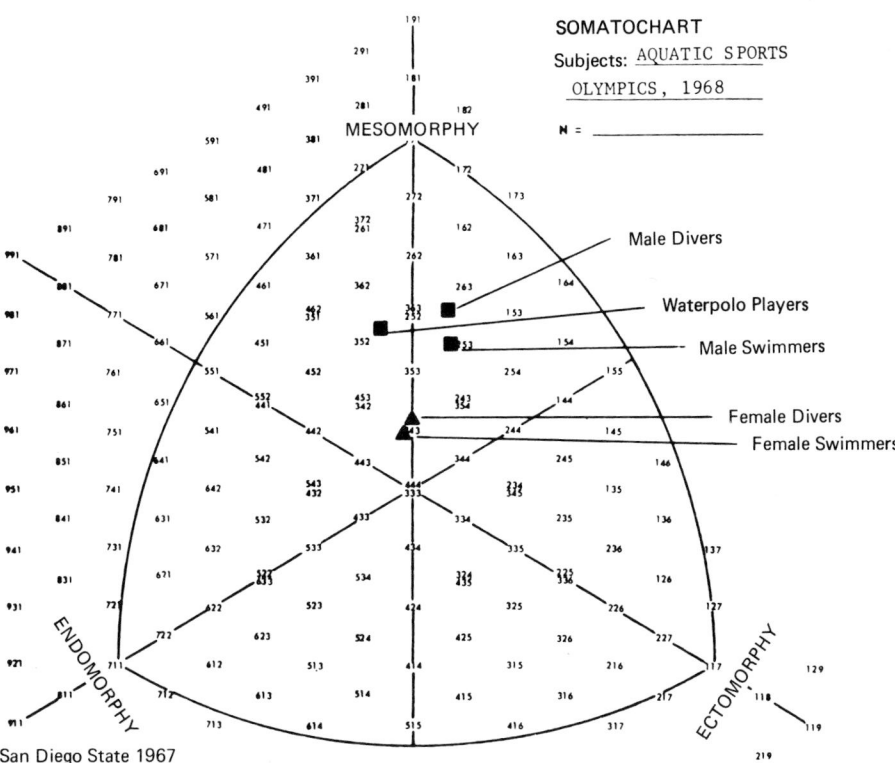

Figure 3.4 Somatoplots for swimmers, divers, and water polo players (see Table 3.2)

type number in the third component row directly under the column in which this value is found is noted. Half numbers such as 3½, 4½, etc., may be used.

Cureton's Simplified Physique Rating

Cureton[13] has described a relatively simple and quick method for rating physique in which external fat, muscular development and condition, and skeletal development are rated subjectively according to the following scales in Table 3.3. External fat is rated on the seven-point scale by pinching the cheek, abdominal, waist, thigh (front and back), and gluteal fat. Muscular development and condition is rated by pushing the fist into the abdomen to appraise the hardness of the abdominal muscles and by feeling the hardness

of the contracted biceps, calves, and thighs. Height is measured to the nearest tenth of an inch while weight is measured to the nearest one-quarter pound. The Reciprocal Ponderal Index is computed by dividing the height in inches by the cube root of the weight. To determine whether a subject is more ponderous or less ponderous than average, a standard score scale is referred to. This rating scale is presented in Table 3.4.

METHODS FOR ASSESSING LEANNESS/FATNESS

The problems associated with direct measurement of fat have been expressed earlier in this chapter. Fortunately, several indirect methods for measuring fat have been developed. A few of these can be utilized in re-

HEATH-CARTER SOMATOTYPE RATING FORM

NAME ....J.B.............................. AGE 45-2 ... SEX: Ⓜ F ... NO: 135

OCCUPATION ....Teacher........................ ETHNIC GROUP Caucasian .... DATE 11 Nov 1966

PROJECT: ...A.T.P.......................... MEASURED BY: L.C.

Skinfolds (mm):		TOTAL SKINFOLDS (mm)
Triceps = 13·0	Upper Limit	10.9 14.9 18.9 22.9 26.9 31.2 35.8 40.7 46.2 52.2 58.7 65.7 73.2 81.2 89.7 98.9 108.9 119.7 131.2 143.7 157.2 171.9 187.9 204.0
Subcapular = 15·3	Mid-point	9.0 13.0 17.0 21.0 25.0 29.0 33.5 ⟨38.0⟩ 43.5 49.0 55.5 62.0 69.5 77.0 85.5 94.0 104.0 114.0 125.5 137.0 150.5 164.0 180.0 196.0
Supraliac = 9·9	Lower Limit	7.0 11.0 15.0 19.0 23.0 27.0 31.3 35.9 40.8 46.3 52.3 58.8 65.8 73.3 81.3 89.8 99.0 109.0 119.8 131.3 143.8 157.3 172.0 188.0
TOTAL SKINFOLDS = 38·2		
Calf = 9·8		
	FIRST COMPONENT	½ 1 1½ 2 2½ 3 3½ ④ 4½ 5 5½ 6 6½ 7 7½ 8 8½ 9 9½ 10 10½ 11 11½ 12

Height (in.) = 67·1		55.0 56.5 58.0 59.5 61.0 62.5 64.0 65.5 67.0 68.5 70.0 71.5 73.0 74.5 76.0 77.5 79.0 80.5 82.0 83.5 85.0 86.5 88.0 89.5
Bone: Humerus = 6·82 (cm)		5.19 5.34 5.49 5.64 5.78 5.93 6.07 6.22 6.37 6.51 6.65 ⟨6.80⟩ 6.95 7.09 7.24 7.38 7.53 7.67 7.82 7.97 8.11 8.25 8.40 8.55
Femur = 9·27		7.41 7.62 7.83 8.04 8.24 8.45 8.66 8.87 9.08 ⟨9.28⟩ 9.49 9.70 9.91 10.12 10.33 10.53 10.74 10.95 11.16 11.37 11.58 11.79 12.00 12.21
Muscle: Biceps 33·0 (cm) = 31·7 - 1·3 - (triceps skinfold)		23.7 24.4 25.0 25.7 26.3 27.0 27.7 28.3 29.0 29.7 30.3 31.0 ⟨31.6⟩ 32.2 33.0 33.6 34.3 35.0 35.6 36.3 37.1 37.8 38.5 39.3
Calf 35·1 = 34·1 - (calf skinfold) ·95		27.7 28.5 29.3 30.1 30.8 31.6 32.4 33.2 ⟨33.9⟩ 34.7 35.5 36.3 37.1 37.8 38.6 39.4 40.2 41.0 41.8 42.6 43.4 44.2 45.0 45.8
	SECOND COMPONENT	½ 1 1½ 2 2½ 3 3½ 4 4½ ⑤ 5½ 6 6½ 7 7½ 8 8½ 9

Weight (lb.) = 147·0	Upper limit	11.99 12.32 12.53 12.74 12.95 13.15 13.36 13.56 13.77 13.98 14.19 14.39 14.59 14.80 15.01 15.22 15.42 15.63
Ht. /∛ Wt. = 12·76	Mid-point	and 12.16 12.43 12.64 12.85 13.05 13.26 13.46 13.67 13.88 14.01 14.29 14.50 14.70 14.91 15.12 15.33 15.53
	Lower limit	below 12.00 12.33 12.54 ⟨12.75⟩ 12.96 13.16 13.37 13.56 13.78 13.99 14.20 14.40 14.60 14.81 15.02 15.23 15.43
	THIRD COMPONENT	½ 1 1½ 2 ⟨2½⟩ 3 3½ 4 4½ 5 5½ 6 6½ 7 7½ 8 8½ 9

	FIRST COMPONENT	SECOND COMPONENT	THIRD COMPONENT	
Anthropometric Somatotype	4	5	2½	BY: L.C.
Anthropometric plus Photoscopic Somatotype				RATER: ....

Figure 3.5 Heath–Carter somatotype rating form (from Mathews, D. K. (Ed.), **Measurement in Physical Education**, 4th ed. Philadelphia, W. B. Saunders Co., 1973, with permission)

search laboratories of physical education departments. Others can be utilized in physical education classes. The indirect methods are of two types. In the first type, the ratio of body weight to body volume is computed to ascertain the percentage of fat. This procedure requires that the subject be totally immersed in water and consequently requires specialized equipment. The second method involves either measurement of girth or circumference of several body parts such as the forearm, upper arm, abdomen, buttocks, thigh, or calf or measurement of skinfold thickness at several points such as at the triceps, below the scapulae, above the hip bone, or on the thigh. This procedure is described in Chapter 14.

Hydrostatic Weighing

The first method makes application of the principle discovered by Archimedes that an object, when immersed in water, will displace a volume of water equal to its own volume. The volume of water displaced can be measured and its weight is known. Denser objects will displace less water per unit of weight. For example, one pound of bone or lean meat will displace less water than will one pound of fat. By weighing an object on land and while

Table 3.3 Cureton's Simplified Physique Rating Scale

Scale for Rating Endomorphic Characteristics		
1 2	3 4 5	6 7
Extremely low in adipose tissue and relatively small anterior-posterior dimensions of the lower trunk	Average tissue and physical build of lower trunk	Extremely obese with large quantities of adipose tissue and an unproportionately thick abdominal region
Scale for Rating Muscular Development and Condition		
1 2	3 4 5	6 7
Extremely underdeveloped and poorly conditioned muscles squeezed or pushed in the contracted states (biceps, abdominals, thighs, calves)	Average in skeletal muscular development and condition	Extremely developed with large and hard muscles in the contracted state, firm under forceful squeezing
Scale for Rating Skeletal Development		
1 2	3 4 5	6 7
Extremely thick and heavy bones, short and ponderous skeleton with relatively great cross section of ankle, knee, and elbow joints	Average-size bones and joints in cross section and length	Extremely thin frail bones, tall linear skeleton with relatively small cross section of ankle, knee, and elbow joints

With permission of T. K. Cureton.

totally submerged, its density can be ascertained. This is accomplished by computing the object's *specific gravity*.

$$\text{specific gravity} = \frac{\text{weight of an object}}{\text{weight of an equal volume of water}}$$

Because an object's loss of weight in water equals the weight of the volume of water it displaces, specific gravity can also be defined as the ratio of the weight of an object in air over its loss of weight in water.

$$\text{specific gravity} = \frac{\text{weight of an object in air}}{(\text{weight in air} - \text{weight in water})}$$

Experiments have established that fat has a specific gravity of 0.90; in other words, its weight for a specific volume is less than the weight of a like volume of water. These same experiments have also established that fat-free tissue has a specific gravity of 1.10. Because animal bodies, including man's, consist of fat and fat-free tissue, their specific gravity must range between 0.90 and 1.10.

Specific gravity is a measure of the weight of an object in relation to its volume or its density.

$$\text{density} = \frac{\text{weight}}{\text{volume}}$$

From the preceding, it becomes obvious why a person's specific gravity is basically a measure of the proportion of fat to lean tissue in his body. The following equation is used to determine the percent of body fat:

$$\text{percent body fat} = \frac{495}{\text{body density (or specific gravity)}} - 450$$

The weight of the total body fat is determined by multiplying the total body weight by the percent of body fat. Subtracting weight of body fat from total body weight will give the lean weight.

Table 3.4 Rating Scale for the Somatotype Numbers and Reciprocal Ponderal Index (Arranged for the Appraisal of Young Men)

Classi-fication	Letter grade	Standard score	Percentile	Reciprocal ponderal index	Somatotype numbers
Superior	A+	100	99.87	14.57	171
		95	99.65	14.42	172 271
		90	99.18	14.26	173 262 261 371
Very good	A	85	98.2	14.11	163 265 263
		80	96.4	13.96	165 264 362 361 363 472
		75	93.3	13.80	365 364 363 464 463 462 461
Above average	B	70	88.4	13.65	253 352 252 453 452 451
		65	81.6	13.49	454
		60	72.6	13.34	354 353 563 562 561
Average	C+	55	61.8	13.19	356 245 243 355 455 445 343
		50	50.0	13.03	244 344 444
		45	38.2	12.88	235 445 545 544 554 433 543 542 443 442
Below average	C	40	27.4	12.72	335 234 553 552 551
		35	18.4	12.57	435 334 434 663 662 661
		30	11.5	12.42	246 346 446 534 533 532
Poor	D	25	6.7	12.26	136 236 336 436 535 651 653 652
		20	3.6	12.11	325 645 644 643 642 641
		15	1.8	11.95	225 424 634 633 632 631
Very poor	E	10	.82	11.80	126 326 426 415 425 523 524 522 624 623 622
		5	.35	11.65	514 613
		0	.14	11.49	117 127 216 217 316 515 612 731 744 712 711

From Cureton, T. K., 7-Point Scale, "Simplified Somatotype Plan," Chapter XV, *Physical Fitness Workbook*. The C. V. Mosby Co., St. Louis, Mo., 1947, pp. 103–106, with permission.

In the practical application of the above-described principles, two corrections must be applied to the computations. These are for water temperature and residual lung volume. The density of water varies according to temperature. As water's temperature increases, its density decreases or, stated another way, a cubic yard of water would weigh less at a higher temperature. Thus, when measuring the volume of water displaced to determine body density, a correction for temperature must be introduced into the formula. Standard density of water is at 39.2 F. Obviously, warmer water is used when immersing subjects to determine specific gravity. Therefore, a correction factor is always used.

Although the subject is instructed to make a maximal forced exhalation before complete submersion under water, some air always remains in the subject's lungs while submerged. This residual air will increase buoyancy and cause the person to weigh less while being weighed under water. Consequently, the residual lung volume must be subtracted from the underwater weight. Residual lung volume is computed before the subject enters the tank. The formula for computing body density becomes:

$$\text{body density} = \frac{\text{weight in air}}{\left(\dfrac{\textit{weight in air} - \text{weight in water}}{\text{water temperature correction}}\right) - \begin{array}{l}\text{residual} \\ \text{lung volume}\end{array}}$$

ASSESSMENT OF BODY COMPOSITION THROUGH GIRTH AND SKINFOLD MEASUREMENTS

Pryor Width-Weight Tables

Pryor[14] was the first to give consideration to bony framework and body structure as well as to sex, height, and age in assessment of nutritional status. She devised a test that included measures of the width of the pelvis and the thoracic diameter. She prepared tables that gave consideration to all these factors—age,

height, sex, and bony framework or body structure.

The ACH Index

Franzen and Palmer[15] proposed a procedure for screening children between seven and twelve years of age for medical examinations. This procedure was called the ACH Index, the initials signifying the measures that were to be taken—arm girth, chest depth, and hip width. The three measures were regarded as most significant from among numerous anthropometric measures made on over 10,000 children. The measures included shoulder breadth, hip width, chest depth and width, height, weight, arm and calf girth, size of the deltoid, and thickness of subcutaneous tissue over various parts of the arms and legs.

The Wetzel Grid

The Wetzel Grid (Figure 3.6) is an ingenious device for recording a child's growth in height and weight that facilitates appraisal of the quality of the growth while permitting each child to serve as his or her own standard of comparison. A record of the child's height and weight is kept on the grid. The child's height is located on the horizontal axis while weight is located on the vertical axis. A dot is placed on the grid where these two measures intersect. This point is in one of the nine channels running diagonally across the grid. Each channel represents a physique or body type. Stocky types are located in channels A3 and A2; those of medium build in A1, M, or B1; the slender in B2 and B3; the extremely thin to the right of channel B4; and the obese to the left of channel A4.

Height and weight are measured and recorded each month. These measures indicate the child's body size and place him at a certain developmental level within his channel indicated by a line running across all channels. The child should advance a level line

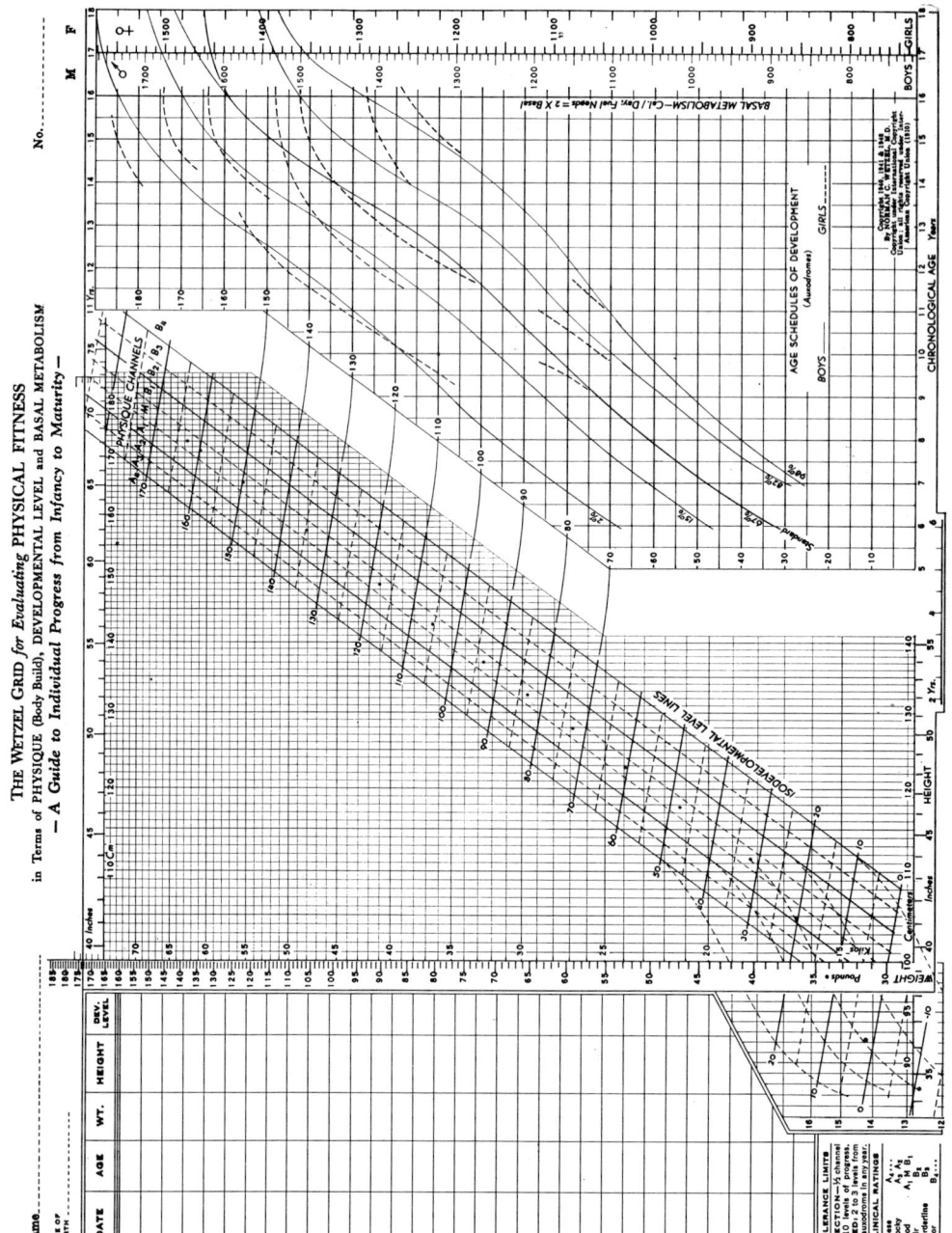

Figure 3.6 Wetzel grid

each month in his established channel. The lines representing developmental levels run over to a grid on the right side of the Wetzel Grid. By following this line horizontally across the right-hand grid to the vertical line representing the child's age, a point will be located within one of five standard "auxodromes." Auxodromes are age schedules of development and represent the percentage of children reaching the various levels throughout their period of growth. For example, a child who is 65 inches tall and weighs 120 pounds will be found to have a developmental level of 149 (plotted on the left-hand grid). If he is 13 years old, he is in the auxodrome that indicates that 15 percent of the children reach this level or above by age 13. This enables the teacher to determine whether the child is advanced, average, or below average in physical growth.

Wetzel contends that the grid facilitates early recognition of malnutrition. A child should not depart more than one-half channel per ten levels of advancement from the main direction of his channel. A child should not deviate by more than one or two levels, or three at the very most, from his expected position as determined by projecting this auxodrome forward and parallel to the standards for a distance equivalent to the time interval in question. The progress of children in channels A4, B2, or B3 should be closely monitored. The Wetzel Grid also includes panels for determining estimates of basal metabolism and caloric needs, which are not normally used by teachers.

Circumference Measurements

Katch and McArdle[16] have developed a system for predicting body fat from three circumference measurements. Different girth measurements were secured according to sex and age. The best measures for young women were of the abdomen, the right thigh, and the right forearm; for older women, the abdomen, right thigh, and right calf; for young men, the right upper arm, the abdomen, and the right forearm; and for older men, the buttocks, the abdomen, and the right forearm. The investigators worked up conversion constants for a range of possible measures for each of the four categories for all girths to be measured. These conversion constants can be found in reference 16 at the end of this chapter. Three measures are converted into constants while the third constant is subtracted from the total of the other two to secure percent of body fat. The weight of body fat is found by dividing 100 × body weight into percent of body fat. Lean body weight is found by subtracting weight of fat from body weight.

Katch and McArdle point out that although utilization of this procedure resulted in predicted values within 2.5 to 4.0 percent of values determined through hydrostatic weighing, the method may not be valid when applied to athletic young men and women or for very large or small people who are thin or obese.

EFFECTS OF BODY DENSITY AND SOMATOTYPE UPON PERFORMANCE

In sports in which the body must be lifted, hurled, or carried such as in gymnastics, diving, pole vaulting, jumping, dancing, ice skating, or running, we can suspect that high body density is one of the prerequisites for success. Fat is not only dead or nonfunctional weight that must be carried, but it also must be nourished and oxygenated, thereby placing a greater load upon the cardiovascular-respiratory system.

Karpovich and Sinning[17] reported that average fat values for athletes participating in spring sports at Springfield College varied according to the sport. Track team members possessed 9.4 percent fat; middle and long distance runners, 8.0 percent; baseball players, 12.1 percent; tennis players, 14.6 percent; and football players, 14.5 percent.

In sports in which a heavy implement or an opponent must be manipulated, such as in the hammer throw, the shot put, the line position in football, and the unlimited weight class in weight lifting or wrestling, body density is generally lower because, within limits, fat increases body weight thereby presenting an advantage in these activities. However, it must be emphasized that in all sports muscular strength is essential to success although excessive muscle size is a deterrent to success in some sports. Muscles, like fat, must be nourished, and if their size is beyond that needed to accomplish the task, they provide extra weight to be carried and increase the load upon the cardiovascular-respiratory system. Distance and marathon runners have small muscles. Sprinters, on the other hand, are generally well muscled. Sprinting is a power event with powerful muscular bursts repeated only a few times. It is an anaerobic activity, which permits repayment of the oxygen debt after the event has been concluded. The sprinter need not have an oxygen uptake equal to the demand for oxygen during the event as does the distance or marathon runner.

A large body mass can make it more difficult for an opposing lineman or wrestler to move the athlete as well as being an advantage in pushing against the opponent. Heavy and dense bones are disadvantageous in activities that require agility or in which one's body must be carried, hurled through space, or lifted as in dancing, diving, gymnastics, high or broad jumping, distance or marathon running, pole vaulting, or hurdling.

Individuals high in mesomorphy, unless they are unusually obese or also high in endomorphy, have greater body density because of large muscles and large, dense bones. Carter[8] reported in his study of the somatotypes of Olympic athletes that he found the mean somatotype for marathon runners as 1.4-4.3-3.5; pole vaulters 1.5-4.8-3.2; and swimmers, 2-5-3. It should be noted that for athletes in these sports, the rating for ectomorphy was higher than that for endomorphy. Earlier, Carter had found that the mean somatotype of football players was 4.2-6.3-1.4, which is endo-mesomorphic.

The relationship between strength and body type in boys 10, 13, and 16 years of age was studied.[19] After dividing 722 boys into high-, average-, and low-strength groups as indicated by scores on the Strength Index, the boys were somatotyped; it was found that the high-strength group had the highest ratings in mesomorphy.

Everyone has noted that outstanding athletes in certain sports are usually average or below average in height while in other sports outstanding athletes are tall. In the latter category are basketball and volleyball players because achievement of the objectives in basketball and volleyball requires that players be able to reach higher than their opponents. In the former category are gymnasts, divers, and weight lifters. In gymnastics and diving, great height increases the difficulty of establishing and controlling rotation around the axes of the body. In weight lifting, the taller the competitor, the higher the weight must be lifted and the longer the resistance arm in the human levers.

Those high in endomorphy, because of their relatively short arms, forearms, and fingers, are not likely to find success in throwing activities. Longer arms provide a longer lever for throwing. Longer levers provide greater distance through which to generate speed and momentum in throwing a ball, football, discus, or javelin. Those high in endomorphy have relatively short legs and forelegs and small feet. For this reason, they are handicapped in running, jumping, and hurdling events. However, because of their above average amounts of fat, they have good buoyancy and can enjoy recreational aquatic activities. They can apply a larger proportion of the thrust of arms and legs to propel themselves forward through the water since they need not apply as much downward thrust to keep themselves at the surface.

Those above average in ectomorphy, because of their more frail and delicate body structure and bones of small diameter, are more prone to suffer fractures and joint injuries in contact sports such as football, hockey, boxing, and wrestling. Because of their relatively longer arms, forearms, thighs, and lower legs, they are more likely to excel in jumping, hurdling, and middle and long distance running. Study of the skeletal characteristics of high jumpers concluded that they have longer legs, greater height, and broader feet.[20] The following formula was developed for predicting the height a high jumper could achieve:

$$\text{Height of jump (cm)} = 0.494 \text{ (height in cm)}$$
$$+ 1.522 \text{ (length of legs in cm)}$$
$$+ 0.338 \text{ (breadth of foot in mm)}$$
$$+ 57.818$$

The crural index (ratio of lower leg length × 100 to the length of the thigh) is higher in jumping animals such as rabbits and kangaroos than in nonjumping animals. It is certain that athletes with higher crural indexes have an advantage in jumping.

RACIAL AND ETHNIC SOMATOTYPE CONSIDERATIONS

It was pointed out earlier that certain somatotype characteristics provide an advantage in certain sports. When the athletes of one country repeatedly excel in Olympic events, as the Japanese have in recent years in gymnastics or as the Finns had from 1912 until 1928 in the 10,000 meter run, the temptation is great to attribute their repeated success to peculiarities of racial body type. However, a check of the national origin of Olympic winners since the Modern Olympic Games began in 1896 reveals that over the entire span of the Games men and women from many different countries have won the various events. Many factors combine to determine which nations' athletes win the event. To mention only a few, these factors are developmental training programs, emphasis the sport receives in the country (popularity), quality of coaching, scientific research on the sport, facilities provided, psychic and material rewards accruing to the successful participants, and number of national participants.

To what degree does race and country of national origin influence performance in motor skills? Are there differences in body composition and dimensions among people of different race and nationality? These questions are common ones and have elicited considerable discussion. However, surprisingly little research has been completed to answer these questions.

Instructors of swimming have long noted the difficulty experienced by blacks in floating horizontally. In one study 17 anthropometric measures of 69 white and 52 black male students between 17 and 27 years of age were made.[21] All 6 of the white group nonfloaters and 33 of the 35 black nonfloaters were swimmers of varying ability; consequently, their inability to float could not be attributed to fear of the water. The study showed that black males are anthropometrically different. The black nonfloater was taller, had longer legs, wider shoulders, a larger chest, narrower hips, larger arms and legs, weighed less, and had less fat and smaller breathing capacity than the floater group.

The results of this study carry important implications for teaching methods and evaluative criteria in beginning swimming classes containing black males. Floating and sculling requirements should either be deleted or modified for these students.

Skinfold and other anthropometrical measurements (height, weight, chest girth, upper arm girth, thigh girth, and bi-iliac diameter) of 647 Italian, Jewish, and black preadolescent boys 10 to 12 years old were compared.[22] It was found that the largest skinfold measurements were scored by the Jewish boys followed by the Italian boys, while the black boys showed the smallest skinfold measurements. Jewish boys were the heaviest and had the largest upper arm and thigh girth and bi-iliac diameter. The Jewish boys were followed in these measures by the Italian and black boys, in that order.

Another study, although not a study of the relationships between race or ethnicity and anthropometrical measure, points out the influence of heredity upon measures that influence performance in athletics.[23] The researchers evaluated the heritability estimate in monozygous and dizygous twins of both sexes with regard to maximal oxygen uptake (VO_2 max), maximal muscular power, maximal isometric strength, and fibertype distribution of skeletal muscle. The subjects were 14 monozygous and 16 dizygous pairs of both sexes ranging in age from 15 to 24. The authors secured the following results:

1. The male monozygous twins showed less variation in VO_2 max between pairs than did the dizygous twins. In females, the intrapair variances did not differ significantly between the two twin types.

2. Maximal muscular power was almost identical in the monozygous twins.

3. Muscle fiber distribution (percentage of slow twitch vs. fast twitch fibers) in the monozygous twins was almost identical in both sexes. The dizygous twins showed great intrapair variances.

The authors concluded that genetic factors are operative in the monozygous twins, especially in the males, and that these factors are important in determining capacity to perform muscular exercise.

EFFECT OF EXERCISE UPON SOMATOTYPE

Somatotype is genetically determined at conception. Exercise, diet, rest, climate, altitude, or other environmental factors have no influence upon somatotype. Those high in endomorphy can undergo hard conditioning programs and/or reducing diets and decrease body fat, but they will still be high in endomorphy. Those high in mesomorphy can (and often do) overeat and secure insufficient (for them) amounts of exercise and become obese so that they look like endomorphs, but they are still high in mesomorphy. Their outward appearance has changed but their skeletal proportions have not been altered. Somatotype is based on the dominance of the visceral area, muscle, or surface area (skin). The determining factor is whether the endoderm, the mesoderm, or the ectoderm is dominant during the development of the egg cell. This produces differences in the skeletal structure that determine the somatotype.

Exercise and diet can change the density or the specific gravity of the body through reduction in the depot fat. However, this does not change body type. This is why body type should be a consideration when advising students in physical education classes and when counseling students for selection of sports activities. The various body types have differing exercise and diet needs, respond differently to physical activities, experience success in different sports, and have varying health problems.

EFFECT OF AGE ON SOMATOTYPE AND PERFORMANCE

Body density, dimensions, and shape do change because of muscle atrophy and accumulation of fat. The amount of fat need not increase with increased age if exercise is continued throughout life and proper dietary habits are maintained (see Chapter 14 for more detailed information). Continuation of vigorous physical activity throughout life is especially important for those high in mesomorphy if they are to avoid cardiovascular and related health problems. Of all three somatotypes, mesomorphs adapt best to physical activity, profit most from it, and need it most in order to maintain organic efficiency. Endomorphs, because of their tendency toward obesity, and because of the resultant health problems, must make strenuous efforts to control body weight if they are to experience a healthy and vigorous middle age and years of senescence. Ectomorphs, because of their smaller body volume producing a smaller load upon the heart muscle, experience a smaller incidence of cardiovascular problems.

As people age, the proportion of fat deposited in the trunk increases.[24-27] However, several studies have indicated that the distribution and nature of fat in physically active individuals is different from that in individuals who are sedentary.[28,29] Cellular aging occurs when active tissue, such as muscle, is replaced by metabolically less active fat and connective tissue. From youth to old age, the basal metabolic rate declines about 25 percent. At the same time, strength declines as measured by grip strength tests. The typical person achieves his maximum strength at age 17, maintains this level to about age 45, and then declines about 15 percent by age 65. Women follow a similar pattern, except that maximal strength is reached at the onset of puberty.

The rate of physiologic aging can be decreased through a lifelong and regular exercise program. A higher body density, due to a decrease in fat, can be maintained as well as a reduction in serum cholesterol, triglyceride levels, and blood pressure. Increased collateral circulation in the heart muscle, increases in the number of red blood cells and in blood volume, and improved fibrinolytic capability are other benefits of physical activity for the middle-aged and the aging. Individuals who exercise regularly are also found to have a lower incidence of low back pain, ulcers, diabetes, and emotional problems, less neuromuscular tension, and greater flexibility, strength, and breathing capacity.

Among adult and aging men who do not exercise, a number of changes occur in physiologic processes that account for decrements in their performance in physical activities. (See Chapter 14 for more detailed information.) Along with changes in body composition, systolic and diastolic pressures increase 10 to 15 mm Hg and flexibility of the thorax and the elasticity of the lungs decrease, producing decreases in vital capacity, maximal oxygen intake, forced expiratory volume, and maximal ventilation on the order of 20 to 25 percent. A progressive loss in aerobic power occurs from 20 to 60 years of age on the order of 40 and 50 percent. There is also a loss in anaerobic power.

The decrements in performance can be minimal when strenuous physical activity is continued on a regular basis into advanced age. A 52-year-old woman ran 26 miles in 3 hours and 45 minutes.[30] Harry Lewis ran 6 miles almost every day until his death at 106 years of age. Cureton[31] cites the case of Sidney Meadows, who ran 10 miles in 1 hour and 11 minutes at the age of 65.

SPECIAL PROBLEMS OF OBESE CLASSIFICATIONS

All heavily muscled athletes are overweight if the standards by which they are judged are the widely used height-weight tables—even those that list different weights for small, medium, and large frames. The height-weight charts are computed from a large number of weights at each specific height. These standards are averages. They are not ideal weights. At the same time, authorities estimate that approximately one-fourth of the people in the United States are obese. Many whose weight is correct for their height according to the height-weight charts are too fat because an excessive proportion of their total weight is fat rather than muscle. At near ideal weight, muscle makes up roughly 45 percent of total body weight in men and 36 percent in women. Ideally, fat should account for about 10 percent of the total weight in men and 15 percent in women. Observation of many different people tells one that the percentage of total body weight made up of fat and of muscle varies greatly. It should be obvious that more sophisticated methods are required to correctly appraise an individuals's ideal weight.

A number of different methods have been devised for assessing body composition. These can be classified into two general procedures. One procedure measures body composition directly, by chemical analysis. This method is inappropriate for use in physical education because it requires not only highly specialized laboratory equipment but, more importantly, the use of cadavers. Use of cadavers presents both legal and ethical problems. Nevertheless, the few studies that have been done with cadavers have provided the information that has served as the basis for the second and more widely used procedures, those of indirect measurement through hydrostatic weighing, circumference measurements, or skinfold measurements. The body composition of only a few cadavers has been studied. From these few studies, however, it has been learned that differences in total weight are accounted for principally by fat, and to a lesser degree by muscle. The weight of the dry, fat-free skeleton was found to be remarkably similar in all the cadavers. Furthermore, the percentage of water in fat-free tissue was found to be similar in the cadavers regardless of the amount of adipose tissue. Water makes up about 72 percent of the body when all the fat is removed. A study done with rats showed that the percentage of body water in the fat-free tissues varied by less than one percent even when the amount of fat on the rats varied by as much as 300 percent. These findings point out that differences in body weight are due principally to differences in fat.

Body fat is classified into two types. *Essential* fat is the fat stored in the marrow of bones and in such organs as the heart, kidneys, liver, lungs, spleen, intestines, brain, and spinal cord. Essential fat accounts for about 3 percent of total body weight in men and about 10 to 12 percent in women.[32] It is suspected that reduction of total fat below these limits will impair physiologic functions and exercise tolerance. Studies have shown that international level male marathon runners have total fat content in the range of 4 to 8 percent.[33] The caloric cost of marathon runs and the conditioning programs these athletes undergo is so great that this cost insures maintenance of minimal body weight. Minimal body weight may also be affected by an increase in muscle mass. Body builders, weight lifters, and athletes in heavy resistance sports such as wrestling and field events in track, are well acquainted with this phenomenon.

The eminent nutritionist Jean Mayer is convinced that the most important factor accounting for the high incidence of overweight in modern Western societies is inactivity. He writes:

Natural selection, operating for hundreds of thousands of years, made men physically active, resourceful creatures, well prepared to be hunters, fishermen, or agriculturists. The regulation of food intake was never designed to adapt to the highly mechanized sedentary conditions of modern life, any more than animals were made to be caged. Adaptation of these conditions without development of obesity means that either the individual will have to step up his activity or that he will be mildly or acutely hungry all his life. The first alternative is difficult, especially as present conditions, especially in cities, offer little inducement to walking and are often poorly organized as regards facilities for adult exercise. Even among the young, highly competitive sports for the few are emphasized at the expense of individual sports which all could learn and continue to enjoy after the high school and college years are over. But if the first alternative, stepping up activity is difficult, it is well to remember that the second alternative, i.e., lifetime hunger, is so much more difficult that to rely on it for weight control programs can only lead to the fiascos of the past.[34]

Dr. Mayer exposes the fallacy of the belief that an increase in the amount of physical activity is followed by an increase in food intake. On the other hand, if physical activity is decreased below a certain point, appetite not only does not decrease correspondingly but in many individuals increases. When this occurs, fat accumulates. Individuals high in mesomorphy, who during their youth and early adulthood had been physically active and who drastically reduce their physical activity due to the responsibilities of marriage, a family, and professional or business responsibilities, are especially prone to this syndrome. Those individuals high in mesomorphy must continue to be physically active throughout their lifetimes if they are to avoid accumulation of excessive fat. Dietary habits, especially with regard to caloric quantity, are difficult to change. Young, active mesomorphs can ingest large quantities of food without becoming obese, but when they decrease their activity and continue eating the same amount of food, they accumulate fat.

In experiments with mice in activity cages with unlimited availability of food, it was found that mice that did not become obese were 50 to 100 times more active than those that did become obese. It was found that the characteristic of inactivity preceded obesity rather than the other way around. Like people, some mice are sedentary by nature. These mice, it was found, were not only less active but also consumed greater quantities of food and, as a consequence, became obese.[35, 36]

Some individuals high in endomorphy are genetically obese. Experiments with genetically obese mice have shown that their weight gains can be drastically reduced by treadmill exercise.[37]

The amount of different kinds of strenuous activities one would have to do to lose a pound of fat has been computed. To lose a pound of fat, one would have to walk for 36 hours, split wood for 7 hours, or play volleyball for 11 hours. Many sedentary individuals used these figures to rationalize their inert state by pointing out the impossibility of losing weight through exercise, since few would walk continuously for 36 hours, chop wood for 7 hours, or play volleyball continuously for 11 hours. It is surprising that they failed to realize that if one chops wood for only a half hour each day, in 14 days he will lose one pound and in a year he would lose 26 pounds. Furthermore, the caloric cost of the same dosage of physical activity is greater for the obese than it is for the thin individual because the obese person has more weight to carry. Since the energy cost of physical activity is proportional to body weight, overweight of 20 percent will increase the caloric cost of an exercise or sport participation by 20 percent. This is why physical activity is the most effective normalizer of body weight. The underweight will gain in weight due to development of muscle mass while the overweight will lose weight. Reduction of weight through exercise is of greater permanence than through diet. Mayer[38] experimented with sedentary rats in activity cages subjecting them to varying amounts of exercise. He found:

1. With moderate intensity of exercise for short periods (20 minutes to 1 hour), food intake decreased slightly but significantly. Body weight also decreased.

2. With longer exercise periods (1 to 6 hours) intake increased but weight remained constant.

3. With very long exercise periods (above 6 hours), the rats lost weight and their physical condition deteriorated.

Fat Cells

Excess calories are stored in the body as fat either through *hypertrophy* in existing fat cells, through *hyperplasia* (the formation of new fat cells), or through a combination of both hypertrophy and hyperplasia. The relationships between body weight, fat, fat cell size, and number of fat cells in obese and nonobese subjects was studied by Hirsch and Knittle.[39] In their subjects, the body weight of the obese subjects was more than twice that of the nonobese and the total fat was three times that of the nonobese. The amount of fat within each fat cell of the obese was 35 percent greater than in the nonobese. The total number of fat cells in the obese was about three times that in the nonobese. It appears that fat cell number rather than size of fat cells is the principal factor in obesity. The average person has 25 to 30 billion fat cells, the moderately obese 50 billion, and the extremely obese up to 237 billion.

During weight reduction in obese adults, the size of fat cells decreases (if the subject reduces to normal weight) to a size even smaller than in adults who have never been obese; however, there is no decrease in the number of fat cells. This means that the obese person who reduces his body weight will still have the same number of fat cells sending messages to the appetite control center in the brain asking for more food. If the formerly obese adults are to retain normal weight, they must be perpetually hungry. The number of fat cells increases rapidly during the first year of life, being three times greater at one year than at birth. The number increases more gradually after the first year until about age 10 and then accelerates again during the adolescent growth spurt until adulthood. It is not known at the present time whether the number of fat cells that develop in humans can be controlled. Experiments with animals show that early nutritional deprivation does have an influence upon both fat cell size and number. Rats from large litters who, after weaning had unlimited access to food, showed fewer and smaller fat cells than rats from small litters.

Effects of Exercise upon Fat Cell Size and Number

The effects of physical activity and food restriction early in the growth period of rats has been studied.[40] The experimental group had free access to food but was forced to swim for 15 minutes progressing to 6 hours by the end of 4 weeks. They continued to swim for 6 hours per day for 6 days a week for the 12 weeks of the experiment. During the same period, there were two control groups, one a sedentary group with free access to food and the other a group with restricted amounts of food. The sedentary, free-eating group showed the greatest weight gain and the exercise group with free access to food the least weight gain. Further, the exercise group possessed both smaller and fewer fat cells. It is highly probable that exercise programs for children will delimit the number of fat cells as well as their size and, consequently, limit the amount of total fat. Further experiments with rats have confirmed the suspicion that exercise during the growth period has a permanent infuence upon the total body fat cell size and number of fat cells. Follow-up showed that these effects remained through the adult life of these rats.[41]

It is apparent that exercise programs before adulthood can be especially effective in causing a reduction in the incidence of overweight. Exercise programs during childhood will help to keep weight within normal limits even after these children become adults. The evidence indicates that early prevention of obesity through exercise and diet is more effective than correction of obesity after it has arrived. Exercise and diet begun during the adult years can decrease the total body fat but they cannot decrease the number of fat cells. The number of fat cells will have a permanent influence upon the amount of body fat. Exercise and diet programs during the growing years will also, probably, influence the amount of body fat throughout the individual's lifetime.

SEGMENTAL BODY WEIGHTS

The relative weight of various body segments can be either an advantage or a disadvantage in specific athletic events. Massive muscular arms, shoulders, and thorax present the marathon or distance runner with a greater load upon his cardiovascular system as well as upon the muscles of his legs. Large feet and heavily muscled legs and buttocks present the gymnast with the problem of moving this weight, which is nonfunctional while circling the side horse or swinging on the parallel bars, horizontal bar, or still rings. We have never seen a world class soccer forward with the total muscular development of Russia's Vassili Alexeiev, 1972 and 1976 Olympic champion in the super heavyweight division in weightlifting. One of such muscular proportions would not be likely to possess the agility required to perform well as a soccer forward.

In selecting students for participation in various sports, and when prescribing weight training exercises, consideration must be given to the relationships between the weight and size of various body segments. Gymnasts should not execute low repetition-high resistance weight training exercises for the muscles of the legs. Jumpers and middle distance or distance runners should avoid exercises that develop bulk in the arms and shoulders.

Probably the greatest use that can be made of knowledge of segmental body weights and center of gravity is in the design of prostheses. The closer the center of gravity and the mass of the prosthesis approaches that of the missing limb, the more nearly normal will be the movements with the prosthesis, everything else being equal.

One of the more outstanding studies on body segment parameters was made by Dr. W. T. Dempster of the University of Michigan. Eight cadavers were disjointed into eight limb segments (head, trunk, upper arm, forearm, hand, thigh, lower leg, and foot), each segment was weighed, and its center of gravity was determined. The center of mass for each segment was located, and the distance from this point to the end of the segment was measured. Table 3.5 presents a summary of these findings.

Leveau[42] points out that in kinematic analysis of human motion, it is the total mass of the segments turning about the joint axes that is important and not the bones. Axes are not located precisely at the junctures of bones. This is shown in Figure 3.7. The central straight line that extends between two axes of rotation is called a "link." In some cases, the links are longer and in other cases shorter than the bones. This is an important consideration for accurate computation of the moment of inertia and radius of gyration in dynamic studies. Readers who need additional information on this topic are referred to Leveau,[43] Dempster,[44] Hanovan,[45] Miller and Nelson,[46] and Plagenhoef[47] studies.

SUMMARY

A brief history of somatotyping, as well as the derivation of the words *ectomorph, endomorph,* and *mesomorph* and the physical characteristics of the three extreme body types has been presented. Although, theoretically, 343 different body types are possible, in

Table 3.5 Average Weight of Body Segments for 150 lb Man. Percentage of Total Body Weight and Location of Center of Mass

Segment Weights and Percentage of Total Body Weight for 150 lb Man	Location of Centers of Mass
Head: 10.3 lb (6.9%)	*Head.* In spheroid sinus, 4 mm beyond anterior inferior margin of sella. (On lateral surface, over temporal fossa on or near nasion-inion line.)
Head and neck: 11.8 lb (7.9%)	*Head and neck.* On inferior surface of basioccipital bone or within bone 23 ± 5 mm from crest of dorsum sellae. (On lateral surface, 10 mm anterior to supratragal notch above head of mandible.)
Head, neck and trunk: 88.5 lb (59.9%)	*Head, neck, and trunk.* Anterior to eleventh thoracic vertebra.
	UPPER LIMB
	Upper limb. Just above elbow joint.
Arm: 4.1 lb (2.7%)	*Arm.* In medial head of triceps, adjacent to radial groove; 5 mm proximal to distal end of deltoid insertion.
Forearm: 2.4 lb (1.6%)	*Forearm.* 11 mm proximal to most distal part of pronator teres insertion; 9 mm anterior to interosseus membrane.
Hand: 9.9 lb (0.5%) Upper limb: 7.3 lb (4.9%) Forearm and hand: 3.31 lb (2.2%)	*Hand* (in rest position). On axis of metacarpal III, usually 2 mm deep to volar skin surface; 2 mm proximal to transverse palmar skin crease, in angle between proximal transverse and radial longitudinal crease.
	LOWER LIMB
	Lower Limb. Just above knee joint.
Thigh: 14.5 lb (9.7%)	*Thigh.* In adductor brevis muscle (or magnus or vastus medialis) 13 mm medial to linea aspera, deep to adductor canal; 29 mm below apex of femoral triangle and 18 mm proximal to most distal fibers of adductor brevis.
Leg: 6.3 lb (4.5%)	*Leg.* 35 mm below popliteus, at posterior part of posterior tibialis; 16 mm above proximal end of Achilles tendon; 8 mm posterior to interosseus membrane.
Foot: 2.1 lb (1.4%) Lower Limb: 23.4 lb (15.6%) Leg and foot: 9.0 lb (6.0%)	*Foot.* In plantar ligaments, or just superficial in adjacent deep foot muscles; below proximal halves of second and third cuneiform bones. On a line between ankle joint center and ball of foot in plane of metatarsal II.
	Entire body. Anterior to second sacral vertebra.

*Based on Dempster, 1955; value for head weight was computed from Braune and Fischer, 1889. Center of mass loci are from Dempster except those for entire limbs and body. (With permission of Barney Leveau and W. B. Saunders Company.) From: Leveau, Barney, *Biomechanics of Human Motion*, W. B. Saunders Company, Philadelphia, Pa., 2nd ed., 1977, p. 207.

actuality, the extreme types rarely occur. Sheldon described 76 body types of which 50 are seen fairly frequently.

The relationships between somatotype and performance in different sports was discussed. In all sports, successful athletes are

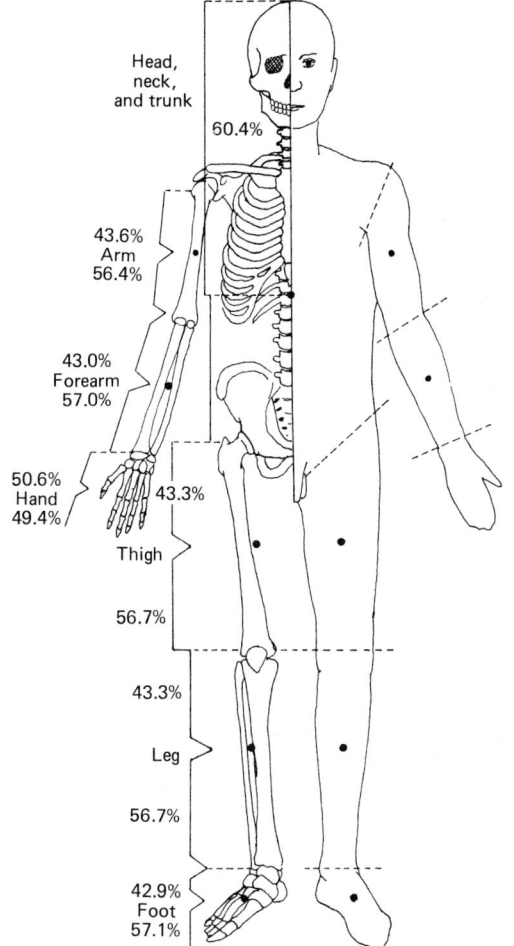

Head,
neck,
and trunk

60.4%

43.6%
Arm
56.4%

43.0%
Forearm
57.0%

50.6%
Hand
49.4%

43.3%

Thigh

56.7%

43.3%

Leg

56.7%

42.9%
Foot
57.1%

Figure 3.7 Location of link boundaries or center of rotation of body segments and percentage of center of gravity of the segments from link boundaries (from Leveau, B., **Biomechanics of Human Motion**, 2nd ed. Philadelphia, W. B. Saunders Co., 1977, p. 206, with permission)

shot put, it is advantageous to be above average in endomorphy. Body type is an important consideration when counseling students for selection of interscholastic sports participation and recreational activities, as well as when evaluating performance in selected physical education activities.

Height–weight charts are inadequate indices of ideal weight because they do not take into consideration relative proportions of muscle and fat, nor do they give adequate consideration to skeletal structure. Fat stored in the bones and organs accounts for 3 to 12 percent of total body weight and is termed *essential* fat. *Storage* fat accumulates in fat pads and as subcutaneous tissue. Storage fat accounts for about 12 percent of body weight in men and for about 15 percent in women. Excess storage fat is called obesity.

Excess calories are stored in the body in fat cells. Extremely obese people may have as much as 10 times the number of fat cells found in the average person. The number of fat cells in obese people after a weight-reduction program remains the same as it was before the weight loss. A decrease in the size of the fat cells occurs, however. During adulthood, the number of fat cells remains constant. If people with large numbers of fat cells are to avoid becoming obese, they must be constantly hungry since the individual fat cells must remain small and, consequently, these fat cells will be sending messages to the appetite control center demanding more food. Evidence seems to indicate that exercise programs during childhood serve to delimit both the number and size of fat cells. Further, the limitation on the number of fat cells seems to be permanent.

Endomorphs usually carry considerable storage fat while ectomorphs carry very little. Mesomorphs require large amounts of physical activity throughout their lifetime if they are to control their body weight.

Three methods for determining somatotype are described. These are the methods

above average in mesomorphy. However, in sports in which endurance is important to success or in which the body must be propelled through space as in jumping, pole vaulting, or gymnastics, it is advantageous to be above average in ectomorphy. In sports in which body mass is helpful, as in the line position in football, the hammer throw, or the

used by Sheldon, Heath and Carter, and Cureton.

Several methods for assessing leanness and fatness are described. These include hydrostatic weighing and a variety of methods utilizing measurements of skinfold, girth, width, and diameter. The latter includes the Pryor Width-Weight Tables, the Wetzel Grid, the method of Katch and McArdle, and several skinfold techniques.

It has been pointed out that surprisingly little research has been done on the relationships between race or nationality and somatotype. It has been found that black males have a greater body density and, consequently, a greater proportion than among whites are unable to float. Also, blacks have a larger crural index (relationship between the length of the lower leg and the thigh) than do whites, which presents an advantage in jumping and running. In a study comparing skinfold and girth measures of Jewish, Italian, and Negro boys, it was found that Jewish boys had the largest skinfold measures, were heaviest, and had the largest upper arm, thigh girth, and bi-ileac diameter measures. The Italian boys ranked next and the Negro boys last in all these measures.

Exercise and age have no influence upon somatotype but do influence body density and performance. The decrements in physical performance due to aging can be considerably retarded through an exercise program continued into advanced age. Most of the decrements in performance witnessed with increasing age are due to decreased physical activity.

Finally, the studies of Dempster on segmental body weights is discussed. The importance of this study to accurate computation of the moment of inertia and radius of gyration in the study of human movement and in the design of prostheses is pointed out. Differences in the relative weights of various body segments of world class athletes in different sports are readily observed.

REFERENCES

1. Kretschmer, E., *Physique and Character*. London: Kegan, Paul, Trench, Trubner and Co., 1936.

2. Sheldon, W. H., Stevens, S. S., and Tucker, W. B., *The Varieties of Human Physique*. New York: Harper and Brothers, 1940.

3. Davenport, C. B., "The Crural Index," *American Journal of Physical Anthropology*, Jan.-March, 1933, pp. 333-353.

4. Carter, J. E. L., "Somatotypes of College Football Players," *Research Quarterly*, 39:476, 1968.

5. Clarke, H. H., and Broms, J., "Differences in Maturity, Physical, and Motor Traits of High, Average, and Low Gross and Relative Strength," *Journal of Sports Medicine*, 8:143, 1968.

6. Lauback, L. L., and McConville, T. T., "Muscle Strength, Flexibility, and Body Size of Adult Males," *Research Quarterly*, 37:384, 1966.

7. Jones, H. E., "The Relationships of Strength to Physique," *American Journal of Physical Anthropology*, 5:29, 1947.

8. Carter, J. E. L., "The Somatotypes of Athletes—A Review," *Journal of Human Biology*, V, 42:4, Dec., 1970, pp. 535-569.

9. Carter, J. E. L., Stepnicka, Jiri, and Clarys, Jan P., "Somatotypes of Male Physical Education Majors in Four Countries," *Research Quarterly*, 44:361-374, Oct., 1973.

10. Sinning, Wayne E., and Lindbert, Gary D., "Physical Characteristics of College Age Women Gymnasts," *Research Quarterly*, 43:226-234, 1972.

11. Sheldon, William H., *Atlas of Men*, New York: Harper and Brothers, 1954.

12. Carter, J. E. L., and Heath, B., "Somatotype Methodology and Kinesiology Research," *Kinesiological Review*, A.A.H.P.E.R. Washington, D.C., 1971, pp. 10-19.

13. Cureton, Thomas K., *Physical Fitness Appraisal and Guidance*. St. Louis: C. V. Mosby, 1947, p. 120.

14. Pryor, Helen B., *Width-Weight Tables*. California: Stanford University Press, 1940.

15. Frazen, Raymond, and Palmer, George, "The ACH Index of Nutritional Status," New York: American Child Health Association, 1934.

16. Katch, Frank, and McArdle, William D.,

Nutrition, Weight Control, and Exercise. Boston: Houghton Mifflin, 1977, pp. 120–121.

17. Karpovich, Peter V., and Sinning, Wayne E., *Physiology of Muscular Activity*, 7th Ed. Philadelphia: W. B. Saunders, 1971, p. 311.

18. Carter, J. E. L., *op. cit.*, 1970.

19. Clarke, H. H., and Broms, J., *op. cit.*

20. Krakower, H., "Skeletal Symmetry and High Jumping," *Research Quarterly*, 12:218–227, May, 1941.

21. Lane, Elizabeth C., and Mitchem, John C., "Buoyancy as Predicted by Certain Anthropometric Measurements," *Research Quarterly*, 35:21–28, March, 1964.

22. Piscopo, John, "Skinfold and Other Anthropometrical Measurements of Preadolescent Boys from Three Ethnic Groups," *Research Quarterly*, 33:2:255–264, May, 1962.

23. Komi, P. V., Vitasolo, T. T., Haver, M., Thorstensson, A., and Karlsson, J., "Physiological and Structural Performance Capacity: Effect of Heredity," *Biomechanics V-A* (edited by P. V. Komi). Baltimore: University Park Press, 1976, pp. 118–123.

24. Garn, S. M., "Selection of Body Sites for Fat Measurement," *Science*, 125:550–551, 1957.

25. Garn, S. M., "Fat Accumulation of Aging in Males and Females," *The Biology of Aging*, 6:176–180, 1960.

26. Garn, S. M., and Harper, R. V., "Fat Accumulation and Weight Gain in the Adult Male," *Human Biology*, 27:39–49, 1955.

27. Quit, William B., and Golding, Lawrence A., "Equations for Estimating Percent Fat and Body Density of Active Adult Males," *Medicine and Science in Sports*, 5:4:262–266, 1973.

28. Parizkova, J., and Kuta, I., "Impact of Age, Diet, and Exercise on Man's Body Composition," *Annals of New York Academy of Science*, 131:661–674, 1963.

29. Parizkova, J., Kuta, I., and Ducka, J., "Muscle Strength and Lean Body Mass in Old Men of Different Physical Activity," *Journal of Applied Physiology*, 29:168–171, 1970.

30. Harrison, H., *Physical Fitness Research Digest*, President's Council on Physical Fitness and Sports, Series 7, No. 2, April, 1977, p. 10.

31. Cureton, Thomas K., "A Case Study of Sidney Meadows," *Journal of Association for Physical and Mental Rehabilitation*, 19:2:36, March–April, 1965.

32. Katch, Frank I., and McArdle, William D., *Nutrition, Weight Control, and Exercise*. Boston: Houghton Mifflin, 1977, p. 104.

33. Benke, A. R., and Royce, J., "Body Size, Shape, and Composition of Several Types of Athlete," *Journal of Sports Medicine*, 6:75, 1966.

34. Mayer, Jean, "Exercise and Weight Control," Chapter 16, p. 308, in *Science and Medicine of Exercise and Sports*. Warren R. Johnson, ed. Copyright©1960 by Warren R. Johnson. Reprinted by permission of Harper and Row Publishers, Inc.

35. Mayer, Jean, "Decreased Activity and Energy Balance in Hereditary-diabetic Syndrome of Mice," *Science*, 1953, pp. 117, 504.

36. Mayer, Jean, "Genetic, Traumatic, and Environmental Factors in the Etiology of Obesity," *Physiological Review*, 33:472, 1953.

37. Mayer, Jean, et al., "Exercise, Food Intake and Body Weight in Normal Rats and Genetically Obese Adult Mice," *American Journal of Physiology*, 177:544, 1954.

38. Mayer, J., *op. cit.*

39. Hirsch, J., and Knittle, J., "Cellularity of Obese and Nonobese Human Adipose Tissue," *Federation Proceedings*, 29:1518–1519, 1970.

40. Oscai, L., et al., "Effects of Exercise and of Food Restricton on Adipose Tissue Cellularity," *Journal of Lipid Research*, 13:590, 1972.

41. Oscai, L., et al., "Exercise or Food Restriction: Effect on Adipose Tissue Cellularity," *American Journal of Physiology*, 227:902, 1974.

42. Leveau, Barney, *Biomechanics of Human Motion*. Philadelphia: W. B. Saunders, 1977, pp. 206–212.

43. *Ibid.*, p. 206.

44. Dempster, W. T., "Space Requirements of the Select Operator," Wright-Patterson Air Force Base, Ohio (WADCTR 55–59), 1955.

45. Hanovan, E. P., "A Mathematical Model of the Human Body," Wright-Patterson Air Force Base, Ohio (AMRTR 64–102), 1964.

46. Miller, D. I., and Nelson, R. C., *Biomechanics of Sport*. Philadelphia: Lea and Febiger, 1973.

47. Plagenhoef, S. C., "Methods for Obtaining Data to Analyze Human Motion," *Research Quarterly*, 37:103–112, 1966.

4

FOUNDATIONAL NEURAL, PHYSIOLOGICAL, AND MOTOR LEARNING ELEMENTS OF MOVEMENT

CONCEPTS

1. The quality of human motor performance depends upon the structural and functional integrity of the central and peripheral nervous systems.

2. The brain is the control center of the nervous system and the site where sensations are received and interpreted.

3. Modulation of motor movements and coordination is a prime function of the cerebellum.

4. Motor movements function at three neural levels: (1) spinal cord level, (2) lower brain level, and (3) higher brain or cortical level.

5. Neurons are classified according to function. Sensory neurons convey signals to the spinal cord and brain, whereas motor neurons carry impulses from the brain and cord to effect muscular contraction or relaxation.

6. The cerebral cortex of the brain in a young adult contains approximately 10 billion neurons, and about 100,000 nerve cells are lost each day.

7. Exteroceptors, interoceptors and proprioceptors are sensory receptors that provide neural feedback information about the internal and external environment of the human organism.

8. Proprioception is particularly applicable to movement because of its special effect upon the quality of execution of motor skills.

9. Sophisticated motor skills are learned through the phenomenon of the conditioned reflex mechanism.

10. Reciprocal innervation permits the coordinated innervation and inhibition interplay of agonist and antagonistic muscles.

11. The motor unit, which consists of a single neuron, and all the muscle fibers that are innervated by the composite parts of the motor nerve, is considered a functional entity in the muscular contractile process.

12. Skeletal or voluntary muscles contract or relax at will, whereas heart and smooth muscles are governed by involuntary neural mechanisms.

13. The all-or-none-law of contraction applies to the muscle fiber in a motor unit, and not the muscle as a whole.

14. Motor learning includes performance tasks of all types, from the fine dexterity of knitting to the skill of athletic sports.

15. Maturation is a growth parameter and must be considered in determining a readiness to learn various skills.

16. The nature of the learner and complexity of a task must be considered before selecting the whole or part method of teaching motor skills.

17. Practice in one particular motor skill task does not transfer to a similar skill unless the neuromuscular requirements are directly related.

18. Speed and accuracy should be stressed concurrently in the early learning stages when these variables are inherently part of a successful performance.

19. Kinesthesis is an internal sensory receptor mechanism that provides an awareness of position about the whole body or its segments.

GENERAL NEURAL AND PHYSIOLOGICAL CONSIDERATIONS

The following presentation does not attempt to include a comprehensive review of neurology and physiology. We have selected those topics relevant to the understanding of neuromuscular aspects of human movement.

The integrity of the nervous system is basic to muscular contraction and to the myriad of motor patterns in human movement. Muscular response depends upon the structural and functional quality of the *central nervous system* (brain and spinal cord) and the *peripheral nervous system* (nerves, ganglia, and end organs), which interconnect and interrelate from stimuli to response. The brain may be considered the control center of the nervous system as a whole. Here sensations are received and interpreted from inside and outside the body. Nervous impulses travel the interconnected nervous network by way of *afferent* fibers to the central nervous system; and via *efferent* neurons from the brain and cord to the muscles and periphery of the body.

The peripheral component is further divided into *somatic* and *autonomic* systems. The somatic division carries peripheral sensations to the spinal cord or brain and integrates impulses from these nerve centers that result in muscular action. The autonomic component is divided into (1) *sympathetic* and (2) *parasympathetic* classifications. These categories are completely involuntary, with the sympathetic regulating such mech-

anisms as heart action, ductless gland secretion, arterial blood flow, and vital functions of the stomach and intestines. Parasympathetic nerve fibers work in concert with the sympathetic division and assist in the maintenance of neurological homeostasis (steady state). The human nervous system governs sensations and motor movements by transmitting neural messages. These messages are conveyed bioelectrochemically in a wavelike impulse fashion via *sensory* and *motor* neurons. Sensory neurons forward sensations about pain, pleasure, pressure, and emotions to the brain; motor neurons provide the vehicle for conducting impulses from the central nervous system to the muscles initiating movement.

THE CENTRAL NERVOUS SYSTEM

Brain

The brain may be considered the core or the central focus of the nervous system with its component parts: *cerebrum, cerebellum, pons,* and *medulla oblongata.* The integrity and function of this organ change with age; sensory perception and motor responses lessen, particularly when devoid of mental and physical stimulation. The brain weight is greatest at 20 years of age and then decreases 7 to 11 percent in poundage between the ages of 20 and 96 years with a loss of about 100,000 nerve cells each day.[1]

Cerebrum. The cerebrum is the chief portion of the brain, occupying the entire upper part of the cranium. It consists of right and left hemispheres. Usually one side is dominant, e.g., certain motor activities of one side of the body as throwing, batting, kicking, etc., in right-handed individuals are controlled by the left hemisphere. The external gray layer of the cerebrum is called the cortex and is considered the seat of reasoning and intelligence. The cortex is responsible for intellectual decision-making and conscious thinking in solving cognitive and motor learning problems.

Cerebellum. The cerebellum is located at the inferior part of the brain, lying below the cerebrum and above the pons and medulla. The general function of the cerebellum is associated with the modulation of motor movements. Specifically, this portion of the brain (1) regulates muscle tone, (2) governs certain mechanisms that influence balance, and (3) coordinates body motor activity. The cerebellum is especially vital to the control of very rapid muscular activities such as running, typing, playing the piano, and talking. The motor areas of the cortex and the proprioceptors of the muscles and joints are also connected with the cerebellum. These nerve interconnections allow transmission of circuit messages pertaining to the amount and extent of muscular force required for a motor performance. Destruction or lesion of the cerebellum drastically impairs the adjustment role of this portion of the brain. The coordinating function of the cerebellum is evident from observations of patients with cerebellar lesions. Such injuries result in a loss of coordination, poor equilibrium, and poor muscle tone. Although complete normal functioning of motor movements is impaired by cerebellar damage, severity of mobility and balance abnormalities can be reduced through brain compensatory mechanisms with appropriate exercises and motor activities concentrating upon reeducating unused and undamaged neurons of the cortex and cerebellum. Certain activities that focus on relaxation and coordination are further discussed in Chapter 8.

Pons Varolii. The pons varolii is composed of nerve fibers linking up the different parts of the brain from and to the spinal cord. It forms the white matter and is made up of small masses of nerve cells consisting of gray matter, irregularly scattered through the white matter. Structurally, the pons is part of the brain stem, which also includes the medulla oblongata and connects the spinal cord with the cerebrum. The pons also serves as an integral part of the vasomotor center, which controls respiration, heart beat, swallowing, and dilation or constriction of blood vessels.

Medulla Oblongata. The medulla oblongata is the transition stage between the spinal cord and brain; its diameter increases as it ascends upward to the cerebrum. The medulla performs the important function of regulating breathing and ventilation of the lungs, which is accomplished by alternation between inspiration and expiration. The inspiration or enlargement of the chest results from the contraction of the respiratory muscles followed by expiration, when the thorax returns to normal circumference at rest with air forced from the lungs. These muscles are controlled by a group of nerve cells in the medulla oblongata. Contraction and relaxation are governed by nerve impulses from these respiratory centers, which regulate the rate of breathing.

Spinal Cord

The spinal cord is part of the central nervous system. Contained within the vertebral canal, it extends from the medulla oblongata at the lower part of the head to the beginning of the second lumbar vertebra. The cord is about 18 inches long and, like the brain, contains both white and gray matter. It measures approximately one-half inch in diameter. Three protective membranes cover the cord. These are (1) *dura mater*, (2) *arachnoid mater*, and (3) *pia mater*. These layers also surround the brain. The cord contains neural cells that transmit impulses to and from the column to all parts of the body. Figure 4.1 exhibits important parts of a cord section.

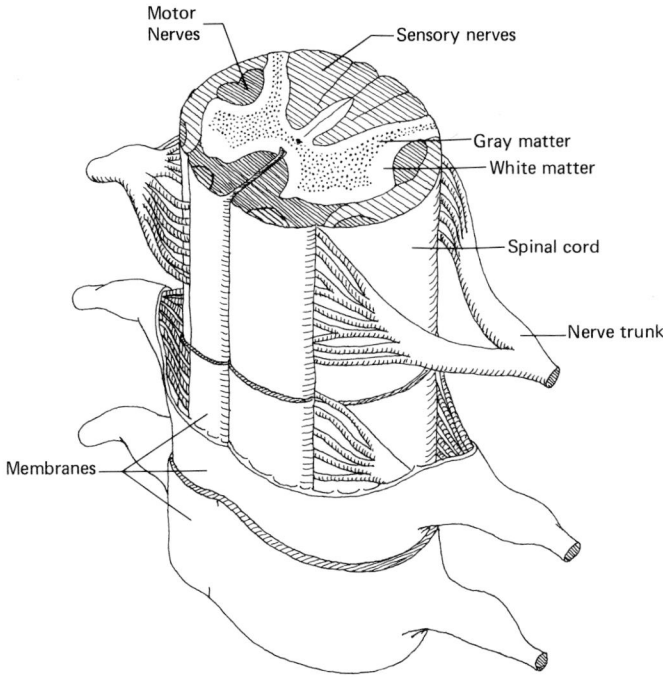

Figure 4.1. Internal and external spinal components

Spinal Cord Support Factors. Enclosure of the spinal cord within the backbone provides remarkable protection to its sensitive component parts. Spinal stability emanates from two sources: (1) *intrinsic* and (2) *extrinsic*. Intrinsic stability arises from the vertebral disks and ligamentous support. Extrinsic stability is provided by the muscles, especially of the abdominal and thoracic area. Since the spine is capable of motions in all planes, with greatest mobility occurring at the cervical level, exposure to injury is a likely threat whenever excessive hyperflexion and/or hyperextension is executed. Most sport injuries to the spinal column are related to (1) hyperflexion, (2) hyperextension, and/or (3) spinal compression.[2, 3] The combined intrinsic and extrinsic support capabilities of the spinal column can withstand great forces similar to the function of an elastic rod. However, aging causes a significant reduction in elasticity in the vertebral disks. Disk compression tests reveal that the disks behave normally up to a maximum pressure of 635.0 kg (1398.67 lb) in specimens from young adults and 158.8 kg (349.77 lb) in samples from older persons.[4] The implication of this study is that elderly people should avoid excessive ranges of spinal movement since they can cause trauma to the cord.

Levels of Nervous System Function

Three levels of motor functions have been identified from evolutionary development that have functional significance. These levels are (1) *spinal cord level*, (2) *lower brain level*, and (3) *higher brain* or *cortical level*.

Spinal Cord Reflexes. Motor responses at this level do not involve higher brain function but entail receptor-effector reactions such as the knee reflex shown in Figure 4.2. Sensory signals are received through the spinal nerves to the cord and are relayed to effector nerves, causing a localized muscular response. The knee tap activates the sensory neuron, which sends its message to the anterior horn of cord gray matter where a motor neuron is stimulated to activate the quadriceps, causing a sudden extension of the knee joint.

The knee jerk reflex is a classic example of coordinated muscular movement without conscious thinking. The response is accomplished automatically by sensory-motor nerve stimulation of the spinal cord and responding muscles. Although the simple jerk responses are not learned, such reciprocal muscular movement does indicate the quality of nervous feedback mechanism and is used as an index to determine the general state of the nervous system. The *withdrawal reflex* is another example of a spinal cord level reflex,

Figure 4.2. Spinal cord reflex action

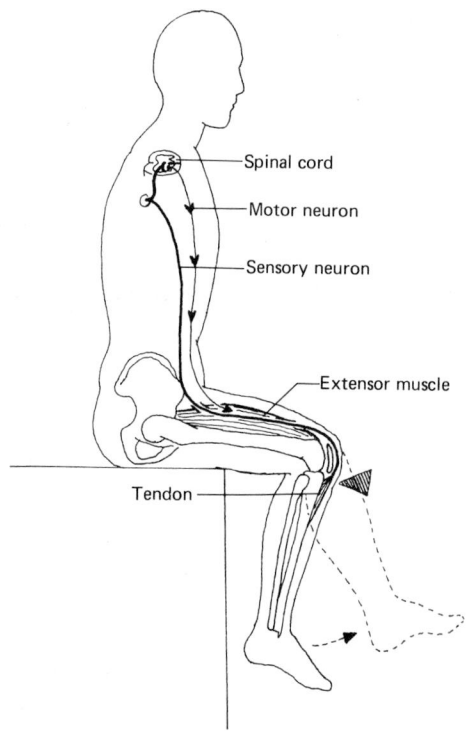

Spinal cord

Motor neuron

Sensory neuron

Extensor muscle

Tendon

which represents a protective function. This reflex involves the withdrawal of any part of the body from an object causing pain, such as removing the hand from a hot stove or quick flexion of the knee resulting from stepping on a tack. The *upright posture reflex* illustrates a static type of reflex action where the extensor muscles remain in a state of partial contraction to counteract the downward pull of gravity.

Lower Brain Level. Certain subsconscious motor activities are governed by the lower portions of the brain (pons, cerebellum, thalamus, and basal ganglia). Such vital functions as respiration, cardiac activity, vasomotor control, and secretion are programmed and automatically controlled by internal needs of the body. These functions usually operate at the subconscious level. Normal performance of these activities requires intact neural structures, and certain movements and processes can occur without the higher brain components. Study of the vital functioning of body needs entails a treatise of normal and pathological neurological nuances beyond the scope of this text. However, certain equilibrium control mechanisms of the cerebellum do fall within the realm of neuromuscular performance. Understanding of these mechanisms is advisable for people in the allied health professions. Chapter 8 contains an expanded discussion of the physiological aspects of balance and equilibrium.

Higher Brain or Cortical Level. The cerebral cortex contains an estimated 10 billion neurons.[5] Some individuals may have more neurons than others. This should increase their potential in motor performance. As previously mentioned, the cortex is the seat of reasoning and intelligence. The cognitive or intellectual aspect of motor performance is the prime function of this higher brain center.

While the subcortical and spinal levels control internal physiological needs and reflex characteristics of life, the cortex serves as a reservoir for storing information. Memories of past experiences are stored in the gray matter and are called upon when information is needed for controlled motor performance. The cortex contains sensory areas that receive an infinite number of messages, which are sorted out, organized, interpreted, remembered, and transmitted to other subareas of the brain and stem. The "thinking" process of the brain may be considered the primary function of the higher cortical level.

THE PERIPHERAL NERVOUS SYSTEM

The parts of the peripheral nervous system consist of (1) *somatic division* (cerebrospinal) and (2) *autonomic division* (which includes sympathetic and parasympathetic components). The somatic aspect, interconnected with the brain and cord, involves sensory and motor neural responses of the general skeletal body musculature. The autonomic component is divided into the sympathetic division (two nerve cords outside the spinal column with ganglia at the solar plexus, near the heart, neck, and abdominal areas) and the parasympathetic division (nerve fibers extending from the brain stem and sacral region of the spinal cord). The sympathetic aspect regulates actions of the heart, endocrine gland secretion, and other body responses previously indicated. The parasympathetic component serves as a check-and-balance mechanism upon the sympathetic division.

Impulses arising from the sensory end organs are carried toward the central nervous system via *afferent* (sensory) fibers. *Efferent* (motor) fibers convey stimuli from the central nervous system to the muscles and other body organs. The somatic fibers, both sensory and motor, are typified by neurons found in bones, skeletal muscles, and skin. The autonomic division also contains both types of neurons (sensory and motor), which influence internal body organs, vessels, and mucous membranes.

Somatic Relationships

The peripheral nervous system contains 12 pairs of *cranial nerves* and 31 pairs of *spinal nerves*. These structures function dependently upon one another. They also communicate with the sympathetic and parasympathetic divisions. At the outset, it should be noted that the spinal nerves are of greater significance to gross motor movement than the cranial nerves, which innervate muscles of the face, eyeball, tongue, throat, and inner ear.

Autonomic Relationships

As the name implies, the autonomic portion of the nervous system is automatic, since its function is not under voluntary control of the individual. The two subdivisions of the autonomic part—(1) sympathetic and (2) parasympathetic—differ structurally and physiologically. The sympathetic part mobilizes energy for sudden activity such as manifested in rage; e.g., pupils dilate, heart beats faster, blood vessels constrict, blood pressure rises. The parasympathetic component strives toward reestablishing the reserves by contracting pupils, slowing down the heart rate, and reducing blood vessel pressure levels. Some evidence suggests that emotional states affect posture movements through the autonomic system. Fear and pain trigger "flexion patterns" of human movement, the "extension pattern" position is exhibited in anger, while the unique relaxed "bowed-back" flexion posture is manifested in grief or depression.[6] Cognizance of probable autonomic influences, caused by certain emotional conditions, upon the quality of movement patterns certainly has implications for instructors of physical education and therapeutics.

NEUROMUSCULAR MECHANISMS

Movement in man is entirely dependent upon excitation and stimulation of the basic cell structure of a *neuron*. The quality of muscular tone and movement arises from neurogenic sources of nerve fibers. Flaccidity and ultimate muscle atrophy result when signals fail to transmit electrochemical excitation from nerve fibers to muscle contractile tissue.

The human body is endowed with an astonishing number of neurons to serve its voluntary and involuntary motor response needs. The sensory and motor unit components of the body carry an estimated 2.5 million fibers (bundles) to and from the central nervous system; of these, 2 million are sensory fibers, while the remaining 0.5 million are motor fibers.[7] Characteristics that all fibers share are keen sensitivity to stimulation and the special function of transmitting nerve impulses.

Neurons

A neuron is defined as a complete nerve cell, including the *cell body, axon,* and *dendrites.* Neurons are situated in the brain and spinal cord, as well as in the peripheral and autonomic systems. Neurons vary in size and shape in different parts of the body. Generally, a neuron has but one axon, which may be more than 2 feet long. Neurons are generally classified according to their functioning role. Afferent (sensory) neurons receive sensations from sense organs at the periphery of the body, or may originate in the brain. Sensory neurons convey signals to the spinal cord and brain. Motor or efferent neurons carry impulses from the brain and spinal cord to produce muscular contraction or relaxation depending upon the movement at hand. Figure 4.3 exhibits the major structural elements of typical sensory and motor neurons.

The nervous system contains approxi-

Figure 4.3. Typical neurons: (a) Motor, (b) sensory (from Clayne R. Jensen and Gordan W. Schultz, **Applied Kinesiology**, McGraw-Hill, New York, 1977, p. 41, with permission)

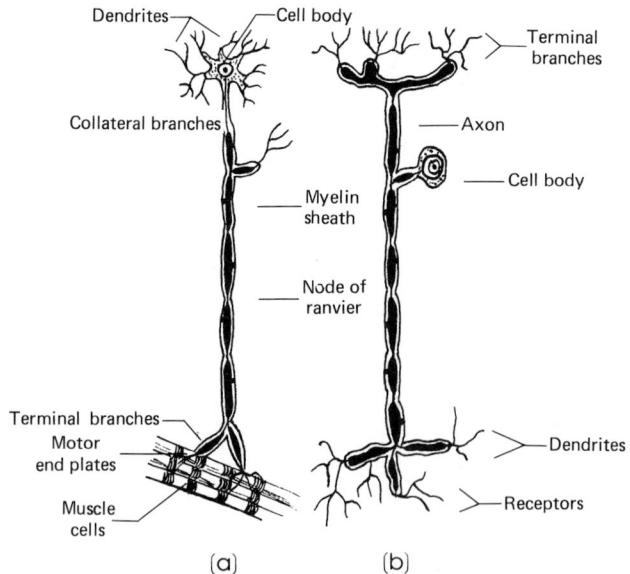

mately 10 billion independent neurons (cells). More than 90 percent of these units are located in the brain. A third type of neuron is termed *internuncial* or *interneuron*. These nerve cells are contained within the brain and spinal cord for the express purpose of serving as connectors and integrators between the sensory and motor neurons.

Medullated Nerve Fiber. Certain neurons contain myelin and a cellular membrane called the *neurilemma* sheath. Neurons placed in this sheath are termed *medullated nerve fibers*. This sheath contains a nucleus called the *Schwann cell*, which is of particular importance for the regeneration of peripheral nerves whenever these fibers are damaged. The general component parts and their location are shown in Figure 4.3. Medullated neurons are found in the voluntary muscles but are not present in the brain and cord.

The component parts of a neuron are:

Axon
Axis cylinder, one axon to each neuron, bound into bundles to form a nerve and conducting the impulse lengthwise to receiving tissues or other neurons.

Cell Body
Body of gray cytoplasm that contains the vital center of core (nucleus) of the neuron from which project multiple cytoplasmic extensions called dendrites that receive impulses traveling toward the cell body.

Myelin Sheath
A fatty white substance that covers the axon and serves as an insulator.

Nodes of Ranvier
Indented intervals of the sheath that allow the axon to contact intercellular fluids necessary for the electrochemical flow of nerve conduction.

Neurilemma Sheath
A cellular membrane that encloses the myelin

and is deemed a vital factor in regeneration of peripheral nerve fibers.

Motor End Plate. This component is a specialized end structure of motor neurons called a myoneural or neuromuscular junction. It is at this point that the motor nerve makes functional and transmission contact with a muscle cell. Figure 4.3 shows the connecting linkage typically found at the motor end plate junction.

Synapse. The synapse is a region of communication between neurons or the point at which an impulse passes from an axon of one neuron to a dendrite or to the cell body of another. The impulse travels along the axon to the dendrites through the cell body to the dendrites of another neuron, in one direction. The synaptic connections are of two types: (1) *excitation* and (2) *inhibition*. A process of membrane depolarization entailing a release of a chemical substance called acetylcholine gives rise to the excitatory response. Also, an inhibitory element may be released, which increases membrane permeability thereby preventing the transmission of a neural impulse. It becomes evident that the function of the synapse may be such as to facilitate or to inhibit the passage of impulses from one neuron to another. This is well illustrated by the phenomena of *reciprocal inhibition* and *reciprocal innervation*, which are discussed in later sections of this chapter.

Neural Conduction of Impulses

Neural stimulation may originate from physical, chemical, or electrical sources. Once neurons are activated, a bioelectrochemical process of transmission occurs within the neuron, setting the impulse into motion at a velocity of 1 to 350 feet per second. The speed depends on the size of a particular nerve fiber and the thickness of the myelin covering. Large fibers with thick myelin sheaths are faster impulse conductors than smaller non-medullated nerves. The transmission of the impulse may be described as an electrical-chemical phenomenon whereby the membrane covering the neuron is polarized with positive sodium and chloride ions on the outside and negative potassium ions on the inner surface of the neuron's cylindrical structure. When the axon is stimulated, a fuse-like ignition is fired, and a process called *membrane depolarization* occurs, as shown in Figure 4.4.

A polarization state in a resting membrane contains a higher concentration of sodium and chloride ions on the outside while the potassium ions are higher on the inside. Therefore, a resting state of membrane polarity contains an unequal distribution of ions between the outside and inside axon membrane.

Neural transmission obeys the *all-or-none law*, which means that conduction begins when stimulation intensity reaches a minimum level. The intensity of the stimulus does not affect the quality of the impulse; however, it may spread to other nearby neurons. A very brief pause exists following the passage of a nerve impulse, representing a point at which initiation of a new stimulation can be effected. This pause or resting state is termed a *refractory period*. It lasts for several milliseconds. Polarity of the neuronal membrane quickly follows, and the nerve fiber is ready to transmit a new impulse.

SENSORY RECEPTORS

The quality of human motor performance is affected by the functioning of three types of sensory mechanisms termed (1) *exteroceptors*, (2) *interoceptors*, and (3) *proprioceptors*. These physiological parameters provide feedback information to the human organism and are intimately involved in learning simple and complex motor skills. Exteroceptors and proprioceptors supply external sensory clues about outside environmental conditions. Interoceptors furnish sensory clues from internal organs of the body. Skillful

Figure 4.4. Conduction of nerve impulse (from Clayne R. Jensen and Gordan W. Schultz, **Applied Kinesiology**, McGraw-Hill, New York, 1977, p. 53, with permission)

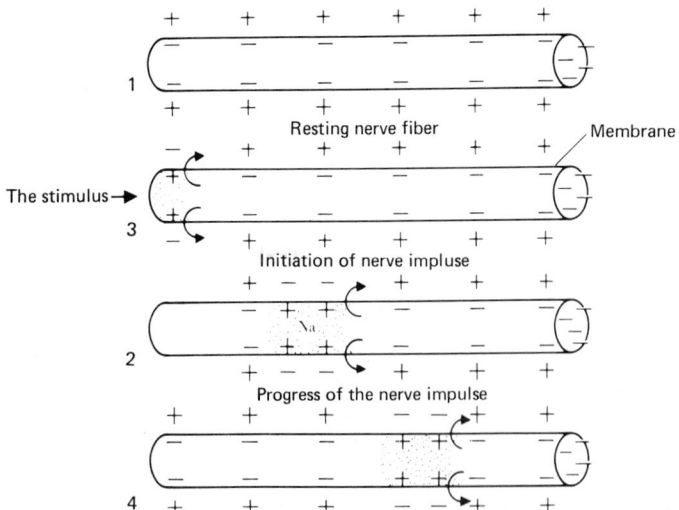

movement entails the integrative and cooperative functioning of these sensitive receptors.

Exteroceptors

The exteroceptor is an end organ in or near the skin or a mucous membrane that receives stimuli from the external world. The enjoyment of the five senses — taste, smell, hearing, sight, and touch that respond to the numerous changes that occur in our external environment are classified as exteroceptors. Certain exteroceptors, called *telereceptors*, function as distance receivers, i.e., sensations from a stimulus not in contact with the body. Vision, hearing, and olfactory senses are telereceptors. Other receptors, such as touch and taste, entail the reception of stimuli by direct communication and are called *contact receptors*. Each receptor is specialized. Heat receptors react to warm and hot signals, whereas others respond to cold exclusively. Exteroceptors may function in concert with each other by communicating sensation about time, space, equilibrium, and other external environmental changes. For example, a blind person may improve kinesthetic and neuromuscular control by developing touch acuity. Individuals with impaired hearing can utilize visual telereceptors to effect movements of the lips for a spoken word.

Interoceptors

The site of these sense organs is located within the viscera of the body. They are also called *visceroceptors*. Interoceptors respond almost exclusively to internal visceral changes. Sensations of digestion, excretion, and circulatory adjustments involve the transmission of internal stimuli to the cortex. Pain or stomach cramps induced by indigestible food is signaled via visceroceptors. The practice of avoiding heavy meals prior to competitive contests requiring all-out muscular effort is based upon sound neural feedback-mechanism principles.

Proprioceptors

These sensory receptors greatly influence physical performance. They are of particular interest to students of kinesiology. Although an intact proprioceptive feedback system is part of the normal organism, the quality of function varies greatly and is manifested by the skill level of the individual. Skilled athletes generally possess acute proprioception, characterized by superior qualities of balance, neuromuscular coordination, and kinesthesis. Proprioception is also referred to as one's "muscle sense." The ends of proprioceptive nerves are situated in muscle spindles. Balance and equilibrium are also intimately associated with this receptor; they are discussed further in Chapter 8. *Proprioception* provides an awareness of movement derived from muscle, tendon, joint, and internal ear receptors. As pointed out in Chapter 8, proprioception is an integral component of all motor skills entailing balance. The reader is referred to Figure 8.12 illustrating the neural pathway of proprioceptive transmission from nerve endings to the brain.

Proprioceptors are categorized in three groups: (1) *muscle receptors*, (2) *joint and skin receptors*, and (3) *inner ear and neck receptors*.

Muscle Receptors. This group of receptors is found within the muscle, specifically in the *Golgi tendon* at the insertion of the tendon into the muscle and the muscle spindle located among the tendon and fiber bundles. Golgi tendon organs are responsive to the degree of tension within the muscle whether this tension is produced by a stretch or a contraction. In this regard, mucles are protected from excessively high contractions by Golgi receptors exerting an inhibitory effect on the motor neurons. The tendon organ is composed of myelinated nerve fibers and is arranged in series with extrafusal muscles fibers as shown in Figure 4.5. The structure of nerve and tendon fiber is so arranged that it

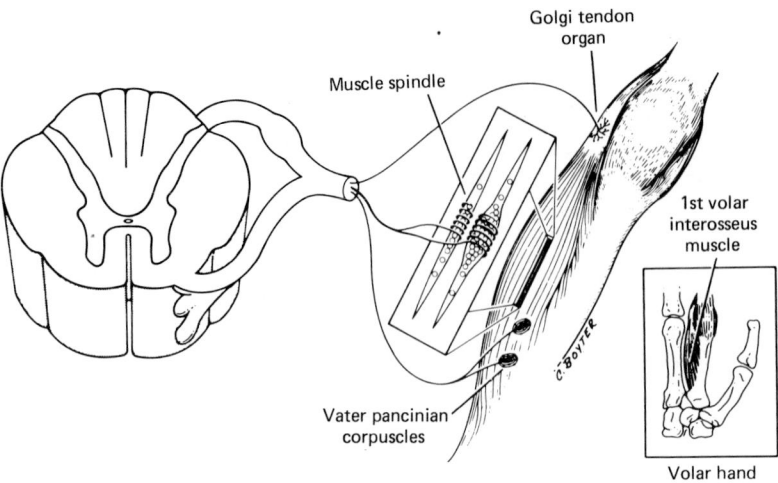

Figure 4.5. Proprioceptive monitoring of skeletal muscle (from Whitney R. Powers, "Nervous System Control of Muscular Activity," in Howard G. Knuttgen (Ed.), **Neuromuscular Mechanisms for Therapeutic and Conditioning Exercise**, University Park Press, Baltimore, 1976, p. 15, with permission)

can record tension changes in muscles, thus serving as a specific safety device in preventing muscular injury. The limits of physical strength may be determined in large measure by the control exerted by the Golgi tendon organs.

In summary, muscle spindle feedback receptors provide primarily the continuous adjustment in the magnitude of force generated by the muscles to conform to the amount of work load or motor skill. Light or heavy muscular effort and coordination are governed by these specialized proprioceptors. O'Connell and Gardner make the following point about the Golgi tendon organs relative to muscular effort:[8]

> . . . immediate relaxation of muscles when volition ceases;—In Indian wrestling, the loss of the contest usually occurs abruptly, when mounting tendon organ inhibition finally overcomes the voluntary effort to maintain contraction;—the "breaking point" in muscle strength testing is probably due to tendon organs and, if this is so,

it suggests that maximal strength is dependent upon the individual's ability to voluntarily oppose the inhibition of his own tendon organs . . . .

Joint and Skin Receptors. Structures located in the deep layers of the skin, connective tissues of the joints and ligaments, and fascia that surround the muscle and tendons contain intrinsic receptors called *Pacini* and *Ruffini* corpuscles. Pacinian corpuscles are considered "touch" receptors and are bountiful in the hands, feet, and joints. Functionally, Pacinian bodies are sensitive to vibration and pressure. When situated in ligaments, they are very sensitive to quick movement or vibration. Structurally, the corpuscle is composed of onionlike connective tissue surrounding a nonmyelinated nerve fiber. The Ruffini corpuscles are receptors located in joint capsules and the dermis. Together with the Pacini forms they signal joint position. These receptors are of particular significance in performing intricate motor skills requiring exact precision of joint extension such as maintaining a one handstand shown in Chapter 8. Thus, joint receptors provide feedback information about necessary pressure and angle of movement around a joint.

Cutaneous receptors may function as proprioceptors or exteroceptors since these skin sense organs respond to touch and pressure. These sensitive receivers are also associated with various inborn reflexes such as the extensor thrust reflex, withdrawal reflexes, and certain other basic movements that do not involve the cerebral cortex.

Inner Ear and Neck Receptors. These two groups of proprioceptors are intricately involved with movement orientation of the head and balance movements. Inner ear receptors are specialized receivers situated in the labyrinth of the inner ear. The neck receptors emanate from the cervical spine and, in concert with inner ear mechanisms, feed signals to the trunk and limb muscles for the purpose of maintaining normal posture and body alignment.

The "righting reflexes" and vestibular receptors, associated with the important function of balance and equilibrium, are discussed further in Chapter 8. Proprioceptive activity also occurs within the fluid-filled labyrinth, the semicircular canals, and the utricle of the inner ear. The canals are oriented to the plane coordinates of the body and contain ciliary hairs called the *otoliths*. Movements of the head and/or body cause a shift in otolith position, resulting in maintenance of stability and poise without cortical consciousness.

Inner ear and neck receptors deal with movements of the head.

Receptors located in each of these structures are stimulated whenever movement affecting upright posture and/or equilibrium of the body is negotiated. The tendency for beginners to hyperextend the head in performing a simple front dive, which often results in a "belly flop," may be attributed to

labryinthine or inner ear righting reflexes, which tend to resist the "head-down-hips-up" position necessary for a successful head-first dive. Sport and physical activities provide immeasurable opportunities for the stimulation and development of inner ear and neck reflexor mechanisms, which can improve the individual's quality of motor performance in work or play.

REFLEXES AND MOTOR PERFORMANCE

Reflex movement is part of daily living and, as defined earlier, involves motion of the body without cerebral intervention. Basically, two types of reflexes are classified: (1) *innate reflexes* and (2) *conditioned reflexes.*

Innate reflexes do not involve any learning process and are typified by spinal responses such as the knee jerk and withdrawal reflex patterns described earlier in this chapter. The conditioned reflex is more complicated than the mechanism found in the innate reflex arc action. *Learned* or *conditioned actions* utilize cortical processing before automatic responses are elicited.

Innate Reflexes

The *stretch reflex* is a vital innate type of response that is stimulated by proprioceptive endings located in the muscle spindles. Such movements as the knee jerk response and maintenance of upright posture are largely achieved by a reflex contraction in response to a pull or stretch on the affected muscle(s). The stretch reflex is also called the *myotatic reflex*, and these terms are frequently used synonymously. DeVries[9] points to the relationship between ballistic stretching exercises and the myotatic reflex phenomenon. Quick, jerky type of ballistic exercise may invoke undue contractions that interfere with the development of flexible joints and muscles. On the other hand, a firm steady static stretch calls forth an inverse reflex that brings about inhibition, not only of the muscle whose tendon organ is being stretched, but of the entire functional group of involved muscles. This reflex phenomenon certainly has direct application for physical education and fitness specialists designing and formulating flexibility exercise programs.

Maintaining an erect posture involves the stretch reflex mechanisms. Extensor muscles provide primarily the power source against the pull of gravity. For example, a person falling asleep in a sitting position begins to flex the head forward—the sudden forward contraction of the neck triggers the stretch reflex embedded within the muscle spindles of the extensors and consequently causes a return of the head to the upright posture. The *extensor thrust reflex* is effected by pressure against the sole of the foot from stimulation of the Pacinian corpuscles. The significance of this reflex helps the individual to assess the necessary pressure required in jumping, landing, and/or balancing maneuvers. A third type of innate reflex is called the *withdrawal (flexor) reflex.* This response serves as a protective mechanism and is typified by the immediate flexion of the lower limb after stepping on a sharp object. Innate reflex responses serve as a means of clinically evaluating inherited and clinical functioning of the nervous system. Achieving high levels of skill performance requires an intact structural and physiological base. An understanding of automatic innate reflex responses can help physical educators to ascertain which motor movements can be learned, as well as those actions that are automatically built into our neural reflex mechanisms.

Conditioned Reflexes

Conditioned reflexes are learned behaviors and/or motor responses that initially entail cortical activity. These motor responses are voluntary, and the quality of performance is governed by multiple feedback from extero-

ceptive, interoceptive, and proprioceptive stimuli. Highly skilled athletes develop a keen sensitivity of sensory receptors that ultimately transfers conscious thinking of "how" to move for a given motor skill to unconscious cerebellar modulation of skeletal muscles. For example, a novice learning a handstand thinks about the relative position of body parts in relation to the center of gravity of the body over its supporting base and strives to attain a predetermined body arch magnitude, elbow extension, and a certain posture in head position. Correct biomechanical principles for successful execution of a handstand apply that mandate keeping the line of gravity within its supporting base. Continuous practice of this motor skill then becomes conditioned to the point where the performer disregards the intellectual aspect of the cortex and performs, free of conscious thinking. During the initial stages of learning a motor skill, mental judgments and processes are involved in the cortex of the brain. The performer "thinks" about the required "firmness" or "tension" of skeletal muscles for a specific motor task. However, upon repetition through correct practice, the feedback control mechanism gradually assumes increasing responsibility and relieves the higher brain centers of this function. Of particular importance to the physical educator, this entails the role of proprioceptors in conditioned reflex movements. The acuity of these receivers can be sharpened through sport performance to a point where a "smash" in badminton or "polished entry" in diving is executed automatically without conscious control. The cortex, at the level of refined motor performance accomplishment, merely monitors the total response, standing ready to impose changes or modification in the event an error in skeletal motion is made.

Sophisticated motor skills are learned through the phenomenon of the conditioned reflex. The coordinated effort is projected from the cortex and is subsequently transmitted to the cerebellum and the subcortical and spinal centers of the cord itself. Appropriate innervation and/or inhibition of specific muscles necessary for a particular skilled motor performance can be conditioned. Unskilled motor patterns can be transformed to skilled movements by applying the conditioned reflex mechanism. The performer learns to correct innervating and/or inhibitory skeletal responses as a part of the conditioning process. It appears that once a certain conditioned reflex is learned, longstanding qualities of performance remain. It is not uncommon for individuals to perform skills, such as diving or hand balancing, in their 60s and 70s, provided other fitness parameters are maintained. Conditioned reflexes seem to be of a permanent nature. Mastery of correct voluntary reflexes in early childhood is a sound principle for retaining efficient neuromuscular control of sport skills throughout life.

Reciprocal Innervation

A reflex mechanism that permits the coordinated interplay of agonist and antagonist muscles entails the phenomenon of *reciprocal innervation*. This mechanism implies that when agonist muscles are stimulated, inhibitory action of the opposing or antagonist muscles is effected. The term *reciprocal innervation* is also identified with *reciprocal inhibition*. Actually, both terms are part of the same concept. For example, during the pull-up, flexion of the biceps brachii (agonists), which automatically triggers impulses to the triceps brachii (antagonists) result in relaxation or inhibition, and a free-flow dynamic movement of the elbow joint. The *cross extensor reflex* is another example of the reciprocal innervation principle; withdrawal or flexion of the foot, after stepping on a tack, causes concurrent relaxation of the extensor muscle and an extension of the opposite leg in support of the body weight during the flexion reflex. Kabat[10] points out that reciprocal innervation is a useful mechanism for inhibi-

tion of reflexes that interfere with voluntary movement, such as spasticity, reflex spasm, and flexion reflexes. Inhibition of the antagonist is augmented when the agonist is contracted against resistance, since "the stronger the contraction, the greater the reciprocal inhibition." A specialized technique for relaxation of spasticity, called *proprioceptive facilitation*, combines reciprocal innervation with voluntary relaxation of spastic antagonists. The spastic muscle is placed in the lengthened range and is contracted voluntarily against manual resistance great enough to prevent motion. The patient is then requested to relax and follows this with voluntary contraction of the agonist against resistance. This therapeutic technique offers a useful application of the reciprocal innervation mechanism for the improvement of voluntary movements of individuals with certain neuromuscular impairments.

The functional muscle relationship of agonist and antagonist can be applied to sport. For example, the desired even free-flowing movement of the arm action in the crawl stroke is enhanced by the deliberate effort of a swimmer flexing and relaxing the flexors and extensors during appropriate phases of the arm stroke, thus contributing to greater efficiency with less energy expenditure. The principle of reciprocal innervation, broadly conceived, coordinates muscles by allowing alternate movements of ipsilateral (same side) and contralateral (opposite side) limbs, as well as mutual interchanges between forelimbs and hindlimbs. Figure 4.6 illustrates the neural pathway of reciprocal inhibition of the flexor and cross extensor reflexes stimulated by a receptor in the hand.

Postural Reflex

Maintaining the upright postural position is basically a *stretch reflex* mechanism. Activation of the receptors in the muscle spindles, together with balance mechanisms within the inner ear, eyes, and cerebellum continually

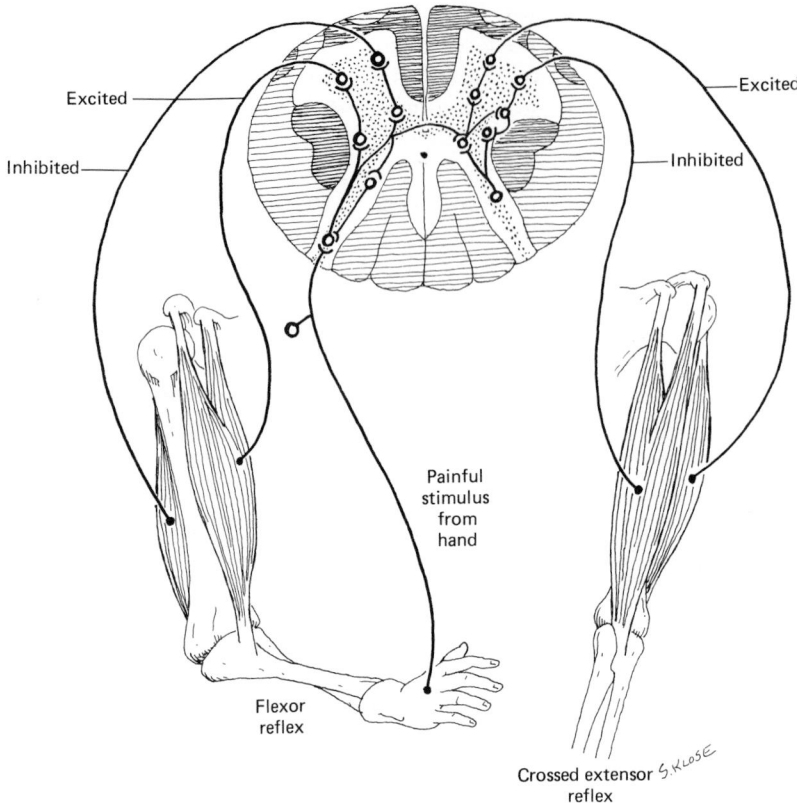

Excited

Inhibited

Excited

Inhibited

Painful
stimulus
from
hand

Flexor
reflex

Crossed extensor S.KLOSE
reflex

Figure 4.6. The flexor reflex and crossed extensor reflexes and the reciprocal inhibition effect (from Arthur C. Guyton, **Basic Human Physiology**, W. B. Saunders, Philadelphia, 1977, p. 525, with permission.)

innervate the antigravity or extensor muscles. Therefore, the basic ingredient for the control of posture is neurological and requires an intact reflex feedback system. However, proprioceptive awareness can be improved through conscious effort and training. Sport activity such as fancy diving, gymnastics, and dance reinforce neural pathways involved in the stretch reflex and ultimately enhances upright postural stance by improving muscular tonicity of the antigravity muscles. Postural reflex appears to diminish with age. Hasselkus and Shambs[11] selected a group of young and older females (ages 20 to 80 years) and found significantly larger posture sway in older persons than younger adults when assuming the upright stance. This may be partially due to the changes in muscle tone, equilibrium, and reflex patterns that tend to decrease with aging. The mechanical aspects and other external factors affecting posture are discussed in Chapter 12.

THE MOTOR UNIT

Functional Role

The neuron represents a *structural* entity of the neuromuscular system. The motor unit, which contains the neuron, is regarded as the *functional* unit of the stimulus/response contractile process. The motor unit consists of a single neuron and all the muscle fibers that are innervated by the composite parts of the motor nerve. The number of fibers within a motor unit varies, depending upon its location and function. Muscles that control fine movements and adjustments, such as those attached to the ossicles of the ear and to the eyeball, have the smallest number of muscle fibers per motor unit; large coarse-acting muscles, e.g., those in the limbs, have more fibers per motor unit. Certain muscles that move the eye have units with less than ten fibers per unit.[12] Figure 4.7 schematically illustrates the components of a motor unit.

Two major types of motor units are identified: (1) *alpha* and (2) *gamma*. Alpha motor units are further divided into two subdivisions called *alpha fast-twitch* neurons and *alpha slow-twitch* neurons. Fast-twitch neurons contain large axons and innervate pale or phasic (rapid and brief duration) extrafusal muscle fibers. These pale motor units are geared toward power and mass activity production. The slow-twitch neurons are identified by small neurons and innervate tonic or red muscle fibers. These red fibers are able to make sustained contractions such as those supporting the body in the upright position. The neural pathway of fast- and slow-twitch axons are shown in Figure 4.7.

Gamma units are found in the intrafusal muscle spindle and are part of the intrinsic feedback (servomechanism) mechanism of skeletal muscle. These fibers are smaller and transmit impulses more slowly to the muscle fibers. Gamma efferent fibers supply the motor control to the spindle and keep it operative no matter what length the muscle may assume. They exhibit a persistent low level of impulse firing to the spindle.[13]

The neurological characteristics of muscular fibers have interesting implications for exercise performance. It appears that we preferentially recruit slow-twitch units in low-tension, slow-moving, or enduring exercises, while we involve fast-twitched units in fast movements. The soleus muscle, which con-

Figure 4.7. Components of a motor unit. (a) Fast twitch, (b) slow twitch: the anterior horn cell, its axon, and all the muscle fibers the cell innervates (from Whitney R. Powers, "Nervous System Control of Muscular Activity," in Howard G. Knuttgen (Ed.), **Neuromuscular Mechanisms for Therapeutic and Conditioning Exercises**, University Park Press, Baltimore, 1976, p. 4, with permission)

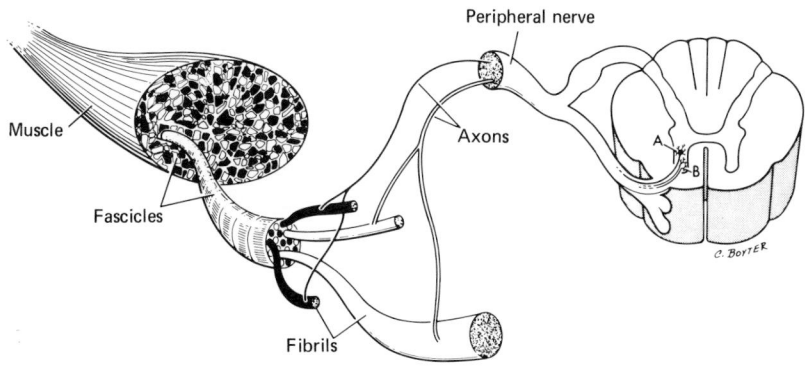

sists of a high proportion of slow-twitch fibers, fatigues at a slower rate than the gastrocnemius, which is a fast-twitch muscle; thus the soleus is more naturally used in longer enduring types of exercises.[14]

The notion that individuals are genetically endowed with a predominance of one type fiber over another and that training programs might be developed to accommodate this natural difference is suggested. For example, sprint swimmers may possess a predominance of fast-twitch fibers. This theory lends credence to training based upon fiber types. Caution is advised, however, before assumed generalizations are used to train according to morphological fiber characteristics of individuals.

All-or-None Law

Motor neurons abide by the all-or-none law, which implies that when a stimulus exceeds a threshold level, the neuron will transmit the impulse over its axon to the fibers it serves. The law states that the stimulus must be of a certain threshold intensity or the nerve will not react at all. This law also applies to the muscle fiber; that is, the fiber contracts to its maximum ability once stimulated or remains at rest. Therefore, the activation of muscular contraction depends upon how many complete motor units are required for a given task at hand. Light tasks require fewer motor units, whereas heavy work loads demand greater recruitment in numbers of motor units. This phenomenon is called *gradation of muscular contractions*. A well-conditioned muscle generally uses fewer motor units than a weak, flaccid one. The concept of the all-or-none law applies to strength development. Strength increases depend upon supplying impulses of sufficient intensity to recruit the maximum number of motor units, and consequently the greatest number of muscle fibers. It must be remembered that this law applies to the motor unit, and not to the entire muscle. The response of the whole muscle is based upon the number of motor units necessary to perform a task, which consequently depends upon the degree and qualitative functioning of nervous and muscular systems.

MUSCULAR TONE

Muscle tone is a condition of muscular firmness that stems from two principal sources: (1) *neurogenic* and (2) *myogenic*. Neurogenic tone is related to a constant state of nerve impulse transmission to the fibers, which maintains the muscles in a condition of partial contraction typified by postural tonus. Myogenic tone pertains to the degree of muscular firmness developed through exercise.

Neurogenic Tone

Neurogenic tone is that portion of tonus that provides a continuous barrage of low-level impulses that enhances firmness. If the muscle is deprived of its nerve supply for a long period of time, flaccidity and ultimately atrophy of the muscle will occur. It would seem that muscles are never in a complete state of rest; however, electromyographic studies by Basmajian[15] suggest that complete relaxation of normal human striated muscle at rest can abolish electrical activity. Thus, tone of a muscle is determined both by the passive elasticity or turgor of muscular (and fibrous) tissues and the active contraction of muscle in response to neural stimuli. At complete rest, a muscle has not lost its tone, even though electric activity is absent. Neurogenic tone probably applies most directly to posture and the myotatic stretch reflex phenomenon. Erect posture automatically triggers the contraction of antigravity or extensor muscles, which provide tone or a continuous state of readiness preventing the body from collapsing. An interesting instrument designed to measure tone called a *myotonometer* was utilized by Gordan.[16] The device determined the degree of hardness in a resting muscle by measuring the muscle's resistance to applied pressure. The major findings of this study indicated that the device differentiates normal from flaccid muscles, and suggests that moderately flaccid muscles recover firmness more rapidly than severely flaccid muscles. Although this instrument may not be as precise as electromyographical evaluation, it does have some practical value as an evaluative tool in rehabilitative medicine for estimating recovery from muscle flaccidity or determining various degrees of muscle relaxation that stem from neuromuscular hypertension.

Myogenic Tone

Residual firmness when a muscle is at rest, resulting from the effects of exercise, is termed *myogenic tone*. Myogenic tone is affected by the type, duration, and intensity of exercises performed. For example, prolonged hard, heavy, resistive-type exercise may induce a condition called *hypertonicity*. The effect of this state of musculature can result in muscle rigidity. In extreme contrast to hypertonicity, soft, flabby, underdeveloped muscles exhibit a condition called *hypotonicity*. The ideal norm for myogenic tone development seems to rest between the extremes of hyper and hypo levels. It appears that a balance between resistive-type exercise, such as manifested by weight lifting and gymnastics, and stretching/suppleness types of movements found in swimming and dance is a logical approach toward gaining desirable levels of myogenic tonus.

Tonus provides shape and contour to muscles. The exact neurological mechanisms that cause muscular differences in appearance is controversial. A sensible explanation appears to embrace the concept of confluency between neurogenic and myogenic elements affecting resting muscle tone. The neurogenic factor provides the basic reflex blueprint, and the myogenic element serves to enhance optimum levels of established neurogenic tone in opposition to flaccidity.

MECHANICAL AND KINETIC CHARACTERISTICS OF MUSCLES

Muscular tissue makes human movement possible and comprises up to 50 percent of body weight in adults. Functionally, muscle contains three important characteristics: (1) *contractility*, (2) *extensibility*, and (3) *elasticity*. Contractility permits fibers to shorten and change their shape, which makes possible such movements as flexion of the biceps and expansion of the chest. *Extensibility* refers to the elongation or stretching quality of muscles. The range from complete contraction to full extension is termed *muscle amplitude*. Amplitude is a significant factor in the flexibility component of fitness. *Elasticity* of muscular tissue relates to the ability of fiber bands to return to their normal resting length following a state of maximum stretching.

Muscle Force-Length Relationship

Muscles pull toward their middle (belly) from points of origin and insertion. The maximum force the muscle can generate is determined, in part, by the contracted muscle's length with respect to its resting length. Generally, as muscles shorten, they become weaker in tensile strength. A curve of the relative contributions of a muscle's contractile force and its inherent elastic resistance to stretch is shown in Figure 4.8. Therefore, a muscle that has shortened loses some of its active tension. Muscles must be stretched from their resting length for most effective action. For example, flexing the knees before jumping from one point to another is necessary before external movement occurs. This places the quadriceps on a stretch. The concept of placing a muscle on a stretch, within normal

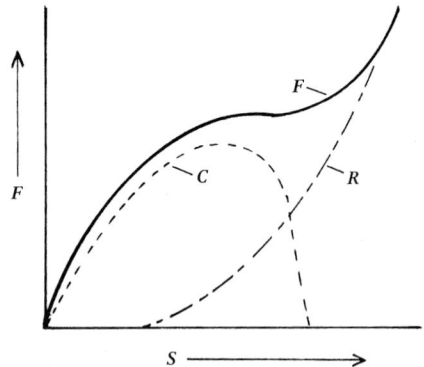

Figure 4.8. Stress–strain curve of skeletal muscle. C: the contractile force that tends to increase to a maximum as the muscle is stretched, and then fall off; R: the passive, elastic resistance to stretch; F: the combined force, which is the pull exerted on the muscle attachments. The vertical axis is the force of muscle pull, the horizontal its length (stretch) (from J.M. Frost, **An Introduction to Biomechanics**, Charles C. Thomas, Springfield, Ill., 1967, with permission)

physiological limits, to obtain its greatest internal force is sound. However, such factors as joint angle must also be considered in determining the effective pulling force of muscles performing external work.

Changing Angle of Pull

In addition to the length–tension relationship, the muscle's angle of pull must be considered in the production of internal work. As the joint angle decreases and angle of pull increases, internal muscular force decreases owing to a weakening of tension created by the shortening process of fibers. Changing the joint angle alters the muscle length. Other biomechanical aspects of rotary and stabilizing components are further discussed in Chapter 7.

Force-Velocity Relationship

Another element that influences muscular contraction is the force-velocity relationship.

The velocity of shortening is greatest when there is no resistance and it diminishes progressively with increasing load or resistance. Figure 4.9 indicates the relationship between contraction velocity and load.

Increased load decreases the velocity of contraction to a point where resistance equals force, resulting in an isometric contraction with zero velocity.

Hypertrophy

Hypertrophy is the antithesis of atrophy. Muscular hypertrophy is an increase in the size of fibers resulting from continued resistive-type exercise training regimens. The mistaken notion that muscles "grow in numbers" probably emanated from the precept that the subunit of the fiber called *myofibrils* increase in number. However, it should be remembered that individual fibers that represent the basic entity in the muscle structural hierarchy do not multiply numerically. The diameters of the individual muscle fibers increase, and the fibers gain in total numbers of myofibrils (actin and myosin filaments) as well as in various nutrient and intermediary metabolic substances such as ATP and glycogen.[17] Therefore, the formative development of new fibers (hyperplasia), as indicated by contemporary evidence, does not occur. Clarke[18] suggests that there is an increase in *packing density* of the small contractile elements within a cell, as well as a change in the ratio of actin to myosin. This hypothesis partially explains the increase in muscle size and change in shape.

Increased muscle size may or may not be accompanied by increased strength. Studies by Wilmore[19] provide some evidence that strength in the upper body of women can be improved up to 30 percent with only a slight increase in muscle size; and a comparable study of males showed slightly less gain in strength but more than double the increase in muscle size. According to Wilmore, muscular hypertrophy is not a necessary consequence of such activities as weight training. It is generally acknowledged that the average male is considerably stronger than the typical female to levels up to 40 percent.[20] This is most likely due to genetic differentials, i.e., more muscle fibers and larger cross section among men than women. It may be postulated, "Everything else being equal (and it very rarely is!)—muscles that contain more fibers should yield greater strength indexes." It should be noted that high levels of muscle bulk are not always followed by increased strength. Females can develop high levels of strength without bulk. This probably results from the predominance of estrogens in females as compared with males. Notwithstanding the androgen–estrogen ratio differential among the sexes, it is now generally recognized that both males and females can equally benefit in strength gains from resistive-type exercise regimens such as weight training.

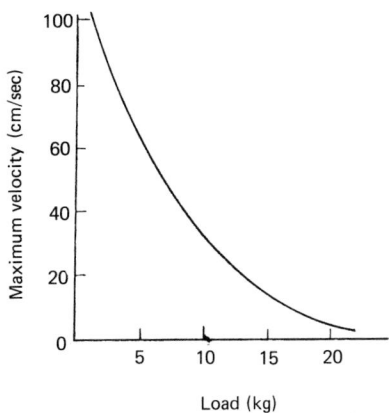

Figure 4.9. Hypothetical relationship between contraction velocity and load (from S. Bouisset, "EMG and Muscle Force in Normal Motor Activity," in **New Developments in Electromyography and Clinical Neurophysiology**, Vol. 1, J.E. Desmedt, (Ed.), Karger, Basel, 1973, pp. 547–583, with permission)

GENERAL MOTOR LEARNING CONSIDERATIONS

The process of acquiring controlled skills— simple or complex, gross or fine movements, athletic or nonathletic—is termed *motor learning*. At the outset, the authors are aware of the magnitude of motor learning theories, studies, and research, ranging from mental emphasis to perceptual-motor problems of the learner. Although a complete treatise on motor learning is not within the scope of this text, certain salient concepts about the learning of skills do have a bearing on the biomechanics of human physical performance. Several selected topics and theorems are presented to provide the reader background information with implications for the study of human movement. The names given to motor learning often depend upon the investigator's field of expertise. For example, the behavioral psychologist concerned with motor learning might be expected to use the term *psychomotor*. The experimenter in physiology may refer to *sensory-motor* learning patterns, and those engaged in cognitive problems refer to nonverbal behavior responses in the specialty of *perceptual-motor* learnings. The biomechanics specialist looks at motor learning in relation to correct application of *kinematic* and *kinetic* principles and laws. Irrespective of orientation, the authors believe that motor skill learning occurs holistically since man functions as a total organism. Dualistic segmentation separating intellectual processes and motor performance is defunct. Motor learning is complex, entailing confluent and integrated mental, emotional, and physiological mechanisms.

Motor skills are frequently thought of as being the exclusive domain of athletic prowess. On the contrary, motor ability and learning connotes movements of all types including knitting, typing, playing a piano or guitar as well as performing a winning "smash" in badminton. Certain individuals possess high levels of motor ability or the capacity to learn skills quickly; others, for a variety of internal or external environmental reasons, struggle to acquire foundational movement patterns. The experienced kinesiologist recognizes that the quality of motor performance is facilitated when constitutional factors and environmental learning elements are coordinated in the learning process.

MATURATION AND MOTOR SKILL LEARNING

Human maturation is the timing and growth rate of biological, psychological, and sociological developmental patterns. In terms of motor skills, it determines *readiness to learn.*

Biological Elements

Maturation is not simply a matter of calendar or chronological age. The concept that individuals mature at different rates is a central precept in learning motor skills. *Skeletal maturation* is one gauge for determining biological maturity. The articulations in the hand and wrist are generally used as an index to bone maturity because of their numerous interconnections, accessibility, and standardized data at different growth periods. Bone growth is of particular concern to coaches involved with adolescents in athletics. The adolescent is subject to several complications in bone injuries. Among these is premature epiphyseal closure. With respect to the upper extremities, injury can result in inflammation of the bone and cartilage.

Knowledge of bone growth maturity and the vulnerability of bone to injury can help to prevent unnecessary trauma as the active youngster participates in sports during the growing years.

Certain body types may be more prone to injury during the growth spurt. For example, the tall, uncoordinated adolescent is more vulnerable to injury than his compactly built counterpart. Individuals so identified should be closely supervised when participating in contact sports such as football.

The development of *phylogenetic* activities (grasping, reaching, turning, crawling) in children appears to proceed according to maturation. *Ontogenetic* activities, such as manipulating objects, swimming, bicycling, and skating rely primarily upon appropriate training and practice. Optimum motor learning develops in children when skills are taught at the right time (maturation-readiness) and in the proper manner (experiences-practices).

In young children, the rate and timing sequence of phylogenetic activities is individualistic. Lockhart[21] points out that although maturation rates vary, the general *sequence* and *direction* of early growth in all children is very similar and orderly. This sequence is as follows: (1) Development proceeds from head to foot (cephalocaudal principle), i.e., control from upper body before lower segments (throwing before kicking); (2) development proceeds from inside to outside (proximodistal principle) control from the center outward (manipulate upper arm before handling objects); and (3) development proceeds from the mass to the specific (large, gross movements before refined patterns). The implication of these maturation series is especially relevant for teachers of young learners. For example, big muscle activities such as tumbling, jumping, and swimming should precede such sports as fancy diving or archery where precision in form and accuracy is required.

Strength and endurance increase with growth and maturity. Therefore, those activities that require these parameters should be considered in the process of motor learning, particularly those movements that demand force for supporting the body or moving its weight from one point to another. Maturation is one variable, among others, i.e., genetics, training, nutrition, nervous integration, which affects the ability and the rate of learning motor skills. The evidence is quite clear that certain strength qualities are necessary for many gross muscular movements. The question of "how much strength" is necessary for the assorted tasks in everyday living and the myriad of athletic sports remains unanswered.

Chronological age is the least accurate in assessing biological maturation. Motor learning activities should be geared to individual characteristics rather than group norms. Each person follows his/her own growth pathway and may not behave in patterns shown by group averages.

Motor skill and learning process probably relate more to maturity than any other single variable, barring pathological growth dysfunctions.

PROGRESSION AND MOTOR LEARNING

The human organism learns motor skills with greater effectiveness when they are presented in progressive order. For example, a forward roll is a progressive step that should precede any attempt in learning a forward somersault. Mechanically, the movement pattern of each stunt is similar, i.e., rotation in a sagittal plane around a frontal-horizontal axis; however, the difficulty and complexity of each maneuver is quite different. The forward somersault requires greater force on the take-off, followed by high-speed rotation in an aerial maneuver; a forward roll simply necessitates rudimentary balance and turning skills without leaving the ground. Fundamental motion patterns should be taught before complex motor skills are introduced. Another type of progression in learning motor skills is progression from the simple to the complex when performing inverted static balance skills. The fundamental squat head balance is mastered before proceeding to the forearm or "tiger" stand; the headstand is learned next, and finally the handstand is attempted. Each of the skills requires progres-

sively greater balance precision. Precision of balance movement is refined gradually with correct practice whereby the learner discovers sensory and motor feedback clues inhibiting extraneous motions and/or accenting other body maneuvers. Basmajian[22] hypothesizes that the perfection of motor skills is largely dependent upon controlling undesired muscular contractions by learning to inhibit non-useful motor neural activity.

A variety of activities can be successfully learned by a sequential gradation process. Push and glide skills precede coordinated arm/leg stroking in swimming, and lead-up games comprised of baseball handling skills precede participation in sophisticated sports and games such as basketball or baseball. Progressive skill teaching should not be confused with whole, part, or whole–part methods of teaching. The simple-to-complex continuum pertains to a particular skill as a whole, whereas the whole or part methods of teaching deal with the segmentation of an activity or skill to be learned.

MOTOR LEARNING FACILITATORS

Motor learning is a self-discovery process producing growth and change in motor performance. Growth and change in motor skills normally occur when the learner actively participates and correctly practices skills through assorted repetitive training designs related to the task at hand. The well-known cliché "learning by doing" is a central concept that is vital in the learning process. Successful development of skills cannot take place unless the learner is intimately involved in utilizing neural mechanisms of the nervous pathways and body movements of the skeletal and muscular systems, The learner must want to learn before changes can effectively occur. The following topics may be termed as *facilitators* for the enhancement of motor skills. These topics do not represent an exhaustive list, but reflect our view of salient areas that affect the learner.

Whole and Part Learning

Should a skill be presented as a whole or should it be broken down into its constituent parts? Categorical answers cannot be made because of the complexity of skill learning. In addition to reorganizing maturation of the learner, the complexity of the skill to be learned should be considered before deciding upon segmental or whole teaching procedures. Complicated motor skills, entailing subunits of basic movement, need some sort of a breakdown for effective learning. For example, teaching the coordinated timing of leg kick and arm action in swimming can be taught separately, and then presented as a whole after rudimentary learning has been achieved. An early study by Shay[23] provides some evidence that the whole method is superior to the progressive-part method. The kip-up on the horizontal bar was taught in progressive series: (1) arch on forward swing, (2) hip flexion on the backward swing, and (3) hip extension on the forward swing. Shay reported that the whole method of presenting the skill was superior because relationships between parts of the movement (timing) are learned simultaneously with body positions.

Studies on whole and part learning demonstrate mixed preferences.[23,24] It appears that the whole method is preferred over the part approach. However, the evidence is not conclusive. In certain sports, the whole method is preferable when the activity is composed of continuous or serial movements that form a chained sequence and in activities where speed and timing are fundamental to the basic pattern. This rationale appears to support the logic of teaching a successive movement such as juggling via the whole method. The skill to be learned should not always be presented as a whole except when the performance requires its practice as an entity for successful execution. Whenever the part method is used, it should always relate in some fashion to the whole. In a skill such as the breaststroke, correct kicking action or arm pull taught in separate parts will not assure the learner of proper timing; however, these subskills do have individual unit integrity and can be learned separately without destroying the pattern of the total stroke. The unification of arm pull and leg kick to produce effective propulsion is a skill unit in itself and can be effectively taught after the constituent leg and arm actions are satisfactorily learned. Complexity of the skill is one variable that, in certain instances, demands the whole approach and, on the other hand, requires a segmental breakdown depending upon the individual components of the skill to be learned and other factors such as the nature and characteristics of the learner.

Specificity versus Generality

In particular instances, athletic sport and motor skills may be related, but on other occasions similar skill characteristics are not connected. For example, although an individual may be expert in badminton, that person may not possess the same level of skill in tennis. Body builders with symmetrical physiques and high levels of muscle hypertrophy may not have the neuromuscular qualities necessary for gymnastics. On the other hand, divers often transfer their acrobatic skill to the trampoline—yet, from one of the author's (Piscopo) gymnastic and swimming coaching experiences, skilled trampolinists seldom become champion divers. Are successful pole vaulters fast rope climbers? What are the motor learning relationships between gymnastics, tumbling, pole vaulting, and diving? *Specificity of practice* implies that practice in one particular motor task does not transfer to a similar skill unless the neuromuscular requirements are directly related. Some confusion exists about the specificity of learning a skill and specificity of performance ability. For example, similar skills in tumbling might well transfer or enhance one's ability to learn fancy diving skills; however, since springboard diving primarily entails head-first entries preceded by an approach and the intricate mechanics of a run, hurdle, take-off, execution, and entry, specific proficiency in ground tumbling may not directly transfer to the graceful technique of completing a forward one-and-one-half somersault (performance ability).

Sports and athletic events are composites of specific skills that contain similar and, in certain instances, identical movement patterns. For example, a full twist employs the same mechanical motions whether it is performed on a trampoline or in diving; the principal difference is landing in water or on the webbed. The actual twisting mechanic can be transferred from one sport to another. But, as indicated previously, trampoline specialists may not exhibit the graceful and precise qualities required of a diver. Other factors such as the approach and entry into the water present significant differences that alter definitive conclusions favoring the general motor learning and ability concept. There appears to be scant evidence supporting the transfer of skills from one sport to another. Many variables enter the scene, such as motivation, physique, teacher effectiveness, and similarity of movements within and between skills. Several questions and further research concerning the relationship between and among various types of dynamic and static balance categories are discussed in Chapter 8.

Although certain studies point to the general acceptance of task-specificity, the authors believe that specificity of skills is one variable involved in the transfer process that can positively or negatively affect learning depending upon the *nature of the learner, environmental influences,* and *teacher effectiveness.* Each of these variables has a combined effect upon the others that makes it ex-

tremely difficult to quantify data objectively without segmentation of the holistic concept of human movement. The reader is referred to "Individual Differences in Motor Performance and Learning," by R. G. Marteniuk[25] for further analysis of the topic.

Distributive versus Mass Practice

One of the authors (Piscopo) utilized a verbal principle of repetition with his divers by repeating the phrase, "The first 500 times of performing the forward 2½ somersault will be hit and miss—the 501st execution will be of championship caliber!" Of course, the objective was to arouse and motivate the diver to practice continuously with belief in the premise of the well-known cliché, "practice makes perfect." Such a statement assumes that the performer practices the *correct* application of mechanical principles. Practice does not make perfect unless certain conditions are nurtured together with proper mechanics. Two variables that have been studied by psychologists and physical educators are (1) practice over a period of time and (2) practice with concentrated or massed repetition with little or no rest. The effects of distributive and mass practice are explored with implications for the acquisition and performance of motor skills.

The evidence as to whether distributive practice is more effective than massed practice on motor learning is inconclusive. Some research favors short distributive practice sessions over mass concentrated practice periods.[26,27] Similar to the issue of generality versus specificity, the effect of practice factors are multifold. Such elements as *motivation, rest, complexity of skill, individuality of the learner,* and *teacher effectiveness* can influence distributive or mass practice results.

Whether massed or distributive practice procedures are used, it is important to remember the purpose of the task at hand. Where a peak level of an already learned motor skill is sought, massing practice may be desired, provided adequate rest and the avoidance of "staleness" is considered. Long, boring repetitive-type skills probably can best be learned via distributive practice models. Sage[28] has proposed several principles that appear logical, but are subject to exceptions depending upon variable conditions:

1. Distributed practice is more efficient when the task has energy demands and is complex, the length of task performance is great and not meaningful, and motivation of the learner is low.

2. Massed practice is preferable when the skill level is high, and peak performance on a well-learned skill is needed.

3. Massed practice may be effective when the skill is highly meaningful, motivation is high, and a considerable transfer is present from previously learned tasks to the new task.

Speed and Accuracy Aspects

What effect do speed and accuracy have on motor skill learning? Should a skill be learned at low speed and then increased to high speed after acquisition is attained? At what point in the learning process should precision or accuracy be stressed? These questions are continuously raised by physical educators about teaching motor skills. It is generally accepted that when speed and accuracy are necessary for successful performance of the skill to be learned, then these two factors should be stressed simultaneously in the initial stages. Conversely, if the ultimate performance does not specifically rely upon these variables, a slower pace, executing the skill in gross accuracy and form is effective. However, whether speed and accuracy are stressed depends upon other factors as well, such as the nature of the learner and the goal to be attained. In certain instances, speed should not be initially emphasized. For example, a nov-

ice gymnast, practicing the hip and back extension and flexion sequence of a backward handspring quickly learns that "rushing" or hastening the initial backward swing to the hands causes a backward somersault movement, rather than the back-bend motion, to the hands. Initial learning proceeds best, in this instance, by practicing the extension move slowly, until the student learns the kinesthetic feel of hip flexion. After the performer has learned the "timing" sequence at a slower pace, speed of the whole backward handspring will increase at a rapid rate, assuming that the proper mechanics are applied. In contrast, a performer attempting to negotiate a low or high hurdle must consider a minimum threshold of speed in straddling the hurdle. Speed of movement should be emphasized in the early learning stage since this variable is inherently part of successful execution.

In skills in which both speed and accuracy are important to successful performance, emphasis on both speed and accuracy yields the most desirable results. Some evidence stresses the value of emphasizing speed and accuracy when these variables are part of the desired polished performance such as targeting an object while moving the entire body. This would also include a skill such as fencing. Emphasizing accuracy and speed simultaneously is contrary to *Poppelreuter's law of practice* (PLP),[29] which advocates the development of accuracy before speed is emphasized with the hypotheses that accuracy is gained more effectively at a low rate of speed and that accuracy obtained at low rates is sustained when speed is increased. Although this law may not apply to the sport of tennis, the authors believe that in certain activities PLP has value, as discussed in the gradual build-up of speed in teaching the backward handspring. The attainment of speed, which is one criterion of high-level performance in this particular motor skill, will normally occur after the correct form is reasonably learned according to correct biomechanical principles.

Mental Practice and Motor Learning

Mental practice, whereby the individual passively mimics or images the performance of a particular movement, generally facilitates the acquisition of skills. However, it should be noted that mental practice is more effective when the learner has experienced the actual physical practice of the motor task at hand. Mental practice can be used to facilitate learning of high-level skills by providing a "thinking" mechanism of reviewing the actual performance in the "mind's eye." For example, a diver "thinks about" raising the hurdle leg for greater board depression in attaining maximum height, which sequentially will allow more time for a graceful execution of the water entry. Mental practice probably has greater value in activities that require fine motor control such as diving, high jumping, pole vaulting, gymnastics, golf, and complex movements found in individual and team sports.

FEEDBACK MECHANISMS AND MOTOR LEARNING

Feedback connotes the return of information from external or internal environmental sources; which results in perception awareness and correction adjustment, if necessary, to produce a skilled motion pattern. Information can be received from *external sources*, which include changes occurring outside the body and picked up by the sense organs such as hearing and vision. This type of feedback provides information and knowledge about the outside world. For example, a performer is utilizing an extrinsic feedback mechanism for the improvement of a specific skill. A diver speeding up his approach and takeoff resulting from a "quick" or "stiff" board is receiving external clues and feedback. *Internal feedback* stems from receptor organs that record the information and affect the necessary movement to create the desired body action. Proprioceptive feedback, which is an integral constituent of kinesthesis, is one type of internal retriever. For example, the "right amount of grip," in relation to a flat drive shot in tennis, is signaled from the proprioceptive nerve endings located in the periphery of the hand. Internal and external feedback is vital for the development and facilitation of motor skills.

Kinesthesis

A highly skilled movement pattern is characterized by a kinesthetic fluency, or ease of motion with superb efficiency and form. The ultimate in sophisticated motion is devoid of rigidity and errors and is the hallmark of the champion athlete. The term *kinesthesis* is of Greek derivation: *Kinesis* = motion, and *asthesia* = to perceive; medical clinicians classify kinesthesis under *bathesthesia*.[30] The receptors of kinesthesis emanate from muscle spindles, tendons, and inner ear sources as described in Chapter 8.

It should be pointed out that *kinesthesis* and *proprioception* are often used as synonyms. The authors view proprioception as part of kinesthesis. The term *kinesthesis* was invented by Bastian in 1883.[31] Bastian included the labyrinth mechanism of the inner ear because of its role in balance. Historically, kinesthesis and proprioception may be classified differently; however, from a functional view, these sensory modalities overlap and, together, serve to contribute feedback information about body position. This motor sense has been studied by physiologists and psychologists. Psychologists generally view kinesthesis from the behavioral response perspective. For example, they explore the effect of various kinesthetic cues upon attention, memory retention, and perceptual skills. Physiologists study this sensory modality from a neurological aspect with a focus on evaluating its inherent medical soundness in structure and function. Physical educators are primarily interested in the application of psychological parameters and physiological characteristics of kinesthesis for the development and improvement of motor and athletic skills. The ensuing discussion accents kinesthesis from a motor-learning and skill-development perspective, which is considered a central concern of all health and physical education professionals.

Several curious questions arise about the role of kinesthesis from a motor development point of view. At what point in motor learning does this sensory modality contain its greatest impact—early or late stages? Is kinesthesis specific or general? Can this quality be measured accurately? How is balance and equilibrium interwoven with kinesthetic sensitivity? Does this quality diminish with age? Several of these topics are examined in the following sections.

Specific or General. Kinesthetic receptors respond to such movement qualities as (1) *duration, direction, velocity and amplitude;* (2) *body positions;* (3) *muscular tension;* and (4) *relative positions* of the total body. It can be seen at once from the above responses that the quality of kinesthetic control entails an integrative functioning of the skeletal, muscular, and nervous systems. The authors contend that one's optimum "position sense" or "motor sense" results from a combination of exteroceptive and proprioceptive (kinesthetic cues) functioning in concert and includes such components as balance, flexibility, muscular tonus, and, indirectly, the five sense organs. Input from other sensory modalities shape the physiological and psychological response of what we call *kinesthesis.* Scott[32] conducted an extensive analysis in 28 mea-

sures of kinesthesis including such items as static balance, dynamic balance, body sway, walk and turn, push and pull, weight lifting, flexion and extension movements, all of which relate to kinesthetic functioning. This investigator concluded:

1. Tests in general show little interrelationship, leading one, at present, to assume considerable specificity of function.

2. Several combinations of tests appear to have validity value for further use.

3. The sensation of kinesthesis is made up of many elements or forms of response. There is little or no evidence that it might be of a general capacity.

Contemporary evidence does support the specificity of kinesthesis; however, the exact method of functioning of the mechanism is relatively unknown. One's "position sense" is a remarkable body control mechanism that indirectly receives input from other sensory organs to fulfill its role of indicating "where" and "how" we are postured in the realm of human movement.

Kinesthetic Perception Tests

Various practical tests of kinesthetic perception have been identified to determine, at least in part, measurement of this sensory feedback modality. Johnson and Nelson[33] describe several tests that can be used in a classroom or gymnasium setting and recommend a combination of specific tests to form a battery, since no single kinesthetic test has a high enough validity coefficient to warrant its exclusive use. The reader is referred to reference 33 for detailed instructions for the administration of specific test batteries.

Kinesthetic perception training is an important concern in programs for the mentally retarded. An interesting modified test of horizontal and vertical linear space was devised by Beter and Cragin[34] to determine specific

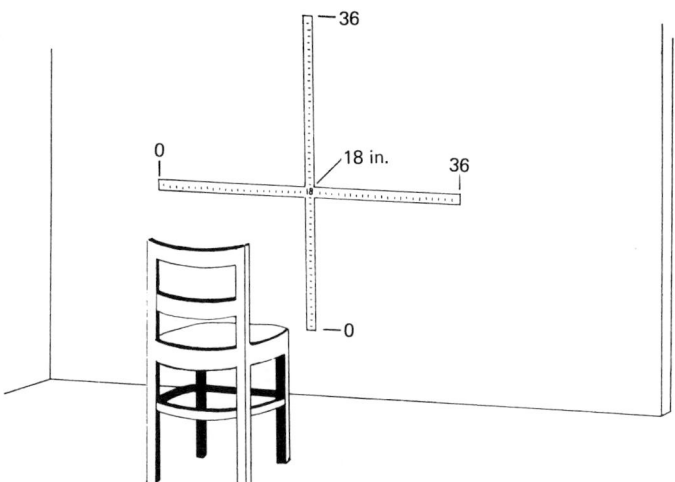

Figure 4.10. Modified test of horizontal and vertical linear space (from Thais R. Beter and Wesley E. Cragin, **The Mentally Retarded Child and His Motor Behavior**, Charles C. Thomas Co., Springfield, Ill., 1972, p. 71, with permission)

positions of the arm along horizontal and vertical lines. Figure 4.10 illustrates the equipment and general arrangement for administering the test.

The procedure requires a chart placed on the wall in front of the seated individual so that the 18-inch mark is at eye level. The person is instructed to point to the 18-inch mark, look at it, and try to sense the position of the arm. The individual is then blindfolded and instructed to point to the same spot again. Scoring is based upon three trials, and on each trial, deviations in both vertical and horizontal positions are recorded. All deviations in the vertical plane are then totaled, and all deviations in the horizontal plane are also totaled.

The above test combines the horizontal and linear space tests and has an advantage in saving time in test administration. Most test batteries assessing kinesthesis include a balancing item that entails a given sensitivity measure when blindfolded, which requires the performer to discount visual clues.

Kinesthetic Learning Points

At what point can kinesthetic clues be best utilized in motor learning? Research evidence does show that athletes generally possess better kinesthetic characteristics than nonathletes. The question arises regarding source of acquisition of kinesthesis. Does it improve as a result of continuous training? When should kinesthetic practice by introduced in the skill-acquisition sequence? The blueprint of constitutional individual differences provides the mold for development. Kinesthesis can be improved through gross and fine motor activity, and, conversely, motor skills can be quickly learned depending upon inherent kinesthetic qualities. It appears that kinesthesis has great impact both early and late in the motor skill developmental process. Piscopo[35,36] utilized the trampoline to help develop a sense of "body relocation," which in effect is kinesthesis. Many programs for exceptional populations such as schools for the deaf, blind, and mentally retarded employ the "rebounding" skill used in trampolining for the enhancement of kinesthesis.

Although some research indicates that kinesthetic cues are significant at early learning stages, some evidence shows that kinesthesis clues are more important in later stages of motor skill learning.[37] We do know that kinesthesis affects the development of motor skills; however, the exact manner of "how" and "when" remains unclear. Whenever a conflict exists between visual clues and kinesthetic reception, vision dominates over the latter in skill learning.[38] The authors believe that the nature of the skill has a significant impact concerning this point. In certain instances visual clues may cause neural conflicts with kinesthesis when both feedback receptors are operating. This even can occur in such highly complex skills typified by a one-hand stand whereby balance (a component of kinesthesis) may be lost, if the performer overdepends upon eye focus at a particular reference point.

Several conclusions are advanced; however, it should be pointed out that not all experts are in agreement with the statements listed:

1. Kinesthesis is considered specific — composed of a number of elements, directed to a particular motor skill and/or body area.

2. Kinesthesis appears to be related to low and high motor skills with uncertain effects upon the so-called average level skill proficiency.

3. Visual clues may or may not conflict with motor skill learning, depending upon the task and level of the learner.

4. Practice can improve kinesthetic perception.

5. Balance and equilibrium are integral components of kinesthesis.

Knowledge of Results (KR)

Knowledge of results is considered a member of the *extrinsic* feedback family. Most au-

thorities on motor learning agree that knowledge of results must be provided to sustain motivation and facilitate learning. Certainly, teachers and coaches use the principle of KR in their everyday teaching and practice experiences. For example, a diver awarded a score of 8 in the performance of a forward one-and-one-half somersault is receiving immediate information feedback. The performer stores this result in his memory bank, thinking how to reduce his errors and improve his diving award on the next dive. Electronic instruments such as television and video tape provide feedback information in a variety of ways, some of which are discussed in Chapter 15.

Feedback is an integral part of the teaching–learning process, and the authors believe that if KR is poorly utilized, little or no learning will occur. However, when this extrinsic mode is appropriately employed, augmentation in improving motor skills to the desired outcome can happen. For example, positive reinforcement can result when the coach keeps split times on a swimmer attempting to establish a certain pace for each length in the 200-yard event and informs the swimmer immediately following a trial. Negative learning can occur when the same swimmer is given inaccurate time for his actual performance. Two important variables alter the effectiveness of KR: (1) *timing and frequency* of receiving information feedback and (2) *accuracy of results.*

Timing and Frequency of Receiving Information Feedback. "Strike while the iron is hot" — this cliché has been said many times, and has particular relevance to KR in motor learning. Research evidence is rather unclear about exact delay-time intervals between performance and results; however, the authors subscribe to the notion that, "the longer the delay in delivering knowledge of results to the performer, the less effect the KR has in augmenting the learning of motor skills." Of course, exceptions always occur. This generalization becomes clear when the delay is extensive. For example, if a swimmer is turning to the right as he enters the water with the right arm leading in a somersault turn, and knowledge of this error is delayed over several days, correction of his performance is retarded since the swimmer may not be aware of his error. On the other hand, the coach who informs the student quickly allows extrinsic feedback to operate with minimum probability of the individual "forgetting" the performance error.

Accuracy of Results. How precisely should the results of a performance be related to the learner? Should the instructor analyze and point out specific quantitative information, or should remarks be made in general terms? For example, the instructor may say: That was a "good" forward roll, or that was a "poor" execution in the turning phase of the roll. Some research points to accuracy of results as a critical factor. If the information is precise, better performance will result.[39] The practical conclusion to KR precision points to a greater value of indicating results of a performance with some degree of specificity of "how and why" rather than the vague comment of such remarks as "well done" or "good job."

Several basic principles from assorted studies on the topic of KR follow.[40] It should be remembered that these principles are not absolute, and exceptions may occur depending upon the nature of the task at hand and the characteristics of the learner responding in a particular environment.

1. Learning is proportionally greater as the quality, exactness, and precision of this playback of knowledge results increases.

2. With a delay of knowledge of results, performance declines.

3. Performance deteriorates when knowledge of results is withdrawn.

4. Precise supplemental aids (graphs, films of action, etc.), which provide a more precise knowledge or make apparent the differences between the learner's performance and those of better performers, seem to increase learning.

5. Feedback of incorrect information retards learning in direct proportion to the amount of misinformation.

Knowledge of Mechanical Principles

Mention should be made about knowledge of mechanical principles in the acquisition of motor skills. Evidence appears to indicate that analytical emphasis during the teaching-learning can enhance skill development. Timing and introduction of such information is important. For example, the authors utilized the principle in the mechanics of buoyancy in teaching: *tuck, prone,* and *supine* back floats. Cognitive aspects of discussing the relationship between the center of gravity and center of buoyancy, body composition, and their effect on floating were introduced in the classroom. The mechanical principles were subsequently presented in the pool with participating students applying the lever principle of rotating around the center of buoyancy. The impact of combining the "why" and "how" has been extremely effective with the majority of students learning their most efficient floating position. The following guidelines are recommended when employing mechanical principles in teaching motor skills:

1. Consider the appropriate time for the introduction of mechanics. Beginners in any skill need initial practice before complicated theories on force, velocity, momentum, and leverage are presented.

2. Select principles carefully. One or two concepts that have *direct* relevance to the performance at hand should be presented.

3. Allow students time to test out the principle presented. For example, flexing the knees and extending the arms overhead will concretely demonstrate the balancing effect of the first-class lever in the supine horizontal floating position.

4. Increase the sophistication in use of mechanical terms according to: (1) intellectual level, and (2) skill level of the performer.

5. Use mechanical terms to arouse motivation and interest when appropriate; however, do not substitute verbal analysis for practice time, particularly among beginner level students.

MANUAL AND MECHANICAL GUIDANCE

Manual Guidance

Manual guidance refers to leading or directing the learner by assisting and guiding the limbs or whole body through a motor skill. For example, the young learner is manually guided when the instructor places one hand behind the neck area and the other hand on the upper leg assisting the student to keep the head "down" and hips "up" as the neophyte experiences the kinesthetic sensation of a forward head-first dive.

Experimental evidence has revealed conflicting results about the effectiveness of such practice.[41] Some experts conclude that this procedure facilitates learning while others hold a contrary view. It is true that certain individuals are annoyed by physical assistance and prefer to discover for themselves how the motor skill "feels." It has been the authors' experience in teaching beginning swimming and gymnastic skills that such guidance is helpful when the student is experiencing difficulty with fundamental mechanics or execution. Another example of utilizing manual guidance is when the instructor assists the learner with extension of the hips at the proper moment during the execution of a floor kip-up from the mat. Certain individuals will learn a motor skill with a verbal explanation and demonstration. Learners must percep-

tually experience the kinesthetic feel of a motor skill task in a self-directed way and manual guidance merely gives the student a gross idea of a successful performance. Manual guidance probably has greater value in teaching *closed-type skills*, i.e., performance executed in a fixed environment such as found in gymnastics, golf, bowling, etc., as opposed to *open-type skills*, where environmental surroundings are continually changing, typified by basketball, tennis and softball.

Mechanical Guidance

Mechanical guidance implies the use of devices such as safety belts in tumbling and trampoline, swim fins, or pitching machines in baseball. The intent of such mechanical aids is to direct the performer through the correct movement and, at the same time, provide a measure of safety. For example, the gymnast learning a complex skill such as the double backward somersault on the trampoline can concentrate on the correct mechanics of the skill with a margin of safety provided by a trained safety belt operator. Individuals experiencing difficulty in learning the forward propulsive movement of the flutter kick in swimming can be significantly assisted through use of swim fins. Fins allow the swimmer to "feel" the correct undulating action of the legs as the body is thrust forward through the water. Piscopo utilized a combination of hand and foot swim fins with cerebral palsied individuals. Some of these students learned to swim a width of the pool with the aid of fins. Likewise mechanical guidance probably has greater significance for young learners, and to those older individuals where the ability to develop coordinated neuromuscular movements is not at optimum levels.

The principal benefit of manual and mechanical guidance procedures is that they allow the learner, experiencing difficulty with a motor skill, to "feel" or develop a kinesthetic awareness of how a particular movement is executed. If the learner moves through the learning sequence with success, then these types of techniques should be employed; however, if the student becomes frustrated and manifests little or no progress, manual and/or mechanical guidance should be discontinued.

REACTION TIME AND MOTOR LEARNING

Inevitably, physical educators and coaches discover distinct differences in motor behavior responses among their charges. Certain performers are typed as "quick movers," others identified as persons with "slow reflexes." These metaphors are commonly utilized to describe an individual's reaction time. A vast amount of research has been completed on reaction time and the speed of movement in relation to motor performance in the fields of physical education, psychology, and physiology. *Reaction time* may be defined as the period from the presentation of a stimulus to the beginning of the response. This motor behavior parameter is of paramount interest to athletic coaches because of the traditional positive relationship between fast reaction time and athletic performance. In certain sports reaction time can make the difference in winning or losing a race. For example, swimmers competing in the 50 yard event must respond immediately to the starter's gun since this particular racing event is often decided within a tenth of a second. Reaction time should not be confused with *movement time*, which is the actual time from the beginning of the response to a stimulus through the accomplishment of the motor task. It would seem that individuals who possess fast reaction time also exhibit fast movement time; however, studies show that a low relationship exists between these two variables.[42,43] Simply stated, although an individual may immediately react to a stimulus, quick perception does not insure fast

muscle movement to complete a motor task. Many factors enter the performance scene.

Individual differences and particular characteristics of a motor task are probably the most significant variables affecting the quality of reaction and movement times. Several important points that have implications for motor skill development are summarized[44]:

1. Reaction time varies according to the type of stimulus (visual, auditory, tactile, olfactory, gustatory, and pain).

2. Sometimes the strength and/or duration of the stimulus influences the reaction time.

3. Another factor influencing reaction time is readiness for response; i.e., whether the subject is warned before the response, the length of time before warning, and the actual stimulation presentation.

4. Reaction time also seems to improve to a point with age in the younger years and then worsens during old age. (This point varies greatly among older persons. The student is referred to Chapter 14 for a detailed discussion of reaction time as relates to aging).

5. Finally, reaction time varies as to the physiological and psychological state of the subject. If the subject is fatigued, sick, worried, and so on, reaction time will probably be influenced.

MOTOR SKILL CLASSIFICATIONS

An outline of motor skill analysis usually contains a descriptive and/or unique list of characteristics of the motor task under study. Several physical education skills are briefly explored and considered with relevance to skill development.

Closed and Open Skills

Skills may be classified in accordance to their environmental situations. Those skills in

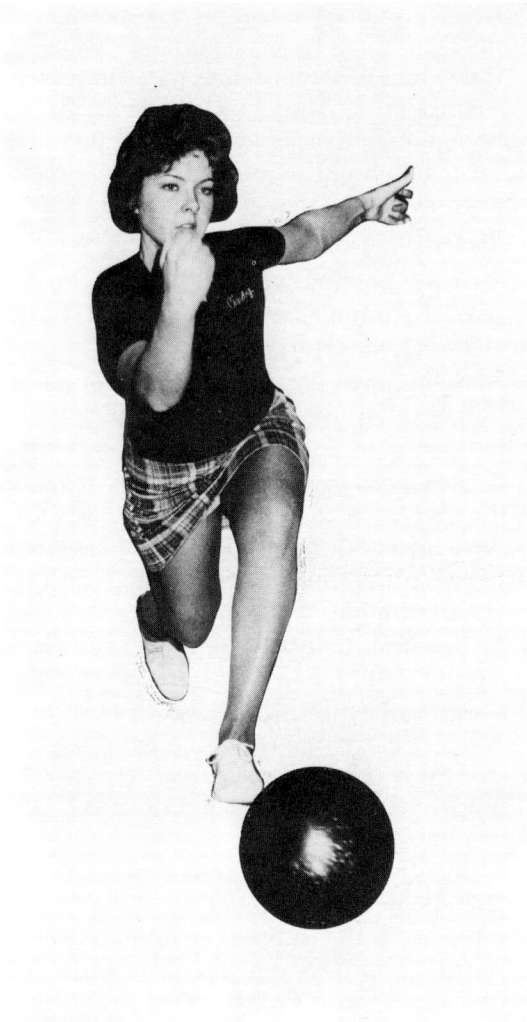

Figure 4.11. Bowling—closed motor skill

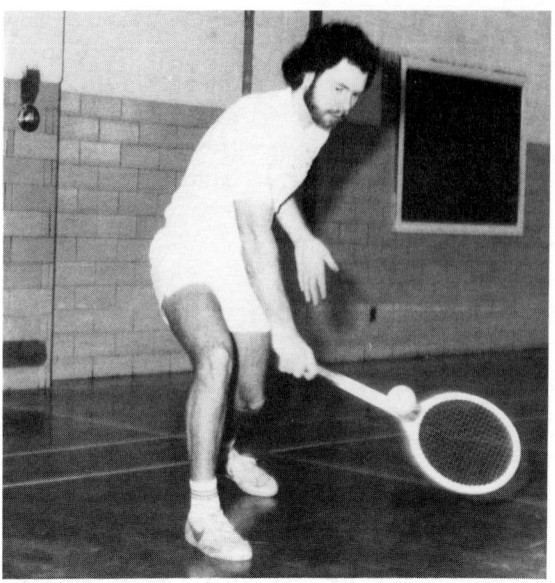

Figure 4.12. Tennis—open motor skill

which the critical cues for performance are fixed or static in one position are called *closed skills* (see Figure 4.11). For example, such skills as bowling, golf and gymnastics are closed skills.

Skills performed in an environmental setting that is continually changing are termed *open skills* (see Figure 4.12). Skills such as basketball, tennis, and football typify open skills.

Open skills are conducted in an environment that is constantly changing. Open skills are not predictable, and correct motor response depends upon meeting changing environmental conditions that, in part, are usually determined by the opposing competitor. Dual and team sports are reflective of open skills. On the other hand, closed skills are predictable. For example, a gymnast practicing a kip-up on the parallel bars can repeat the same movement over again without the stress of change, and the skill can be executed the same way a number of times with the performer sharpening his own precision and form with the correct application of laws of motion. Closed skills can be quantified and evaluated in an objective fashion more easily than an open skill because the pattern is fixed while the action pattern of open skills is changing every moment.

The principal difference between open and closed skills lies in response behavior. Closed skills operate in a constant environment and skill improvement is enhanced with correct practice and repetition; open skills are very

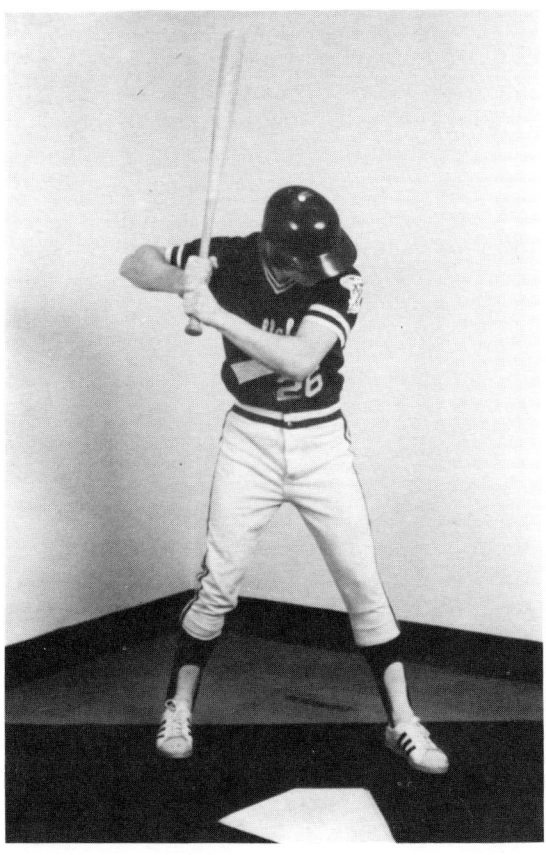

Figure 4.13. Hitting a baseball—a discrete motor skill (from **The Athletic Journal**, 59:23, 1979, Evanston, Ill., with permission)

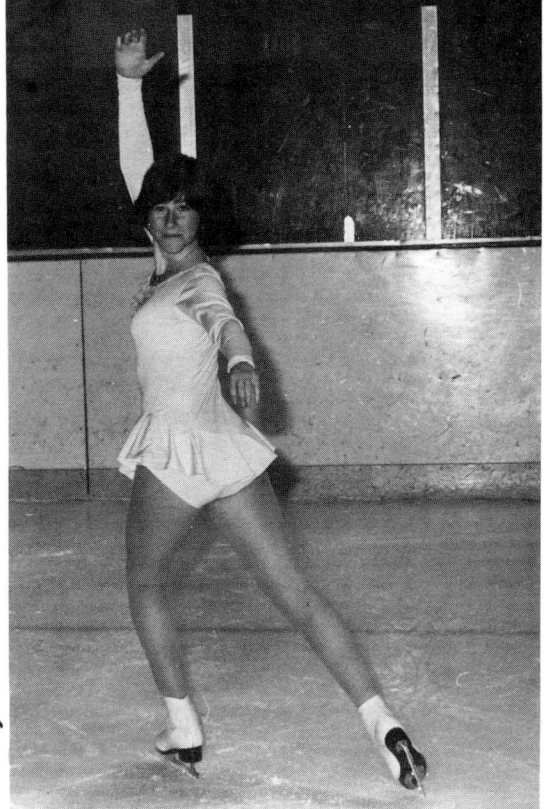

Figure 4.14. Skating—a continuous skill

rarely duplicated in the same manner. Flexibility and a multitude of varied motor responses are needed for a successful performance.

Discrete and Continuous Motor Skills

Another way in which motor skills can be categorized is through movement flow. Certain skills begin and end with a definite effort. For example, tossing a bean bag into a marked circle or hitting a baseball may be termed a *discrete skill* (see Figure 4.13). Other motor tasks do not abruptly end, but continue in a series over a long period of time and are usually repetitive in nature. Activities such as running, bicycling, swimming, and skating are called *continuous skills* (see Figure 4.14). Discrete and continuous skill types relate to the retention of motor performance. Such skills as walking, swimming, and skating are retained indefinitely once the skill is learned well. Skill retention applies most directly to continuous or serial-type activities. On the other hand, discrete skills are not remembered as well, unless continuous practice is sustained. For example, proficiency is lost for performing a discrete task such as a handstand or shooting a basketball or a net shot in badminton, after an extended period of time without practice.

The identification of motor skills as discrete or continuous types has implications for learning and retaining proficiency in motor performance. Many continuous skills are easily recalled after long terms of practice abstinence, particularly in those sports that do not require acute qualities of speed, accuracy, or precision. Many lifetime sports are of the continuous type: bicycling, walking/jogging, swimming, skating, etc.; therefore, those individuals who learn these skills well early in life have a better opportunity to recall and perform these skills without undue complications than those persons attempting to perform an underlearned sport skill.

Gross and Fine Motor Skills

Motor skills may also be classified as *gross* or *fine* muscular responses. *Fine motor skills* entail delicate or precise movements of the body and/or body parts requiring sensitive neuromuscular coordination. Activities such as typing, handwriting, dart throwing, and target shooting are fine motor skills. Gross motor skills are "big muscle" activities such as jumping, running, and ball throwing that require full body motion, in either manipulation or movement from one point to another. It should be remembered that many big muscle activities contain elements of fine motor skills. For example, the precision of a superb entry in diving requires fine neuromuscular coordination and body adjustments, including small and large muscle groups. Gross motor skills, expertly performed with precision, accuracy, and superlative form very often contain the elements of fine skill characteristics. Therefore, motor skills can be analyzed from two perspectives; (1) large or small muscle involvement, and (2) coarse or refined performance quality. Cratty[45] identifies a group of activities that entail large and small muscle groups, shown in Figure 4.15.

Many of the manual or manipulative skills, such as aiming, finger dexterity, or arm-hand steadiness, require precision and accuracy and are considered fine motor skills as compared with the large muscle activity typified by a forward roll and other multilimbed skills such as swimming, running, and jumping. In the study and analysis of skills, it is important to keep in mind the advantages in proceeding from the simple to the complex. Whether gross or fine skills are classified from a muscle-magnitude or refined-quality perspective, motor learning also proceeds from large to small muscle involvement.

SUMMARY

The nervous system operates a network of bioelectrochemical impulses that initiate and direct the body's mental, emotional, and physical activities. Voluntary functions fall primarily within the domain of the central nervous system, composed of the brain and spinal cord. The peripheral nervous system, comprised of nerves, ganglia, and end organs, responds to involuntary or automatic needs and functions of the body. The somatic and autonomic sectors are subunits of the peripheral system.

The basic unit of the nervous system is the neuron. Neurons are grouped into three general classes: (1) sensory, (2) motor, and (3) interneurons.

The brain is the central core of the nervous system; with its component elements including the cerebrum, cerebellum, pons, and medulla oblongata, the brain governs the intellectual aspects of the mind and modulation of motor movements.

Stability of the spine arises from intrinsic and extrinsic sources. Most sport injuries to the spinal column are related to excessive movements beyond normal ranges of motion and/or extreme spinal compression.

Motor responses that do not involve the brain, such as the knee jerk, are at the spinal cord level. Subconscious motor activities such as respiration, cardiac activity, and vasomotor control are governed at the lower

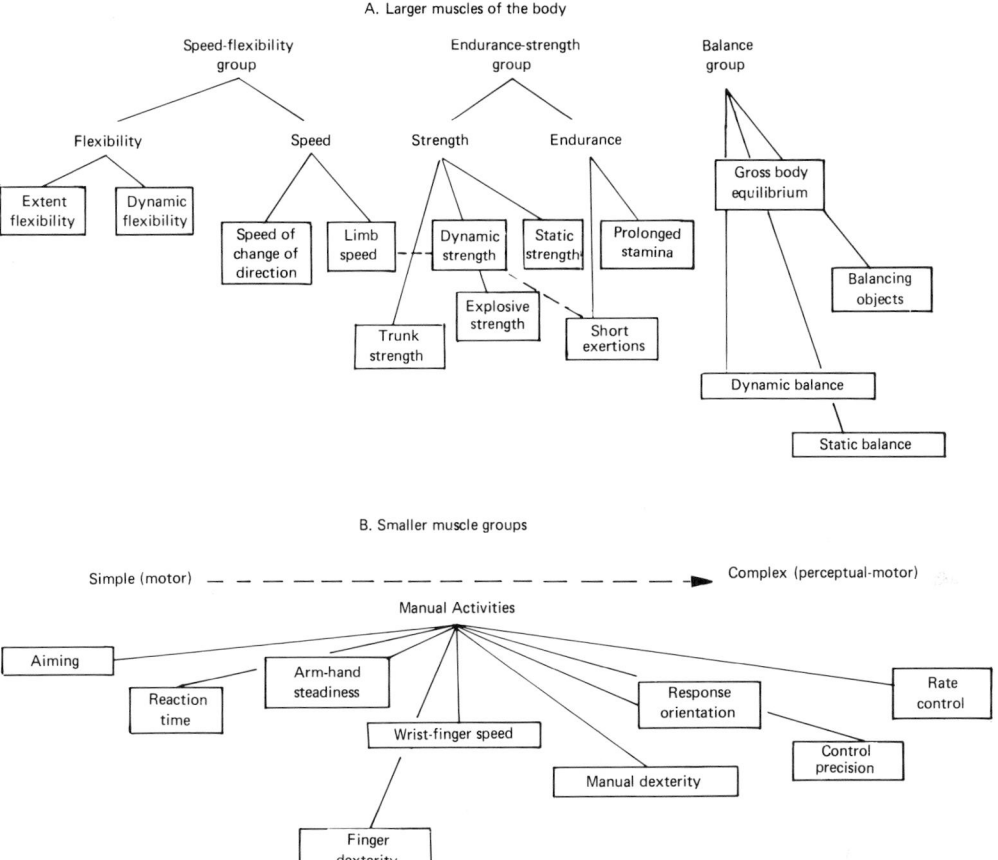

Figure 4.15. Motor ability traits—large and smaller muscle groups (from Bryant J. Cratty, **Movement Behavior and Motor Learning**, 3rd ed., Lea and Febiger, Philadelphia, 1973, p. 210, with permission)

brain level. Cognitive and intellectual functions such as reasoning and intelligence are controlled at the higher brain level.

A neuron is the basic unit necessary for the stimulation and transmission of neuromuscular activity from gross to refined motor movements. Medullated neurons contain a neurilemma sheath, related to the regenerating ability of peripheral nerves. Most fibers of the brain and cord are not medullated and cannot regenerate.

Nerve impulses are transmitted from nerve to nerve via the synapse and are conveyed from nerve to muscle through the motor end plate. The transmission of nerve impulse is a bioelectrochemical process of membrane polarization and depolarization.

Sensory receptors termed (1) *exteroceptors,* (2) *interoceptors,* and (3) *proprioceptors* provide feedback information about the human organism and affect the quality of motor performance.

Proprioceptors have particular relevance to the study of kinesiology because the quality of complex motor patterns, which include balance, kinesthesia, and neuromuscular coordination required in sport and physical education, depend upon the acuteness of proprioceptive organs located in the muscular, tendinous, articular, and vestibular (ear) receptors.

Reflex movement pervades every part of our daily living and consists of innate and conditioned types. The stretch or myotatic reflex represents an innate response and is particularly significant for the prescription of stretching and flexibility exercises. Advanced skills are learned through the process of a conditioned reflex.

Reciprocal innervation is the reflex mechanism that allows the interplay of agonists and antagonists to function in rhythmic coordination.

The motor unit represents a structural entity of the neuromuscular system and consists of a single neuron and all the muscle fibers that are innervated by the composite parts of the motor neuron.

Motor units comply with the all-or-none law and recruit units according to the phenomenon of gradation of muscular contraction.

Functionally, muscles contain three important characteristics: (1) *contractility,* (2) *extensibility,* and (3) *elasticity.* These qualities allow the body to assume numerous changes in muscular shape and body configurations.

Muscles pull toward their middle (belly), and generally become weaker in tensile strength as the shortening process occurs. Placing a muscle on a stretch, within normal physiological limits, to obtain its greatest internal force is recommended.

Force–velocity relationship influences muscular contraction. The velocity of shortening is greatest when there is no resistance and diminishes progressively with increasing resistance.

Motor learning is the process of acquiring controlled motor skills and includes movement of all types from the fine dexterity of

knitting to the prowess of the athlete executing a smash in badminton.

Maturation is the timing and growth rate mechanism that implies a readiness to learn. Biological maturation includes such factors as skeletal maturity; phylogenetic and ontogenetic development; strength and endurance.

Sound progression proceeds from simple to sophisticated motor tasks in the learning sequence. Progressive skill teaching implies the utilization of lead-up activities before complicated movements are presented.

Motor learning facilitators are modalities that, when employed properly, will enhance the learning and development of motor skills.

"Learn by doing" is the *sine qua non* of skill acquisition, and motor learning facilitators can increase the magnitude and rate of learning depending upon how and when these modalities are employed.

The complexity of a skill and nature of the learner must be considered before selecting the whole or part method. Whenever the part method is used, it should always relate in some integral fashion to the whole, especially with difficult movement patterns. The whole method is preferable when the activity is composed of a continuous or serial motion that forms a chained sequence, with speed and timing basic to the total pattern.

Skill practice does not lead to perfection unless performance conditions are considered. These include use of correct mechanics, motivation, difficulty of skill pattern, individuality of the learner, and teacher effectiveness. Distributive practice is probably more effective than mass practice under certain conditions, particularly when the motor task is boring, repetitive, and complex.

In skills where speed and accuracy are important for successful performance, emphasis on both speed and accuracy should be stressed in the learning stages.

Mental practice may have particular value at high skill levels where retroactive inhibition (excessive forgetting between practice and performance) can be prevented, thus sustaining efficient performance levels.

Kinesthesis is an internal sensory receptor mechanism that provides the sensation by which one is aware of position about the total body or its segments. Kinesthesis and proprioception overlap and together provide feedback information about body position. Evidence indicates that kinesthesis is a specific quality rather than a general characteristic; however, some investigators suggest that several related kinesthetic qualities may exist. Visual clues become less important as the kinesthetic ability of the performer improves.

The amount of teaching success attributable to an explanation of applicable principles for the acquisition of motor skills depends upon the manner and timing of application. Factors such as relevance, intellectual maturity, motivation, and teacher effectiveness are important considerations when employing mechanical precepts to facilitate learning and performance.

Manual guidance, whereby the instructor physically assists and/or guides the performer through a skill, may enhance learning among certain students; however, this procedure is not effective for all learners and may have greater value in teaching closed skills such as golf, bowling, and gymnastics as contrasted with open skills typified by basketball, tennis, and softball.

Reaction time is the period from the presentation of a stimulus to the beginning of the response. The speed of neural impulses in reaction time testing is different from the speed of movement time. Although an individual may be able to react quickly to a stimulus, quick perception does not ensure fast muscle movement to complete a motor task.

Skills in which cues for performance are fixed or static in one position are called *closed skills*. Motor tasks performed in a continuously changing environment such as basketball and tennis are termed *open skills*. Closed skills are predictable, whereas open skills are unpredictable.

Skills that begin and end with a definite effort such as tossing a bean bag or horse shoe are termed *discrete skills*. Activities that continue over a long period of time and that are usually repetitive in nature, such as running, bicycling, and swimming, are called *continuous skills*. Open skills are most resistant to "forgetting." Many continuous skills such as ice skating are easily recalled after long terms of practice abstinence.

Fine motor skills entail body movements such as dart throwing, typing, and handwriting. *Gross motor skills* are "big muscle" activities that require full body motion such as jumping, running, and throwing. Gross skills may also be analyzed from a refined or precision category depending upon the acuteness of performance.

REFERENCES

1. Harris, Raymond, "Fitness and the Aging Process," in Harris, R., and Frankel, L. J. (Eds.), *Guide to Fitness After Fifty.* New York: Plenum Press, 1977, p. 4.

2. Bolton, Jacques E., "Athletic Head and Neck Injuries," *Virginia Medical Monthly,* 96:79-83, February, 1969.

3. O'Boyle, Catherine M., "Sports Injuries in Adolescents: Emergency Car," *American Journal of Nursing,* 75:1732-1739, October, 1975.

4. Morris, James M., "Biomechanics of the Spine," *Archives of Surgery,* 107:418-423, September, 1973.

5. Harrison, Virginia L., "Review of the Neuromuscular Basis for Motor Learning," *Research Quarterly,* 33:59-69, March, 1962.

6. Cratty, Bryant J., *Movement Behavior and Motor Learning.* Philadelphia: Lea and Febiger, 1964, pp. 58, 67.

7. Powers, Whitney R., "Nervous System Control of Muscular Activity," in Knuttgen, Howard G. (Ed.), *Neuromuscular Mechanisms For Therapeutic and Conditioning Exercise.* Maryland: University Park Press, 1976, pp. 3, 5, 6.

8. O'Connell, Alice L., and Gardner, Elizabeth B., *Understanding the Scientific Bases of Human Movement*. Baltimore: The Williams and Wilkins Co., 1972, pp. 208-209.

9. deVries, Herbert A., *Physiology of Exercise* (2nd ed.). Dubuque, Iowa: William C. Brown, 1974, pp. 434, 441.

10. Kabat, Herman, "Proprioceptive Facilitation in Therapeutic Exercise," in Sidney Licht (Ed.), *Therapeutic Exercise* (2nd ed.). Baltimore: Waverly Press, 1965, pp. 327-343.

11. Hasselkus, Betty R., and Shambs, Georgia M., "Aging and Postural Sway in Women," *Journal of Gerontology*, 30:661-667, 1975.

12. Basmajian, J. V., *Muscles Alive*. Baltimore: Williams and Wilkins, 1967, p. 9.

13. Clarke, David H., *Exercise Physiology*. Englewood Cliffs, N.J.: Prentice-Hall, 1975, pp. 33, 57, 63, 66-68.

14. Edington, D. W., and Edgerton, V. R., *The Biology of Physical Activity*. Boston: Houghton-Mifflin, 1976, pp. 56, 61.

15. Basmajian, J. V., "Electromyographic Analyses of Movement Patterns," in Wilmore, J. H. (Ed.), *Exercise and Sport Reviews*, Vol. I. New York: Academic Press, 1973, pp. 261-262.

16. Gordan, Alan H., "A Method to Measure Muscle Firmness or Tone," *Research Quarterly*, 35:482-490, December, 1964.

17. Guyton, Arthur C., *Basic Human Physiology* (2nd ed.). Philadelphia: W. B. Saunders, 1977, pp. 133, 546.

18. Clarke, David H., "Adaptations in Strength and Muscular Endurance," in Wilmore, J. E. (Ed.), *Exercise and Sport Reviews*, Vol. I. New York: Academic Press, 1973, pp. 73-102.

19. Wilmore, Jack H., "Body Composition and Strength Development," *Journal of Physical Education and Recreation*, 46:38-40, January, 1975.

20. Harris, Dorothy V., "The Female Athlete: Strength, Endurance and Performance," in Burke, Edmund J. (Ed.), *Toward an Understanding of Human Performance*. Ithaca, N.Y.: Mouvement Publications, 1977, pp. 42-43.

21. Lockhart, Aileene S., "The Motor Learning of Children," in Corbin, Charles B. (Ed.), *A Textbook of Motor Development*. Dubuque, Iowa: William C. Brown, 1973, pp. 151-157.

22. Basmajian, John V., "Motor Learning and Control: A Working Hypothesis," *Archives of Physical Medicine Rehabilitation*, 58:38-40, January, 1977.

23. Shay, Clayton, "The Progressive-Part versus the Whole Method of Learning Motor Skills," *Research Quarterly*, 5:62-67, December, 1934.

24. Lawther, John D., *The Learning and Performance of Physical Skills* (2nd ed.). Englewood Cliffs, N.J.: Prentice-Hall, 1977, pp. 131-132, 150-154, 155.

25. Marteniuk, Ronald G., "Individual Differences in Motor Performance and Learning," in Wilmore, J. H. (Ed.), *Exercise and Sport Sciences Reviews*, Vol. 2. New York: Academic Press, 1974, pp. 103-130.

26. Kleinman, Mathew, "The Effects of Practice Distribution on the Acquisition of Three Discrete Motor Skills," *Research Quarterly*, 47:672-677, December, 1976.

27. Austin, Dean A., "Effect of Distributed and Massed Practice Upon the Learning of a Velocity Task," *Research Quarterly* 46:23-30, March, 1975.

28. Sage, George H., *Introduction to Motor Behavior: A Neurological Approach*. Reading, Mass.: Addison-Wesley, 1971, pp. 218, 245.

29. Solley, William H., "The Effects of Verbal Instruction of Speed and Accuracy Upon the Learning of a Motor Skill," *Research Quarterly*, 23:231-240, May, 1952.

30. Smith, Judith, "Kinesthesis: A Model for Movement Feedback," in Brown, Roscoe C. and Cratty, Bryant J. (Eds.), *New Perspectives of Man in Action*. Englewood Cliffs, N.J.: Prentice-Hall, 1969, p. 32.

31. Adams, Jack A., "Response Feedback and Learning," in Christina, R. R., and Shaver, L. G. (Eds.), *Biological and Psychological Perspectives in the Study of Human Motor Behavior*, Dubuque, Iowa: Kendall/Hunt, 1972, p. 319.

32. Scott, Gladys, M., "Measurement of Kinesthesis," *Research Quarterly*, 26:324-341, October, 1955.

33. Johnson, Barry L., and Nelson, Jack K., *Practical Measurements in Physical Education*. Minneapolis, Minn.: Burgess, 1979, Chapter XVIII.

34. Beter, Thais R., and Cragin, Wesley E., *The Mentally Retarded Child and His Motor Behavior*. Springfield, Ill.: Charles C Thomas, 1972, pp. 71-73.

35. Piscopo, John, "Clues to Safety on the Trampoline," *Journal of Health, Physical Education and Recreation*, 37:51–52, 61, April, 1966.

36. Piscopo, John, and Hennessy, Jeff, "Safety Update: The Trampoline," *Journal of Physical Education and Recreation*, 47: 33–36, April, 1976.

37. Fleishman, Edwin, A., and Rich, Simon, "Role of Kinesthetic Spatial-Visual Abilities in Perceptual-Motor Learning," *Journal of Experimental Psychology*, 66:6–11, July, 1963.

38. Kerr, Beth, and Klein, Ray, "Vision, Kinesthesis, Consciousness and Skills," *Journal of Physical Education and Recreation*, 47:46–49, November/December, 1976.

39. Newell, Karl M., "Knowledge of Results and Motor Learning," in Veogh, J. and Hutton, R. S. (Eds.), *Exercise and Sport Sciences Reviews*, Vol. 4. Santa Barbara, Calif.: Journal Publishing Affiliates, 1976, pp. 195–228.

40. Lawther, *op cit.*, p. 155.

41. Lockhart, Aileene, "Communicating with the Learner," *Quest*, Monograph VI: 57–67, May, 1966.

42. Smith, Leon E., "Reaction Time and Movement Time in Four Large Muscle Movements," *Research Quarterly*, 32:88–92, March, 1961.

43. Oxendine, Joseph B., *Psychology of Motor Learning*. New York: Appleton-Century-Crofts, 1968, p. 318.

44. Singer, Robert, *Motor Learning and Human Performance* (2nd ed.). New York: Macmillan, 1975, p. 248.

45. Cratty, Bryant J., *Movement Behavior and Motor Learning* (3rd ed.). Philadelphia: Lea and Febiger, 1973, pp. 95, 210, 244–245, 400.

PART 2 MECHANICAL ASPECTS OF HUMAN MOTION

5

CONCEPTS

1. Motion is classified into two general types: rotary and translatory or rectilinear.

2. During rotary motion, the axis may lie either within the body or outside the body.

3. To initiate rotary motion, a force must be applied off-center and at an angle to the radius of rotation.

4. To initiate translatory motion, a force of sufficient magnitude to overcome the pull of gravity must be applied at the object's center of gravity.

5. The best angle of projection varies according to whether the objective is distance, speed, or maximal time in flight.

6. The momentum of a moving object is equal to its mass times its velocity.

7. The momentum of a part may be transferred to the whole.

8. The momentum of one object is transferred to another upon impact.

9. In movements involving the action of several body joints, generally, each joint action should be initiated at the point of greatest speed and least acceleration of the preceding joint action.

10. Newton's second law dealing with the relationships between force, acceleration, and mass, states: "The acceleration of a body is directly proportional to the force exerted on the body, is inversely proportional to the mass of the body, and is in the same direction as the force."

11. The energy cost of muscular contraction varies with the cube of the speed of contraction.

12. The flight path of the center of gravity of the body is determined at the moment of lift-off by the relationship of the center of gravity to the point of application of force and the direction of thrust of the feet.

13. Newton's third law of motion, the law of action and reaction, states: "Whenever one body exerts a force upon a second body, the second exerts an equal and opposite force upon the first."

14. When a circling object is released, it will follow a path that is at a right angle to the radius of rotation at the moment it was released.

15. Impulse is the product of force and the time over which it acts.

16. The greater the momentum of an object, the greater the impulse required to accelerate, decelerate, or change the direction of the object.

17. The initial upward velocity of an object is equal to its final downward velocity.

18. The greater the flight velocity of an object, the greater the air resistance.

19. Every individual possesses his or her own unique rhythmic pattern of motion.

GENERAL CONSIDERATIONS

The branch of the science of physics of greatest importance to students of human motion is *mechanics*. Mechanics includes the study of the effect of forces on bodies and the motion of bodies. All people working in areas that require an understanding of force, matter, space, and time, such as astronomers, navigators, engineers, builders, mechanics, designers of airplanes and spacecraft, and those involved in communications must possess an understanding of mechanics.

Biomechanics is that part of mechanics that is concerned with the study of the motion of all living organisms. *Kinesiology* investigates the motion of animal bodies, particularly human bodies. The study of animal motion draws on anatomy and physiology as well as mechanics.

Statics is that part of mechanics that studies bodies in a state of equilibrium when all forces acting on a body are balanced. The reader is referred to Chapter 8 for an expanded analysis of balance and equilibrium. An understanding of statics is essential in analyses of posture, static balance positions in gymnastics, pyramid building, many circus stunts, and "set" positions preparatory to movement in many sports. An understanding of statics facilitates the understanding of levers and problems involving the center of gravity and the center of buoyancy. *Dynamics* is the study of objects in motion that are under the influence of unequal forces. Principles dealing with energy, work, and acceleration arise out of the study of dynamics. These terms are discussed and applied to motion with examples in Chapter 6. Dynamics offers explanations and predicts results of unequal forces upon changes in direction or speed.

Dynamics is subdivided into *kinematics* and *kinetics*. Kinematics is the study of displacement, velocity, and acceleration. It is not concerned with the forces that produce motion. Kinetics studies mass, force, and energy and their influence upon motion. Kinematic and kinetic parameters with specific reference to forces affecting motion are discussed in the next chapter.

MOTION DESCRIPTIONS

Motion is classified into two general types: rotary and translatory. In rotary or angular motion, any point on the object moves in a circle or arc of a circle around an axis. This axis is at the center of the circle described by the moving part. *Spinning, twisting, angular motion,* and *turning* are synonyms for rotary motion. The center of rotation, or axis, may lie within the body, as when a skater pirouettes on the top of one skate. The center of rotation may also be located outside the body, as when a gymnast or diver executes a jackknifed front somersault or a layout back somersault. Many other examples of rotary motion can be provided. During running, walking, or kicking, the thigh undergoes rotary motion around the hip joint, the lower leg undergoes rotary motion around the knee joint, and the foot describes rotary motion around the ankle joint. Together, these rotary motions produce linear motion of the entire body when walking or running. In executing a jackknifed forward somersault, the trampolinist's body undergoes rotary motion around an axis that is located outside the body in front of the hips between the trunk and the extended legs.

Repetitive Angular Movements

Repetitive angular movements, such as those of a pendulum or of the forearm in hammering a nail, are called *oscillation*. The three parts of the legs (thighs, lower legs, and feet) undergo repetitive angular movements or oscillation during walking and running.

Rotary Motion

An object will rotate, if it is freely movable, when a force is applied off-center. The further away from the center of gravity the force is applied, the more effective it will be in producing rotation. This is why, when initiating somersaults and spins, the arms should be extended. However, after the somersault or spin has been initiated the arms are flexed and brought against the body. An object will also rotate when it is free to move only in a rotary path regardless of where the force is applied. A door will rotate on its hinges regardless of where one pushes against it. Similarly, when the force generated by muscular contraction acts on body levers, they will rotate. However, the nearer the point of application of force to the axis of rotation, the greater will be the force required to produce rotation.

Translatory Motion

In translatory or rectilinear motion, the entire object moves from one place to another, in a more or less straight line. All parts of the object move the same distance. Translatory movement may be of two types: *linear* or *curvilinear*. When motion has occurred in a more or less straight line, it is said to be linear motion. The movement of the body during walking and running is called linear motion even though it is well known that the center of gravity of the body moves forward and backward, laterally, and up and down while walking or running. The fist, in a straight right cross, is said to move linearly even though it may not move in a perfectly straight line.

Curvilinear Motion

During curvilinear motion, the object moves in a more or less curved pathway. While curvilinear motion may occur in a perfectly circular pathway, it is distinguished from rotary motion since the axis of rotation in curvilinear motion is not within the object as found in angular or rotary motion. A thrown ball undergoes curvilinear motion. The shot during the shot put describes a curvilinear pathway.

When force is applied at the center of gravity of an object, the object will undergo translatory motion if it is freely movable. If the object is free to move only in a linear path, as when a bullet moves through the barrel of a gun or in the case of a sliding mirror in a medicine cabinet, force applied at any point will produce linear motion.

Relationships Between Angular and Linear Motion

All linear movement of the body as a whole (as in walking, swimming, or jumping) or of parts of the body (like the hand in a jab in boxing or the thrust in fencing, or the foot in the vertical jump or a karate kick) are the result of angular movements of one or more body parts. Further, many movements in sports such as the flight of projectiles are at first linear but become curvilinear as air resistance and gravity act upon them. A ball thrown with great force will leave the hand in a linear path but will eventually be pulled to the ground by the force of gravity, which begins to act on the ball the moment it leaves the hand.

Optimum Projection Angles

In many situations in sports, the sole objective is to project the object (discus, shot, javelin) as far as possible. In other situations, it may be advisable to keep the object in the air for a longer time, as in a punt, in order to give teammates time to get to the receiver. In other situations, distance may be sacrificed to speed, as in baseball when a fielder throws to the shortstop, who throws to the second baseman to "pick-off" a runner. Consequently, the trajectory of the projectile must vary according to the requirements of the situation.

Formulas for determining the distance an object will be projected, the height it will reach, and the time it will remain in the air demonstrate that the best angles of projection are different for different objectives. To achieve greatest distance, the best angle of projection is between 37 and 45 degrees. To achieve greatest height, the best angle of projection is 90 degrees. To move the ball fastest horizontally, an angle of projection of 30 degrees is better than one of 45 degrees.

Where R = horizontal distance; V = initial velocity of the projectile; Θ = angle of projection; and g = acceleration of gravity, the following formulas are used:

$$R = \frac{V_2 \sin 2\Theta}{g}$$

$$\text{height} = \frac{(V \sin \Theta)^2}{2g}$$

$$\text{time in the air} = \frac{2V \sin \Theta}{g}$$

NEWTON'S THREE LAWS APPLIED TO HUMAN MOTION

Some 300 years ago three laws of motion were discovered by Sir Isaac Newton (1642–1727). These laws are followed by all objects on the earth, the earth itself, the sun, the moon, and the stars. The movements of man in sports and all other activities are executed most efficiently when performed according to these laws. From these classic precepts, we can derive a number of principles of motion.

Newton's first law of motion is commonly known as *the law of inertia*. It may be stated in the following way: *A body continues in its state of rest or uniform motion unless an unbalanced force acts on it.* This law refers to resistance to any change relating to motion. Force is required to initiate motion of an ob-

ject or to stop, retard, accelerate, or change the direction of motion of an object. Resistance to change of motion is called *inertia*. The amount of resistance varies directly with the mass of the object. Less force is required to overcome the inertia of a small car than that of a truck because the truck has considerably greater mass. Catching a shot put is not recommended because of its great mass and consequent great inertia. A softball can be caught with relative safety. The heavier the sprinter, the greater the force he must exert in order to decelerate after crossing the finish line.

Momentum and Mass

We have stated that resistance to change in motion or inertia varies directly with the object's mass. When an object is in motion, its resistance to change in motion is determined by its velocity as well as by its mass. *Mass times velocity equals momentum.* The greater the momentum of an object, the greater its inertia. When two opposing football players collide, the player with the least momentum will be knocked down. Since a player cannot readily change his mass, he must increase his velocity in order to hit with greater force. The greater the momentum of an athlete, the greater the force necessary to change the direction of motion. The greater the degree of change in direction, the greater the force necessary. Muscles provide the force necessary to initiate, stop, decelerate, accelerate, or change the direction of motion. The degree of success of sprinters, successful "broken field runners," soccer players, basketball players, and other athletes in sports requiring agility or quick changes in direction or velocity will be proportional to the strength of the involved muscles relative to body mass (other factors being equal). Increase in strength can improve agility run times. Baley[1,2] found that college freshmen who increased their leg strength via isometric exercises also improved their performance in the agility run.

The greater the momentum of a baseball bat, the farther the ball can be batted. If the batter possessed sufficient muscular force to swing a bat as large as a telephone pole with sufficient speed and control, he could bat the ball outside the city limits. In actual practice, the batter must select the size bat that his available strength permits him to swing with accuracy and speed.

The momentum of a body part may be transferred to the whole. The longer and heavier the body part and the greater its speed, the more momentum it transmits to the entire body.

In the neck and head spring, the rotary momentum generated in the legs during the extension of the hips is transferred to the entire body when the hips reach the hyperextended position. The trunk is then rotated upward and forward toward the upright position to complete the move. In the front handspring, the rotary momentum generated in the arms and trunk, as they are swung downward, is transmitted to the legs when the hands contact the mat. This causes the legs to rotate upward and around to complete the move. In the high jump, the arms and swing leg are swung upward, and their momentum is transferred to the entire body to gain greater height.

Lever Length and Momentum

In the neck and head spring, the legs should be held in an extended position as the hips are extended. In the handspring, the arms should be in an extended position as they are swung downward. In the high jump, the swinging leg and the arms should be extended during the lift. The longer the lever the greater the velocity at the end of the lever at a specific number of revolutions per second.

By holding the body parts extended, the tumbler and high jumper increase velocity and thereby momentum in order to transmit greater momentum to the entire body.

Techniques for Increasing Momentum

In many sports skills, translatory and rotary motions are combined in order to generate greater velocity (and consequently momentum) and to apply thrust against an implement through a greater distance. This principle is nicely illustrated in the discus, javelin, and baseball throw, the tennis drive, and the forward somersault. In the discus throw, the athlete moves forward within the throwing circle while rotating his body. In addition, the force of the rotation of his arm at the shoulder joint is added to the other two movements. In the javelin throw, the athlete sprints forward in linear motion and, before releasing the javelin, rotates his body as well as his arm at the shoulder joint. The baseball pitcher adds the linear motion of his body to the rotary motion of his trunk and arm by taking a long forward step. In the tennis drive, several linear movements are added to the rotary movements. The weight is shifted to the rear foot and then to the forward foot as contact with the ball is made. The trunk is flexed laterally toward the rear foot before initiation of the arm swing. During the arm swing, the trunk is laterally flexed in the direction of the drive. These linear movements increase the distance through which the racket head can accelerate. In the forward somersault, the gymnast runs forward to generate momentum and then translates this forward momentum to upward momentum by means of "blocking" action, landing with his legs angled backward preparatory to the leap. Rotary motion is added at the moment of lift-off through flexion of the neck and hips and extension of the arms (arms swing downward).

Sequence to Joint Actions

In practically all sports skills, two or more consecutive joint movements contribute to movement of the body or implement in the desired direction. When timing and body mechanics are correct, the force of each subsequent joint action is added to that of the preceding one.[3] Generally, each joint action is initiated at the point of greatest speed and least acceleration of the preceding joint action. Hesitation between successive movements results in loss of momentum. The movements in the standing broad jump provide a relatively simple demonstration of this principle. First, the feet are plantar flexed. Next, the knees and then the hips are extended. Finally, the vertebral column is extended. The snatch event in weight lifting competition also provides a good illustration of this principle. In this lift, the barbell is hoisted in one continuous movement from the floor to arms' length position overhead. First, the knees are extended to start the barbell on its way upward. Then the hips are extended. After the barbell has upward momentum, the knees are flexed slightly and extended again to maintain an efficient angle of pull for the quadriceps muscle. The shoulders are elevated and then the elbows are flexed to pull the barbell to chin height. At this time, the hips and knees are quickly flexed in the squat style or the legs are straddled in the split style to drop under the upward moving barbell.[4] The wrists are rotated to place the hands under the barbell, and the elbows are quickly extended while the barbell still has upward momentum. If there is hesitation in extension of the elbows, momentum will be lost and the lift will fail. In the shot put, discus, and javelin throw and many other skills, hesitation between sequential joint actions may not lead to failure, but the distance achieved will be considerably less than the athlete's potential permits. If each successive joint action is to make its maximal contribution, the joints below must be stabilized.

Newton's second law, or *law of acceleration*, is concerned with the relationships between force, acceleration, and mass. The law is as follows: *The acceleration of a body is directly proportional to the force exerted on the body, is inversely proportional to the mass of the body, and is in the same direction as the force.* In the metric-kilogram-second, or MKS system, the term used is *newton* (nt). This is the force required to accelerate one kilogram of mass at the rate of one meter per second squared (1 kg m/sec^2). In the centimeter-gram-second or CGS system, the force required to accelerate one gram of mass at the rate of one centimeter per second squared is called the *dyne*. In the English variation, called the foot-pound-second, or FPS system, the mass that will be accelerated at the rate of one foot per second squared when a force of one pound acts upon it is called the *slug*. It should be noted that the newton and dyne are units of force since the mass and acceleration are stipulated, while the slug is a unit of mass since the force and acceleration are stipulated. However, all three terms serve as units for measurement of acceleration.

Velocity and Acceleration

Acceleration is a vector quantity; therefore, both its magnitude and direction are required for its complete description. The direction and magnitude of a vector can be illustrated graphically by means of a line with an arrowhead. The length of the line indicates the magnitude of the vector quantity while the direction of the line and its arrowhead indicates the direction. Acceleration may be either an increase or decrease in velocity. Velocity is a measure of the distance covered in a unit of time. When we say a car's speed or velocity is 60 mph, we mean that the car will be displaced from point A to point B 60 miles distant in one hour. Force must be applied to an object to cause it to accelerate. If the force is in the direction of movement, the object's velocity will be increased. If the force opposes the direction of movement, a decrease in velocity will result. The greater the mass of the object, the greater the force must be to produce the same amount of acceleration. During city driving, velocity is constantly changing, requiring more force to traverse a specified distance. This increases gas consumption. The same phenomenon applies to the human body. This is why a steady pace in distance running and swimming events is more economical in terms of expenditure of energy. In practice, the first lap is often done a little faster than the others due to nervous energy, while during the last lap or two, the remaining energy reserves should be depleted.

This physical law also explains why the greater the strength relative to body mass, the better the performance in agility events or events requiring a decrease and/or an increase in velocity. Muscles provide the force necessary to change the velocity of the body.

All objects, including the body, are subject to the force of gravity. Gravity brings the jumper, gymnast, and pole vaulter to the ground. It also causes the skier to move down the mountain at increasing speed. Wind, air resistance, and friction are other factors that influence sports performance.

Implications for Efficient Sports Performance

Several principles for effective and efficient performance in sports can be drawn from the law of acceleration. Maximum acceleration is achieved most effectively when all available forces are applied sequentially at the proper time and in the desired line of motion with all unnecessary body actions reduced to a minimum. An example of the sequential application of forces is provided in the swimmer's racing start after the swimmer has dropped to the horizontal position with his knees and hips flexed to right angles and with the shoulders hyperextended in preparation for the arm swing (see Chapter 10). The arms are driven forward against the extending hips, which apply force against the extending knees, which apply force against the plantar flexing feet, which apply force against the

starting platform. The sequential actions are initiated in the arms and progress to the feet. All of these actions must be directly forward. If the arms are driven sideward, the flight through the air will be shortened.

An example of the need to eliminate extraneous actions is provided in swimming the crawl. Beginning swimmers are seen to lift the head above the surface, roll the body, bob up and down (due to excessive downward thrust during the arm pull), and weave the body from side to side. All of these movements are wasteful of energy since they contribute nothing to forward propulsion. (They also create eddies that retard forward motion.) The reader is referred to Chapter 10 for a detailed discussion of swimming and forward propulsion.

The relatively wider pelvic girdle of females places them at a disadvantage in the sprint because their arms tend to swing diagonally across the body rather than directly forward in the direction of movement. This action is wasteful of energy. For this reason, females must practice more diligently in swinging the arms directly forward.

Energy Cost of Acceleration

In endurance events, rapid acceleration may be contraindicated because the energy cost of muscular contraction varies with the cube of the speed of contraction. When a muscle contracts twice as fast, the energy cost is eight times greater. When it contracts three times as fast, the energy cost is 27 times greater. A constant velocity is most economical of energy. This is as true when propelling the body as when driving a car.

Radius of Rotation

The speed of rotation of the body, as in somersaults or spins, is accelerated by shortening the radius of rotation and decelerated by lengthening the radius of rotation. The greater the number of somersaults executed by divers or gymnasts, the tighter the tuck. A one-and-one-half backward somersault in layout position is ranked higher in difficulty than is one in jackknifed position. The somersault in jackknifed position ranks higher in difficulty than one in tucked position. When the diver or gymnast has completed the desired number of somersaults, the hips and knees are extended to lengthen the radius of rotation to decelerate the speed of rotation. When the desired number of spins have been executed, the arms (or the leg in the case of certain skating maneuvers) are extended to slow down the rate of rotation. Greater resistance to rotation is present with a long radius of rotation than when the radius of rotation is short.

The radius of rotation should be in a lengthened position when rotation is being initiated in order to generate greater force in the direction of rotation. For example, the arms are extended when a somersault is initiated. Greater force is required to initiate the arm swing when the arms are extended because the resistance arm is longer. However, more momentum is generated when the arms are extended because the arc through which the hands move is longer. The hands move through this longer arc in the same time as they would if the arms were flexed and they moved through a shorter arc. The hands, therefore, move more rapidly when the arms are extended (see Figure 5.1). Momentum is a measure of force; it equals mass times velocity. Consequently, when the arms are extended as a somersault is initiated, greater momentum is generated and greater force is applied to initiate rotation. Although the mass of the arms is the same in both the flexed and extended positions, the velocity at the distal end of the arms is greater when they are in the extended position.

As soon as rotation has been initiated, the arms must be wrapped around the body and the body must be tucked in order to shorten

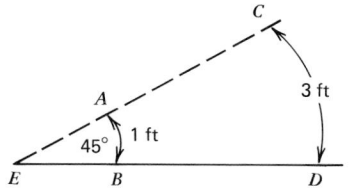

Figure 5.1 Relationships between length of lever and length of arc of movement. Arc CD is longer than arc AB. If lever ED rotates 45 degrees, points B and D will reach their new positions at A and D at the same moment; however, point D will have moved through a greater distance and consequently will have moved at greater velocity

the radius of rotation. This will accelerate the speed of rotation. The circumference of a circle equals pi (3.14) × (2 radii). The hands and distal parts of the body will continue to move at the same rate of speed and complete more revolutions per second since the circumference of the circle becomes shorter when the body is tucked and the arms are pulled close to the body.

This principle can be dramatically illustrated by tying a weight to one end of a string, then passing the opposite end of the string through a hollow cylinder, giving the weight a spin, and pulling downward on the opposite end of the string. This shortening of the radius of rotation will accelerate the speed of rotation. If the radius of the circle is 12 inches and the weight makes one revolution per second, the weight is moving at the rate of 6.28 ft/sec. If we pull on the string so that the radius becomes 6 inches, the weight will continue to move at the rate of 6.28 ft/sec, but the new circle will have a radius of only 6 inches or half that of the original circle and the weight will make two revolutions per second (see Figure 5.2).

In swinging movements, the radius of rotation should be shortened on the upswing to increase the speed of rotation. On the other hand, the radius of rotation should be lengthened on the downswing to increase the velocity and, consequently, the momentum of the

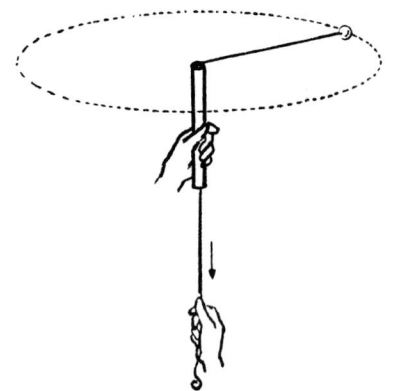

Figure 5.2 Shortening the radius of rotation increases the speed of rotation

more distal parts of the body. In giant swings on the horizontal bar (Figure 5.3), shoulder rolls on the parallel bars (Figure 5.4), and swings on the still rings, the body should be fully extended (neither flexed nor arched) during the downward swing. As the body begins to swing upward from the bottom of the swing, the radius of rotation should be shortened through appropriate flexion of the hips and, in the giant swing, extension of the shoulders. [Extension of the shoulder, it will be recalled (see page 69) is a downward movement of the humerus in the sagittal or anteroposterior plane.]

Trajectory of the Body

When the body is in flight, movements of the arms, legs, head, or trunk may cause the body to rotate, but its flight path or trajectory will remain unaffected. The trajectory is determined at the moment of takeoff and nothing the trampolinist or diver does after leaving the diving board or bed of the trampoline will alter the trajectory.[5] The trajectory is determined by the angle of inclination of the body and direction of push of the feet against the surface at the moment of takeoff. In the running broad jump, athletes often kick their legs and swing their arms during

flight. These actions have no influence upon their trajectory, flight path, or distance jumped. Examples applied to springboard diving are described in Chapter 10.

Action and Reaction in Twisting

Although most twisting actions are initiated from the supporting surface because this method is less complicated, a twist or spin may be initiated after the feet have left the supporting surface. When initiating a twist from the supporting surface, the reaction is against the supporting surface, which is heavier than the body and consequently will not move. When initiating a twist after the feet have left the supporting surface, actions are initiated with one part of the body to produce the desired reactions in other parts of the body. In one method, the arms are extended directly forward at shoulder height after the feet have left the supporting surface and are then swung vigorously to the right at shoulder height. The body reacts by turning to the left. When the left arm runs into the chest, no more torque or force can be applied. In order that a twist of the body will not occur in the opposite direction when the arms are brought back into position, they are either dropped to the sides or lifted overhead in line with the body. This action also shortens the radius of rotation, thereby increasing the speed of rotation. To combine the twist with the somersault, the arms are lifted slightly above the horizontal and the head and trunk are thrown backward to initiate simultaneously rotation around the horizontal axis and the vertical axis.[6] For a more detailed discussion, see Chapter 10.

Newton's third law of motion states: *"Whenever one body exerts a force upon a second body, the second exerts an equal and opposite force upon the first."* This law is often stated in the following manner: For every action there is an equal and opposite reaction. When one pushes against the ground as

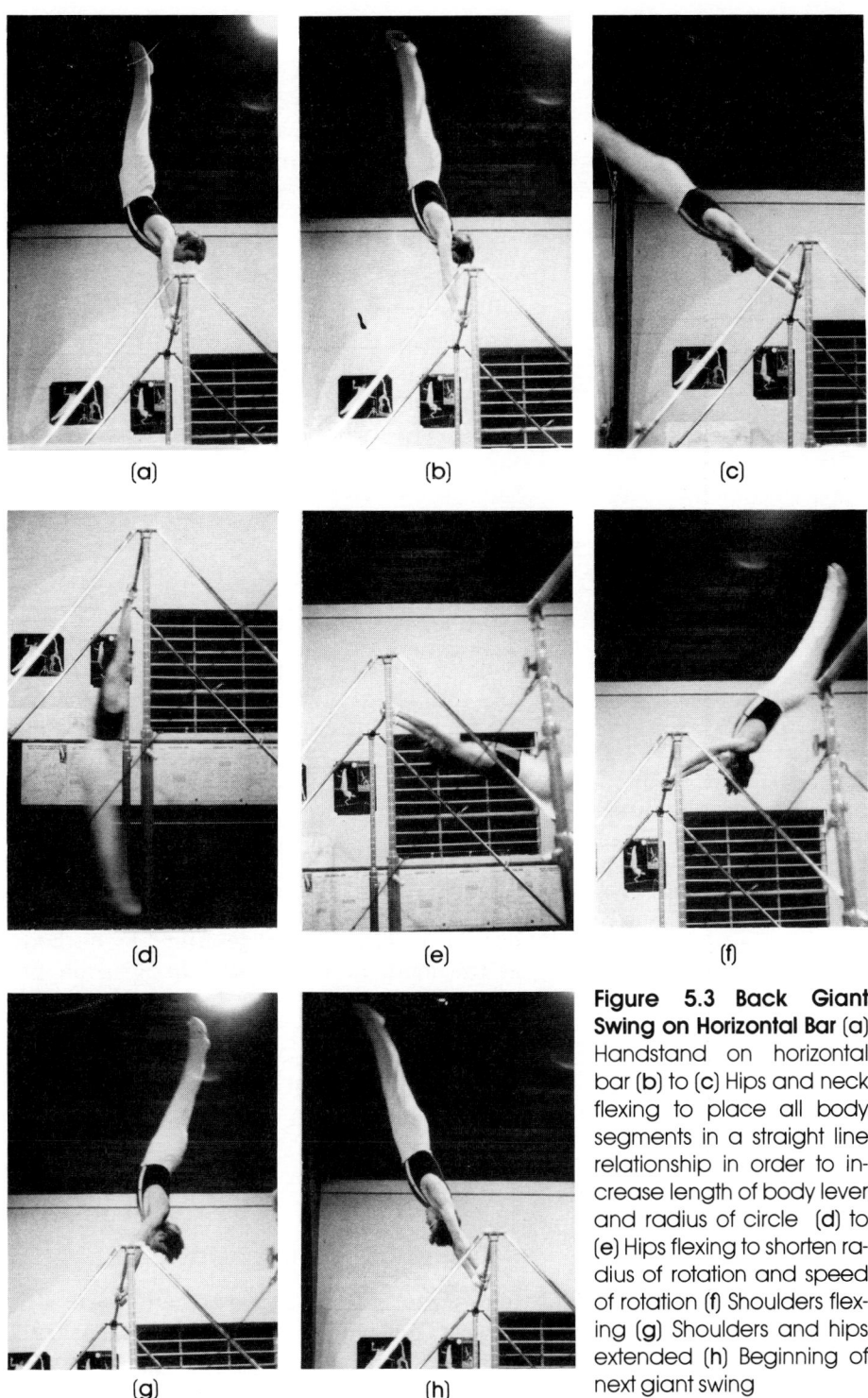

(a)

(b)

(c)

(d)

(e)

(f)

(g)

(h)

Figure 5.3 Back Giant Swing on Horizontal Bar (a) Handstand on horizontal bar (b) to (c) Hips and neck flexing to place all body segments in a straight line relationship in order to increase length of body lever and radius of circle (d) to (e) Hips flexing to shorten radius of rotation and speed of rotation (f) Shoulders flexing (g) Shoulders and hips extended (h) Beginning of next giant swing

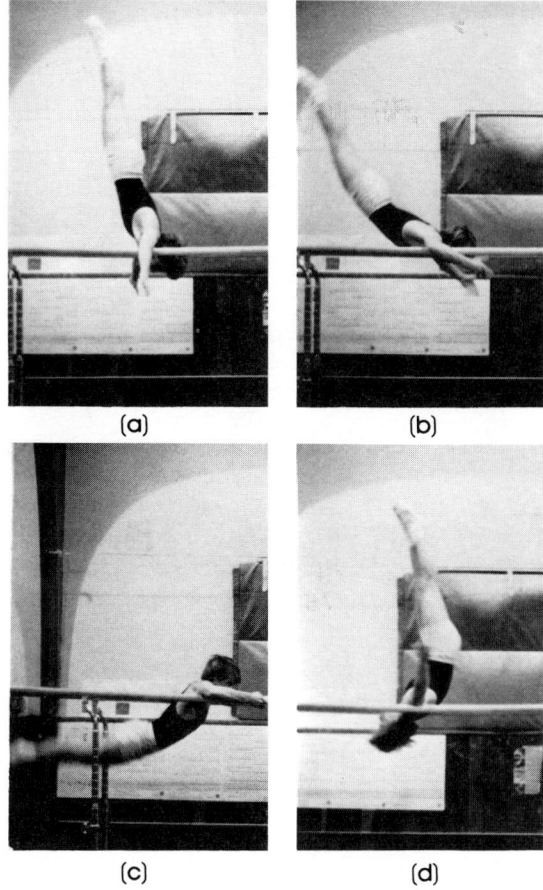

(a)   (b)

(c)   (d)

Figure 5.4 Shoulder Roll on Parallel Bars (a) Hips extended for longest possible lever in order to generate greatest possible momentum. Note downward pressure of arms (b) Hands grasping bars (c) Hips beginning to flex to shorten radius of rotation (d) Hips extending to complete the move

in walking, running, or jumping, the ground pushes back against the foot with equal force and in a directly opposite direction. The higher one wishes to jump, the greater the force exerted against the ground must be. If one wishes to jump directly upward, the push must be directly downward. If one wishes to jump directly forward, the push against the ground must be directly backward.

Thrust in Somersaults

If one wishes to execute a forward somersault off the diving board, the push against the board must be downward and slightly forward. The downward thrust will cause the body to be propelled upward. The slightly forward thrust will drive the hips backward over the head to contribute to forward rotation. Clearance of the end of the diving board will be accomplished as a result of forward momentum established during the approach and through forward inclination of the body at the moment of lift-off. In reverse dives, the thrust of the feet must be downward and slightly backward. The backward tangent of force is necessary so that the reaction will drive the feet upward in front of and around the head.

Direction of Projectiles

A baseball struck with a bat will leave the bat at a tangent at a right angle to the long axis of the bat at the moment of impact (Figure 5.5). The flight of a discus or a hammer will be in a path at a right angle to the radius of the circle being described by the implement at the moment of release. The flight of the gymnast in executing a flyaway from the horizontal bar will be at a right angle to the radius of the circle being described by his body at the moment he released his grip on the bar. If he releases the bar too soon, his flyaway will be low and long, and he may not complete the somersault. If he releases the bar too late, he will strike the bar. The release should be made slightly before the body reaches the horizontal position in the upward swing.

Stability of the Reacting Surface

In order to secure maximal reaction, the supporting surface must be stable and firm. When the supporting surface "gives" on receiving a force, the counterforce or reaction

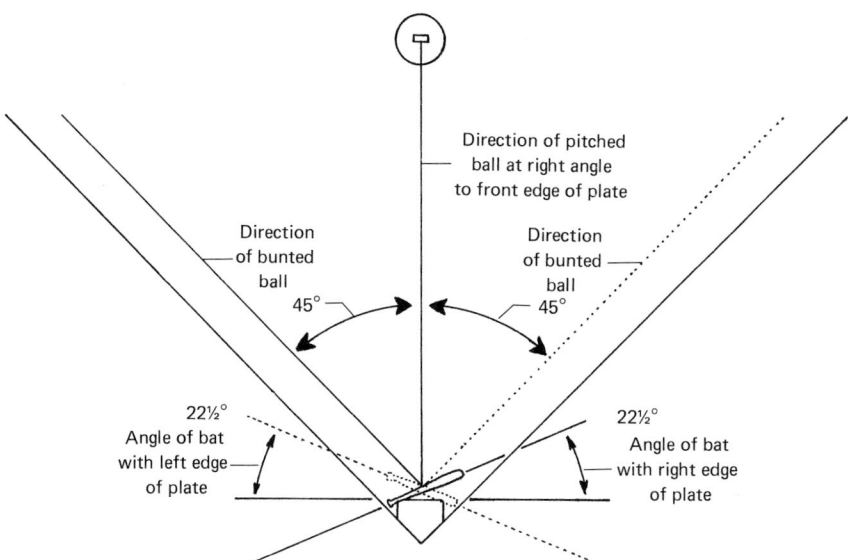

Figure 5.5 Angle of flight of ball relative to long axis of the bat at the moment of impact

is diminished. It is more difficult to run on sand or ice. It is more difficult to propel oneself in water than on land because water is less firm than ground. An orange crate may support an individual's weight while standing, but if the person attempts to jump upward from the crate, it will break. The individual will be unable to jump upward because he will receive inadequate reaction or counterforce from the crate as he pushes downward against it. The strength of the crate will be sufficient to provide a counterforce equal to the weight or downward force of the individual. However, its strength will be insufficient to provide the additional force imposed upon it when the person attempts to jump off.

The force with which an implement, the body, or one of its parts strikes another implement or body is dependent upon the combined momentum of the two implements or bodies. The greater the velocity of the bat, ball, or both, the farther the ball can be batted, all other factors being equal. The greater the mass of the bat, the farther the ball can be batted, all other factors being equal. The problem for the batter is to select a bat of maximal weight that can be swung with accuracy and speed. A bat of optimum weight must be selected.

Absorption of Impact

Flexibility in the striking implement reduces the propulsive force unless the object is both firm and highly elastic as in the case of a tennis racquet, trampoline, or diving board. When striking a ball with a bat or racquet, the grip must be firm and all body joints between the wrist and the supporting surface (floor or ground) must be firm or the force of the impact will be diminished due to the absorption of force. In the bunt, the bat is held loosely and the body joints are relaxed to help absorb the impact of the ball upon the bat. Boxers learn to absorb the impact of a punch by giving with the blow. A safety skill on the trampoline called "kill spring" involves the absorption of impact by flexing the knees and hips at the moment of impact. This action stops the rebound immediately.

FUNCTIONAL TERMS AND PRECEPTS

Velocity

The terms *speed* and *velocity* commonly have the same meaning. In physics and, consequently, in kinesiology, they have definite and separate meanings. The speed of an object indicates how fast it is moving. The term *speed* does not indicate direction of travel or displacement. *Velocity* is the rate of motion in a specific direction or the rate of displacement. The term *velocity* indicates both speed and direction of movement. Speed and velocity will be the same if the movement is in the same direction. They will be unequal if the direction of travel zigzags. Motion is said to be *uniform* when velocity is constant. If either speed or the direction of travel is changed, motion is said to be *variable*.

Velocity is a vector quantity because it is, by definition, the rate of displacement, and displacement is a vector quantity. Parallelograms may be utilized in the solution of problems involving vectors. A football punted so that it flies through still air with a velocity of 300 mph eastward will move at 315 mph if the wind is blowing eastward at 15 mph. If the ball is kicked into a 15 mph wind, it will move at 285 mph. This is illustrated through the use of vectors (Figure 5.6).

If a football is kicked eastward at a velocity of 100 mph and a southward wind with a velocity of 40 mph is blowing, what is the resultant velocity of the football? To find the answer, a parallelogram is constructed utilizing the two velocities as vectors forming two sides of a parallelogram. The respective direction and velocity of the two vectors will be represented by the direction and length of the lines. The other two sides of the parallelogram are drawn and a line is drawn connecting the corner of the parallelogram representing the point of application of force and the diagonally opposite corner of the parallelogram. This diagonal line represents the resultant velocity and direction of the football (Figure 5.7).

If the punter wishes to make a field goal with the wind blowing southward at 25 mph, the angle of the kick can be determined through the use of a parallelogram. The vector representing the force and direction of the wind is used as one side of the parallelogram while the vector representing the desired direction and velocity of the football is used as the diagonal of the parallelogram. Points S and R are connected to form the second side of the parallelogram. Side OE is drawn parallel to and equal in length to side SR. Points E and R are connected to form the fourth side of the parallelogram. Line OE represents the direction and velocity the football must have to score a field goal under the circumstances described (Figure 5.8).

Figure 5.6

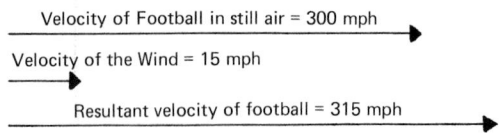

Velocity of Football in still air = 300 mph

Velocity of the Wind = 15 mph

Resultant velocity of football = 315 mph

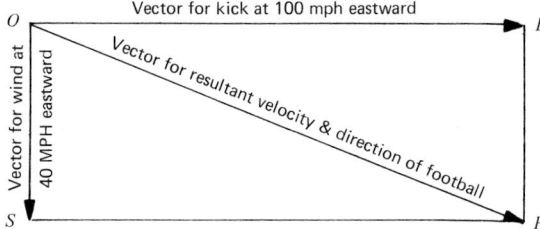

Figure 5.7 Utilization of parallelogram to determine resultant direction of an object when it is acted on by two forces. **O** = point from which football is kicked; **OS** = vector indicating direction and velocity of wind; **OE** = vector indicating direction and velocity of kick; **OR** = resultant direction and velocity of football

Velocity is the amount of displacement per unit of time or the rate of displacement. A soccer player may be dazzling due to his speed, agility, and ball handling, but if he fails to displace the ball from his position toward the goal line, he is not making progress toward scoring a goal. The formula for computing average velocity is:

$$V = \frac{s}{t}$$

where $\overline{V}$ is average velocity, s is displacement, and t is time. Few human movements are at a uniform rate of displacement; therefore, av-

erage velocity is most meaningful when describing human motion. Average velocity may also be computed from initial and final velocities. Where u represents initial velocity and V final velocity,

$$V = \frac{u \mathrm{T} V}{2}$$

Angular Velocity

Angular velocity refers to the rate of rotatory displacement. The symbol for angular velocity is ω (omega). Angular velocity is the angle through which a radius turns divided by the time taken for the displacement and is expressed as degrees per second, revolutions per second, or radians per second. A full circle of 360 degrees in one second is an angular velocity of 360 degrees per second, one revolution per second, or 6.2832 radians. The term *radian* arises from the term *radius*. The circumference of a circle is equal to $2\pi r$, where r is the length of the radius and π is a constant value of 3.1416.

It is obvious that an object moving at an angular velocity of one revolution per second

Figure 5.8 Use of parallelogram to determine direction and velocity of punt necessary to correct for wind

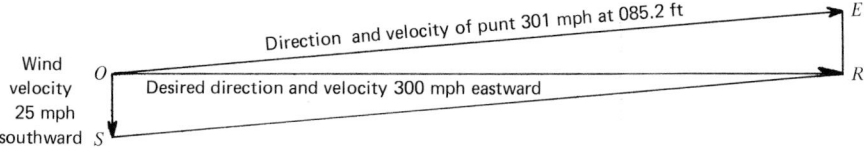

in a circle with a long radius will be moving faster than one moving at the same angular velocity in a circle with a short radius. The circumference of the circle with the longer radius is greater than the circumference of the circle with the shorter radius. Expression of rotatory motion in linear units of velocity presents the problem of varying velocities of points on the radius. Points farthest from the axis of rotation on the radius are displaced a greater distance than are the proximal points. For example, in linear terms, the feet of the gymnast while executing a giant swing are being displaced a greater distance per unit of time than are his elbows, even though the angular velocity of his feet and his elbows is the same. The linear velocity for a point on a radius can be determined by computing the circumference of the circle, or the part of the circle it describes, and dividing this measure by the time required to traverse this distance.

Angular velocity is determined through the formula:

$$\omega = \frac{\Theta}{t}$$

where ω represents angular velocity, Θ represents the angle through which the radius has turned in degrees, and t represents time. A change in angular velocity is called *acceleration*. Angular acceleration is the rate of change of angular velocity. The formula for computing angular acceleration is:

$$a = \frac{\omega y - \omega u}{t}$$

where α (alpha) represents angular acceleration, ωy represents final velocity, ωu is initial velocity, and t is time. If the angular velocity is 1000 degrees per second and accelerates to 2000 degrees per second and the time for this acceleration is 0.12 seconds, the angular acceleration is 8333.3 degrees/second/second (assuming that the velocity increased at a uniform rate).

Linear Acceleration

The rate of change of velocity is called acceleration. Where a = acceleration, Vf = final velocity, Vi = initial velocity, and t = elapsed time, the equation for acceleration is:

$$a = \frac{Vf - Vi}{t}$$

Acceleration is a vector quantity. When acceleration is constant over each succeeding time period, it is called *uniformly accelerated motion*. When acceleration is different during each succeeding time interval, it is known as *variable accelerated motion*. When the velocity of an object decreases with each succeeding time interval, the value of the acceleration is negative. This is called *negatively accelerated motion, retarded motion,* or *decelerated motion*. Retarded motion may, like accelerated motion, be variable or uniform.

Acceleration is the rate of change of a rate of motion. Therefore, time enters into the unit twice. Typical units for acceleration are ft/sec/sec or mi/hr/sec. When the two units of time are the same, the term used is ft/sec/sec or ft/sec². If the two time units are different, acceleration is usually expressed as mi/hr/sec.

It has been stated that the equation for computing acceleration is:

$$A = \frac{Vf - Vi}{t}$$

where A = average acceleration, Vf = final velocity, Vi = initial velocity, and t = time during with the change in velocity occurred. If a sprinter accelerates from 0 ft/sec to 30 ft/sec in 10 sec, his acceleration is:

$$A = \frac{Vf - Vi}{t}$$

$$A = \frac{30 \text{ ft/sec} - 0 \text{ ft/sec}}{10 \text{ sec}}$$

$$A = \frac{30}{10}$$

$$A = 3 \text{ ft/sec/sec}$$

Note: This is true only if the acceleration is uniform throughout the time period. This is seldom true in sports.

To determine the sprinter's velocity at any given time, the rate of acceleration is multiplied by the elapsed time and added to the original velocity. The sprinter's velocity at six seconds was:

V = rate of acceleration $\times$ time plus original velocity

$$V = At + Vi$$

$$V = (3 \text{ ft/sec} \times 6) + 0$$

$$V = 18 \text{ ft/sec}$$

If an object undergoes uniform acceleration, its displacement equals the sum of its initial velocity times the elapsed time plus one-half the acceleration times the square of the elapsed time. The equation for displacement is:

displacement (s) – initial velocity $(Vi) \times$ time (t) + 1/2 acceleration (A) $\times$ square of time (t^2)

If our sprinter accelerates at the rate of six feet per second, in ten seconds he will run 100 yards or:

$$s = Vi\,t = \frac{At^2}{2}$$

$$s = 0 \times 10 = \frac{6 \times 10^2}{2}$$

$$s = 0 + \frac{600}{2}$$

$$s = 300 \text{ ft or 100 yds}$$

When an object starts from rest, as our sprinter in the above illustration, the following equation may be used:

$$s = \frac{At^2}{2}$$

$$s = \frac{6 \times 10^2}{2}$$

$$s = \frac{6 \times 100}{2}$$

$$s = \frac{600}{2}$$

$$s = 300 \text{ ft or 100 yds}$$

Angular Acceleration

In measuring rotary motion, the same concepts are utilized as for measuring linear motion except that answers are expressed in degrees or radians rather than in feet. A rotating object moves through a certain number of degrees or radians of an arc or makes a certain number of revolutions in a unit of time. (A radian is equivalent to 57.3 degrees.) Where Θ = angular displacement in radians, ω = average angular velocity in radians/sec, and t = time:

$$\Theta = \omega t \text{ or } \omega = \frac{\Theta}{t}$$

The equation for determining angular acceleration is:

$$a = \frac{\omega f - \omega i}{t}$$

where A = angular acceleration in radians/sec^2, ω = angular velocity in radians/sec, and t = time. If a gymnast executes a giant swing in 1.7 seconds, we can compute his average angular velocity in radians/sec and his angular acceleration.

$$\omega = \frac{\Theta}{t}$$

$$\omega = \frac{6.2832 \text{ radians (360 degrees)}}{1.7}$$

$$\omega = 3.694 \text{ radians/sec}$$

$$A = \frac{\omega f - \omega i}{t}$$

$$A = \frac{3.694 - 0}{117}$$

$$A = 2.173 \text{ radians/sec}$$

Momentum

Momentum is the product of the mass of an object times its velocity. When mass is constant, momentum may be increased or decreased by increasing or decreasing velocity. If two opposing football players of equal weight or mass are approaching one another, the one with greater speed will possess greater momentum and will bring down his opponent. The greater the mass of a baseball bat, the farther the ball can be batted, all other factors being equal. If two shot putters can move the shot with equal velocity, the heavier competitor will put the shot further because his body will have generated greater momentum.

The greater the momentum of an object, the greater must be both the force and time over which the force acts to accelerate or to decelerate the object. The product of force and the time over which it acts is called *impulse*. The greater the momentum of an object, the greater the impulse required to accelerate, decelerate, or change the direction of the object. This is illustrated by the formula:

$$Ft = m(Vi - Vf)$$

where F = force, t = the time over which force acts, m = mass, Vi = initial velocity, and Vf = final velocity.

The equation points out why the greater the mass of an individual, the greater the force required to accelerate, decelerate, or change direction. Outstanding gymnasts, who must quickly accelerate or decelerate their direction of motion, are seldom people of great body mass. They also possess outstanding muscular development, which is necessary to provide a sufficiently sizable impulse. The same is true of athletes in other sports that require agility such as diving, soccer, tennis, and the sprints. It will also be noted from the equation that force requires time over which to act. This is why baseball pitchers bend the trunk backward, wind up, take a long step forward, and rotate the trunk. This is also why a long backswing is advised in the drives in tennis, golf, handball, and batting. It is the reason, when catching a ball with great velocity, one should reach forward to decelerate the ball over a greater period of time, or when landing from a height, one bends the knees and hips upon landing and if necessary, rolls, steps, or runs forward. Discus, javelin, and hammer throwers as well as shot putters make every effort to increase the time over which they apply force to the implement.[7]

Conservation of Momentum. When a bat, racquet, club, foot, hand, or other object strikes another object such as a ball, the momentum (mass times velocity) of the ball is changed. Upon impact, the velocity of the striking implement is decreased while the object struck is either accelerated or has its direction of motion changed. The greater the mass or velocity of the striking implement, the greater the velocity of the object struck after impact. In golf, the farther one wishes to hit the ball, the heavier the head of the club selected and the faster the club is swung. The heavier the bat the batter can swing with speed, the farther the ball can be hit (providing the ball is hit squarely). The greater the mass of the object being struck, the more difficult it will be to change its velocity or direction.

The influence of the mass and velocity of one object upon another object's mass and velocity is most obvious when one steps from a canoe to the dock. If the canoe is not held in position or if the foot is thrust too forcefully against the canoe, the laws of action–reaction will insure that the canoe is pushed backward; the canoeist will be convinced that this law should be followed as he splashes into the water. The law is operational when stepping off an aircraft carrier; however, the mass of the aircraft carrier is so much greater than that of the passenger that its velocity is little affected.

All of the preceding illustrates the principle of conservation of momentum. The momentums of the two objects before the force or impact equal their momentums after the force or impact. The more quickly the canoeist steps from the canoe to the dock, the greater will be his momentum (mass times velocity) and the more rapidly the canoe will move backward. The canoe's mass is considerably less than the mass of the canoeist, and consequently it will move backward at a greater velocity than the canoeist will move forward.

The loss in momentum of the striking object is always equal to the gain in momentum of the object struck (unless some momentum is lost through friction or other forces). Mass of both objects generally remains constant. This means that velocity is changed. (momentum = MV). The velocity of the club head is decreased while that of the golf ball is increased so that the total momentum (MV) of the two objects after the impact is exactly equal to the total momentum of the two objects before the impact. In other words, the momentum is conserved.

The momentum of the foot before the ball is kicked minus the foot's momentum after the ball is kicked equals the momentum of the ball before it is kicked minus its momentum after it is kicked or:

$$mfvf - mfUf = mbUb - mbvb$$

where f = foot, b = ball, m = mass, v = ve-

locity after impact, and U = initial velocity. The equation can be rearranged to read:

$$mfUf - mbUf = mfvf - mbvb$$

Conservation of Angular Momentum. Rectilinear momentum, as has been stated, is the product of mass times velocity. Angular momentum is the product of the moment of inertia (J) times the angular velocity (ω) or angular momentum = $J\omega$. The moment of inertia is the sum of the mass of each particle of the rotating object times the square of its perpendicular distance to the axis of rotation. The greater the mass and the greater the distance of the mass from the axis of rotation, the greater will be the moment of inertia. The moment of inertia during a giant swing of a 250-lb student in a gymnastics class will be much greater than that of a 128-lb competitive gymnast. The moment of inertia of the 250-lb student will very probably be so great that he will be unable to hang onto the horizontal bar. If the 128-lb gymnast wore heavy G.I. boots while executing the giant swing, he would increase his moment of inertia considerably more than if he tied them to his chest or wrists because of the shorter distance from the axis of rotation. This, incidently, is why gymnasts wear slippers of light weight.

The angular momentum generated in the hammer throw is obviously considerably greater than that generated in the discus event. This is evidenced by a comparison of the amount of body inclination required in the two events and by comparing the body weights of champions in the two events. The amount of weight and its distance from the axis of rotation in the hammer throw are both considerably greater than they are in the discus throw.

Angular momentum ($J\omega$), once established, will not change unless another force is brought to bear. Angular momentum, like rectilinear momentum, is conserved. When the moment of inertia is decreased by shortening the radius, the angular velocity is increased. It will be recalled that the moment of inertia is determined by multiplying the mass of each particle of the rotating object by the square of its perpendicular distance to the axis of rotation and then adding these products together. Stated in another form, the moment of inertia equals the sum of the mass of each particle times the perpendicular distance of each particle to the axis squared. When the radius is decreased from 3 feet to 1 foot, the moment of inertia is decreased by 900 percent ($3^2 = 9$ and $1^2 = 1$). Since angular momentum is conserved, shortening of the radius will produce an increase in angular velocity. In the case of our illustration, angular velocity will be increased by 900 percent since angular momentum equals the moment of inertia (J) times angular velocity (ω).

The principle of angular momentum is widely used in sports. Its application is seen, for example, in throwing a baseball, pole vaulting, figure skating, dancing, diving, gymnastics, basketball, football, and the tennis serve. (See Chapter 10 for examples from diving.) In pitching a baseball, the arm is extended backward, and as it is swung forward, the elbow is flexed. This increases the speed of the ball, which approaches 100 mph. In pole vaulting, there are two major axes of rotation: (1) of the pole at the bottom of the pole and (2) of the vaulter's body around his hands. As the pole rotates upward, the vaulter pulls his body upward toward his hands and flexes his hips and knees to shorten his radius of rotation, thus increasing his speed of rotation. This brings his body through a 180 degree rotation to the inverted position more quickly and with less effort.

The dancer and the figure skater, when doing pirouettes, extend the arm opposite to the direction of the pirouette and then quickly flex it to bring it closer to the vertical axis of rotation. To slow rotation around the vertical axis, they again extend the arm sideward.

Gymnasts, divers, and trampolinists apply the same principle when executing somersaults with twists. However, since they usually rotate around both the horizontal and vertical axis simultaneously, they must throw the arm upward as well as sideward (in the diagonal plane) when performing backward twisting somersaults.

A diving skill in which a swan dive is executed momentarily followed by a tucked forward one-and-one-half somersault illustrates the great increase in angular velocity as a result of shortening the radius of rotation. Rotation is barely perceptible during the swan portion; however, it is very rapid after the tucked position is assumed.

The tennis serve is executed in a manner very similar to the baseball pitch. However, the arm is flexed during execution to increase angular velocity. In sports such as football, basketball, and soccer, which require quick changes of direction, the radius of rotation around the vertical axis is shortened by pulling one leg and both arms inward. The pulling inward of the arms is seen most readily when the player has the ball in his possession, as in a hand-off in football.

Falling Free in Air

No one has ever been injured while falling through the air. They are injured when the kinetic energy generated during the fall is suddenly absorbed by the body. Obviously, certain parts of the body, such as the head and long bones, are more vulnerable to injury than other segments. The factors that determine the probability and extent of injury are (1) body mass, (2) velocity at the time of impact, (3) portion of the anatomy subjected to the impact, (4) size of the surface area subjected to the impact, (5) time of absorption of the impact, and (6) absorptive qualities of surface upon which impact is made.

Momentum equals mass times velocity. Everything else being equal, the greater the momentum, the greater the probability of injury. Kinetic energy equals $mv^2/2$. A heavy person, although falling no faster, will impact with greater force. Further, his strength relative to his body weight will not be as great as that of a person weighing less, and, consequently, he will not be able to decelerate the impact as effectively.

Another determinant of the force of the impact is the amount of kinetic energy generated during the fall. A falling body accelerates at the rate of 32.2 ft/sec/sec. The greater the height of the fall, the greater the velocity generated and, consequently, the greater the kinetic energy generated. The formula for computing the distance of a fall when the time of the fall is known is:

$$S = gt^2/2$$

where S = space, g = gravity (32.2 ft), and t = time. The time of the fall can be computed from the above formula by rearranging it in the following manner:

$$t^2 = \frac{S}{g/2}$$

Suppose we wished to determine the time of the fall of a parachutist whose chute failed to open. Assume he bailed out at 10,000 feet.

$$S = gt^2/2$$

$$10,000 \text{ ft} = \frac{32.2 \times t^2}{2}$$

$$t = \sqrt{625}$$

$$t = 25 \text{ sec}$$

During the 25th second, just before impact, the person would be traveling 800 ft/sec or 545.4 mph (32 ft × 25 sec = 800 ft/sec). Fortunately, falls in sports and at work do not involve such velocities. However, due to the increase in air resistance with increased speed, the terminal velocity of a freely falling skydiver is 120 mph (176 ft/sec). With a parachute the terminal speed is 12 mph.

Transfer of Momentum

Because of the law of conservation of momentum, just as the momentum of one object is transferred to another upon impact, so is the angular momentum of one body part transferred to other body parts when the momentum of the first part is stopped. In the running front handspring, the momentum generated in the arms and trunk as they are brought downward is transferred to the legs to bring them up, over, and around. In the back dive off the diving board, the momentm generated in the head and arms as they are brought backward is transferred to the rest of the body to cause it to rotate 180 degrees into the inverted position. When a soccer player leaps up and snaps his head forward into the ball, an equal and opposite reaction occurs in the remainder of his body, causing the legs and body to move backward. To avoid the unbalanced position into which this would place him, he flexes his hips, moving his legs forward-upward as he brings his head forward into the ball. The two actions nullify one another if they are in correct proportion. Because of the greater mass of the legs, their forward-upward velocity should not be as great as the forward velocity of the head. The mv of the two forces must be equal and opposite.

The axis of rotation for any rotatory movements may be in any plane, but the reactions will always be in the same or parallel planes. If a trampolinist jumps upward and, after leaving the bed, sweeps the extended right arm to the left in the horizontal plane, his body will turn to the right. Trampolinists have perfected procedures enabling them to utilize this phenomenon in the execution of somersaults with multiple twists. This action–reaction technique is described later in this chapter.

Females, when running, particularly those with relatively wide hips, create a rotatory force around the vertical axis, producing a reaction of the trunk in the opposite direction. This is detrimental to running speed and efficiency since, ideally, all of the thrust should be directly forward. To balance out the reactive twist produced by the legs, the arms are swung forward in opposition to the legs. The more massive the legs and the greater their velocity, the more vigorous the arm movements must be.

PARABOLIC FLIGHT PATH

Any object projected into the air, whether it is one's own body, an implement such as a shot or soft ball projected through the body levers, or an implement such as an arrow projected by the recoil of the bow, a stone projected by a slingshot, a bullet projected by explosion of gunpowder, or a nuclear warhead projected by nuclear fission, is acted on by the force of gravity. The downward acceleration due to the pull of gravity is 32.2 ft/sec/sec regardless of the weight or size of the object. The downward pull of gravity is independent of the horizontal or vertical force with which the object had been projected, except that greater time in flight gives gravity greater time to accelerate the object downward. If a ball is dropped from the top of the New York World Trade Center and, at the same instant, another ball is thrown horizontally from the same point, both balls will strike the ground at the same instant (if the elevation at both points of impact is the same). How far the thrown ball will travel before striking the ground is dependent upon its velocity at the moment it leaves the hand since it has a predetermined amount of time in which to travel. In other words, it will be projected as far as it can travel forward in the time it takes gravity to pull it to the ground from the height at which it was released. An object projected horizontally begins a downward-curved path as soon as it is released due to the force of gravity.

The horizontal distance the object will travel can be computed through the formulae:

$$S = Ut + at^2/2$$

where S = space or distance, U = initial velocity, a = downward acceleration due to gravity (32 ft/sec/sec) and t = time. Although U or initial velocity will vary according to throwing technique, strength, length of body levers, and speed of muscular contraction, t or time will be constant at a specfic height since the acceleration downward due to gravity does not change; it is always 32 ft/sec/sec. Gravity begins accelerating the ball downward the moment it leaves the hand.

Projectile problems can be resolved through the use of vectors. The *horizontal vector* represents the force imparted to the projectile in a horizontal direction. *Horizontal velocity* is uniform because no opposing force is present (except air resistance). It becomes apparent that the horizontal distance covered is the product of the horizontal velocity and the time in flight. The downward pull of gravity is represented by the vertical vector (Figure 5.9).

In the above illustration, the ball was thrown horizontally from a height of 16 ft. At the end of one second it was falling at a velocity of 32 ft/sec. It fell 16 ft by the end of the first second since its downward velocity was zero at the initiation of the throw. The distance the ball falls per unit of time can be computed by the formulas:

$$S = \tfrac{1}{2} \times at^2$$

$$S = \tfrac{1}{2}(32 \text{ ft} \times 0.1^2)$$

$$S = \tfrac{1}{2}(32 \text{ ft} \times 0.01)$$

$$S = \tfrac{1}{2}(0.32)$$

$$S = 0.16 \text{ ft}$$

Following this procedure, we find that the ball falls 0.64 ft at 0.2 sec, 1.44 ft at 0.3 sec, 2.56 ft at 0.4 sec, 4 ft at 0.5 sec, 5.76 ft at 0.6 sec, 7.84 ft at 0.7 sec, 10.24 ft at 0.8 sec, 12.96 ft at 0.9 sec, and 16 ft at 1 sec. It now becomes obvious that the greater the height from which an object is projected horizontally and the greater its velocity, the farther it will travel.

When an object is projected vertically upward, its velocity continues to decrease until it reaches a point when the force of the velocity upward is equal to the downward pull of gravity. Gravity then pulls the object downward at a velocity accelerating from zero at 32 ft/sec/sec. The greater the projecting velocity, the higher the object will travel and, consequently, the greater will be its velocity when it returns to earth. That the initial upward velocity equals the final downward velocity can be shown through substitution in the formula:

$$V^2 = U^2 + 2as$$

where V = final velocity, U = initial velocity, a = acceleration, and s = space or distance. Assume a ball is thrown upward to a height of 20 ft. When the ball is thrown upward, final velocity or $V = 0$. When it starts downward, its initial velocity or $U = 0$.

Computation for Final Downward Velocity	Computation for Initial Upward Velocity
$V^2 = U^2 + 2as$	$V^2 = U^2 + 2as$
$V^2 = 0 + (2 \times 32 \times 20)$	$0 - U^2 + (2 \times 32 \times 20)$
$V^2 = 1280$	$U^2 = (2 \times 32 \times 20)$
$V = \sqrt{1280}$	$U^2 = 1280$
$V = 35.777088$ ft/sec	$U = \sqrt{1280}$
	$U = 35.777088$ ft/sec

The greater the upward velocity of the ball, the higher it will travel. The higher the ball goes, the more time gravity is afforded to accelerate the ball during its downward plunge.

The greater the initial upward velocity, the more time the object will remain in the air.

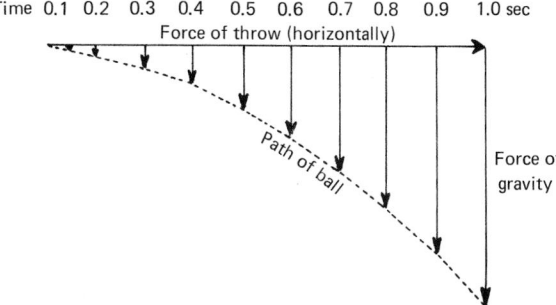

Time 0.1 0.2 0.3 0.4 0.5 0.6 0.7 0.8 0.9 1.0 sec

Force of throw (horizontally)

Path of ball

Force of gravity

Figure 5.9 Influence of the force of gravity upon displacement of a horizontally projected object

The higher the lift-off of trampolinists, divers, and gymnasts, the more time they are afforded in which to complete somersaults and twists. This is why coaches urge divers to secure as nearly a vertical lift-off as possible. The kicker in football must endeavor to secure optimal height in the kick, balancing the objectives of maximal distance and time allowing his teammates to get under the ball or, at a minimum, reasonably near the receiver at the moment he catches the ball.

A projectile impacting with the ground at an elevation lower than that from which it was projected will travel farther than one landing at the same elevation. This phenomenon occurs because the projectile has more time in flight. Conversely, a projectile impacting with the ground at an elevation higher than that from which it was projected will not travel as far as one landing at the same or a lower elevation (see Figure 5.10).

It is generally believed that a projection angle of 45 degrees is optimum where greatest possible distance is desired. However, this is true only when the elevation of the point of projection and the landing point are the same, i.e., on flat and level terrain. Cooper and Glassow[8] describe Bunn's procedure for determining the best angle of projection for securing maximum distance. This procedure requires that the velocity of the projection and the difference in elevation between the projection and landing point be known. This

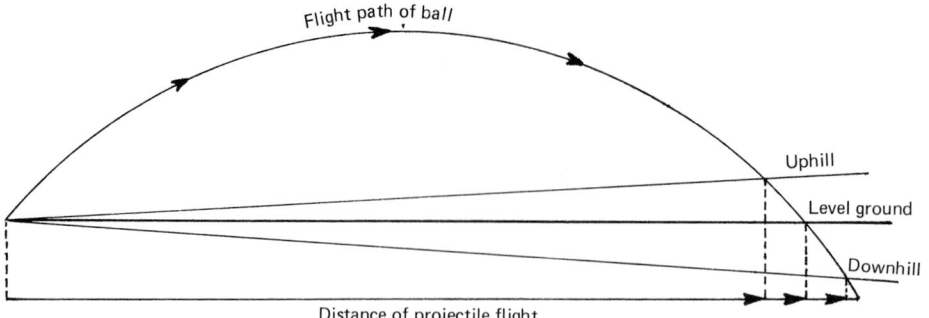

Figure 5.10 Influence of relative elevation between projection and landing points upon flight distance

difference is identified as h in the formula used by Bunn. If the start is higher than the landing point, h will be a negative quantity, while if the start is lower than the landing point, h will be positive. The formula is as follows:

$$\sin^2 = \frac{\text{velocity}^2}{2(\text{velocity}^2 - gh)}$$

The angle for which the derived figure is the sine is found from standard tables. The higher the sine value, the greater the angle. The sine value increases as velocity increases and as h goes from a negative to a positive quantity. From the point of view of application in practice, the greater the initial velocity of the projectile and the higher the landing point with reference to the starting or projecting point, the more nearly should the projection angle approach 45 degrees. Bunn found that in some situations, the best projection angle is as low as 37 degrees. These angulations occur when a projectile's velocity is lower and the landing point is at a lower elevation than the projection point.

In some sports skills, such as the long jump, the center of gravity of the body is lower at the conclusion of the maneuver than it was at its initiation. This is due to different body alignments. In the case of the long jump, the body and legs are extended and the arms are elevated at the initiation of the jump (with the center of gravity about three feet above the ground), while upon landing the hip joints are flexed and the arms are depressed. This lowers the center of gravity approximately 1½ feet, which has the same effect as jumping downhill to an elevation 1½ feet lower than the starting point. This, of course, adds distance to the jump.

Cinematographic studies of various skills are useful in determining the most effective positionings and velocities of the center of gravity of the body in jumping, vaulting, and gymnastic skills. The allied health professions, in recent years, have been making increasing use of these studies.

The parabolic flight path of the center of gravity of the body is determined at the moment of takeoff. The alignment of various body parts can be changed during flight and the body can rotate around one or more of its axes, but the path of the center of gravity cannot be changed.

The flight path of a badminton shuttlecock is known to differ considerably from that of a baseball. The shuttlecock, because it is light and presents relatively greater surface area, is affected by air resistance to a greater degree. The greater the speed, the greater the air resistance. Consequently, a hard hit shuttlecock loses its momentum and drops quickly and almost vertically. As has been pointed out, even heavier objects such as sky divers reach a terminal velocity (120 mph) when the velocity is no longer increased due to increase of opposing air resistance to the point where it equals the accelerating force of gravity.

Although the most effective angle of projection for distance is between 37 and 45 degrees, a golf ball, because of its great speed, must be projected at a considerably lower angle in order to compensate for the greater air pressure. When a discus wobbles, a football turns end over end, or an arrow or javelin quivers, a greater surface is presented, increasing air resistance and, consequently, decreasing the distance of the object's flight.

HUMAN TWISTING MOTION

Gymnasts, divers, dancers, trampolinists, and skaters all utilize twisting movements. An understanding of the application of kinesiologic principles in human twisting motions will facilitate learning and teaching of all skills involving twisting or rotation around the vertical axis (see Figure 5.11).

In all twists, as well as saltos or somersaults, the principle "action and reaction are equal and in opposite directions" is applied. This phenomenon is clearly shown in the "Cat Drop" twist in Chapter 10. In the "direct" twisting method, if the twist is to the left (and without somersaulting action), the horizontally extended right arm is swung forward across the chest, flexing at the elbow during the swing. The elevated flexed left arm is driven backward in the horizontal plane as the head is rotated to the left on its vertical axis. At the same time, the trunk is rotated to the left. These movements constitute the action. This action culminates through the feet against the supporting surface, mat, Reuther board, bed of the trampoline, springboard, ice, or dance floor. The feet push downward to secure lift-off and to the right to initiate the twist. The supporting surface reacts by

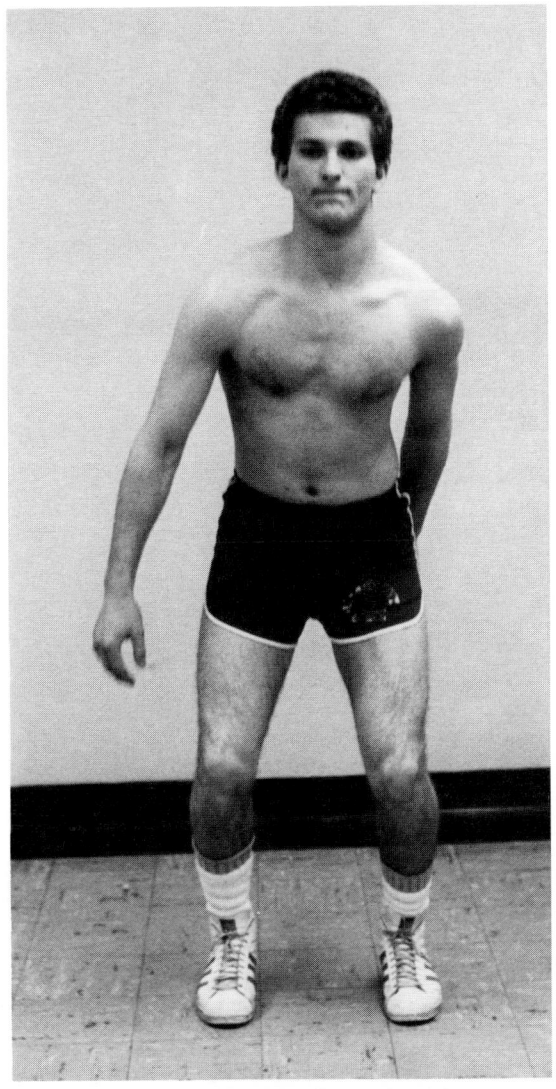

Figure 5.11 Rotation Around the Vertical Axis During a Vertical Jump (a) Knees beginning to extend for the jump and left arm is swinging behind trunk

pushing against the feet in the opposite direction. This force is transmitted through the body segments to cause the body to rotate around its vertical axis and to lift off.

Direct Method

To execute a back salto (somersault) with a twist utilizing the direct method (Figure

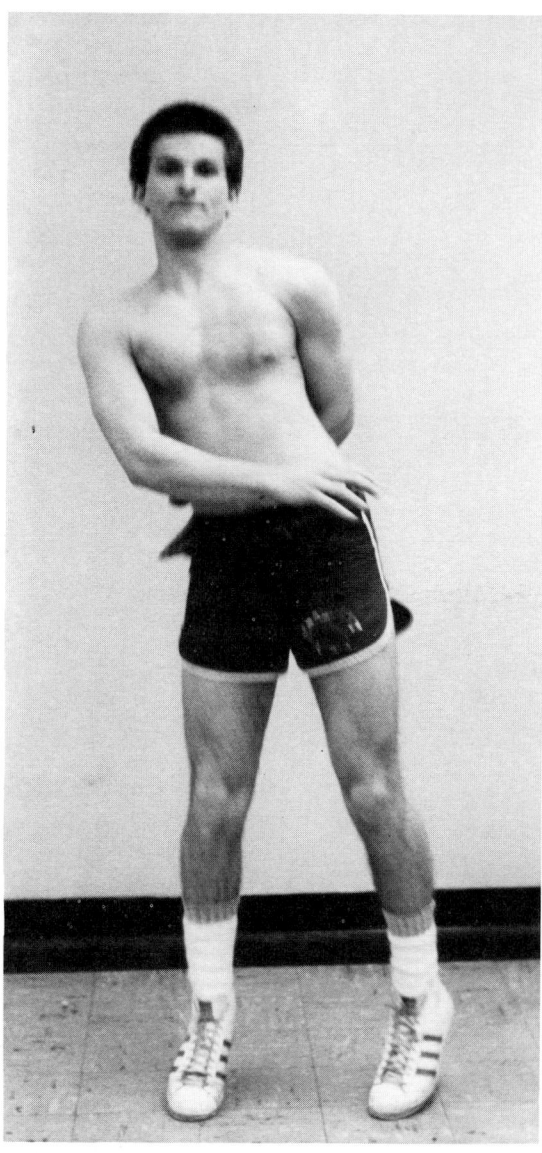

Figure 5.11b Wrap around of arms completed. Note left foot pushing sideward as well as downward.

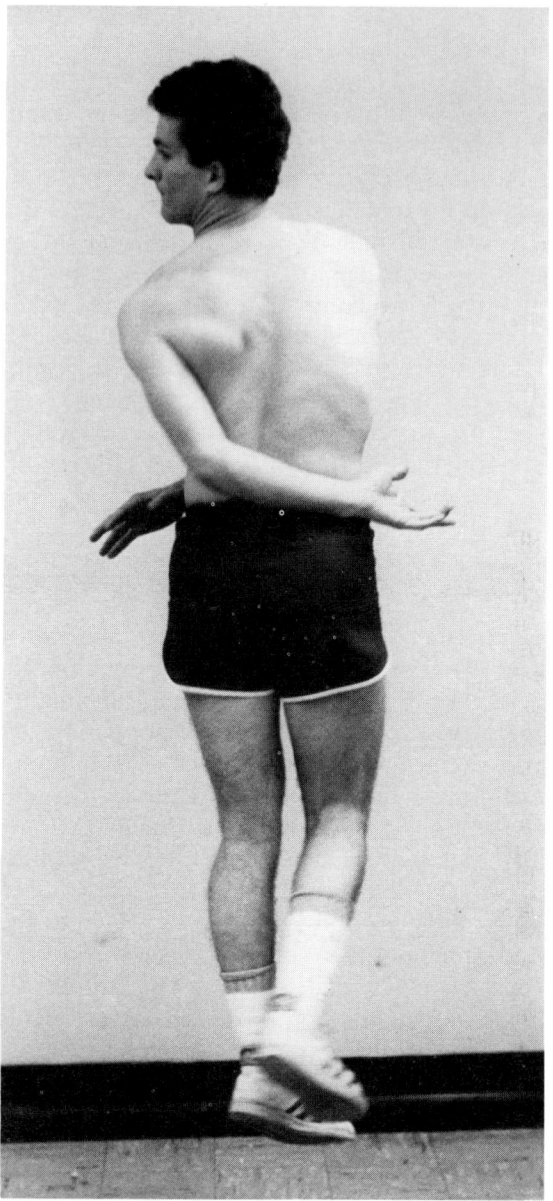

Figure 5.11c Body rotating to left. Note that head is turned to the left

5.12), the performer may lift the left arm vertically overhead to assist in initiation of rotation around the horizontal axis while swinging the right arm upward-sideward until the right hand reaches the area of the left shoulder. Some performers lift the right arm above the head. The head, shoulders, and trunk are thrown backward as well as turned to the left to initiate the salto or rotation around the horizontal axis, which occurs simultaneously with the twist. Figure 5.13 illustrates the forward salto with a direct full twist.

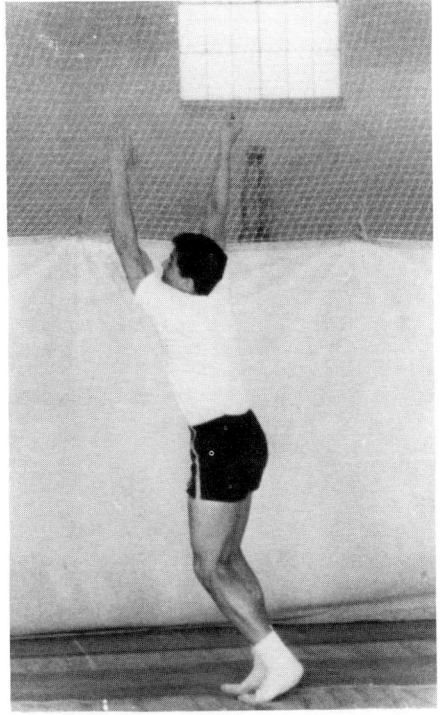

(a)

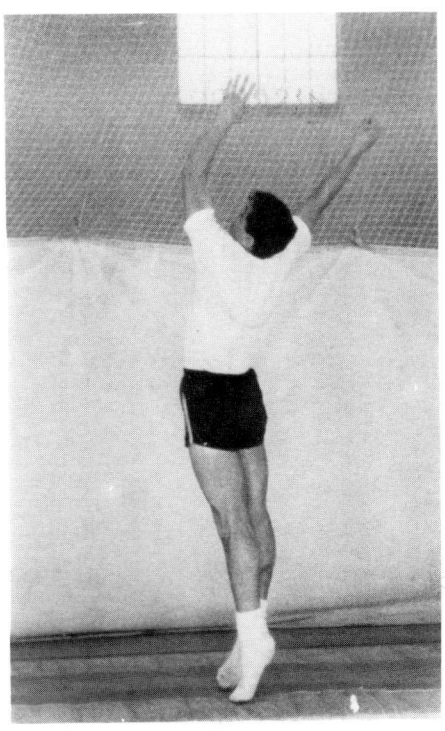

(b)

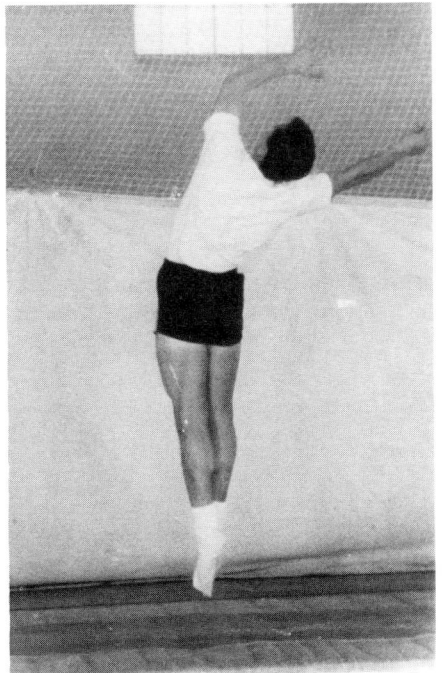

(c)

Figure 5.12 Backward Salto with Direct Full Twist
(a) to (b) Note angle of legs relative to floor (blocking action). Feet pushing against floor unequally to initiate twist. Also not diagonal movement of left arm (c) Center of gravity has moved backward behind the back due to arched back

The role of the reacting surface can be more greatly appreciated if the reader will imagine endeavoring to leap upward and twist from a heavily greased surface, ice, or a pedestal that rotates easily. In this case, the reaction from the supporting surface will be insufficient to facilitate the twist.

Action-Reaction Method

The action-reaction principle also has application in the other two methods of executing

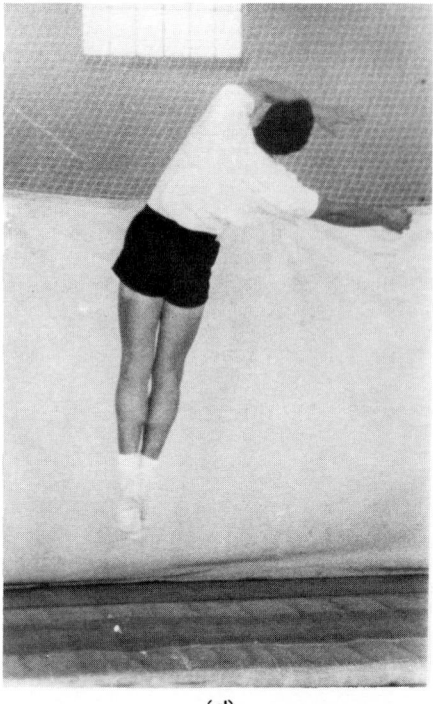

(d)

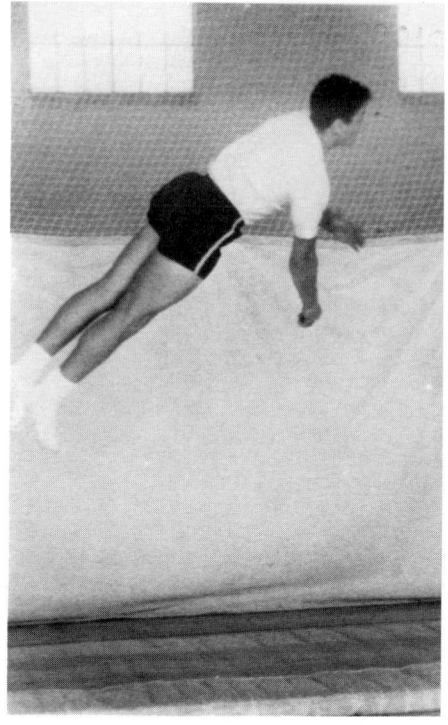

(f)

Figure 5.12d Trunk turning to right. Right arm pulling backward. Left arm pulling across face (e) to (f) Right arm whipping diagonally downward and across abdomen. Hips extend

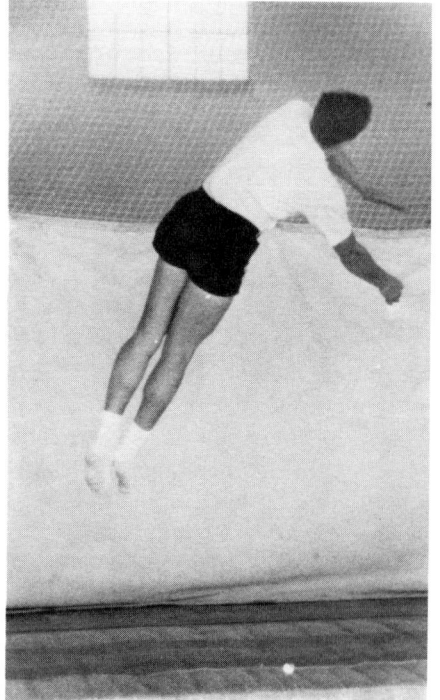

(e)

saltos with twists. The first of these methods is called the *action–reaction twist*. In this method, the action of a rapidly moving small mass, the arms, produces a reaction in a larger mass, the body. It is recommended that the performer first attempt utilization of the method while jumping vertically. In this method, after the feet have left the supporting surface and with the arms extended horizontally forward at shoulder height, the arms are swung vigorously to the right at shoulder height. The momentum of the arms is transferred to the body when they reach the end of the range of their movement. The body

MECHANICAL ASPECTS OF HUMAN MOTION

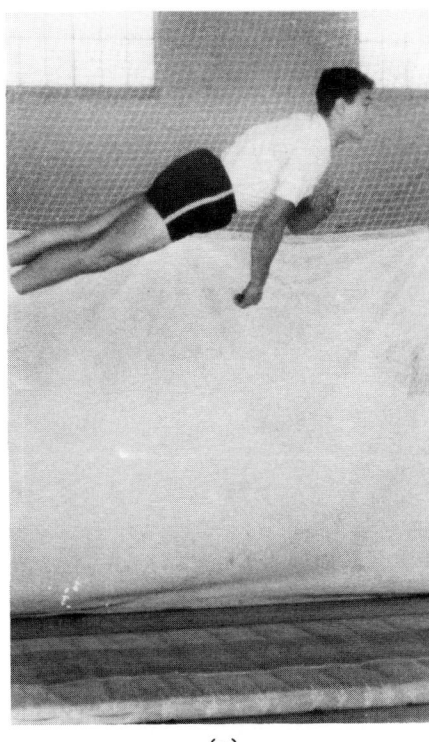

(g)

Figure 5.12g Hips extended

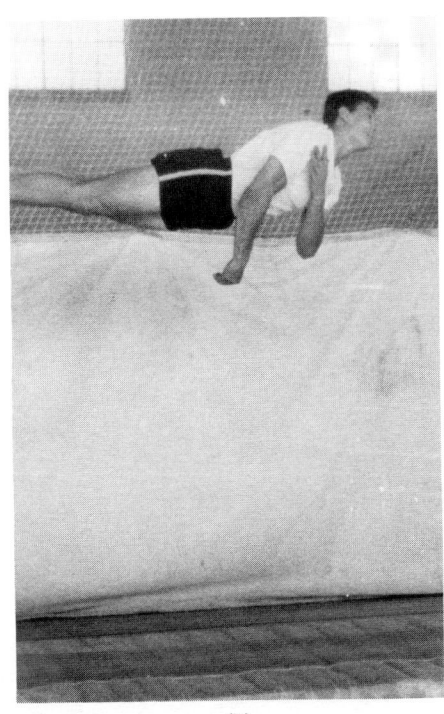

(h)

Figure 5.12h Twist halfway completed. Somersault one-quarter completed

reacts by turning to the left. In order that a twist of the body in the opposite direction will not occur when the arms are brought back into position, they are either dropped to the sides or brought overhead in line with the body. This action also shortens the radius of rotation, thereby increasing the speed of rotation. To execute the back salto with a twist utilizing this method, the arms are lifted forward-upward slightly above the horizontal in order to assist the backward-moving head and trunk in initiating the somersault. The arms are then thrown to the right. Although this method produces a slight side somersaulting motion, it is negligible because the weight of the body is so much greater than that of the arms. In the event additional rotational force is required, the shoulders and head can be squared, the arms extended forward again, and the action repeated.

Twisting from a Pike (or Arch)

The third method of twisting is called "twisting from a pike" or "twisting from an arch." This method, like the "action–reaction twist" is initiated after the feet have left the supporting surface. Like both the other methods of twisting, several kinesiologic principles are utilized. First, momentum is generated in certain body parts. With respect to the twisting mechanics, these parts are the arms, head, and trunk. Second, the momentum of a body part or parts (in the case of the twisting movements, the arms and head) is transferred to the entire body. Third, the speed of rotation around the vertical axis is increased by bringing the arms closer to the vertical axis or by flexing them to shorten the radius of rotation. The more twists desired or the lower the somersault and consequently the

MECHANICAL ELEMENTS OF HUMAN MOTION **201**

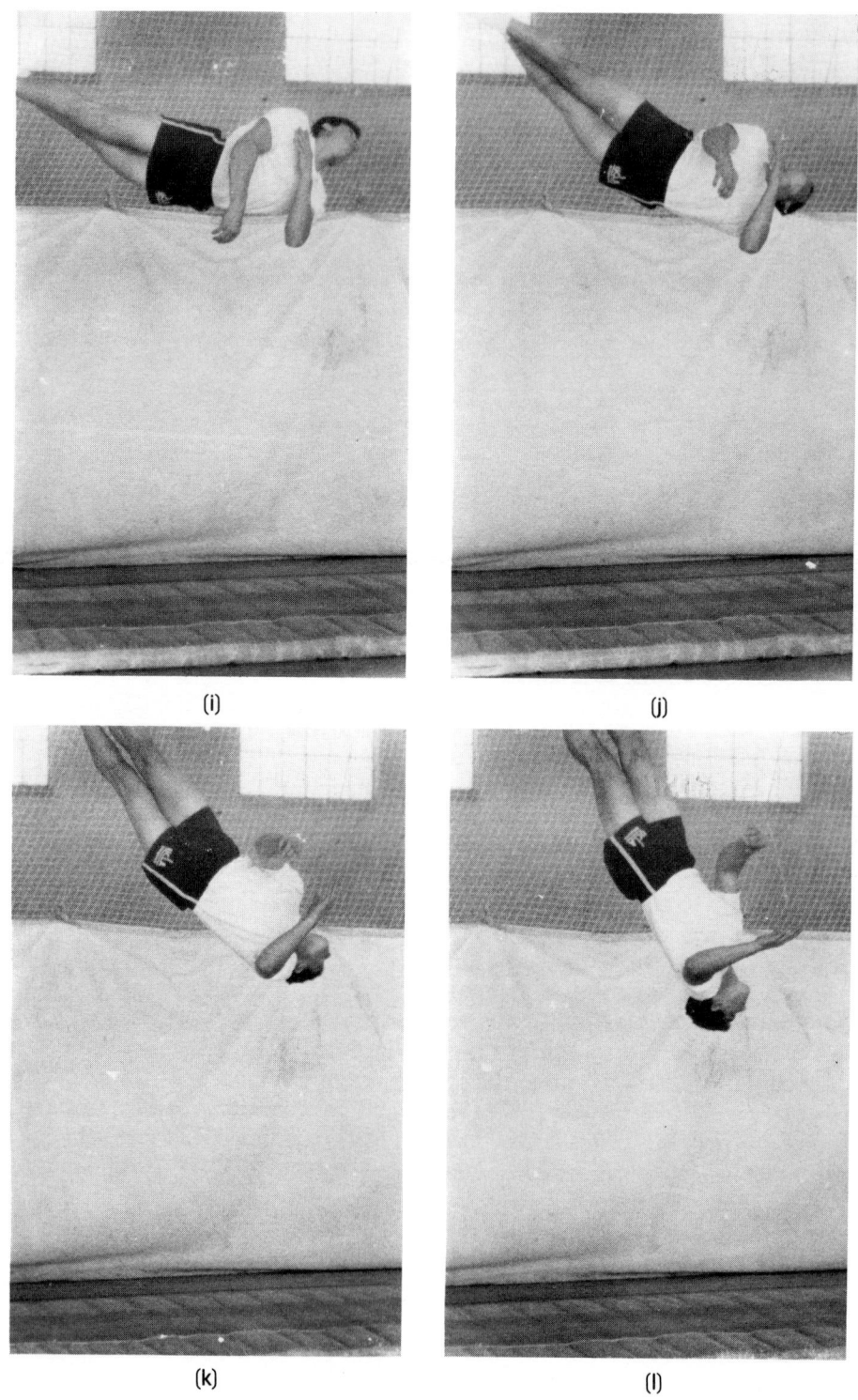

(i) (j)

(k) (l)

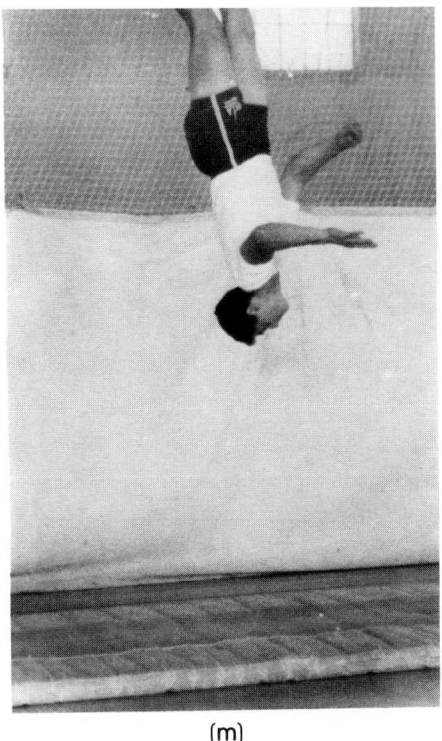

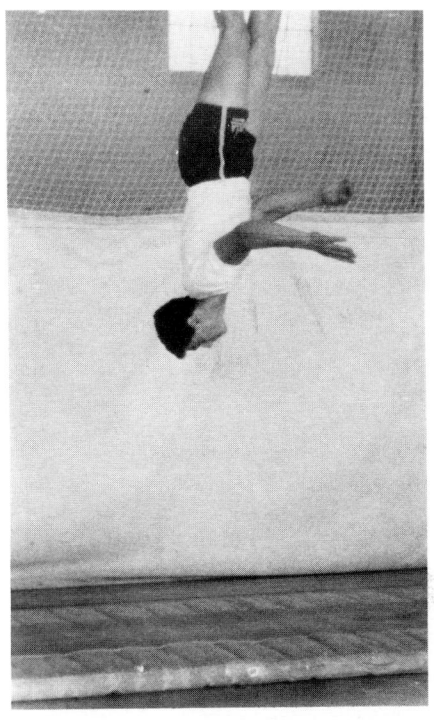

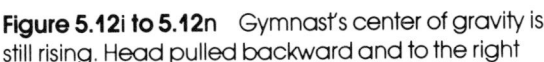

(m)

(n)

Figure 5.12i to 5.12n Gymnast's center of gravity is still rising. Head pulled backward and to the right

Figure 5.12o Twist completed. Arms extended sideward to slow rotation around long axis. Somersault halfway completed

less time to perform a stipulated number of twists, the tighter must be the "wrap-up." To decrease the speed of rotation, the radius of rotation is lengthened by extending the arms sideward, perpendicular to the vertical axis. This is the procedure utilized to slow down the rotation enabling the performer to complete the move facing in the desired direction. Fourth, in all three types of twists, force is applied at an angle to the vertical axis. When rotating only around the vertical axis, this force may be applied at a right angle to this axis. However, when a twist is combined with a salto it is necessary to compromise since it is impossible to throw the arms at

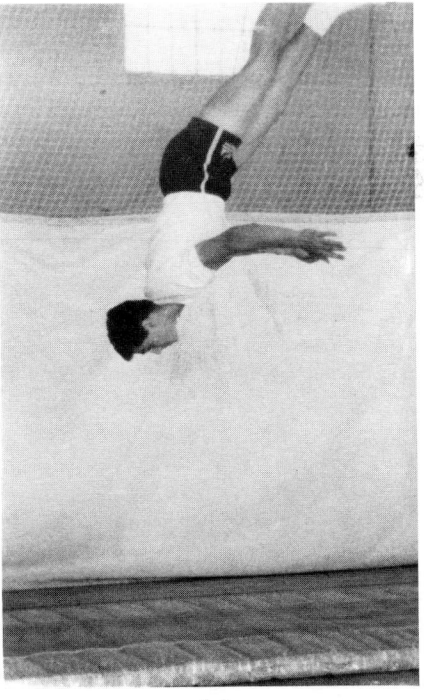

(o)

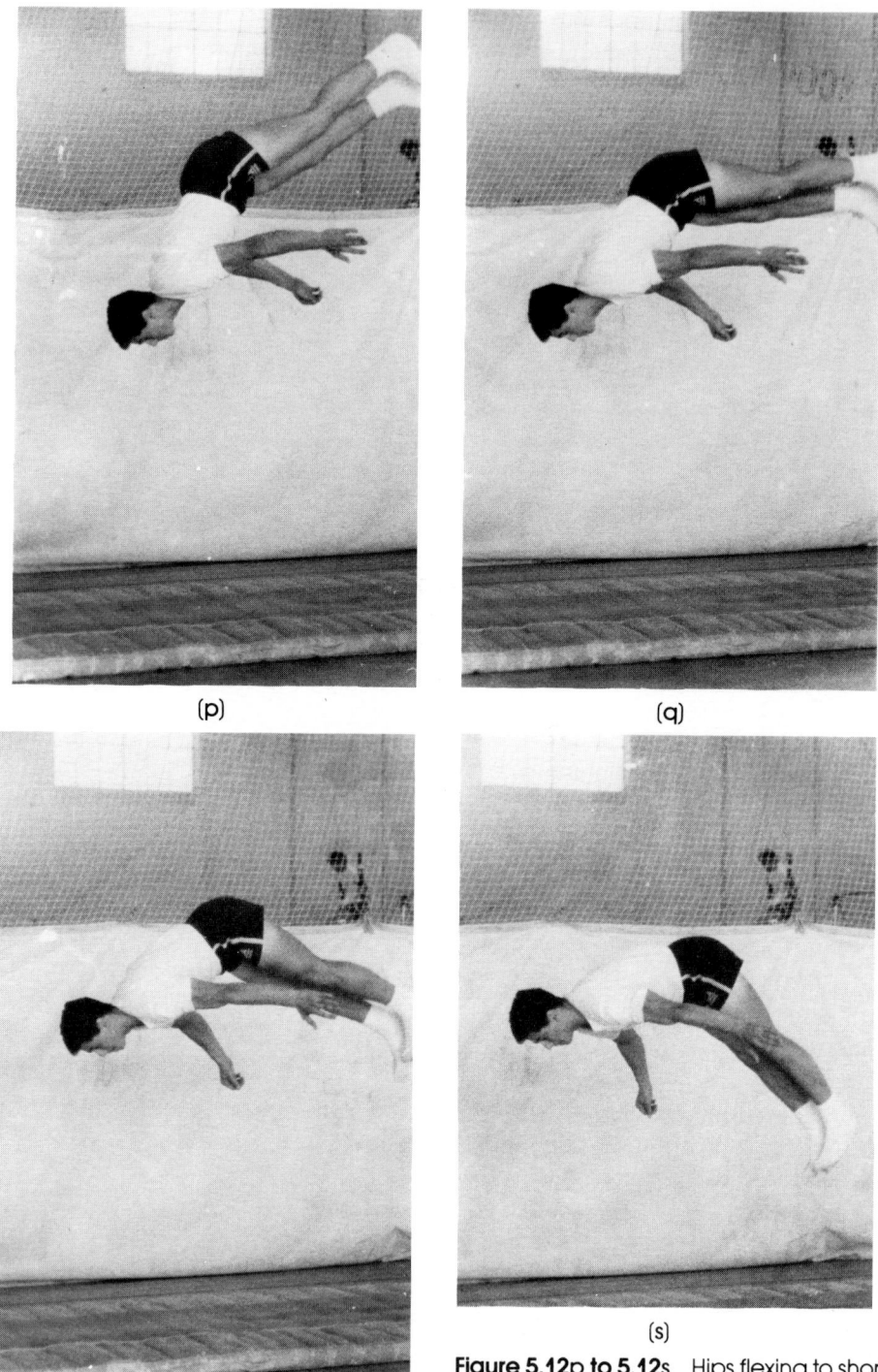

(p)

(q)

(r)

(s)

Figure 5.12p to 5.12s   Hips flexing to shorten radius of rotation around transverse horizontal axis to speed rotation to get feet under the body

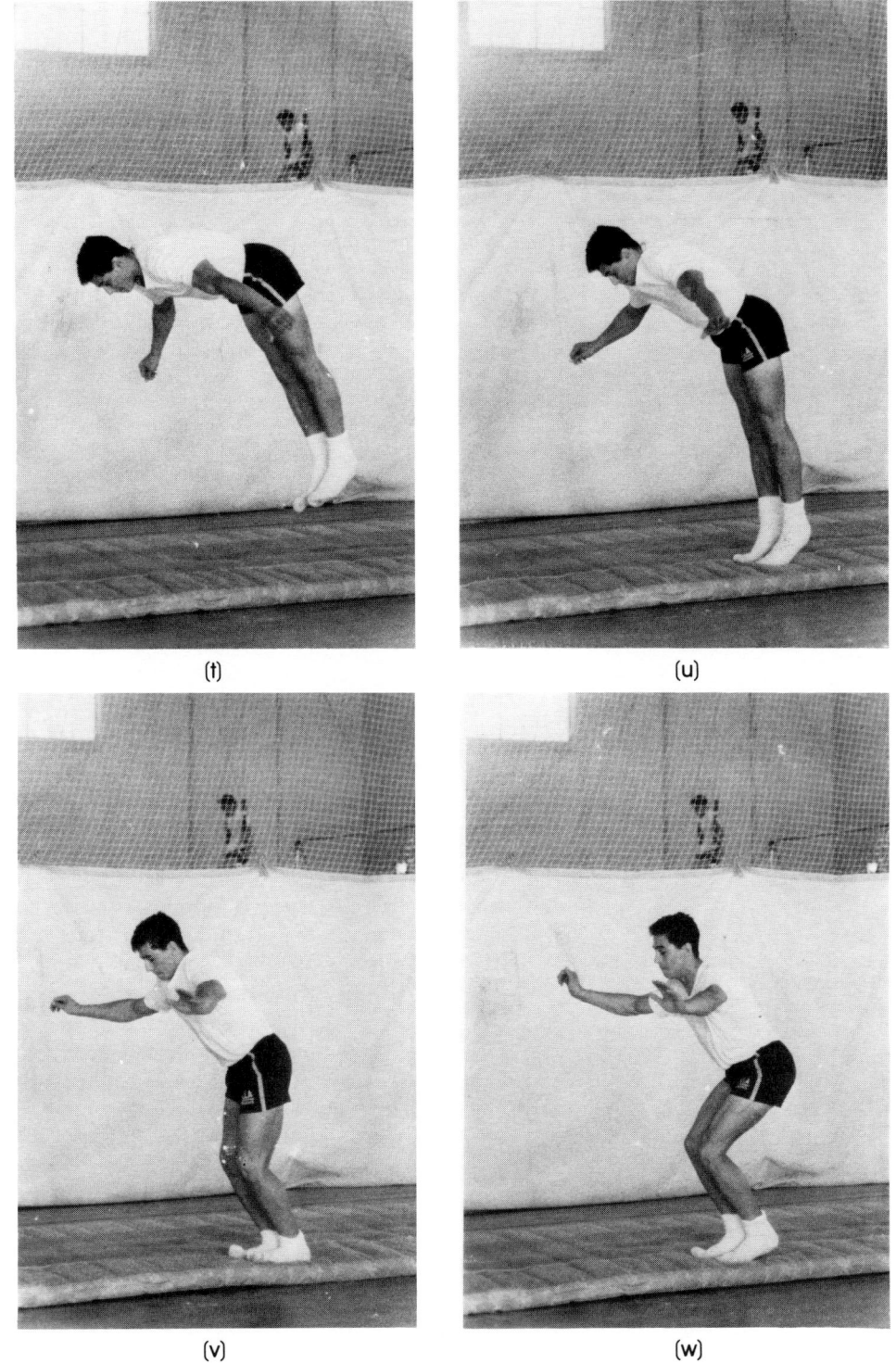

(t)

(u)

(v)

(w)

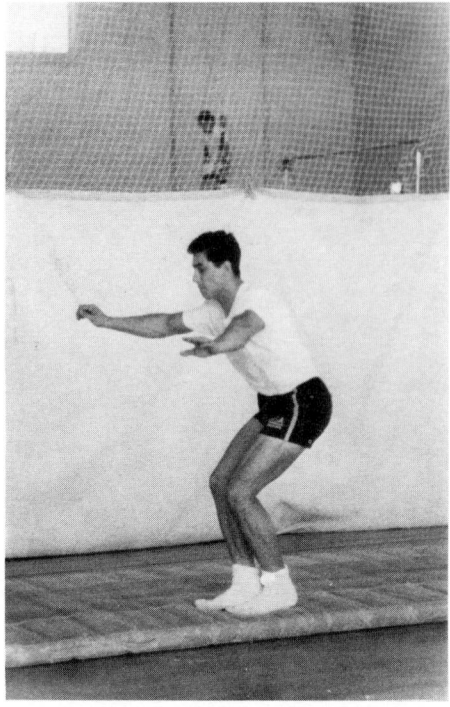

(x)

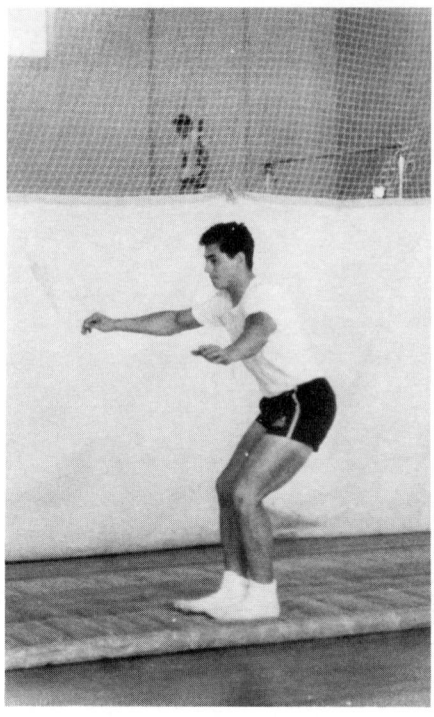

(y)

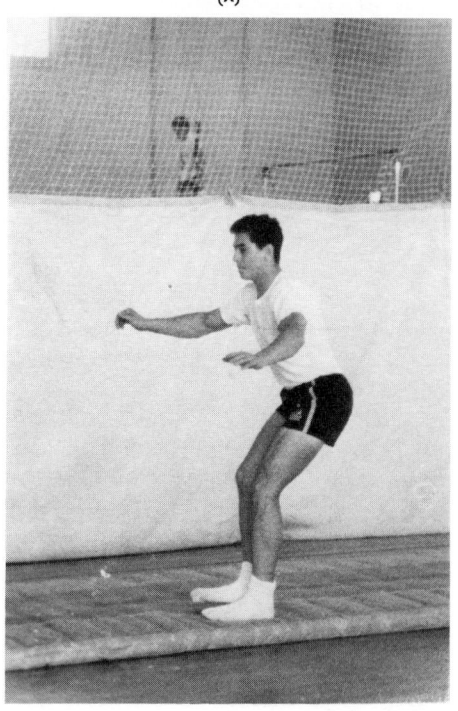

(z)

Figure 5.12t to 5.12z Feet contact mat and knees and hips flex while ankles dorsiflex to absorb impact through eccentric contraction of muscles. Somersault was slightly overspun

right angle to both the horizontal and vertical axis at the same time. Therefore, the arms are thrown diagonally to deliver a force at an angle to both axes. Fifth, to increase the moment of force or torque around the vertical axis, the arms begin their swing around the vertical axis in an extended position. In an extended position, the leverage provided the arms is greater, enabling them to generate greater force.

It is now time to discuss the procedures for "twisting from a pike." The performer leaves the supporting surface, traveling directly upward with no twisting motion. He moves into the piked position (hips flexed and legs extended). When the hips are up with the back and legs forming the sides of a triangle the base (line between head and feet) of which is

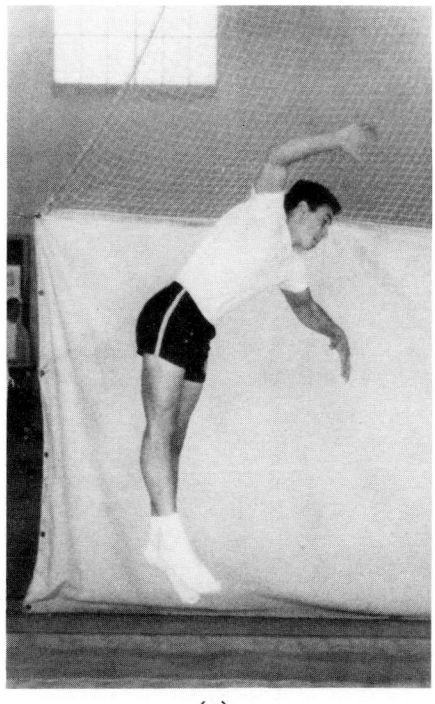

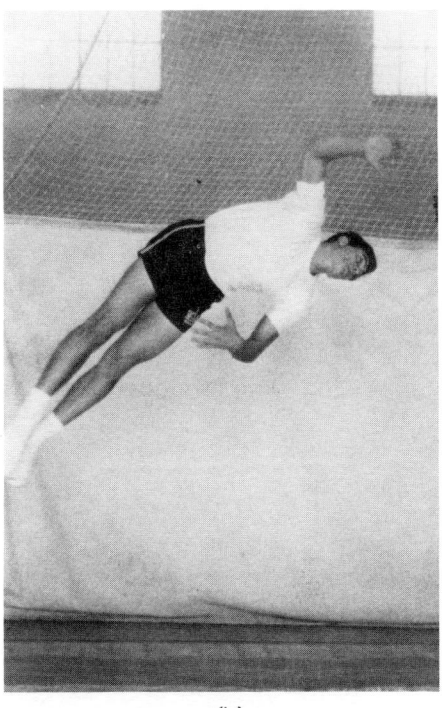

| (a) | (b) |

Figure 5.13 Forward Salto With Direct Full Twist (a) Gymnast has left mat and twist already begun. Note degree of hip flexion

Figure 5.13b Hips extending to facilitate twist (twists easier with body extended). Left arm sweeping across abdomen

horizontal, the right arm is thrown in a line parallel to the plane or in the plane of this base. No reactive twist occurs at this time because the arm movement is parallel to or in the plane of the body's vertical or twisting axis, which at this point is horizontal. The momentum of the arm is transferred to the body, the hips are extended, and the right arm continues to sweep across the chest while the left arm is pulled backward. At the same time, the head is vigorously turned in the direction of the twist. The body follows the arms and head in the same direction during the twist. When the hips are fully extended and the body is straight, the twist accelerates very rapidly. With this method there is a slight rotation around the transverse (front to rear) axis producing a side somersaulting action, but it is so small as to be barely noticeable due to the small mass of the arm relative to that of the body. When the body is in a piked position, the vertical or twisting axis is in front of the hips since the body weight is always distributed equally to both sides of the axis. The movement of the right arm, at this time, is parallel to or in the plane that passes through this axis. When the hips are extended, the vertical or twisting axis moves backward so that it passes through the body from head to toe. At this point, the arm movement is at an angle to the twisting axis and its momentum can produce torque around the twisting axis.

These kinds of actions could not be produced with a ball, javelin, or other object since they cannot change their shape voluntarily as can the human body. The ability of the human body to change its shape voluntar-

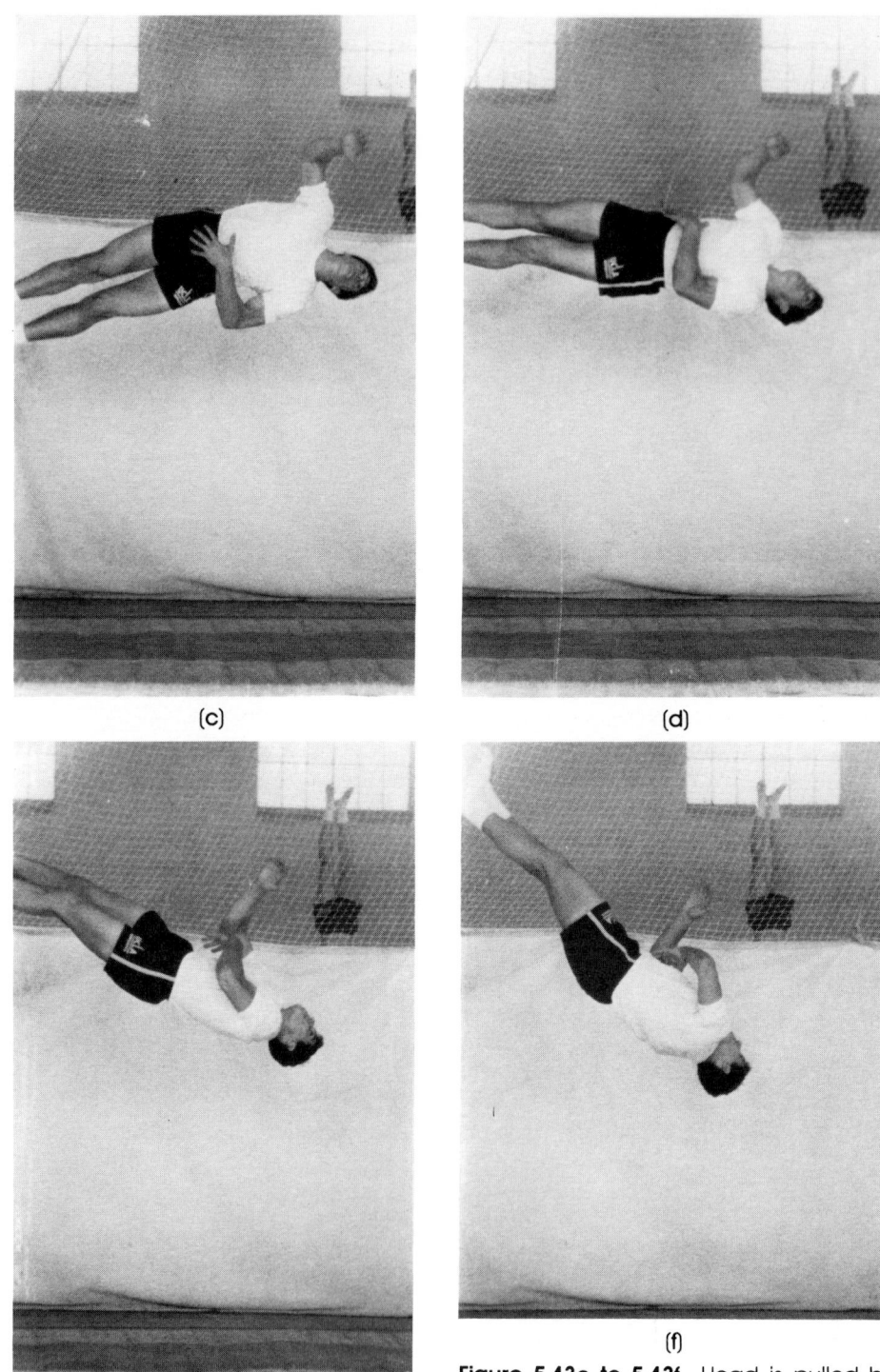

(c)

(d)

(e)

(f)

Figure 5.13c to 5.13f Head is pulled backward
and trunk and legs are in a straight line relationship

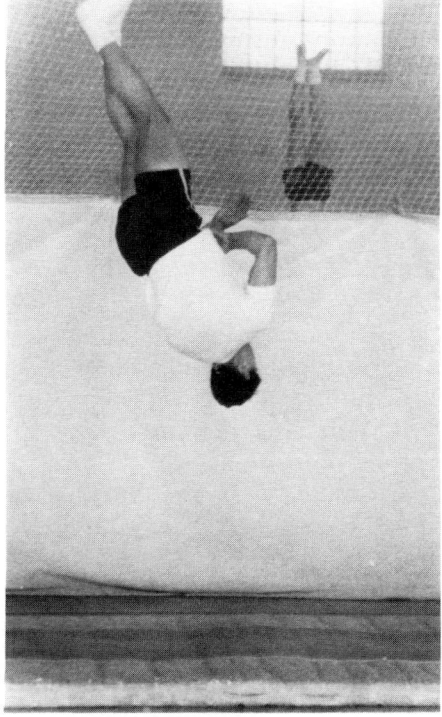

(g)

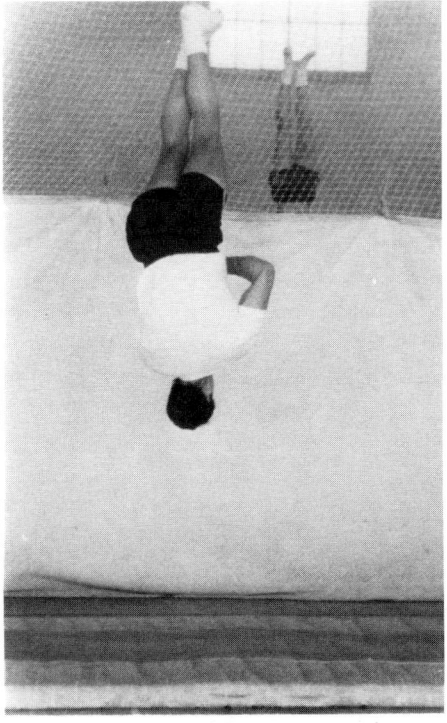

(h)

Figure 5.13g to 5.13i Twist and spin continuing. Hips and knees flexing to accelerate speed of rotation around horizontal axis

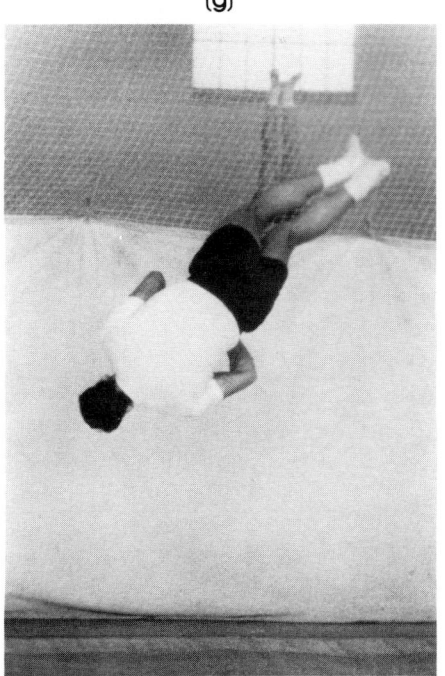

(i)

ily makes possible the accomplishment of many interesting movements—if the performer, coach, or instructor understands kinesiologic principles.

"Twisting from an arch" can also be initiated after the feet have left the supporting surface by applying the same principles and procedures as in "twisting from a pike." The difference is that in the former, the arm action is initiated while the body is arched and the twisting axis is behind the hips, while in the latter the arm action is initiated when the body is piked and the twisting axis is forward of the hips. In twisting from an arch, one arm is swung downward while the other is swung upward parallel to the vertical axis while the body is arched. As the arms wrap around the

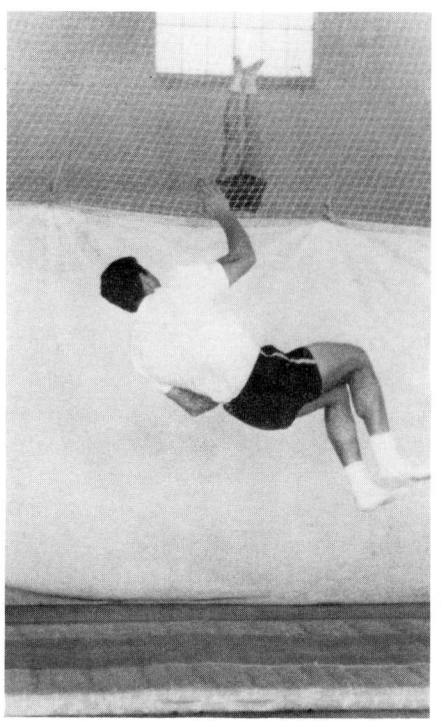

(j)

body to shorten the radius of rotation, the body is extended (made straight), thereby moving the twisting axis forward and placing it within the body. At this point, the arm action is at an angle to the twisting axis and the twist begins and rapidly accelerates.

HUMAN SOMERSAULTING MOTION

Whether doing single or multiple forward, backward, or sideward somersaults, the performer must obey the laws of physics and proceed according to kinesiologic principles. Torque must be applied at an angle to the axis of rotation. This torque must be of suffi-

Figure 5.13j Arms extending to slow twisting action. Knees flexing to speed rotation around transverse horizontal axis and to prepare for landing (k) to (l) Center of gravity moving over feet

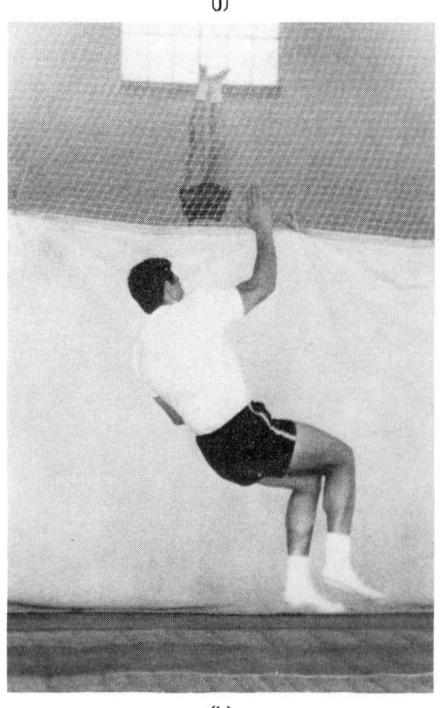

(k)

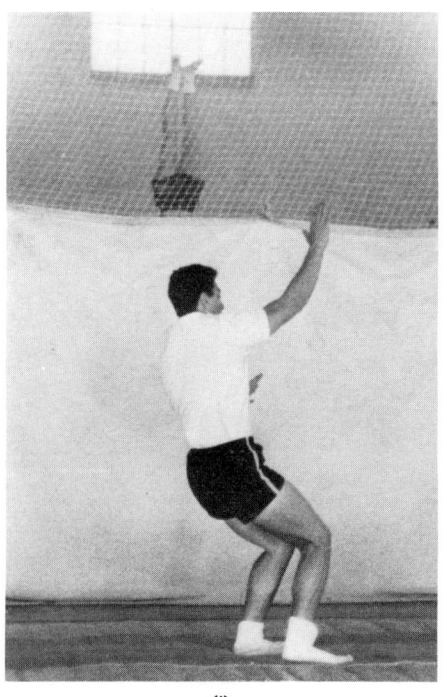

(l)

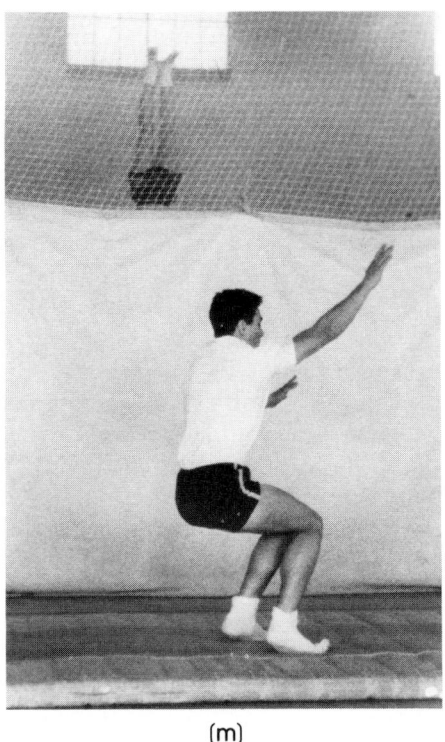
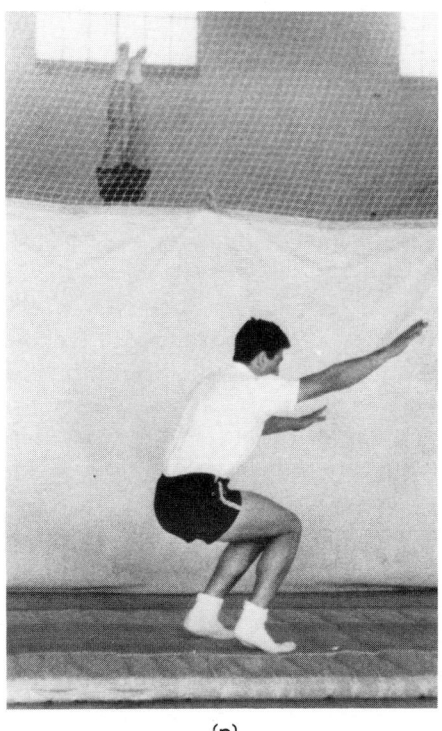

(m)   (n)

Figure 5.13m to 5.13n Knees and hips flexing to absorb impact

cent force to complete the somersault. The smaller the radius of rotation, the faster the rotation. The amount of torque, the length of the radius of rotation, and the height and direction of the lifting force must be in proper relationship to one another to produce the desired amount of rotation to land in the desired position. Further, the trajectory of the center of gravity, rotation of the body around the center of gravity, and the location of the center of gravity with respect to the actions of the legs and arms must be considered.

Front Saltos

At the moment of lift-off, the center of gravity of the body should be in front of the hips and directly over the feet. This requires that the hips be flexed and behind the vertical axis, which will pass from the feet through the back. The hips will also be behind the horizontal axis. The trajectory of the center of gravity is determined at the moment of lift-off. If it is forward of the feet, a low, traveling salto will result. If it is behind the feet, the salto will also be low but it will move backward. Further, greater difficulty will be experienced in completing the move. With the center of gravity directly over the feet, maximum height will be secured, providing more time to complete the somersault. With the hips behind the vertical axis, and flexed, the thrust from the backward angled legs will drive the hips upward more rapidly than the head and shoulders, thereby initiating the somersaulting movement. The push from the feet should be forward-downward. If the body is straight at the moment of lift-off, there will be no rotation.

These principles can be demonstrated with a jackknife opened to 45 degrees, balancing the handle of the jackknife on the fingertip and then pushing it upward. If the handle is vertical at the moment of the push, the jackknife will travel forward. It will travel even further forward if the handle is forward of the vertical. If the handle is angled backward but with the jackknife balanced (center of gravity over the fingertip), the knife will travel directly upward.

In the running front salto, because it is necessary to convert horizontal momentum to vertical momentum, the backward angling of the legs is even more pronounced than when doing the salto from a stand or on the trampoline.

As the feet are leaving the supporting surface, the arms, head, and trunk are thrown vigorously downward to further facilitate rotation by exerting a force at an angle to the axis of rotation. This force must be applied before the feet have left the supporting surface. The greater this force, the greater the rotation. After leaving the supporting surface, the rotational force cannot be increased by forcing the head or arms in the direction one wishes to rotate. This action also shortens the radius of rotation, which speeds up rotation. The shorter this radius, the faster the speed of rotation; therefore, rotation is more rapid in the tucked than in the jackknifed or piked position.

The success of the somersault is determined principally at the moment of lift-off. However, after lift-off the speed of rotation can be increased by tucking or piking more tightly in the event the performer finds he is not rotating rapidly enough or it can be decreased by opening up or extending the body sooner to lengthen the radius of rotation. The performer prepares for the landing by extending the body to decrease the speed of rotation. This extension should place the body

parts in a straight-line relationship, i.e., the head and legs should be in line with the back. If the head is forward or the hips are flexed while the other body parts are in a straight line, the slowing of rotational speed will not be as effective.

Preparation for the landing should be made while in flight. For a feet-first entry into water, the toes should be pointed, the body parts in a straight-line relationship, and the body angled slightly backward on completion of a forward somersault and slightly forward on completion of a backward somersault. A head-first entry into water requires a stretched body with the arms extended beyond the head and in line with the body and with the head between the arms. The entry should be made with the body at a slight angle from the vertical since it will continue to rotate, although more slowly, in the extended position after the feet or hands have entered the water. These positions will provide the most streamlined entry and least resistance from the water.

Landing on the trampoline should be as nearly vertical as possible due to the hazard of rebounding off the bed. Obviously, divers practicing on the trampoline must remember to dorsiflex the feet before landing.

Tumblers should endeavor to land in an extended position just slightly short of the vertical. They should absorb the impact by landing on the balls of the feet and allowing the ankles to dorsiflex and the knees and hips to bend by means of eccentric muscle contractions.

Back Saltos

The same principles apply to execution of a back salto as to a front salto except that the movements are reversed. The center of gravity is directly over the feet at the moment of thrust. The feet push backward and the head and trunk are thrown backward as the arms lift upward and backward to apply rotatory force at the moment of lift-off. If the center of gravity is behind the feet, a low, backward-traveling somersault will result. If it is forward of the feet, a low, forward-traveling (gainer) somersault will result. The trajectory of the center of gravity should be straight up and down. If the arms are driven too far backward too soon and too vigorously, an overspin is likely. This action must be proportional to the height of the lift-off and the desired number of revolutions. The tighter the tuck, the faster the somersaulting action. A back salto may be done in tucked, piked, or layout position. The degree of difficulty is in the order presented. During the layout somersault, the center or axis of rotation is outside (behind) the body. Execution of the back somersault or salto in layout position requires application of greater rotatory force than does the tucked or piked backward salto.

The speed of rotation is decelerated before landing by stretching the body so that the body parts assume a straight line relationship. Landing should be with the body just slightly short of the vertical. Impact of landing should be absorbed through eccentric contraction of the muscles of the feet, knees, hips, and back.

RHYTHMIC PATTERNS OF HUMAN MOTION

Most teachers and coaches of human movement and many regular sports spectators have noticed that each individual performer has his/her own preferred speed of movement. Rasch and Burke[9] point out that the speed and rhythm of an individual's movement patterns are probably the result of the sum of all the kinesiological, physiological, and psychological factors involved and that the individual tends to move at the rate most efficient for him. A study by Ronnholm[10] showed that the ease and efficiency of movement can be increased if it is done to a dis-

tinct rhythm. It is possible that one of the factors determining an athletic team's success is the degree of similarity between the rhythmic patterns of the individual members of the team.

SUMMARY

Throughout this chapter we have discussed selected laws and principles of physics and their application to human movement. Rotary and translatory motion have been defined as the two principal classifications of motion. These are further subdivided into repetitive angular movements and curvilinear motion. Angular or rotatory movements of several body parts may be combined to produce linear motion of other body parts or of implements. Optimum projection angles for achievement of different objectives such as speed, distance, or height vary. Formulas for computing horizontal distance, height, and time in the air have been presented.

Newton's laws of motion—inertia, acceleration, and action and reaction—were reviewed. The roles of force, velocity, mass, momentum, transfer of momentum, and length of levers in various forms of human movement were analyzed. It is necessary to understand the relationships between momentum and impact, force, agility, speed, and strength if maximal potential human movement efficiency is to be obtained. Strength relative to body mass is an important consideration in performance in most sports. Additionally, the heavier the implement used, the more important strength becomes. Great body mass is advantageous in some sports activities but is nonfunctional if strength is inadequate. In many activities, the momentum of the body or its parts is transferred to other body parts, to implements, or to other players. Where maximal rotatory momentum, moment of force, or torque around an axis is desired, the length of the lever arm should be increased. When maximal rotational speed is desired, the radius of gyration should be shortened.

One of the techniques for generating maximal momentum is that of initiating each sequential joint action at the point of greatest speed and least acceleration of the preceding joint action. Other techniques are increasing the distance and, consequently, the time through which velocity is accelerated. This is done by increasing the length of the backswing and the follow-through.

The different systems for indicating acceleration—MKS, CGS, and FPS—have been explained, as have the terms newton (nt), dyne, and slug. The utilization of vectors and parallelograms has been presented.

Energy cost varies with the cube of the speed of contraction. Since rapid acceleration requires fast muscular contractions, rapid acceleration may be contraindicated in endurance events.

The flight path of the center of gravity of the body, like all other objects, is determined at the moment the body leaves its supporting surface. The flight path is determined by the direction of thrust and the relationship of the location of the center of gravity with respect to the point of projection. If the center of gravity is forward of the point of projection, a low, traveling somersault will result. If it is behind the point of projection, a backward-traveling somersault will be the outcome.

The direction of thrust from the feet differs in forward and cutaway (inward) and backward and gainer (reverse) somersaults. A circling implement such as a discus or hammer will fly off in a direction at a right angle to the radius of its circular path at the moment it is released. A ball struck with a bat will leave the circling bat at a right angle to the long axis of the bat at the moment it struck the ball.

The action–reaction law mandates that the reacting surface be firm and stable and pro-vide good traction if force is to be effectively utilized. If maximum momentum is to be transferred from one part of the body to an implement, all the joints between the striking body part and the supporting surface must be stabilized or the force of the impact will be diminished due to the absorption of force.

Motion may be either uniform or variable. Procedures were described for use of vectors in constructing parallelograms to determine the direction and velocity of objects acted on by two different forces or to determine the necessary direction and amount of velocity required to project a missile to a desired point.

Procedures for determination of angular velocity and angular acceleration have been presented, as have procedures for determination of linear velocity. Like velocity, acceleration may be either uniform or variable. Since acceleration is the rate of change of a rate of motion, time enters into the unit twice.

Impulse is the product of force and the time over which the force acts. The greater the momentum of an object, the greater the impulse required to accelerate or decelerate the object. This principle illustrates why the differing objectives of different sports require players of different body mass for successful play. These relationships are fully treated in the body of this chapter. Force × time = mass × (initial velocity − final velocity); consequently, the greater the time during which force is applied, the greater the final velocity. This is the basis for recommending a long backswing, specific landing procedures, use of crash pads, and many other procedures in human movement.

Momentum is conserved, i.e., the total of the momentums (mv) of two objects before impact equals their total momentums after impact. Upon impact one object will lose velocity while the other gains velocity.

Angular momentum is the product of the moment of inertia times the angular velocity. The moment of inertia is the sum of the mass of each particle of the object rotating times the square of the particle's perpendicular distance to the axis of rotation. The greater the mass and the greater the distance of the mass from the axis of rotation, the greater the moment of inertia. Angular momentum is conserved. If the moment of inertia is decreased by moving the mass closer to the center of rotation, the angular velocity will be accelerated so that the product of the moment of inertia and angular velocity will be the same after the mass was moved closer to the axis as before. The application of this principle to a number of different sports movements has been described.

Gravity begins to act on any projectile from the instant it is projected until it returns to the earth. Due to the uniform pull of gravity, all projectiles follow a parabolic flight path. The time the pull of gravity has to act is the sole determinant of the time a projectile will remain in flight; consequently, the initial velocity and the angle of projection are the two factors to be considered when distance is desired. The optimum angle of projection ranges between 37 and 45 degrees depending upon the initial velocity of the projectile and the difference in elevation between the point of projection and the landing point. The implications of these phenomena for throwing various implements and for hurling the body were discussed.

Finally, the individual nature of rhythmic patterns of human movement was pointed out. A person moves most efficiently when movement is according to the individual's own unique rhythmic pattern.

REFERENCES

1. Baley, James A., "A Comparison of the Effects Upon Selected Measures of Physical Fitness of Participation in Sports and in Mass Isometric Exercises Done with a Belt." *The Journal of Sports Medicine*, 7:198-203, December, 1967.

2. Baley, James A., "Effects of Isometric Exercises Done With a Belt Upon the Physical Fitness Status of Students in Required Physical Education Classes, *The Research Quarterly*, 37:291-301, October, 1966.

3. Toyoshima, S., Hoshikawa, T., Miyashita, M., and Oguri, T., "Contribution of Body Parts to Throwing Performance," *Biomechanics IV* (edited by R. C. Nelson and C. A. Morehouse). Baltimore: University Park Press, 1974, pp. 169-174.

4. Roozbazar, A., "Biomechanics of Lifting," *Biomechanics IV* (edited by R. C. Nelson and C. A. Morehouse). Baltimore: University Park Press, 1974, pp. 37-43.

5. Schvartz, Esar, "Effect of Impulse on Momentum in Performing on the Trampoline," *Research Quarterly*, 38:2:300-304, May, 1967.

6. Baley, James A., *Handbook of Gymnastics in the Schools*. Boston: Allyn and Bacon, 1974, pp. 31-32.

7. Kunz, H., "Effect of Ball Mass and Movement Pattern on Release Velocity in Throwing," *Biomechanics IV* (edited by R. C. Nelson and C. A. Morehouse). Baltimore: University Park Press, 1974, pp. 163-168.

8. Cooper, John M., and Glassow, Ruth B., *Kinesiology* (4th ed.). St. Louis: C. V. Mosby, 1972, pp. 290-291.

9. Rasch, Phillip J., and Burke, Roger K., *Kinesiology and Applied Anatomy* (6th ed.). Philadelphia: Lea and Febiger, 1978, p. 464.

10. Ronnholm, N., "Physiologic Studies on the Optimum Rhythm of Lifting Work," *Ergonomics*. 1962, 5:1:51-52.

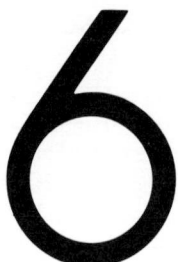

FORCES AFFECTING HUMAN MOTION

CONCEPTS

1. Movement stems from internal and external forces. Internal force is derived from muscular contraction, whereas external force originates from outside mechanical elements.

2. Linear and angular motions, although different, are closely related.

3. A scalar quantity possesses magnitude without reference of direction. A vector quantity contains direction as well as magnitude or mass.

4. A parallelogram may be used as a method of determining the resultant of two forces acting at right angles.

5. A force that pushes or pulls along a translatory line of action is called a linear force.

6. Two equal forces acting on a common point in opposite directions with equal intensity will result in a state of equilibrium.

7. Mechanical advantage is a measure of a machine's efficiency and, as expressed in levers, is the ratio of the resistance overcome to the application of effort.

8. In physics three terms are commonly used to describe muscular activity: work, power, and energy.

9. Conceptually, centripetal force is a force pulling the object or segment toward the center of a circle or arc; and centrifugal force is the opposite force pulling the object away from the axis.

10. Four components regulate the intensity of centripetal and centrifugal forces: Newton's first law of inertia, mass or weight, velocity, and radius of rotation.

11. Friction alters motion and is identified as two types: sliding and rolling.

12. The production and application of force is affected by magnitude, direction, point of application, and time over which force is applied.

13. The force of rebound is contingent upon resistance of contact surfaces, momentum generated by the object, and its coefficient of restitution or elasticity.

14. The angle of incidence is the angle of approach before a ball strikes the surface, while the angle of reflection is the angle of rebound after the ball hits the surface.

GENERAL CONSIDERATIONS

Energy is the ability to produce movement. Energy provides the source of force that may cause a movement or prevent a motion from occurring. Muscular contraction is considered an internal force whereby the body or segment is either moved (dynamic contraction) or stabilized, fixed or neutralized (isometric contraction). For example, contraction of the biceps brachii producing elbow flexion is a motion of the body generated by an internal force of a skeletal muscle. Fixation of the abdominal muscles is also an example of internal muscular force whereby a force is exerted; however, movement does not take place. Therefore, a movement that is generated by the human organism itself is termed *internal force*. The source of internal force in humans stems from the ability and capability of muscles to contract creating a movement or preventing a motion depending upon the nature of the exercise and/or activity. Conversely, a force exerted from sources outside the body, and due to such factors as Newton's laws of motion, gravity, ground contact, or "pushing" or "pulling" producing or preventing a motion is called an *external force*. Forces may also be classified as *linear* or *rotary*.

Biomechanics frequently utilize the terms *kinematics* and *kinetics*. Kinematics, as defined in Chapter 5, deal with the geometry of motion, whereas kinetics considers the forces that produce change of motion. Such parameters as how fast or far a body moves in a straight or linear path are within the domain of *linear kinematics*. The speed of rotation around a horizontal axis such as performing a forward one-and-one-half somersault from a diving board is termed *angular kinematics*.

Kinetics may also be divided into two categories: *linear* and *angular*. A body in motion continues to stay in motion unless an external force acts upon the object to stop or alter its speed and direction. This exemplifies an analysis in *linear kinetics*. The magnitude or degree of tuck tightness, such as executing the forward one-and-one-half somersault dive mentioned earlier illustrates a study of *angular kinetics*. Therefore, it can be seen that linear and angular kinetics are related. Each of these variables affect the rotary quantities of velocity and acceleration in the performance of a somersault dive.

SCALAR AND VECTOR UNITS
Scalar Quantities

A scalar quantity is a unit measure that has magnitude without a reference of direction. Such properties as speed, length, temperature, time, mass, volume, and area are scalars. Magnitude (amount or size) is one variable that affects the quantitative attributes of a body moving under its own initiative or reacting under the influence of an external force. For example, an individual's total body mass and volume affects his/her floating ability. An object placed in water is buoyed up by a force equal to the weight of the water it displaces (Archimedes principle); therefore, individuals who have large surface areas and low mass quantities usually float without difficulty. Conversely, persons with high density and greater mass quantities experience difficulty staying afloat, although factors such as skill and breathing technique (which affects lung volume) also enter the floating scene. Body size and mass probably affects the floating ability of an individual, which is a scalar unit, more than any other single biomechanical variable.

The force exerted upon a body on land is influenced by its mass and weight. Body weight is often used as a measure of mass for practical purposes; however, these terms should be considered separately when quantifying data. Weight is a force with which matter (composition) is drawn toward the earth. For example, when determining the object's weight, we are measuring the attraction of the earth for that body. The weight of a body depends upon (1) mass or quantity of matter it contains and (2) its gravitational pull. Thus, $w = m \times g$, where w = weight, m = mass, and g = force of gravity. It can be seen that mass contains magnitude or size without direction whereas weight not only has magnitude but direction as well. In quantitative terms, mass is a *scalar*; weight is a *vector*, which is described in later paragraphs. The scalar quantity of mass is directly related to Newton's first law of motion (see Chapter 5), which states that inertia is proportional to mass. An object's unit measure of inertia depends upon its packing quality or density described earlier as a "slug." The greater its mass, the more its resistance to motion and/or change in alteration of motion. Mass, when considered as a quantity on land is expressed by the following formula:

$$\text{mass} = \frac{\text{weight (kg)}}{\text{gravity (m/sec}^2)}$$
$$= \frac{\text{weight (kg)}}{9.8 \, \text{m/sec}^2}$$

As shown above, a unit of mass will be accelerated positively at 9.8 m/sec/sec when a force of one kilogram is applied.

The student should keep in mind that mass and weight, although often used as similar concepts—e.g., overcoming the resting inertia in a sprinter's start—are different. The weight of the body involves the pull of gravity on its mass. The above formula is applicable to human performance within the general environs of the earth's atmosphere; however, it does not apply everywhere. Weight changes depending upon the extent of gravitational pull. Slight variation exists at different geographical locations. For example, an individual would weigh slightly less at the equator as compared to his/her weight at the North or South Poles because of a decline in gravitational pull at the earth's poles. This phenomenon is also true when an athlete performs in areas of high sea levels. The weight lessens with increasing height. However, this change is miniscule and probably has an insignificant effect upon the performance of motor or athletic skills. On the other hand, athletes would weigh much less on the moon, where the gravitational pull is about one-sixth that of the earth's attraction. Now that man is ex-

ploring space and moving in states of weightlessness, we may have to consider weight as a vital variable in mobility. However, this consideration is projected into the twenty-first century and entails an entirely different set of biomechanical principles. Whereas the weight of the body can change depending upon location, mass is not affected even though a body may be shifted from one place to another. Although mass and weight differ, there is a clear-cut relationship between the two quantities. An example of a trampolinist weighing 161 pounds at the peak of his flight is explained as follows:[1]

$$F = ma$$
$$w = mg$$
or
$$m = \frac{w}{g}$$

The earth exerts a downward force w on the performer, and as a result, he is accelerated back toward the bed with an acceleration of g. The relationship between his weight, his mass, and acceleration due to gravity is derived from Newton's second law. Thus, it may be seen that a unit of mass (slug) or resistance to change (inertia) is affected by weight and mass as follows:

$$m = \frac{161 \, \text{lb}}{32.2 \, \text{ft/sec}^2}$$
$$= 5 \, \text{slugs}$$

or one of mass 4 slugs to weigh 128.8 lb, viz.,

$$w = 4 \times 32.2$$
$$= 128.8 \, \text{lb}$$

The implication of the scalar quantity of mass simply translated to human performance implies that a lighter object (less massive) requires less force to overcome its inertia, whether it is in a resting state or moving.

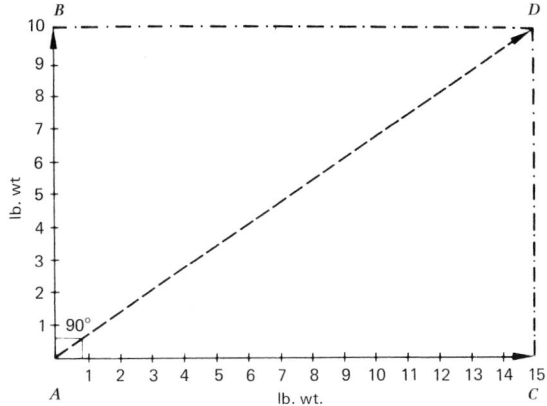

Figure 6.1 Resultant of forces acting at right angles (from F. A. MacDonald, **Mechanics for Movement**, Bell and Hyman Ltd., London, p. 15, with permission)

Vector Quantities

A vector quantity is a unit that possesses *direction* as well as mass. Such measures as velocity, force, acceleration, momentum, displacement, friction, work, and power are vectors because direction is an integral part of the unit. A parallelogram of vectors illustrating a football punt is constructed and an-

alyzed in Chapter 5 (Figure 5.7). This procedure allows the quantification of two forces and represents a vector analysis.

Another example of using the parallelogram procedure to determine the resultant forces acting at right angles is exhibited by Figure 6.1.

As shown in Figure 6.1, two vector quantities are drawn to represent two forces acting at right angles on an object at point A. AB = a force of 10 lb. AC = force of 15 lb. Force AB will tend to pull to B, while force AC will pull to C. As both forces pull at the same time, the object will move along the diagonal of the parallelogram of which the two forces are sides. A rectangle is produced, divided into two right-angled triangles. The geometrical *Pythagorean theorem* states that the square of the hypotenuse of the right triangle is equal to the sum of the squares of the other two sides, therefore:

$$AD^2 = AC^2 + CD^2$$

$$AD^2 = 10^2 + 15^2 = 325$$

$$AD = \sqrt{325} \qquad = 18.03 \text{ lb resultant force}$$

The combination of two or more component vectors results in a new vector quantity. For example, Figure 6.2 shows an object being pushed forward, with a force proportion-

Figure 6.2 Resolution of forces (from F. A. MacDonald, **Mechanics for Movement**, Bell and Hyman Ltd., London, p. 17, with permission)

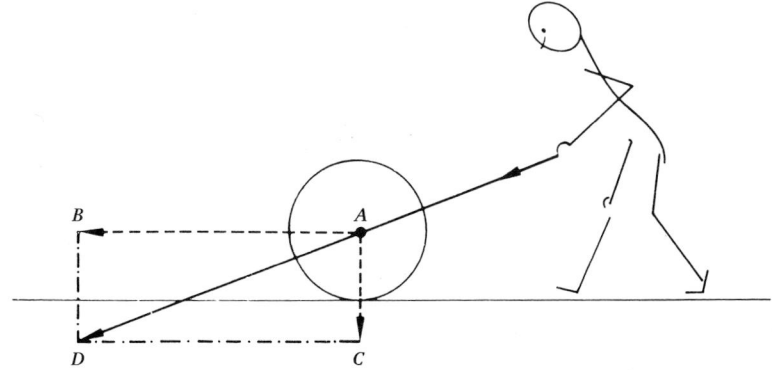

ate to the distance from *A* to *D* (force applied to the handle and transmitted to the axle) broken down into two components: *AB* moves the roller forward; *AC* moves the roller into the ground. The reverse of composing two or more component forces into one force (the resultant) is to separate one force of a given magnitude and direction into two elements. This process is known as the resolution of forces. The resolution of these vectors is illustrated by Figure 6.2, where a single force is separated into two forces (horizontal and vertical components). Generally, these forces act at 90 degrees to each other.

The application of the principle of forces as applied to a long-jumper and exhibited by Figure 6.3 shows the line of action of a force driving him into the air.[2] Two effects of this force project the jumper vertically and forward. The problem is to determine the proportion of forces in each of these two directions. In order to solve this problem, the directions or magnitudes of both components, or the direction and magnitude of one component, must be known in advance. The parallelogram method is used as shown by Figure 6.3.

Horizontal and vertical components are shown as the jumper leaps into the air. A parallelogram is made with the diagonal as the vector of the takeoff force. The length of each of these lines in comparison with that of the diagonal represents the magnitude of the components in relation to the takeoff drive. With a known takeoff force, the line of action can be drawn in units of length corresponding to the units of force, and from the length of the component vectors, the magnitude of the horizontal and vertical forces can be calculated.[3]

Graphic parallelogram of vectors, as described, is a useful procedure to assist the student in the conceptualization of scalar and vector quantities affecting the magnitude and direction of a resultant force in a given performance. Sophisticated trigonometric

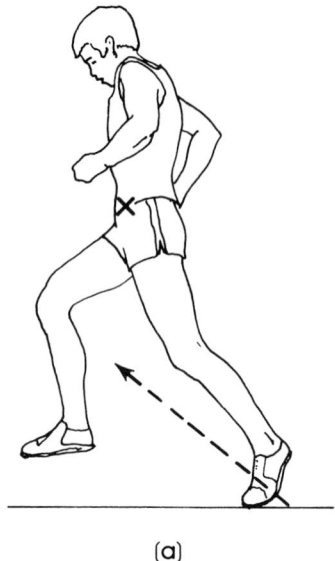

(a)

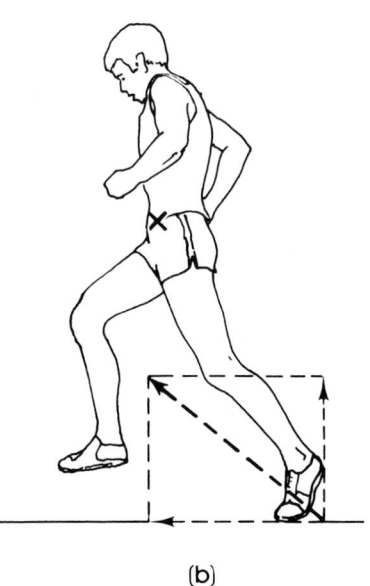

(b)

Figure 6.3 Parallelogram method for determining the resolution of forces in the long-jump (a) Line of action of force driving the athlete in the air. (b) Vertical and horizontal lines producing a parallelogram with the diagonal as a vector (from Geoffrey Dyson, **Mechanics of Athletics**, Hodder and Stoughton Educational, London, 1973, p. 42, with permission)

approaches, which make use of cosine and sine functions, offer a more accurate and precise method in the resolution of vector problems. These procedures are appropriate for research work when exact numerical data are necessary.

FORCE TYPES

It is now apparent from our previous discussion that force is a vector quantity that can produce motion and prevent or neutralize movement. A force that pushes or pulls along a translatory line of action is called a *linear force*, as shown by Figure 6.4 with two persons engaged in a tug-of-war.

A force acting on an object moving in a straight line is called a *single linear force*. An example of this type is typified by pushing a wagon or cart. Two *equal forces* acting on a common point in opposite directions with equal intensity will result in a state of equilibrium. For example, an object placed on a table is in a state of balance. This is because the downward force of the object is opposed by an equivalent upward vertical force from the table with both forces on the same line of action. Forces that lie parallel and in the same plane to each other, but do not act along the same action line are called *parallel forces*. For example, a seesaw motion with

the weight of two individuals, one on each end, constitutes forces in the same direction opposed by the upward force at the fulcrum, as shown by Figure 6.5.

Parallel forces under certain circumstances may cause a turning or rotating action. This action occurs when there are two forces of equal amount and equal distance, and in opposite directions. This force type is called a *couple*. Driving a car with both hands on the steering wheel typifies the coupling forces of the hands as the driver controls the steering mechanism. A parallel force system is also found within the human body. As shown in Figure 6.6, flexion of the elbow joint to the horizontal position contains two lines of action that are parallel and opposite to each other; the force of the arm weight plus gravity pulls downward, and biceps, brachialis, and brachioradialis muscles pull upward.

Forces that act or meet at a point are called *concurrent forces*. Concurrent forces may be applied to the body from different angles from a common point to produce a singular movement. For example, the anterior and posterior fibers of the deltoid muscle flex and extend the humerus in the sagittal plane (forward and backward) when contracting independently or singly; however, when working concurrently, the humerus abducts laterally in the frontal plane.[4]

External concurrent forces are typified by

Figure 6.4 Linear force—pulling in a straight line

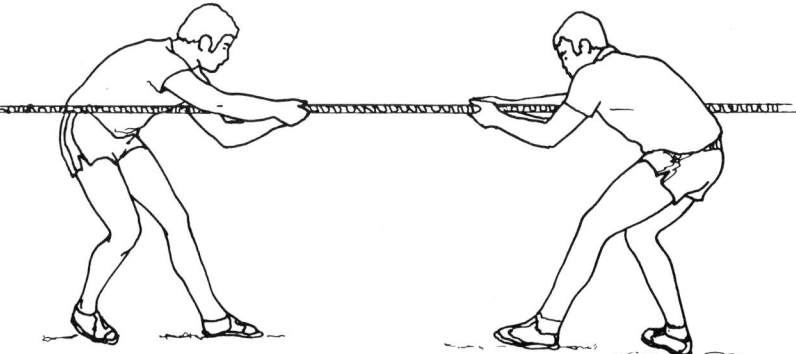

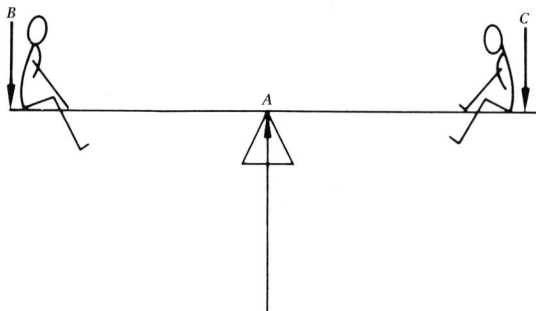

Figure 6.5 Parallel forces exerted in the same plane

two or more football players opposing the ball carrier from different angles, but hitting the player at one point. The resultant of the forces can be determined by applying the parallelogram method described in the pre-

Figure 6.6 Parallel force system causing rotation (from F. A. MacDonald, **Mechanics for Movement**, Bell and Hyman, London, with permission)
a = Distance from center of rotation to the upward line of action
b = Distance from center of rotation to the downward line of action
F = Upward line of action
G = Downward line of action

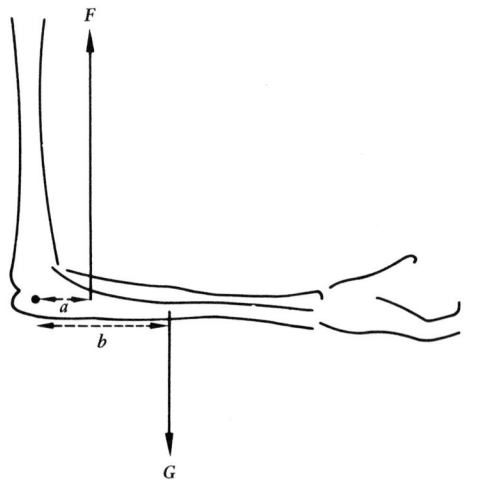

ceding sections of this chapter and in Chapter 5.

TORQUE AND MOMENT ARMS

Many movements of the body involve turning or rotating motions. In fact, all linear movements originate from the lever actions of joint articulations. Whenever a joint rotates, *torque* occurs; and subsequently this action entails the concept of *moment arms*. The turning motion of an applied force is called a *torque* or *moment of force*. The product of the applied force (magnitude) and the lever arm (perpendicular distance from the direction of force to the axis of rotation) determines the torque of an angular movement. The perpendicular distance from the line of force to the axis is called a *moment arm*. It can be seen that torque and moment arm variables are inherent in lever constructs of the body. The composition and characteristics of each lever type are considered in Chapter 7. Our discussion, in this section, focuses on the force aspects of torque and moments, and their applications to motor movements.

The effort required in a given angular movement can be controlled by adjusting the *length of the moment arm* from its fulcrum or axis of rotation or by changing the *magni-*

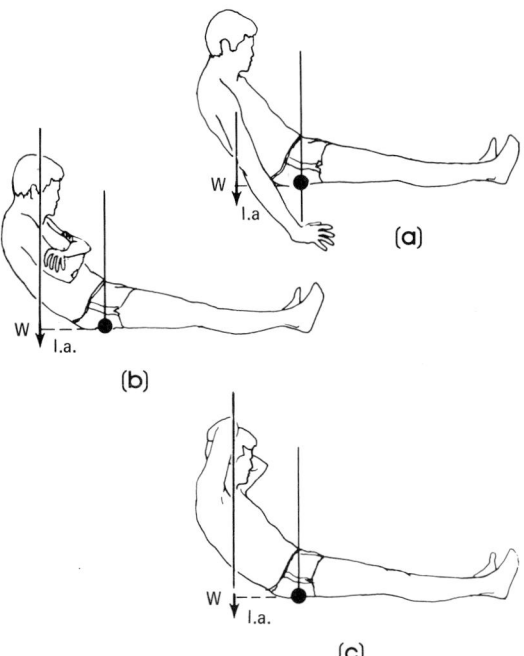

Figure 6.7 Increasing force demands by lengthening the moment or lever arm. (a) Less force required. (b) More force required. (c) Greatest force required. W = weight line. l.a. = lever length

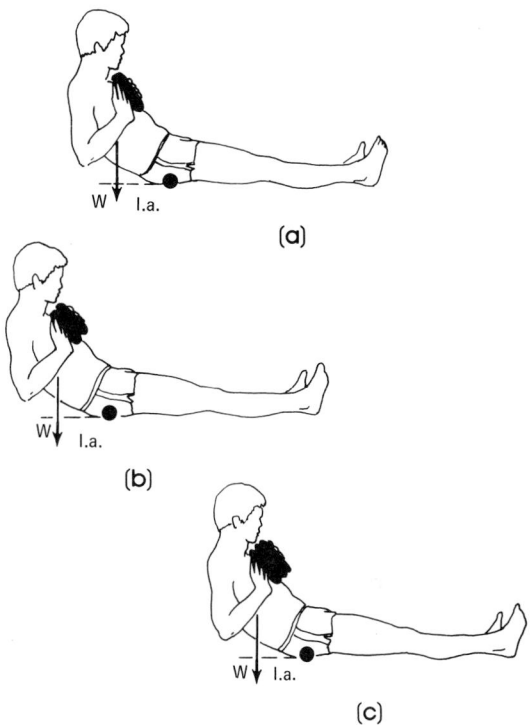

Figure 6.8 Increasing the force demands by adding weight to the moment or lever arm. (a) Five-lb weight. (b) Ten-lb weight. (c) Fifteen-lb weight. W = weight line. l.a. = lever length

tude of the *weight* of the moving segment. Performing a sit-up illustrates a practical application of torque and moment arm concepts. For example, if one executes a sit-up with arms along the sides of the body as shown in Figure 6.7a, the exerciser discovers, very quickly, that this technique is much easier than performing the same movement with hands interlaced and placed behind the head (Figure 6.7c).

The force demand for a sit-up is greater when performing with hands behind the head because of the increased length of the lever arm from its axis of rotation. Another way in which the force demand can be increased is by adding resistance at the end of the lever arm. Figure 6.8a, b, c illustrates a series of progressive loading whereby performing a sit-up becomes more difficult as weights are added to the performer.

It can be seen that muscular requirements in performing the popular sit-up exercise can be altered by changing limb positions and/or by adding weights to the moving segments. The student should keep in mind that as the perpendicular distance decreases from the supine position to the 90 degree or upright sit-up position, less force is required irrespective of the lever length adjustments of the limbs or the weight added to the moving segment. The above torque and moment concepts contain direct relevance for fitness specialists in the development of graded exercises adjusted to the individual's strength condition. Some question can be raised about the validity of norms established for sit-ups at various age brackets. Can we assume that 50 or 75 sit-ups within a specific time period is acceptable as an index to trunk muscle fitness? The authors suggest that consideration be given to the structural differences that affect the mass and weight of the upper torso and the resultant variation in movement. Individuals with long and heavy upper trunks are at a disadvantage when compared with persons of short light upper bodies. Tall persons with greater trunk lengths and weights simply have to exert more force for the same movement of their shorter, lighter cohorts. Thus, arbitrary norms established without consideration, at least to trunk length, can give spurious evidence about abdominal and trunk muscle strength fitness.

MECHANICAL ADVANTAGE

Mechanical advantage is a measure of a machine's efficiency and is expressed, in levers, as the ratio of the resistance overcome to the application of effort. The relationship, in terms of an equation, is formulated as:

$$MA = \frac{R}{E}$$

MA may also be signified as:

$$MA = \frac{\text{force arm}}{\text{resistance arm}}$$

It can be seen from the above formula that the greater the force arm in relation to the resistance arm, the less effort is required to perform a given task. For example, flexion of the biceps in elbow flexion has poor leverage because of its lever arrangement. The force arm is considerably shorter than its resistance arm. Most human body levers possess short effort or force arms and consequently are inefficient with regard to overcoming strength tasks. A machine is considered efficient when the MA is greather than 1. For example, applying the principle of levers, $F \times FA = R \times RA$, discussed in Chapter 7, the

problems below illustrate the concept of mechanical advantage:

Problem A
Given a weight or load of 24 lb and that *FA* and *RA* are both 6 ft. The moment of force of the resistance *mr* (resistance × perpendicular distance from the line of force of *R* to the axis through the fulcrum) is:

$$Mr = R \times RA$$
$$= 24 \text{ lb} \times 6 \text{ ft}$$
$$= 144 \text{ ft-lb}$$

The above needs an equal but contrary moment of force for balancing the lever:

$$F \times FA = R \times RA$$
$$F \times 6 \text{ ft} = 144 \text{ ft-lb}$$
$$F = \frac{144 \text{ ft-lb}}{6 \text{ ft}}$$
$$F = 24 \text{ lb}$$

Problem B
Given a force arm equal to 12 ft whereas the resistance arm stays 6 ft and the weight or resistance is 24 lb as shown below. The moment of force of the resistance is not changed at 144 ft-lb.

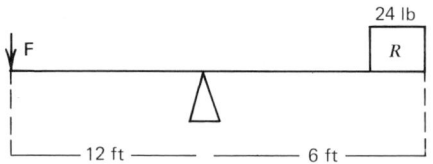

The equation in problem A is substituted as follows:

$$F \times 12 \text{ ft} = 24 \times 6 \text{ ft}$$
$$F = \frac{144 \text{ ft-lb}}{12 \text{ ft}}$$
$$F = 12 \text{ lb}$$

In problem B, 12 pounds of force is required to balance the resistance, which is half the force necessary in problem A, and since the force arm is double the length of the resistance arm, the lever system has a MA of 2. When determining the efficiency of a wheel and axle structure, the equation $MA = R/r$ applies, which is a ratio of the radius (R) of the wheel to the radius (r) of the axle. Examples of wheel and axle arrangements relevant to levers are discussed in the next chapter.

STANDARD MEASUREMENT TERMS

In physics, three terms are commonly used to describe muscular activity and human motor performance: *work, power,* and *energy.* Each of these elements can be measured quantitatively to describe exercise and activity. Knuttgen[5] points out that ambiguities of concepts and definitions have arisen that have become a source of confusion for readers of the scientific literature. Each of these terms is considered with reference to biomechanical analysis of human motion.

Work

Two general classifications of work are generally recognized; *external work* and *internal work. External work* is a force and distance relationship that is the product of the amount of force expended and distance through which the force moves in overcoming a resistance. This quantity may be expressed as:

$$W = Fd$$

It can be seen that external work (W) is accomplished when a unit of force is multiplied by distance. When using the English system, a foot-pound is commonly used; however, with greater universality of metrics, a *joule* (10^7 × one gram of force exerted through one centimeter) is indicated. When the force and distance over which the force acts are known factors, work completed can be calculated. For example, if a high jumper lifts his center of gravity through a distance of 24 inches from a crouch position to a point where his jumping foot leaves the ground, and the force of push is 200 pounds, work completed is as follows:

$$W = 200 \text{ lb} \times 2.0 \text{ ft} = 400 \text{ ft-lb of work}$$

External work may also be thought of as an action that leads to a displacement of the center of gravity.

Internal work is all the work performed by muscles that does not displace the gravity center of the body.[6] Internal work is performed when the muscle contracts *isometrically.* The gravity center is not displaced. Although the distance is zero in static contraction, the energy demands are high and produce fatigue. Physiologically, the work performed internally is definitely related more to developed force times contraction time than force times the displacement.[7] Therefore, work involved in isometrics entails the measurement of energy generated and converted in the form of heat. Other aspects, such as anaerobic (without oxygen) factors and metabolic rate, are also considered when measuring work performance without dynamic movement. Work performed in an isotonic concentric manner is called *positive work.* For example, walking uphill, during which the individual is contracting posterior leg muscles (hamstrings) *concentrically,* involves positive work. Positive work is done by muscles against a resistance such as gravity, and the active muscles *shorten. Negative work* is contrary to positive work, that is, the muscle is *eccentrically* contracting or *lengthening.* For example, since walking uphill is considered positive work, walking downhill is categorized as negative work since the posterior leg muscles are lengthening or contracting eccentrically. Performing a half knee bend also exemplifies the concept of positive work. Moving upward against gravity with concentric contraction of the quadriceps is positive work; on the other hand, flexing to the half squat or knee bend position is deemed negative work. The sum total of work performed is a vector quantity and is the composite of positive and negative work.

Power

The rate of performing work is called power. For example, an individual who performs 20 sit-ups in 10 seconds is considered to be more powerful than a person who completed the same number over twice the time interval. Power may be expressed by the following formula:

$$P = \frac{Fd}{t}$$

or

$$P = \frac{W}{T}$$

P refers to *power*, *W* indicates *work*, and *t* means *time*. Power (English system) is generally defined in horsepower units (1 hp = 33,000 ft-lb/min = 550 ft-lb/sec). The metric system utilizes the following standard:

$$Watt = 1 \ joule/sec$$

There are two types of power in motor activities: *athletic power* and *work power*.[8] Such tests as the broad jump or medicine ball put in which a body or object is propelled through space are expressed as *athletic power*. Such movements as the vertical jump and vertical arm pull, in which measurement is made to eliminate extraneous motions, thus placing maximum effort on a specific muscle group to be studied, is called *work power*. The student is referred to reference 8 for descriptive information about the uses and values of these power tests.

Energy

Two types of energy influence the conduct of human performance: *potential energy* and *kinetic energy*. *Potential energy* is the body's capacity to perform work. This energy is developed from the chemical breakdown of adenosine triphosphate (ATP) to adenosine diphosphate (ADP) and provides the potential energy for muscular contraction. *Mechanical energy* is derived from potential energy of the body plus *kinetic energy* sources. Potential energy (PE) may also be considered gravity energy or position energy and is expressed by the following formula:

$$PE = wh \ or \ mgh$$

Thus, it can be seen from the above equation that potential energy of the body depends upon weight or mass (*w*), vertical height (*h*), and gravity (32.2 ft/sec²). Potential energy represents a reserve capacity of the body that can be changed in a certain manner contingent upon body characteristics and position. For example, a diver can increase his potential energy capability by increasing the height of the hurdle step, thereby causing greater board depression and resultant gain in lifting the body center of gravity from the board. Applying the formula PE = wh, what is the potential energy of a 150-pound diver with a height hurdle step of 2 feet?

$$\begin{aligned} PE &= weight \times distance \ from \ top \ of \ board \\ &= 150 \ lb \times 2 \ ft \\ &= 300 \ ft\text{-}lb \end{aligned}$$

The above example illustrates why diving coaches stress raising the hurdle leg as high as possible without loss of control. Increasing hurdle leg height contributes to a higher parabolic curve, desirable in fancy diving competition. A gymnast attempting an uprise from the hang position to a support on the rings and a high jumper crouching before the leap both have potential energy capabilities that can enhance or retard performance depending, in part, on the application of correct position and technique appropriate to the motor activity or sport.

Kinetic energy (KE) is energy in motion. The magnitude of KE of a given mass depends upon its velocity. Numerically, this scalar quantity may be expressed by the following equation:

$$KE = \frac{1}{2} \text{ mass} \times (\text{velocity})^2 = \frac{1}{2}mv^2$$

For example, applying the above formula, a 140-pound sprinter moving at 40 ft/sec develops a KE of:

$$KE = \frac{1}{2} \ \frac{140 \text{ lb}}{32.2 \text{ ft/sec}^2} (40 \text{ ft/sec})^2 = 3478 \text{ ft-lb}$$

The amount of kinetic energy equals 1/2 the mass times the square of the velocity. Conceptually, KE may be thought of as a driving force generated by mass and velocity. Thus, it can be seen that a heavy person moving at a high rate of speed can develop immense kinetic energy. In certain cases loss of kinetic energy is desirable. For example, killing the bounce on the trampoline by flexing the knees or landing "soft" reduces KE and lessens the probability of injury when the performer desires to stop a rebound. Further considerations for preventing athletic injuries are discussed in Chapter 13.

Conservation of Energy

Energy is characterized in a number of ways: mechanical, chemical, light, nuclear, and magnetic forms. Mechanical energy is of principal concern to the physical educator.

Energy derived to produce motion can never be destroyed or created. Energy is converted from one form to another with a certain amount of waste or decrement in effi-

ciency, but it is never lost. The *law of energy conservation* states that the sum total of kinetic and potential energy is equal to a constant value and expressed by the following equation:

$$PE + KE = \text{a constant}$$

The following example illustrates the law of energy conservation.[9] Assume that a gymnast is swinging on the flying rings in an arc of 63 degrees as shown in Figure 6.9. The gymnast at each high point of his swing has only potential energy and at the lowest point has only kinetic energy. PE + KE at the high point equals a constant, and PE + KE at the low point equals the same constant as follows:

$$PE + KE = PE + KE$$

(top of swing)   (low point of swing)

$$mgh + 0 = 0 + \frac{1}{2}mv^2$$

$$mgh = \frac{1}{2}mv^2$$

(top of swing) = (bottom of swing)

Figure 6.9 Gymnast on flying rings and the law of energy conservation; CG = center of gravity (from Alice O'Connell and Elizabeth Gardner, **Understanding the Scientific Bases of Human Movement,** The Williams and Wilkins Co., Baltimore, Md., 1972, with permission)

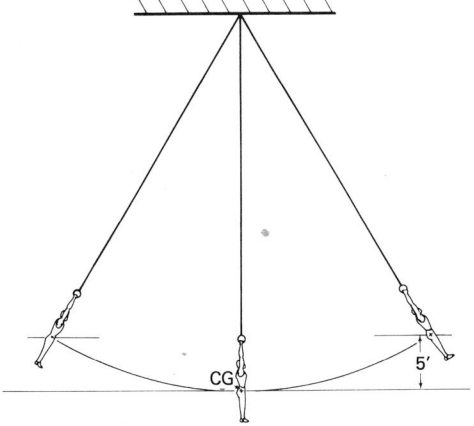

Assuming that the gymnast's center of gravity rises five feet during the swing and that he weighs 140 pounds, the constant is calculated at the top of the swing.

$$(mg = \text{weight})$$
$$PE = 140\,\text{lb} \times 5\,\text{ft} = 700\,\text{ft-lb}$$

Since KE is zero at the top of the swing, 700 ft-lb is the constant for the system. The kinetic energy for a drop of any given distance is as follows: Assuming a drop of one foot, the KE is determined as shown below:

$$PE + KE = 700\,\text{lb ft}$$
$$140\,\text{lb} \times 1\,\text{ft} + KE = 700\,\text{lb ft}$$
$$KE = 700\,\text{lb ft} - 140\,\text{lb ft}$$
$$= 560\,\text{lb ft}$$

The velocity of the swing at that point is calculated as follows:

$$mv^2 = 560\,\text{lb ft}$$
$$\frac{1}{2}\left(\frac{140\,\text{lb}}{32.2\,\text{ft/sec}^2}\right) \quad v^2 = 560\,\text{lb ft}$$
$$\frac{70\,\text{lb}}{32.2\,\text{ft/sec}^2} \quad v^2 = 560\,\text{lb ft}$$
$$v^2 = 560\,\text{lb ft} \times \frac{32.2\,\text{lb ft/sec}^2}{70\,\text{lb}}$$
$$= 8\,\text{ft} \times 32.2\,\text{ft/sec}^2$$
$$= 257.6\,\text{ft/sec}^2$$
$$v = \sqrt{257.6\,\text{ft/sec}^2}$$
$$= 16.0\,\text{ft/sec}$$

The flight path of the gymnast shows that the potential energy at the highest point of the path is a constant for any other point in the arc, and its potential energy (PE) is equal to the maximum kinetic energy (KE) of the system illustrated. It can be seen that energy is not lost, but is changed from one form to another. In the flying rings, swing PE is converted to KE on each swing and vice versa. The higher the swing, the greater the force on the downward swing.

CIRCULAR MOTION

Circular motion is a form of angular motion. An object or body is rotating in a circular path around an axis. For example, a gymnast circling the high bar in a forward swing is a classic demonstration of circular motion. His entire body is revolving in an arc around an axis. A body may also move in a curvilinear manner exhibiting circular motion. For example, hitting a ball with a bat entails a circular motion of the arms moving in an arc at the end of sequential chain of joint actions. Each of these examples involves two basic forces: centripetal and centrifugal. Conceptually, *centripetal* force is the force pulling the body or segment *toward* the center of the circle or arc, and *centrifugal* force is the opposite force pulling the object *away* from the center or axis. These two forces are present in all angular movements of the body where rotation is present, and the correct application of principles governing circular motion is essential for performing motor tasks efficiently and safely.

Components of Centripetal and Centrifugal Forces

A traditional method of producing a functional understanding of circular motion principles is by tying a small object like a metal nut to the end of a string and twirling it with the hand. In this example, centripetal force is supplied by the finger holding the string; the centrifugal force is the tending of the nut to move away from center or axis of rotation.[10] Four components that control the intensity of these forces as the object moves in a circle are identified: (1) Newton's *first law of inertia*, (2) *mass* (or weight), (3) *velocity*, and (4) *radius of rotation*. As stated in Chapter 5, Newton's law indicates that, "a body will continue at a constant velocity in a straight line unless acted upon by an outside force."

Using the above example of the string and

nut, Newton's law of inertia will compel the nut to move in a circular rather than a linear path as long as a constant speed and angular velocity is maintained. When motion in a circular path is not constant, the velocity changes to overcome the pulling-in, or center-seeking, force, and the nut will fly off on a tangent to the circle. This tangential velocity or pulling out tendency is centrifugal force. Thus, Newton's first law can serve to maintain the pulling-in tendency or centripetal force, or it may favor the outward pull depending upon the forces that affect its state. If the nut is increased in weight or speed, then there is a possibility that the circular path may be interrupted. If the nut breaks loose, it will fly off at a tangent as greater force is exerted, causing the object to move at right angles to the radius of the circle. Therefore, it can be seen that increasing the mass (weight) and/or speed of the circular object will also change centripetal and centrifugal forces.

The formula for centrifugal force in a particular situation is:

$$F = \frac{wv^2}{gr}$$

F = centrifugal force
w = weight of the object
v = velocity, in ft/sec
r = radius of the circle
g = force of gravity = 32.2 ft/sec/sec

The following situations illustrate the effect of these circular forces:[11]

Outdoor cinder tracks usually have a radius of about 100 ft. Assume that the runner is traveling 30 ft/sec and that he weighs 175 lb. What force tends to pull him out of his lane at the turn, or how much force is needed to permit him to follow the turn of the track?

$$F = \frac{175 \text{ lb} \times (30 \text{ ft/sec})^2}{32.2 \text{ ft/sec}^2 \times 100 \text{ ft}}$$

$$= \frac{175 \times 900}{32 \times 100}$$

$$= 49 + \text{lb}$$

If the radius is 40 ft, what is the force?

$$F = \frac{175 \times 900}{32 \times 40} = 123 \text{ lb}$$

If the runner is a baseball player who is attempting to make a sharp turn in a radius of 10 ft and is traveling at the rate of 20 ft/sec, what is the force?

$$F = \frac{175 \text{ lb} \times (20 \text{ ft/sec})^2}{32 \text{ ft/sec}^2 \times 10 \text{ ft}}$$

$$= \frac{175 \times 400}{32 \times 10}$$

$$= 218.75 \text{ lb}$$

The preceding problems demonstrate that centrifugal force becomes greater as the radius becomes smaller. This force tends to pull the athlete off course when turning. In order to counteract this force, the runner leans in toward the point about which he is turning as shown in Figure 6.10.

In most cases, it is not necessary for physical educators and health professionals to compute the numerical values of circular motion. However, the following precepts are important for the control of centripetal/centrifugal forces inherent in everyday motor skills and athletics:

1. Mass, speed, and radius of motion govern the intensity of centripetal/centrifugal forces.

2. The law of inertia may decrease or increase either of these circular factors depending upon the mass, speed, and radius of gyration.

3. A greater mass increases the forces more than a lighter one in a circular path.

4. Force exerted is proportional to the square of the velocity, i.e., in doubling the

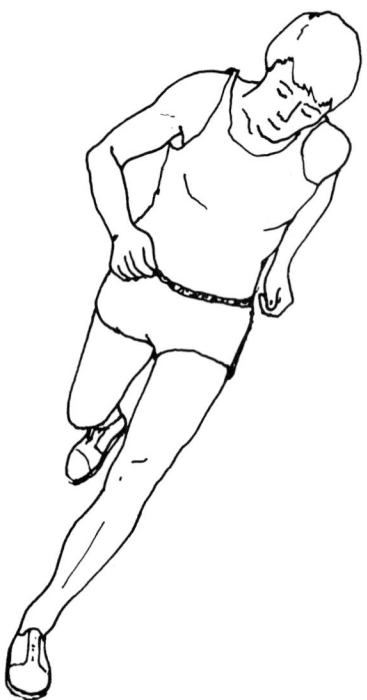

Figure 6.10 Inward lean of runner to counteract centrifugal force

speed, centripetal and centrifugal forces are quadrupled.

5. Force exerted is proportional to the radius of motion at constant angular velocity, i.e., a shorter gymnast will have less centripetal/centrifugal force at the same angular velocity than a taller performer.

Control of circular motion is contingent upon the above precepts. These principles function in concert, one affecting the other, depending upon a given situation. Since all angular motions of the body contain these forces, it is prudent for activity specialists to develop programs that enhance strength. Muscles can contribute to the regulation of centrifugal force, which frequently accompanies vigorous movements of the limbs. For example, Adams[12] found that a child who possessed less than 18 pounds of grip strength was not successful in a traveling exercise across a horizontal ladder, which demands

control of centripetal and centrifugal forces as he moves from one bar to the next.

The game of "crack-the-whip" contains the elements of circular motion demonstrated by the "nut on the string" described earlier. As one end of the line slows, the participants toward the other end begin to run faster, increasing momentum, and therefore their outward pull increases. It becomes more difficult to maintain clasped hands in the line when the centrifugal force becomes greater than the available centripetal force as the grip strength of the weakest person in the line is disconnected. Subsequently, one or more youngsters run off (or are literally thrown off) on a tangent from the circular path. Again, this game also illustrates the importance of developing strength as a means of countering the disconnecting and/or dislocating forces of activities encountered in physical activities.

FRICTION

Friction alters motion. In certain instances, friction enhances the efficiency of motion, and in other circumstances this element may impede performance. For example, shoes that possess high-level gripping strength are desirable in jumping, turning, and dodging activities in the gymnasium; on the other hand the reduction of friction between a swimmer's body and the water fosters speed. This is why some swimmers shave their heads, chest, and limbs before a competitive race. Theoretically, shaved bodies should slide through the water with greater speed and less resistance. Two types of friction have particular reference to human performance: *sliding friction* and *rolling friction*.

Sliding Friction

This type of friction is a force that acts to prevent one object from sliding over another.

The amount of friction is proportional to the force pressing between the two surfaces and is affected by makeup or composition of materials, degree of unsmoothness of contact surface, pressing force between surfaces, and characteristics of actions between surfaces. The equation is:

$$\frac{P}{W} = C$$

The pressing force is represented by W; force required to begin motion is P; and the ratio shown by the above formula is called *coefficient of friction (C)*. The greater the coefficient of friction, the stronger the gripping qualities of the surfaces. Conversely, the smaller this ratio, the more easily objects slide over one another. A coefficient of 0.0 indicates that the surfaces are frictionless. Friction is necessary for the initiation of movement and is also related to stability. For example, the coefficient of friction must be of sufficient levels between the shoe and floor surfaces to prevent slippage. Greater body stability is maintained when the force of friction is high. When supporting surfaces offer low friction such as found on icy pavements, polished floors, and other smooth structures, loss of balance occurs with a resultant fall. Generally, a retarding force on sliding objects is slightly less than the maximum force of friction on stationary bodies. The angle in which a force is applied to overcome the friction also affects the ease or difficulty of moving an object. For example, if an object is pushed forward with an upward angle, movement results with less effort; however, if the force is directed forward at a downward angle, friction is increased, and greater force is necessary to overcome the retarding effect of friction. Some of the practical uses of friction are:

1. Maximize friction for walking, jumping, running, and other activities when changing direction and stability are inherent in the activity.

2. Regulate friction to lessen or intensify resistance in bicycle ergometer work loads.

3. Minimize friction in massage by using lubricants such as oils and powders.

4. Minimize internal friction of muscular contraction by adequate warm-up.

5. Maximize friction when contact between body segments and apparatus or implements is essential, e.g., chalk on hands before using apparatus, golf gloves, rubber handles on racket paddles, etc.

Rolling Friction

Rolling friction is characterized by a golf ball rolling over the lawn or a cart pushed along a hard or soft surface. The resultant friction created depends upon the object rolling and the surface on which it rolls. Hard surfaces generally create less friction than soft surfaces. Smooth surfaces also produce less friction. For example, a bowling ball will roll much more easily on a hardwood floor than on a lawn of green grass. Resistance to movement is considerably less in rolling friction than sliding friction. Rolling friction is approximately 100 to 1000 times less than a sliding friction.[13] Obviously, rolling is of primary importance to athletes using ball-type equipment and instruments. For example, the golfer must consider using greater force when the grass is wet and soft, since the friction on the rolling ball is increased under these conditions. Soccer players examine field conditions to determine the rolling ability of the soccer ball across the field. Whenever a heavy object must be rolled from one point to another, less force will be required if the object is placed upon hard rollers and wheeled on a firm, smooth surface. Physical therapists and corrective therapists can apply this precept in their daily tasks, such as pushing wheelchairs on hard asphalt or linoleum surfaces, rather than on soft, sandy ground. Thus, it can be seen that friction or the lack of friction can help man in a multitude of motor tasks and athletic sports depending upon the nature and objective of the motor performance at hand.

PRODUCTION AND APPLICATION OF FORCE

Force is essential for human movement. As noted earier, force may emanate from internal or external sources. The production of force and its application includes: (1) *magnitude*, (2) *direction*, (3) *point of application*, and (4) *time over which force is applied*. The performance of motor skills depends upon how these variables act and interact to create the desired motion. In certain movements, magnitude of force is highly desirable for a successful performance. For example, a weight lifter must possess a strong component of internal muscular force for elite competition; in other instances, a turning action is desired that entails a certain point where force is applied. Coordinated isotonic concentric muscular force is essential for upward speed in rope climbing, whereas slow isotonic contraction is indicated for controlled downward movements in rope climbing proficiency. Thus, it is obvious that the production and application of these force variables must consider the purposes and objectives of the desired outcome of a specific skill and/or performer.

Magnitude of Force

Magnitude of force deals with the concept of the *amount* necessary to move a given object or propel that body through space. Movement is not possible without a threshold of force magnitude, which may originate internally (muscular) or externally (machine or implement). As indicated earlier by Newton's first law, inertia must be overcome before movement can be initiated. The amount of force required for a given situation is expressed by the following equations:

$$F = ma \text{ or } F = \frac{mv}{t}$$

F indicates force; m = mass; a equals acceleration; v = velocity; and t = time or duration of the acting force. It can be seen from the above formulas that force magnitude is contingent upon the *mass* and *speed* of an object or body imparting the force. For practical purposes, this means that force is determined by the weight of the body segment or the entire human form times its velocity (rate of speed). Force magnitude, therefore, entails overcoming inertia (Newton's first law) and changing speed (Newton's second law). The quantity of force may also be conceptualized in terms of momentum, which is mass times velocity. As stated in Chapter 5, the greater the momentum of an object, the greater its moving inertia. As shown in the above formula, momentum is the product of mass and velocity. When a force of a given amount (magnitude) is directed to an object with a specific mass, that object will change its speed relative to the magnitude of force. For example, when a ball (specific mass) is thrown, the rate of change in speed of the ball (acceleration) is proportional to the amount of force generated.

The magnitude of muscular force (internal) is proportional to the number and size of the fibers in the contracting muscle. From a structural perspective, the larger the cross section of a muscle, the greater its potential magnitude of force. Studies[14] show that human muscles exert a force of 6 to 10 kilograms per square centimeter of their cross section—this is about 85 to 141 pounds per square inch. Therefore, hypothetically, a large person with a great number of fibers should be able to outperform a smaller individual with fewer fibers. Of course, this feat may occur only if fiber number and size alone create force. Other contractile variables also influence the amount of force that can be expended. These are load and velocity curve relationships, as well as the muscle on a stretch principle, discussed in Chapter 4. When a muscle is stretched, greater contraction will result. The implications of this precept in sports are demonstrated by the sprinter stretching the quadriceps at the starting block and the swimmer crouching in a similar position at the starting platform. When explosive power is important to performance, skilled athletes place their muscles on a stretch.

Force magnitude is usually measured in terms of *pounds-weight* (English system), which considers the pull of gravity of 32.2 ft/sec/sec, and by a *newton* when the metric system is employed. Measures of strength are usually determined by various dynamometer and cable tensiometric devices where maximum force is exerted against resistance.

Direction of Force

The direction of a force variable may be considered from two perspectives: (1) external application and (2) internal application.

External Application. A mechanical principle that must be considered when coordinating a motor skill is application of force in the correct direction. Succinctly stated, force should be applied in the direction of the intended movement in order to maximize effort and eliminate wasteful dissipation of energy. For example, high jumpers should address the cross bar in such a way that the upward thrust (vertical component) predominates over the forward thrust (horizontal component) because the goal is to raise the body's center of gravity as high as possible from the ground in order to clear a specified height. Obviously, if all the force is directed upward, the high jumper would have difficulty propelling himself over the bar since force in a forward direction is also necessary. Cooper[15] studied the forces involved in the high jump and hypothesized that 20 degrees is the optimal angle of the approach. He also believes that an approach angle of less than 20 de-

grees would mean that the jumper would have difficulty crossing the bar between the uprights and may land outside the pit. Therefore, the primary thrust for high jumpers should accent the upward vertical component; however, attention should also be given to clearing the bar. The angulation varies according to the style of jumping, but in all styles, the vertical thrust prevails in order to attain maximum height. The student should keep in mind that the upward vertical component is generated by directing the force *downward*, so that the performer is thrown *upward*. In projecting the body or throwing an object, at least two components of force are involved. Such events as the high jump, pole vault, and backward and forward somersault entail vertical and horizontal components or directional forces, which can be calculated using parallelograms discussed earlier in this chapter. When a racket strikes a ball that has a top spin, three forces are involved: (1) effective force from the racket, (2) the rebound force caused by the ball's motion, and (3) the spin force.[16] Therefore, magnitude as well as a diagonal force (resultant of vertical and horizontal components) acts upon the propelled ball. These examples point out the need to analyze the direction of the intended force. After the direction has been ascertained, the performer proceeds to direct his force line mainly in the desired direction. The student should remember that the exerted force must be applied in the direction opposite to the desired motion of his body or its parts, e.g., pushing backward to move forward (horizontally), pushing downward (vertically) to move upward.

Internal Application. Mechanically, muscles pull more effectively when the angle of pull approximates 90 degrees. Two components are acting on turning movements of a joint articulation: stabilizing and rotary. Rotary force is considered the *working force* of the motion, since the stabilizing component does not contribute to external work, but rather provides the internal force necessary to hold articulations together. The majority of muscles in the body are arranged so that the line of pull is almost parallel with the long axis of the lever; therefore, the angle of pull is small. Contrary to this general characteristic is the pectoralis major, which inserts into the intertubercular sulcus (humerus) at almost 90 degrees.[17] The stabilizing component is usually greater than the rotary component at the beginning of the movement.

Although the muscle's angle of pull is a human structural reality that cannot be changed, we can effectively apply the phenomenon of exerting force near the 90 degree angulation when a maximum turning force is desired. The student is referred to Chapter 7 for an expanded discussion of a muscle's line of pull.

Point of Application

Internally, the force point in the lever arrangement of the body is considered the muscle's *insertion point*. The student should remember that the internal line of pull is toward the center of the muscle. The force point is not the belly of the muscle itself. This concept is particularly important when determining lever-type classifications, which subsequently yield the force characteristics of a given articulation under study. Externally, if translatory or linear movement of an object is desired, less force is necessary when the force is applied *directly through its center of gravity*. Therefore, if a tall object has a low weight center, the object will move in a straight line, with less difficulty and effort, if the individual crouches and pushes the object horizontally at a point near the ground. An object will rotate if it is fixed at one point, regardless of where the force is applied. Rotation will occur with less effort if a force is applied at a distant point away from the center of gravity. The practical implications of this principle are multifold. For example, pushing or pulling heavy objects in a horizontal direction indicates the advantage of applying

the force or pressure near or through its heaviest part. Contrarily, if one desires a toppling or turning movement, force should be exerted as far as possible from the center of gravity. Observing these mechanical precepts permits successful work outcomes with the least amount of effort provided other laws of motions and forces such as principle of levers, circular motion, gravity, friction, and Newton's laws are equally observed.

Time Over Which Force Is Applied

The length of time a force acts upon an object affects the amount of force that can be imparted to a body or object. For example, more force can be generated if a badminton bird is held longer on the strings in a smash stroke with a follow-through ballistic action of the wrist (Figure 6.11) than in a quick non-ballistic action whereby the bird bounces off the racket with a locked wrist. This principle entails the concept of *impulse*, which is the product of the force and time over which the force acts (see Chapter 5). Wind-up styles of baseball pitchers and shot putters and exaggerated depression of the hurdle leg before the take-off by divers are attempts to create larger impulses to impart a greater force by increasing the time over which the force is applied.

Field events in track, in which implements such as the discus, shot put, hammer, and javelin are thrown, are sports that utilize techniques in which maximum force is gained when it is applied over long periods of time through preliminary movements before the implement is released. Other examples of impulse are presented in Chapter 5.

REBOUND AND SPIN FORCES

A trampolinist will rebound higher if the bed surface is constructed of tight nylon webbing instead of soft canvas. A ball will spring back or rebound with greater force if it is hard and

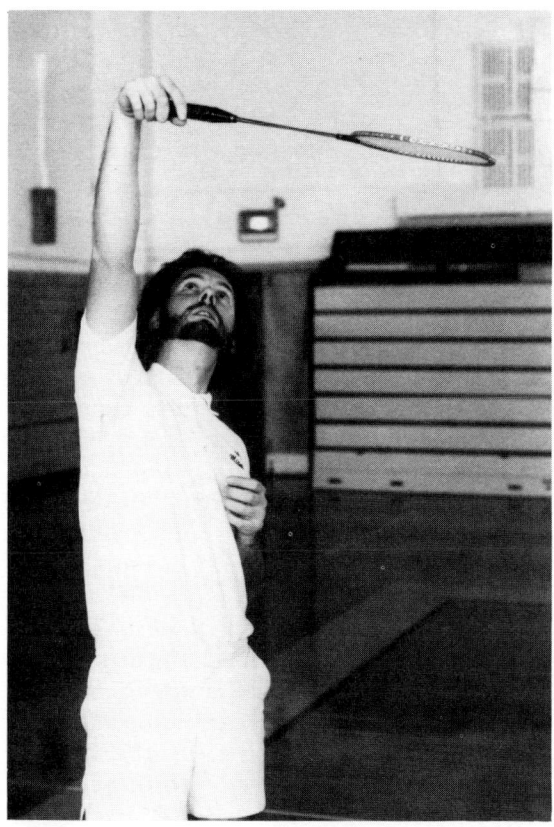

Figure 6.11 Increasing impulse by follow-through motion of wrist in badminton smash

the resistive surface is not soft. If a ball without a spin strikes a hard surface at a 45 degree angle, it will rebound at the same angle. If a ball is spinning forward on contact, it will move downward on the rebound. These examples encompass the mechanical principles of rebound and angle of spin forces.

Rebound Forces

Certain variables affect the way an object rebounds from a surface or another object. The force of the rebound is contingent upon: (1) the amount of *resistance* of the contact surface, (2) the *momentum* generated by the object, and (3) its depression characteristic, called the *coefficient of restitution* or elasticity.

Surface Resistance. A ball falling on a gymnastic crash mat will not rebound because of the mat's impact-absorbing quality. Conversely, a golf ball striking a hardwood basketball floor will reflect to varying heights depending upon momentum and other rebound forces. The less depression that occurs between the bouncing object and the floor or ground, the greater the probability of recoil. Court surface firmness is a critical concern to tennis, handball, squash, and basketball players because velocity is important in game play.

Court surfaces vary from one facility to another. The astute performer should always gauge the velocity of a rebounding ball before beginning competitive play. This assessment will allow the participant to gain an insight to correct pacing and kinesthetic perception of impacting and receiving the ball in the conduct of the game.

Momentum Generated. Ball rebound is greater at higher levels. Therefore, an object moving at maximum speeds (momentum = mass × velocity), excluding other variables, contains high rebounding qualities. For example, if a ball is simply dropped from specified height, the momentum generated is that prescribed by the law of gravity (32.2 ft/sec/sec). The ball would rebound at nominal heights depending on other rebound variables. However, if the same ball is forcefully thrown from the same height, the momentum created will cause the ball to bounce higher in proportion to its speed.

Coefficient of Restitution. When an object strikes a contact surface, a certain amount of depression or distortion takes place on the impacted surfaces. Figure 6.12 illustrates the depression or flattening of a tennis ball as it contacts the strings of the racket. The tendency of contact surfaces to return to normal state or to regain shape is called the *coefficient of restitution* or elasticity.

The coefficient of restitution of a ball re-

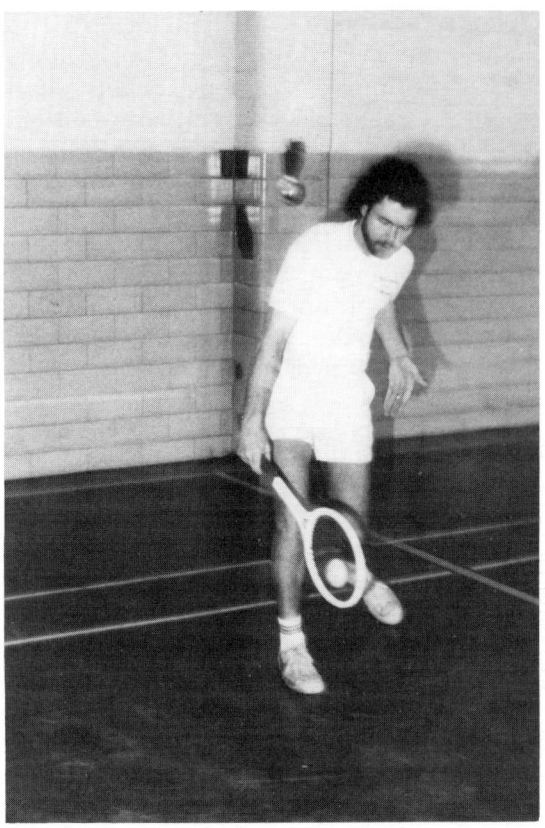

Figure 6.12 Flattening effect of tennis ball and racket on contact

bounding on a specified surface is expressed by the following impact equations:

$$c = \frac{\text{velocity after impact}}{\text{velocity before impact}} \quad (1)$$

or

$$c = \sqrt{\frac{\text{rebound height}}{\text{drop height}}} \quad (2)$$

The first formula requires appropriate measurement equipment; however, the coefficient may be determined by dropping a ball from specific height and applying the second formula. For example, if a ball is dropped 160 centimeters and rebounds 120 centimeters from the bounce, its c is equal to the

square root of 120 cm divided by 160 cm or:

$$c = \frac{120}{160}$$

$$= \sqrt{0.75}$$

$$= 0.866$$

A coefficient of 1.0 means perfect elasticity. Objects with a coefficient of zero do not rebound. The student should remember that c depends upon the impact and elasticity of two bodies. In a given situation of a ball hitting the floor, rebound height is dependent upon the *elasticity* of the ball and floor composition. Tables 6.1 and 6.2 present a sampling of coefficients for different balls dropped from a height of 72 inches and a volleyball from the same height onto various surfaces.

Angle of Rebound. When a ball strikes a rebounding surface, two mechanical precepts are involved: (1) *angle of incidence* and (2) *angle of rebound*. The angle of approach *before* striking the surface is called the angle of incidence; and the angle *after* hitting the surface is called angle of rebound. The angle of incidence and angle of rebound are identical when a ball strikes a surface without a spin, as shown in Figure 6.13.

Spin Forces

Balls and/or objects spinning through the air behave in a prescribed manner serving two important functions: (1) stabilization to keep the ball on course and (2) regulation of the *direction* of the object in flight and/or angle of rebound after striking a surface. For example, spinning keeps the axis of a football on course and prevents it from wobbling. Too much or too little spin may cause the football to fall or rise. The spin in a rebounding basketball can determine its direction. A counterclockwise spin on a basketball before it strikes the floor will cause the ball to rebound to the left. The above examples represent il-

Table 6.1 The Coefficient of Restitution for Balls Dropped from a Height of 72 Inches onto a Hardwood Floor

Type of Ball	Height Bounced (in.)	Coefficient of Restitution*
"Super ball"	56.75	0.89
Basketball	41.75	0.76
Soccer	41.50	0.76
Volleyball	39.75	0.74
Tennis—well-worn	36.00	0.71
—new	32.00	0.67
Lacrosse	27.50	0.62
Field hockey	18.25	0.50
Softball	7.25	0.32
Cricket	7.00	0.31

*Values for the coefficient of restitution vary from 0.0 when the impact is said to be inelastic, because the bodies do not separate after the impact, to a theoretical and never-attained limit of 1.0.

From Hay, James G., *The Biomechanics of Sports Techniques*, 2nd ed. Prentice-Hall, Inc., Englewood Cliffs, New Jersey, 1978, p. 80, by permission.

Table 6.2 The Coefficient of Restitution for a Volley Ball Dropped from a Height of 72 Inches onto Various Surfaces

Type of Surface	Height Bounced (in.)	Coefficient of Restitution
"Proturf"	41.25	0.76
Wood	40.66	0.75
"Uniturf"	40.41	0.75
Steel plating	40.00	0.74
Concrete	39.50	0.74
Tumbling mat (1 in. thick)	32.66	0.67
Gravel	26.33	0.60
Grass	13.50	0.43
Gymnastic landing mat (8 in. thick)	13.00	0.42

From Hay, James G., *The Biomechanics of Sports Techniques*, 2nd ed. Prentice-Hall, Inc., Englewood Cliffs, New Jersey, 1978, p. 81, by permission.

lustrations of flight paths and rebound patterns affected by spin forces. Although a great number of spin designs may be imparted to an object, the mechanics of the most common types will be considered in the ensuing discussion.

Top Spin and Back Spin (around frontal-horizontal axis). Top spin and back spin are typical of flight patterns of a propelled ball with or without an implement. Spinning balls follow *Bernoulli's principle*, which indicates that a ball moving through the air will move

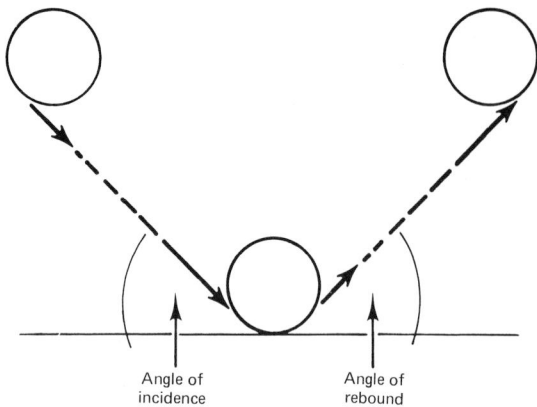

Figure 6.13 Angle of incidence and rebound without a spin

in the direction of least air pressure. When a ball is spinning, it will follow a curved path, as shown in Figure 6.14.

Balls with a *top spin* will move in a *downward curve*, since the air pressure on the balls' underside is reduced by the spin force. Balls with a *back spin* will move in an *upward curve*, as shown in Figure 6.14*b*. The top spin ball drops into a low-pressure area created by the faster moving air as it passes below the ball. The opposite occurs in a back spin, where the ball will rise into the low-pressure area above the ball. Top spins and back spins are typically used in tennis and basketball.

Clockwise and Counterclockwise Spin (sagittal–horizontal axis).

The effect on a football, as viewed from the rear, typifies clockwise and counterclockwise spin. The spin is usually found in the flight of an arrow, bullet, or football pass. Spins revolving around the sagittal–horizontal axis provide stabilization of the propelled object and allow the object, such as a football, to stay on a natural curvilinear flight path. If a football is not spinning fast enough, it will tumble; on the other hand, if it is spinning too fast, the ball will tend to depart from its course and curve excessively with a resultant loss in normal line of flight.

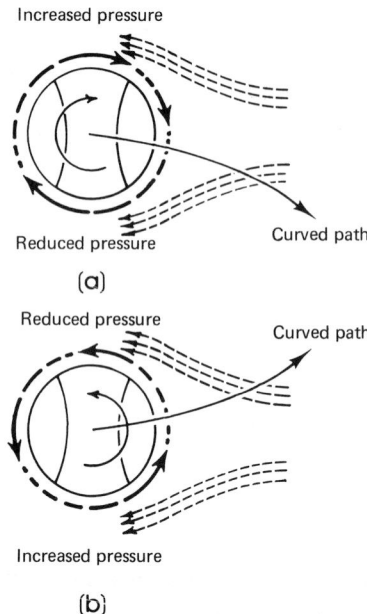

Figure 6.14 Effect of spinning on a propelled ball following a curved path. (a) Top spin. (b) Back spin (from Katharine F. Wells, and Kathryn Luttgens, **Kinesiology**. W. B. Saunders Company, Philadelphia, Pa., 1976, with permission)

Left and Right Spin (around a vertical axis).

Side spins may be left or right when moving around a *vertical* axis, as shown in Figure 6.15.

If the spin is to the left, the ball will curve to the left; if the spin is to the right, the ball will curve to the right. Spins around a vertical axis are typified by the sliced or hooked shot in golf drives.

Spin and Rebound

When a ball bounces on the floor without a spin, the angle of incidence and the angle of rebound (also called reflection) are identical. However, when a spin is added to the ball, the angle of rebound will not be the same as the angle of incidence. The following discussion focuses upon rebound behavior of: top spin, back spin; clockwise and counterclockwise spin; and left and right spin.

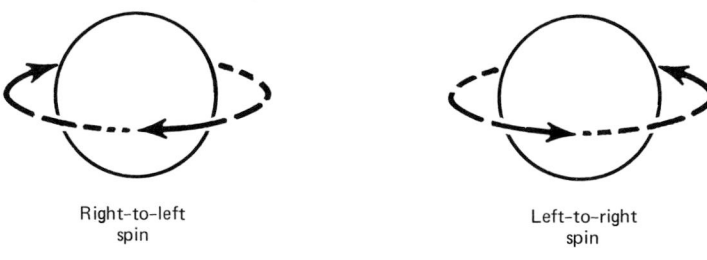

Right-to-left
spin

Left-to-right
spin

Figure 6.15 *Spins around a vertical axis (axis vertical to the ground)*

Top Spin and Back Spin Rebound. Balls propelled with a top spin will rebound in a forward direction at a lower height with greater horizontal velocity. The greater the spin, the faster and lower the rebound from the floor surface. Balls with a back spin will behave in a reverse manner; their pattern will reflect a higher bounce with less velocity in a forward direction depending upon the speed of the spin. A ball may be stopped or reversed if the back spin is of sufficient speed. This maneuver can be demonstrated by a basketball player bouncing a ball with a high back spin resulting in the ball rebounding back to the player's hands. Thus, it can be seen that adjustments in top and back spins can be used to speed up or slow down a ball as well as change its direction. Such maneuvers are especially critical in basketball, in which bounce passes are integral elements of the sport.

Clockwise and Counterclockwise Spin Rebound. The angle of rebound will be to the right when a ball is spinning clockwise upon impact (viewing the ball from the rear of the passer or thrower). If the ball is spinning *counterclockwise* on impact, the ball's reflection will be to the left. As with the top and back spins, spinning around the sagittal–horizontal axis is used extensively in basketball play to manipulate the ball in the bounce pass so that it will move in the direction desired by the passer. Similarly, this type of spin

effect on the ball is used in a basketball lay-up shot, when the ball strikes the backboard to the side of the basket, and a correct spin moves the ball from the side to the basket hoop.

Left and Right Spin Rebound (side spin). The angle of rebound is not affected in right-to-left or left-to-right side spins, since the spin of the ball is neutralized by the backward spin force. When right or left spin is imparted to the ball, the entire ball is depressed; consequently friction against the forward part of the ball is the same as applied to the backward part. These forces are opposite each other and will result in a zero reaction. The ball will not depart from its course on the rebound, as indicted in Table 6.3.

The table summarizes ball response in flight and rebound when different spins are applied. The student should visualize the action of the ball from the rear view.

Each sport contains its own unique characteristics in the application of spins in flight and rebound from floor surfaces. The curve ball, inside, or drop ball is important to the baseball pitcher. Controlling the direction of the bounce pass is a basic skill in basketball using spin mechanics. Attention to the mechanical laws that govern ball behavior allows the learner to develop this aspect of motor skills with a better scientific understanding of "why" objects react in a certain manner in flight and/or rebound from contact surfaces.

Table 6.3 Summary of Ball Response in Flight and Rebound

	Top	Back	CW	CCW	R-L	L-R
Ball in flight will	drop	rise	not react	not react	curve right	curve left
Ball will rebound	fast, low	slow, high	right	left	not react	not react

CW = clockwise spin; CCW = counterclockwise spin; R-L = right-to-left spin; L-R = left-to-right.

From Hinson, Marilyn M., *Kinesiology*, 1977, Wm. C. Brown Company Publishers, Dubuque, Iowa, 1977, with permission.

SUMMARY

Energy provides the source of force for human movement. Movement generated by the human organism itself is termed internal force. A force exerted from sources outside the body that produce or prevent a movement is called an external force.

Forces may be classified as linear and rotary. Kinematics measures temporal (time) variables such as displacement, velocity, and acceleration, whereas kinetics deals with the actions of forces that produce or change a motion.

Scalar quantities such as speed, length, temperature, time, mass, volume, and area are units of measurement that contain magnitude without reference to direction. Vector quantities are measures that possess direction as well: velocity, force, acceleration, momentum, displacement, friction, work, and power.

Parallelograms may be constructed and utilized to determine a resultant force when two forces of differing direction and magnitude act on an object or body at the same time.

A force that pushes or pulls along a translatory line of action is called a linear force. Parallel forces may not always act along the same action line, as on a seesaw, where the weights of the participants, one on each end, exert parallel forces in the same direction opposed by the upward force at the fulcrum.

Concurrent forces may be applied from different angles from a common point to produce a singular movement.

The turning motion caused by an applied force on the body is called a moment of force. The product of the force (magnitude) and lever arm (perpendicular distance from the direction of force to the axis of rotation) determines the torque of an angular movement. The effort required in a given turning movement can be controlled by adjusting the length of the moment arm from its axis, or by changing the magnitude of the weight of the moving segment. Increasing the length of the moment arm and/or weight will increase the force requirement in a torque motion.

Mechanical advantage (MA) is a term used to express a machine's efficiency; it is the ratio of resistance overcome to the effort when applied to lever arrangements.

Work, power, and energy are common terms used to describe and quantify human performance. External and internal work are two general categories. External work describes a precise force and distance relationship. Internal work is energy expended by the muscles that do not displace the center of gravity and is typified by isometrics; that is, the energy generated is converted to heat. Positive work is done by muscles shortening against gravity, whereas negative work is eccentric or lengthening contraction against a gravity force. Power is the rate of performing work.

The conduct of human performance is influenced by potential energy and kinetic energy. Potential energy relates to the body's capacity to perform work, whereas kinetic energy is energy in motion. The concept that energy is converted from one form to another and is never lost is known as the law of energy conservation.

Circular motion is a form of angular motion and contains two elements: centripetal force and centrifugal force. Four components control the intensity of centripetal and centrifugal forces: Newton's law of inertia, mass, velocity, and radius of rotation.

Friction alters the path of motion. In certain instances, friction enhances motion efficiency and in other circumstances it may impede movement. Sliding friction is a force that prevents one object from moving over another.

Generally, a retarding force (kinetic friction) on sliding objects is slightly less than the maximum force of friction on stationary bodies. Rolling friction is characterized by a golf ball rolling over the lawn surface.

The production and application of force depends upon magnitude, direction, point of application, and time over which it is applied.

Force is the energy for producing movement; power involves the time element in performing work. The magnitude of internal muscular force is proportional to the number and size of the fibers in contracting muscle.

Force should be applied in the direction of the intended movement in order to maximize effort and eliminate wasteful dissipation of energy. Externally, a performer should project his or her body or impart an object upward if vertical height is the principal objective in a motor skill.

The length of time a force acts upon an object affects the amount of force that can be imparted to a body or object. This precept is typified by the "smash" in badminton. More force is imparted when the stroke is executed ballistically (follow-through) because the bird is in contact with the strings over a longer period of time.

Rebound performance of objects and/or bodies is contingent upon (1) amount of resistance of the contact surface, (2) momentum, and (3) coefficient of restitution. Ball rebound is greater when momentum is generated at high levels. The tendency of contact surfaces to return to their normal shape is called the coefficient of restitution or elasticity (c). When a ball strikes a rebounding surface, two mechanical precepts are involved: (1) angle of incidence and (2) angle of rebound. The angle of approach is called the angle of incidence, and the angle after hitting the surface is called the angle of rebound.

Balls and/or objects spinning through the air behave in a prescribed manner. This spin has two important functions: (1) stabilization or keeping the object steady and (2) regulation in the direction of the object in flight and/or angle of rebound after striking a surface. Spinning balls follow Bernoulli's principle, which states that a ball moving through an arc moves in the direction of least pressure.

Side spin, left or right, is spinning around a vertical axis. Side spins are demonstrated by the sliced or hooked shot in golf drives.

Spins affect the angle of rebound. The bounce of a ball will not be the same as the angle of incidence or approach, depending upon the direction of the spin.

Clockwise spin rebound (viewed from rear of passer or thrower) will move the ball to the right whereas a counterclockwise spin rebound will move the ball to the left. These types of ball spins are used extensively in basketball in such skills as changing ball direction from one player to another and lay-up shots after the ball strikes the backboard.

The angle of reflection is not affected in side spins, since the spin of the ball is around a vertical axis. The forward spin force is neutralized by the backward spin force upon impact.

REFERENCES

1. Hay, James G., *The Biomechanics of Sports Techniques*, 2nd ed. New Jersey: Prentice-Hall, 1978, p. 63.

2. Dyson, Geoffrey, *The Mechanics of Athletics*. London: Hodder and Stoughton, 1973, p. 42.

3. *Ibid*, pp. 42-43.

4. MacDonald, Francois A., *Mechanics for Movement*. London: G. Bell and Sons, Ltd., 1973, pp. 13-14.

5. Knuttgen, Howard, "Force, Work, Power and Exercise," *Medicine and Science in Sports*, 10:227-228, Fall, 1978.

6. Margaria, Rudolfo, *Biomechanics and Energetics of Muscular Exercise*. Oxford: Clarendon Press, 1976, p. 83.

7. Astrand, Per-Olof, and Rodahl, Kaare, *Textbook of Work Physiology*. New York: McGraw-Hill, 1977, pp. 98-99.

8. Johnson, Barry L., and Nelson, J. K., *Practical Measurements for Evaluation in Physical Education*, 3rd ed. Minneapolis: Burgess Publishing Co., 1979, p. 200.

9. O'Connell, Alice L., and Gardner, Elizabeth B., *Understanding the Scientific Bases of Human Movement*. Baltimore: Williams and Wilkins, 1972, pp. 81-83.

10. Hubbell, Josephine W., "Centrifugal and Centripetal Force," *Journal of Health, Physical Education and Recreation*, 38:78-79, October, 1967.

11. Bunn, John W., *Scientific Principles of Coaching*, 2nd ed. New Jersey: Prentice-Hall, 1972, p. 63.

12. Adams, Fred A., "An Investigation of Grip Strength and Horizontal Ladder Success Among Primary Grade Aged Children," Unpublished Master's Project, State University of New York At Buffalo, 1971.

13. Hay, *op. cit.*, p. 74.

14. Wells, Katharine, and Luttgens, Kathryn, *Kinesiology*. Philadelphia: W. B. Saunders, 1976, p. 294.

15. Cooper, J. M., "Kinesiology of High Jumping," *In* J. Wartenweiler, E. Jokl, and M. Hebbelinck, M. (Eds.), *Biomechanics*. New York: S. Karger, 1968, pp. 291-302.

16. Broer, Marion, *Efficiency of Human Movement*. Philadelphia: W. B. Saunders, 1973, pp. 89-90.

17. MacDonald, *op. cit.*, p. 48.

7 | THE HUMAN LEVER SYSTEM

CONCEPTS

1. Many of the major bones in the human body serve as levers with the fulcrum or axis located at a joint. This is one type of a simple machine.

2. A second type of simple machine found in the body is the pulley. Human pulleys change the direction or line of pull where tendons pass over protuberances.

3. A third type of simple machine found in the body is the wheel and axle.

4. When force is applied to the wheel, the effect is that of a second class lever, while when force is applied to the axle, the effect is that of a third class lever.

5. Levers can be designed or selected to give the advantage either to force or to velocity.

6. Levers are classified as first, second, or third class depending upon whether the axis, resistance, or force is between the other two.

7. Levers are balanced when the force times the perpendicular distance from the line of application of force to the axis is equal to the resistance times the perpendicular distance from the line of resistance to the axis: ($F \times FA = R \times RA$ or $F \times FMA = R \times RMA$, where M = moment, F = force, A = arm, R = resistance.

8. As a joint is flexed, the force moment arm (FMA) increases in length until the joint is flexed to a 90 degree angle. After the angle becomes less than 90 degrees, the force moment arm decreases in length.

9. At the beginning of flexion, most of the muscle's force is used in stabilizing the joint; however, as the joint is flexed, a decreasing proportion of the force is used in stabilization until, after 90 degrees of flexion, the muscle's line of pull is such that its pull tends to dislocate the joint.

10. The smaller the angle of a muscle's pull, the greater the degree of joint movement per centimeter of muscle contraction.

11. The greater the muscular strength, the smaller the probability of a joint sprain or dislocation.

12. Unlike external levers, internal levers can be shortened or lengthened according to the demands of the objective.

13. Shortening of anatomic levers increases angular velocity while lengthening of anatomic levers increases linear velocity.

14. Somatotype bears a relationship to most effective use of anatomic levers because of the relative length of limbs and the distribution of weight or mass over the appendages.

15. Throwing and striking activities can be classified into overhand, underhand, sidearm, and diagonal patterns according to the direction and path of movement of the arm or arms.

243

GENERAL CONSIDERATIONS

All complex machines are merely various arrangements of six kinds of simple machines. The lever, pulley, wheel and axle, inclined plane, wedge, and screw are the simple machines. The lever, pulley, and wheel and axle are used in the human body. All the major bones in the human body serve as levers with the fulcrum located at a joint. An example of one pulley in the human body is provided in the arrangement of the tendon of the peroneus longus muscle as it passes behind and under the external malleolus to change the direction of pull of the muscle from dorsiflexion of the foot to plantar flexion. An example of the wheel and axle in the human body is the pull of the oblique abdominal and iliocostalis muscles on the ribs (wheel) and the force of the multifidi, rotatores, and semispinalis muscles upon the vertebrae (axle) to produce rotation.

A lever is a rigid bar that revolves around a fixed point called a *fulcrum* or *axis* when a force is applied to overcome a resistance. As a result of the relative distances from the fulcrum to the point of application of force and from the fulcrum to the point of application of resistance, the lever can be used either to overcome greater resistance than the force used or to move the resistance a greater distance than the force moves.

Everyone uses levers outside the body (external levers) every day. Some examples of levers are crowbar, claw hammer, wheelbarrow, bottle opener, and scissors. Examples of levers used in sports are tennis racquet, baseball bat, lacrosse stick, and vaulting pole. In the group of examples of levers used around the home, the force end of the lever moves a greater distance than the resistance end, thereby giving the advantage to force. In the group of examples of sports implements, the distance the resistance end of the implement moves is greater than the distance the force point is moved thereby increasing speed.

In the human body, the bone (or several bones) serves as a lever even though it may not have the shape of a rigid bar. The entire trunk, for example, serves as a lever during the dead lift with a barbell. In this lift, the fulcrum is at the hip joint, the resistance point is the shoulder joint, and the force point is the insertion of the muscles that extend the hip joint. When the extended arm is raised, the fulcrum is located at the shoulder joint, the force point is approximately where the deltoid muscle inserts on the humerus, and the resistance point is at the center of gravity of the entire arm. When a weight is held in the hand, the resistance point is then closer to the hand. If a very heavy weight is being lifted, the resistance point, for practical purposes, may be assumed to be at the hand. During a front curl with a barbell, the fulcrum is located at the elbow joint, the point of application of force is the insertion of the biceps, and the resistance point is at the palms where the barbell is held.

The body may be viewed as a system of links articulated at joints. Each link is regarded as a straight line running from the joint at one end of the bone to the joint at the opposite end. This line seldom runs through the center of the bone and in some instances may be wholly outside the bone. This is the case with the femur. A line drawn from the hip to the knee joint will be medial to the femur. The links are functional and, in structure, may bear little resemblance to a bar. The scapulae, head, and thorax are examples of levers that do not look like bars.

LEVER DESCRIPTIONS

Classification of a lever into one of the three types, first class, second class, or third class, is determined by the location of the axis, force point, and resistance point relative to one another. In the first-class lever (Figure 7.1), the axis is between the points of application of

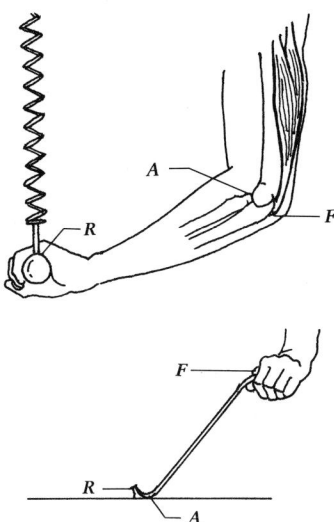

Figure 7.1 First class levers: crowbar and triceps extending elbow

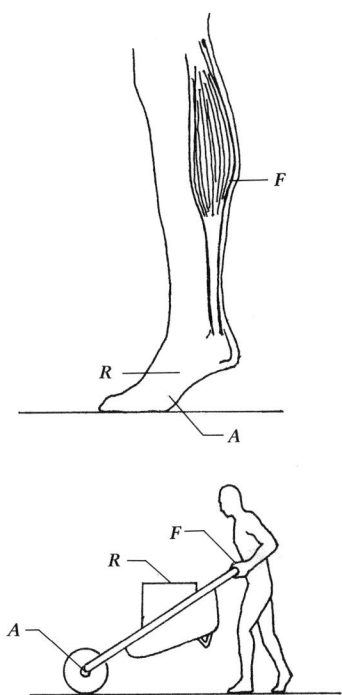

Figure 7.2 Second class levers: wheelbarrow and rise on toes

force and resistance. In the second-class lever (Figure 7.2), the resistance point is between the axis and the force point. In the third-class lever (Figure 7.3), the force point is between the axis and the resistance point. Examples of the three types are:

First class: can opener, crowbar, scissors, seesaw

Second class: wheelbarrow, nut cracker, bottle opener

Third class: lacrosse stick, canoe paddle (when the lower hand pulls faster than the upper hand).

INTERNAL AND EXTERNAL LEVERS

Most external levers are first- or second-class levers because the objective is to decrease the amount of force that must be utilized to overcome a resistance. In the first-class lever, it is possible, by moving the axis closer to the resistance, to increase the difference between the length of the force arm (distance from the point of application of force to the axis) rela-

tive to the length of the resistance arm (distance from the point of application of resistance to the axis). In the second-class lever, the force arm is always longer than the resistance arm. When the force arm is longer than the resistance arm, the advantage lies with force; that is, the amount of force necessary to overcome a resistance will be less than the amount of resistance. This will be noted in the simple machines previously offered as illustrations as well as in many complex machines.

When the resistance arm is longer than the force arm, as it invariably is in third-class levers and may be in first-class levers, the advantage lies with distance or speed at the cost of force. If a 75-pound child sits on one end of a seesaw and a 250-pound man sits on the opposite end, it will be necessary to place the axis or fulcrum of the seesaw very close to the

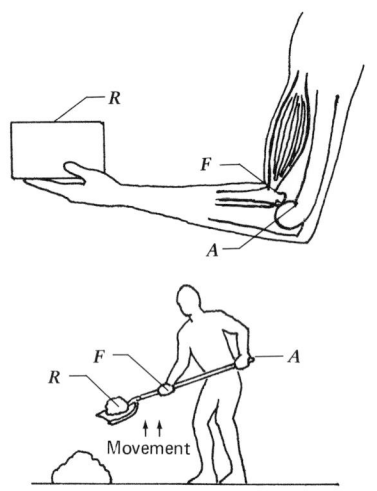

Figure 7.3 Third class levers: use of long shovel and biceps flexing arm

250-pound man in order to balance the see-saw. The distance or arc through which the child moves will be much greater than that through which the man moves because the radius of the child's arc is considerably longer than the radius of the man's arc. Additionally, the child will move at a greater linear velocity than will the man (although angular velocity will be the same). This is true because the child will move a greater distance in the same time.

With sports implements, such as bats, racquets, and paddles, the objective is to increase speed or distance the resistance is moved at the cost of force and distance the force moves. For example, when batting, the wrists are snapped (flexed) at the moment of contact with the ball. If the bat is regarded as a lever (which it is), the axis is at the rear hand, the resistance arm is the distance from the axis to the point of contact with the ball, and the force arm is the distance from the axis to the forward hand. It is obvious that the resistance arm is considerably longer than the force arm and that the end of the bat is moving at greater speed than the forward hand. The same is true in the case of a tennis racquet or table tennis paddle except that the length of the force arm is even shorter—the width of one hand. The sacrifice of force for speed, incidently, indicates why strength is important to success in almost all sports.

Although examples of all three classes of levers can be found in the human body, almost all of them are third-class levers. This means that the human body favors speed at the cost of force and also that in order to overcome even small resistances, the muscles must generate considerable force since the force arms of human levers are very short.

A few examples of first-class anatomic levers can be found. The forearm, when it is being extended by the triceps muscle, is one. The force point is located at the insertion of the triceps muscle on the olecranon process of the ulna at the proximal end of the forearm. The resistance point is the forearm's center of gravity unless resistance to elbow extension is provided, in which case the resistance point would be at the hand. The fulcrum is located between these two points, at the elbow joint. Another example of a first-class anatomic lever is the head during flexion and hyperextension of the neck (Figure 7.4). The axis is located at the atlanto-occipital articulation, which is forward of the insertions of the splenius capitis and semispinalis capitis, the major muscles involved in tilting the head backward, which insert at the base of the skull.

When the head is tilted backward, the center of resistance is located forward of the axis behind the forehead. This resistance arises from the weight of the head and from tension of the antagonist muscles and fascia.

When the head is tilted forward, the axis remains between the points of resistance and force, which change positions. During flexion of the neck, the center of resistance is located in the rear half of the head and behind the axis while the insertion of the muscles that flex the neck is forward of the axis, the atlanto-occipital articulation. These muscles are

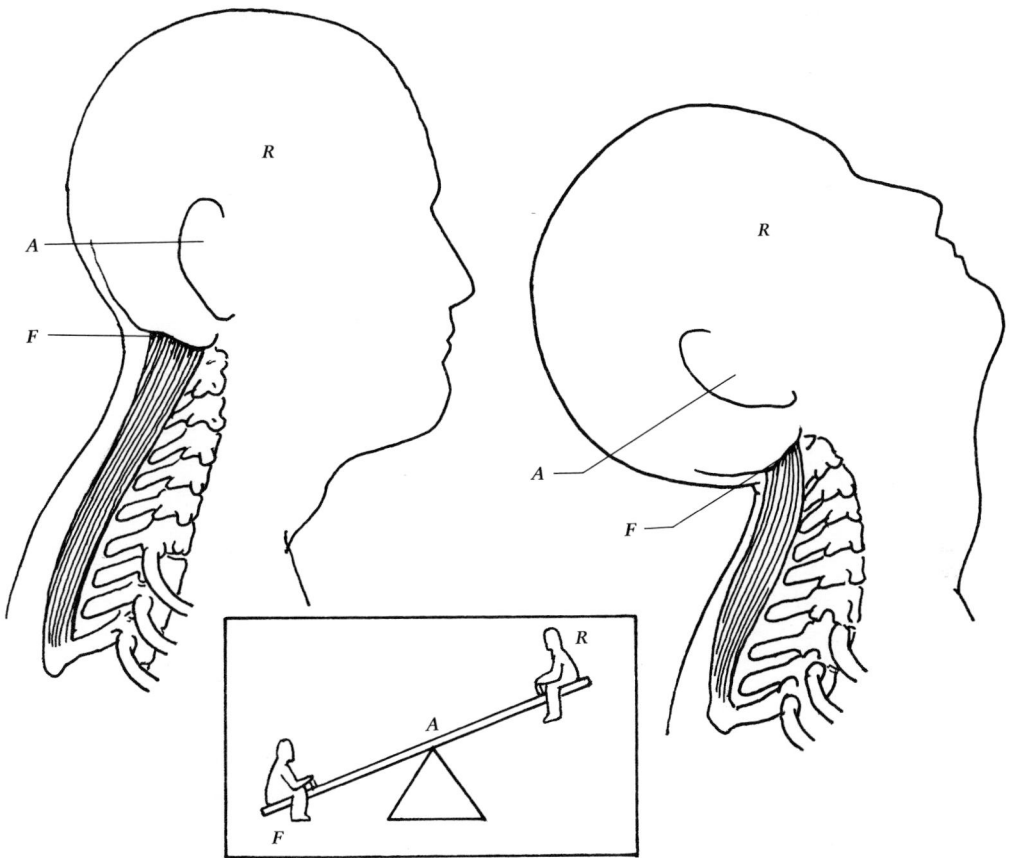

Figure 7.4 Tilting of the head backward as a first-class anatomic lever (cf. inset) showing axis (A), center of resistance (R) and center of force (F)

the longus colli and capitis, rectus capitis, and hyoids, which insert on the occipital bone at the base of the skull.

In second-class levers, as has been pointed out, the resistance point is located between the axis and point of application of force. The opening of the jaw is an illustration of a second-class anatomic lever.[1] The axis is located at the condyle where it articulates with the skull. This is at one end of the lever. The platysma attaches to the opposite end of the lever on the anterior portion of the mandible. This is the muscle that pulls the jaw downward. The resistance is located between these two points.

Karpovich[2] studied the mechanics of rising on the toes (Figure 7.5) and reported that there are two actions in this movement, the first action utilizing a first-class lever and the second action a third-class lever. In rising on the toes, the body is first inclined forward until its center of gravity is forward of the heads of the metatarsal bones where the axis is located at this time. The force is provided by the calf muscles through the tendon of Achilles to its attachment on the calcaneus. This is a first-class lever since the axis is between the points of resistance and force. After the heels have been lifted off the floor, the body is tilted or rotated backward at the talotibial

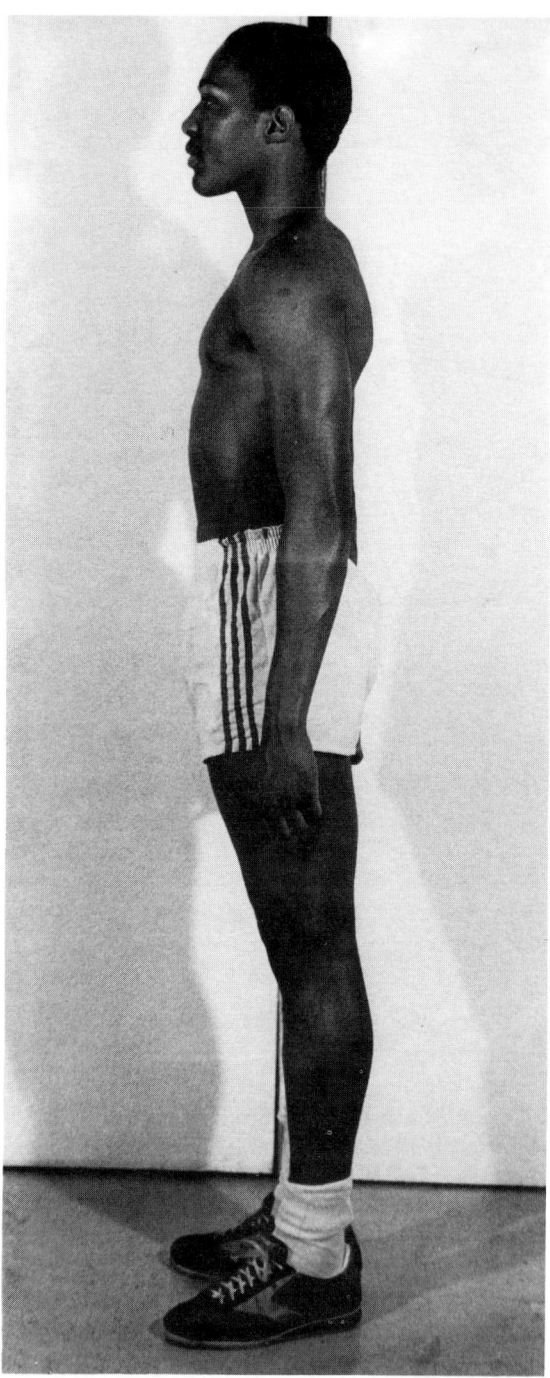

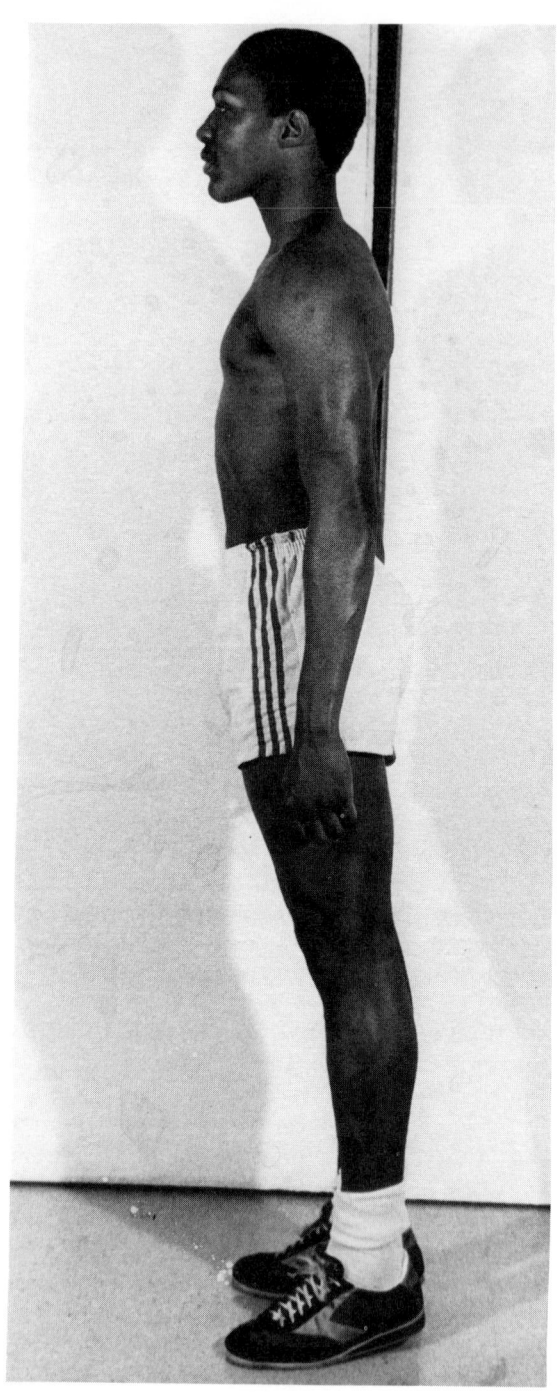

Figure 7.5   Rise on Toes (a) Body in balance. Center of gravity between heads of metatarsals and calcaneus

Figure 7.5b   Body's center of gravity forward of heads of metatarsal bones, which are axis of rotation

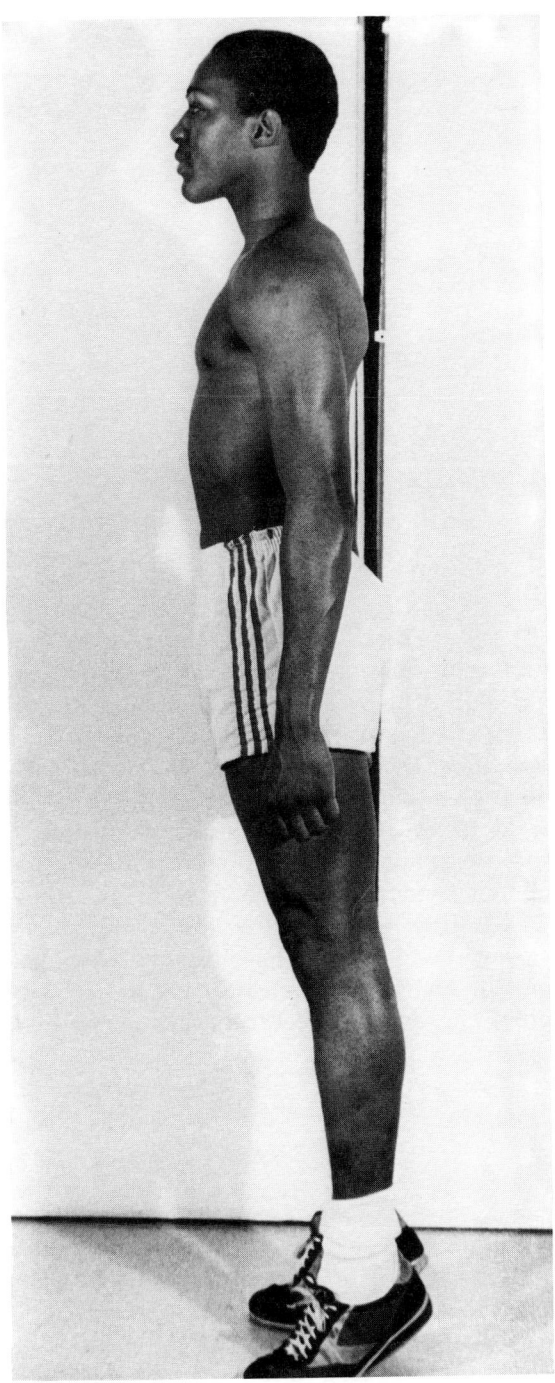

Figure 7.5c Axis of rotation now at talotibial joint

joint to maintain balance. During this action, a third-class lever is utilized. The lever class changes because now the axis is located at the talotibial joint rather than at the heads of the metatarsal bones and the lever is no longer the foot but the lower leg. During this action, the attachment of the calf muscles moves to a point in front of the axis. The resistance, located at the body's center of gravity, is forward of both the axis and the point of force, making this a third-class lever. After the body has been pulled back into balance, the system becomes, again, a first-class lever. The reader is urged to endeavor to rise on the toes while standing with the heels, buttocks, and back in continuous contact with the wall. While the maneuver can be executed, it will be noted that it is easier and more natural to incline the body forward as the move is initiated because the resistance (body weight) is closer to the fulcrum.

In third-class levers, the force point is between the resistance and the axis. Almost all the anatomic levers are of the third class. Examples are the lower leg when the knee is extended, the thigh during extension of the hip, the trunk during sit-ups, the legs during leg raises, the arms in elevation or depression, and the fingers during flexion or extension. Many other examples could be provided. In all of these, the distance from the axis to the point of application of force is considerably shorter than the distance from the axis to the point of resistance. The implications of this relationship can be discovered by comparing the force required and the distance the hand must move when opening or closing a door by the door knob with that required when pushing near the hinges. One could also hold one end of a long-handled and fully loaded shovel still while pivoting the shovel about this axis with the other hand grasping the handle at various points (Figure 7.6). The nearer the second hand is to the loaded end of the shovel, the less force is required. In the case of the illustration with the door, the distance from the axis (hinges) to the door knob is

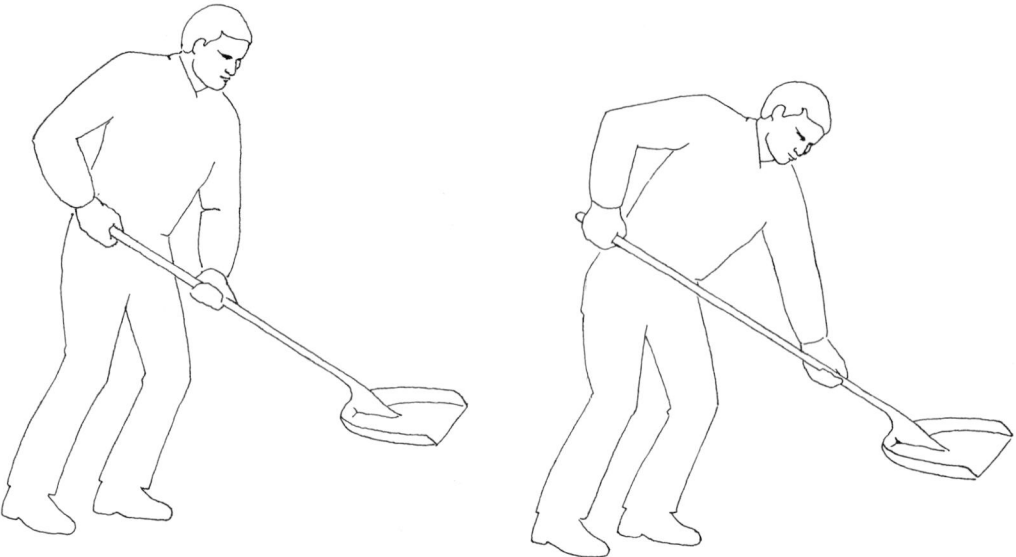

Figure 7.6 Two methods of using a shovel

longer than the distance from the hinges to the center of gravity of the door. The resistance point is between the axis and the force point, making this a second-class lever. When one pushes near the hinges, it becomes a third-class lever with the force point between the axis and the point of resistance. In the case of the illustration with the shovel, the lever was a third-class lever whether the lifting hand was close to or far from the stabilizing hand. However, when the lifting hand was moved toward the loaded end of the shovel, the distance from the axis to the point of application of force (force arm) was increased, increasing the length of the force arm and thereby making it easier to lift the shovel.

PRINCIPLE OF LEVERS

In an earlier illustration, it was pointed out that a seesaw (first-class lever) could be balanced with a 250-pound man on one end and a 75-pound child on the other end if the axis or fulcrum is placed near the 250-pound

man. This is an application of the *principle of levers*, which states that a lever (of any class) will balance when the product of the force times the distance from the point of application of force to the axis (force arm) is equal to the resistance times the distance from the point of application of resistance to the axis (resistance arm) or $F \times FA = R \times RA$. If any three of the four values are known, the fourth can be computed. Assume that the 250-pound man is sitting so that his center of gravity is 3 feet from the fulcrum.

$$F \times FA = R \times RA$$
$$250 \times 3 = 75 \times RA$$
$$750 = 75\ RA$$
$$RA = 10\ ft$$

The child must sit so that his center of gravity is 10 feet from the fulcrum in order to balance the seesaw.

In the preceding illustration, it was assumed that the force and resistance were applied at right angles to the lever. These forces are seldom at right angle to the lever arm. When the forces are applied at other than a right angle, the force is diminished. A more accurate definition of the force arm is: "the perpendicular distance between the fulcrum and the line of force." The specific definition of resistance arm is: "the perpendicular distance between the fulcrum and the line of resistance." These are called the force moment arm (FMA) and the resistance moment arm (RMA), respectively. Consequently, the formula stated earlier becomes: $F \times FMA = R \times RMA$.

Line of Pull

At the beginning of muscular contraction or shortening, when the joint being moved is straight or extended, the line of pull of the muscle involved is almost parallel to the long axis of the bone. The line of pull is altered somewhat by condyles, tuberosities, and sesimoid bones over which the tendon must pass. Nevertheless, at the beginning of the movement, the line of pull of the muscle is considerably less than a right angle. This serves a useful purpose since a portion of the force generated by the muscle is utilized in stabiliz-

ing the joint by pulling the adjacent bones toward one another. This stabilizing force decreases as the need for it decreases as the joint is flexed. After the joint angle during flexion decreases to less than 90 degrees, the muscle's line of pull is such that it tends to dislocate the joint. This is known as *negative stabilization*.

As the joint is flexed due to contraction of the muscle, the perpendicular distance from the muscle's line of pull or the force moment arm (FMA) increases, enabling the muscle to overcome greater resistance with the same force. This explains why it is more difficult to initiate a movement (as in the front curl with a barbell) than it is to continue the movement (see Figure 7.7).

At a small angle of pull, the joint angle will be decreased a greater amount than it will at a large angle of pull with the same amount of muscular contraction or shortening. This facilitates rapid initial flexion but at the cost of force.

The stabilizing component of force in a muscle's line of pull cannot contribute useful work, but if it were not for this construction, dislocations would occur more frequently.

Figure 7.7 Varying lengths of moment arm at elbow during different degrees of elbow flexion

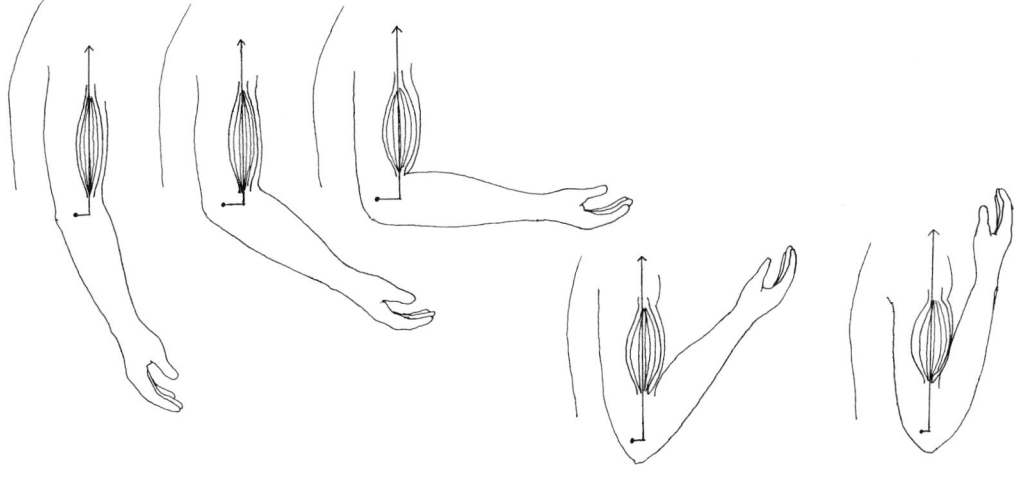

Good muscular development will decrease the probability that an athlete will suffer a dislocation, because the athlete will have greater force available to stabilize the joint and to prevent dislocation. Strong, taut, and large ligaments add to the stability of a joint, as does the depth of the socket in the case of ball and socket joints. In joints normally subjected to large stress, evolutionary modifications have developed that have given these joints great stability. An example is the hip joint with its deep socket and large, powerful ligaments. Other joints, such as the shoulder and knee joints, depend principally upon muscles whose tendons pass over the joint to give them stability. Gymnasts and wrestlers, in particular, need strong muscles in the shoulder girdle, not only to perform skillfully but to withstand forces that tend to dislocate the shoulder. Long diving forward rolls, for example, are contraindicated for those students in tumbling classes with weak shoulder muscles because of the danger of a shoulder dislocation.

The amount of force that muscles must generate to lift a specific weight can be calculated. However, such calculations are almost never computed by practitioners. Because of their complexity, they are made only by specialists in research. In most movements several muscles act on an anatomic lever. Each muscle's line of pull is different from that of others. The line of pull changes constantly during the movement. It is impossible to measure accurately the several muscles' angle of pull, to locate the exact point of insertion of the muscles (in vivo), or to compute the weight of the body segments with accuracy. The studies that have been done in this area all point to the enormous forces that must be generated to lift relatively light weights and the degree to which human anatomic levers sacrifice force for distance and speed. In some activities, such as in the straight leg dead lift, tremendous compressive and shear stresses are imposed upon joints and their cartilage.

Roozbazar[3] compared the effects on compressive stress, shear stress, and bending moment on the intervertebral disk between the fourth and fifth lumbar vertebrae when lifting a 55-kg weight using three methods of lifting. The three methods were: (1) back bent/knees extended (stooped position), (2) back inclined/knees bent, and (3) back vertical/knees bent. Roozbazar indicated that the first method is a back lift while the last two are leg lifts. It should also be pointed out, for our purposes, that in the first method the resistance arm is considerably longer than in the third method. The third method has long been recommended by kinesiologists. The resistance arm is the perpendicular distance from the line of gravity to the axis of rotation located between the fourth and fifth lumbar vertebrae. The differences in this distance in the three methods can easily be perceived by looking at Figure 7.8.

The results of Roozbazar's calculations are shown in Table 7.1:

Table 7.1 Calculations of the Effects of Moment, Compressive Stress, and Tangential Stress on the L4/5 Disk

Method	Moment (kg/cm)	Compressive stress (kg/cm)	Tangential stress on the annulus fibrosus (kg/cm²)
Back bent/knees straight	+ 4224	30	120
Back inclined/knees bent	+ 3003	28.5	114
Back vertical/knees bent	negligible	6	24

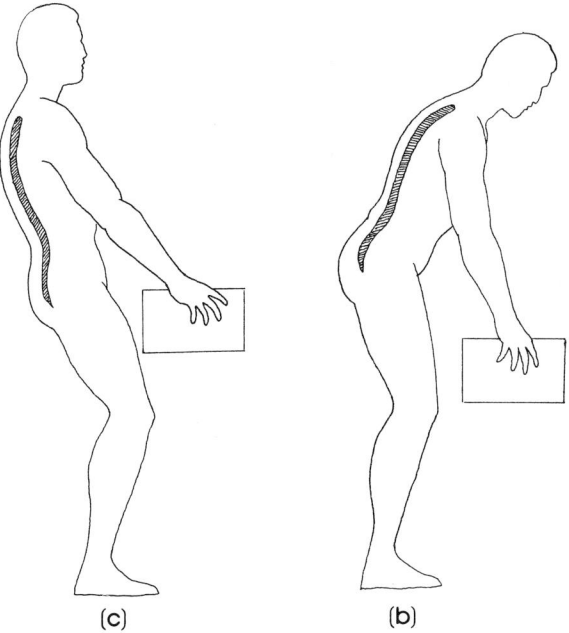
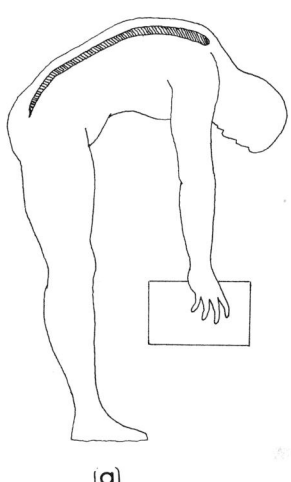

Figure 7.8 The three methods of lifting, **(a)** back bent/knees extended, **(b)** back inclined/knees bent, **(c)** back vertical/knees bent (from A. Rooz-bazar, "Biomechanics of Lifting," Biomechanics IV, edited by R. C. Nelson and C. A. Morehouse, University Park Press, Baltimore, 1974, pp. 37–43, with permission)

Not only can almost three times more weight be lifted using the legs rather than the back, but the danger of suffering an abdominal wall hernia, prolapsed pelvic viscera, torn ligaments of the lower back, or herniated disks is much less. It is the responsibility of all physical educators, coaches, physical therapists, and health educators to teach correct lifting procedures in an effort to decrease the high incidence of lower back problems.

ROTARY MOTION AND LEVERAGE

Every human motion begins as a rotary motion. A combination of two or more rotary movements in the same direction often results in translatory motion. For example, when throwing a punch (a linear motion), the humerus moves through horizontal flexion while the elbow is extended. At the same time, the trunk is rotated. Walking and running (linear motions) are made possible by repeated flexions and extensions of the knee and hip joints as the body's center of gravity is continuously moved forward over the supporting foot.

One of the determinants of success in sports is selection of the implement (bat, golf club, pole, etc.) of the best length and weight. Another determinant of success in sports is selection of the optimum anatomic lever length, utilization of the various levers in the best sequence, and application of the correct amount of force. Unlike implements, human levers can be shortened or lengthened. For example, when kicking a ball, the knee is first flexed and then extended as contact with the ball is made. In gymnastic movements, a lever arm is often shortened to accelerate speed of rotation. A skilled baseball pitcher knows when to lengthen and when to shorten anatomic levers (Figure 7.9). The arm is first brought behind the body to an extended position and then the elbow is flexed while the trunk is rotated and the humerus is brought forward. Finally, the elbow is extended and the wrist is flexed as the ball is released.

In this skill several levers of various lengths are used. Shortening of anatomic levers increases angular velocity while lengthening of levers increases linear speed and range of motion. However, when an anatomic lever is lengthened, the length of the resistance arm is increased while the force arm remains the same length. This requires that greater force

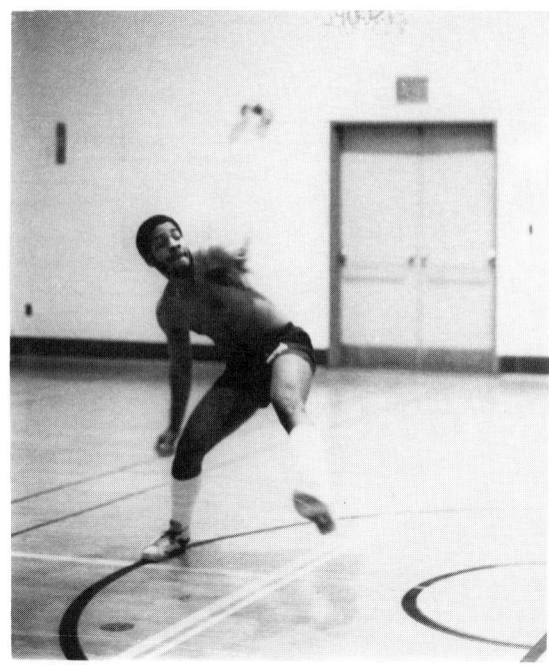

Figure 7.9b Body moving forward to add its momentum

Figure 7.9c Note hyperextension of wrist, flexion of elbow, and outward rotation of humerus

Figure 7.9 Overhand Throw

Figure 7.9a Hip and shoulder levers rotated to increase range of their motion

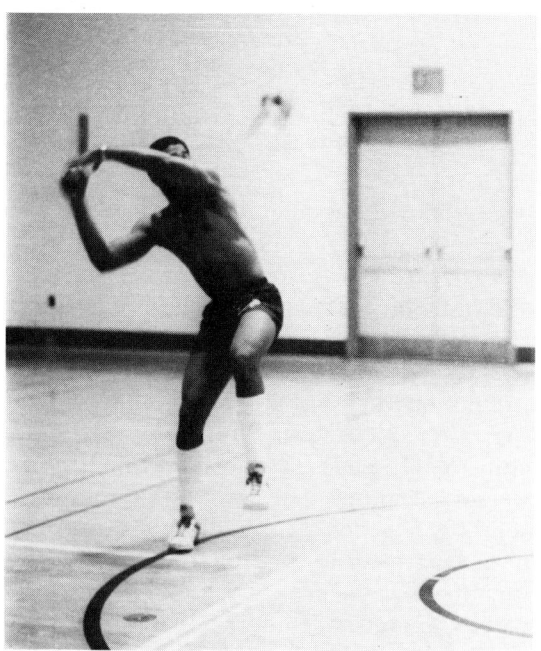

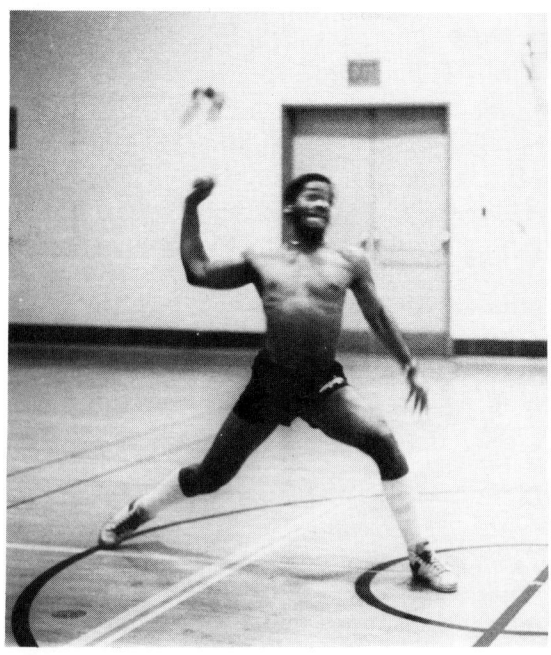

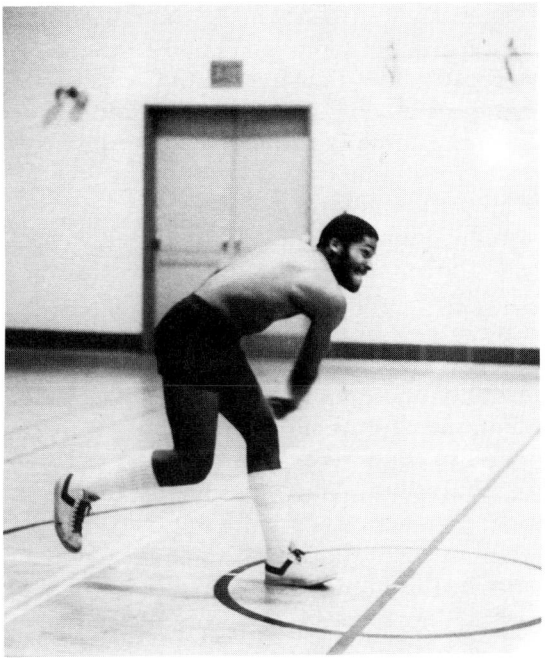

Figure 7.9d Body has moved forward over left foot, shoulders hips, and trunk have rotated counterclockwise, arm is extended, and wrist is flexed

be exerted. Among gymnastic coaches and performers, it is well known that it is more difficult for a tall gymnast to execute strength moves such as planches, the crucifix, and straight body press-ups into handstands than it is for short gymnasts. The reason for this is that the taller gymnasts have levers with longer resistance arms.

The end of a lever moves with greater speed than any other part of the lever simply because the arc of the circle it moves through has a longer radius and consequently, a greater circumference. Although the angular speed of any two points on a lever will be the same, the linear speed of the point closer to the distal end is always greater, because it moves through a greater distance in the same unit of time. For this reason it is recommended that the arm be extended when serving, driving, or smashing a tennis ball, driving a golf ball, bowling, or delivering an

underhand pitch. This is why baseball pitchers extend the arm near completion of the pitch. When gymnasts need to develop momentum ($M = mv$), they extend the body or the involved parts. During the downward swing in giant swings, for example, the entire body and extended arms are the lever. In order to gain greater lever length and, consequently speed and momentum at the end of the lever, the body is made as straight as possible (no arch or flexion at the knees, hips, neck, shoulders, or arms).

Young baseball players who lack the strength necessary to swing the bat with control and speed, "choke-up" on the bat to shorten the lever arm. Some are unable to serve a tennis ball with the arm extended because they are not strong enough. Greater strength is required to use longer anatomic levers because the length of the resistance arm is increased. A contributing factor in the use of shorter levers by young children and some females may be a subconscious awareness of inadequate shoulder girdle and arm strength.

In order to gain maximum speed at the extremity of a system of anatomic levers, as in throwing or kicking, each successive lever used should come into action at the moment the one previous reached its maximum speed. This is a function of the nervous system that can be enhanced through proper coaching and practice. When pushing or lifting against heavy resistance, however, all the levers utilized should be brought into action simultaneously.

In many sports movements, compromises must be made with the objective of gaining maximum speed at the end of the lever on account of other considerations. An example is in batting. Because the maximal speed is at the tip of the bat, one might assume that the greatest distance could be secured by striking the ball with the tip of the bat. However, the greater the distance the ball is struck from the center of gravity of the bat, the more the force of the impact will rotate the bat around its center of gravity. This would cause some of the force of the bat to be lost. The most solid contact will be made when the center of gravity of the bat meets the center of gravity of the ball. However, at this point the bat would not have its greatest momentum. Therefore, the best place to hit the ball is at some point between the end of the bat and its center of gravity. The above also points out why a firm grip is necessary.

There are many instances in sports when it is of greater importance to move the lever through its range of motion quickly than it is to gain speed at the end of the lever. In such instances, the lever arm is shortened. Examples are in volleying at the net in tennis, when the baseball player must move the ball away quickly, or in short, quick passes in soccer or basketball.

Wheel and Axle

The force causing a wheel and axle to rotate may be applied either at the wheel as in an automobile steering wheel or to the axle as in the chain's actions on the rear wheel of a bicycle. Other examples of the wheel and axle are a ship's helm, door knob, water wheel, propeller, meat grinder, pencil sharpener, bicycle sprocket, ferris wheel, and tricycle. When the force is applied to the rim of the wheel, the effect is that of a second-class lever with the fulcrum at one end, the force at the other end, and the resistance in the center. In the second-class lever, force is favored because the force arm is longer than the resistance arm. When the force is applied to the axle, the effect is that of a third-class lever since the axis is at the center of the axle, the resistance is at the center of gravity of the wheel, and the force is applied between these two points, at the rim of the axle. The third-class lever favors speed and distance because

the resistance arm is longer than the force arm. When the force is applied to the axle, the greater the diameter of the wheel, the greater the advantage of speed and distance. When the force is applied to the rim, the greater the diameter of the wheel, the greater the advantage of force.

In the human body, both arrangements are found; however, the third-class type favoring speed is more common. The most obvious example of an anatomic wheel and axle is the thorax and vertebral column. When the oblique abdominals and the iliocostalis pull on the ribs, we have an example of force applied to the wheel. When the spinal rotators, multifidus, and semispinalis contract, the act on the vertebral column (axle).

Other examples of wheel and axle arrangements in the human body are found in the head and neck, arms, and legs. In the neck, force is applied either at the cervical vertebrae (axle) by the splenius capitis and cervicis, suboccipitals, and semispinalis or at the wheel by the sternocleidomastoid and splenius muscles.

SOMATOTYPE AND LEVERS

Although somatotype bears no relationship to total body height, it does bear a relationship to both the length of the appendages and the distribution of weight on the arms and legs. Endomorphs have short upper arms, forearms, thighs, and lower legs relative to their body height. As a result, they are unable to generate as much linear speed at the ends of these shorter levers as are the other two body types. This is a handicap in activities involving throwing, running, jumping, and kicking. Further, their arms taper from "hammy" upper arms to small hands and wrists while, similarly, their legs taper from heavy "hammy" thighs to small ankles and feet. These characteristics place the center of gravity of the arms and legs closer to the joint or axis. As a result, angular momentum of the arms and legs in endomorphs will be less than in the other two body types and they will be able to transfer less momentum to implements such as balls, javelins, and the discus. It will be recalled (see Chapter 5) that angular momentum is the product of the moment of inertia times the angular velocity or angular momentum $-J\omega$. The moment of inertia, which is the same as mass in linear motion, is equal to the mass of each particle multiplied by the square of its distance from the center of rotation. When a mass is whirling around on a string or rope, it is simple to compute the moment of inertia. In human levers, the mass of each body segment is distributed unevenly over the entire lever. To determine accurately the moment of inertia, it is necessary to multiply the mass of each particle by the square of its distance from the axis and then to add all the products. Particles near the axis add less to the moment of inertia and, consequently, less to angular momentum than do particles near the end of the lever, which are further from the axis. The "hammy" upper arms and thighs tapering to small wrists, ankles, hands, and feet of endomorphs prohibit generation of the amount of angular momentum capable of being generated by the other two body types.

Students will recognize that almost all sport implements (which are levers) such as bats, golf clubs, racquets, lacrosse and hockey sticks, which are used to transfer momentum to balls or other objects, have their mass concentrated at the distal end. In addition to their tapering appendages, the small hands and feet of the endomorphs further handicap them in transferring momentum to sport projectiles.

Ectomorphs possess relatively long arms and legs. From the standpoint of leverage, this presents an advantage in throwing, running, jumping, and kicking. However, because ectomorphs are frail and poorly mus-

cled, they are unable to generate the force necessary to perform well in these activities and to take advantage of their relatively long levers.

Although ectomorphs do not perform well in events requiring muscular power or those requiring anaerobic condition such as sprints, hurdling, and games requiring repeated bursts of intensive activity as football, they can excel in the events demanding aerobic endurance such as the mile or greater distances up to and including cross country and marathon runs. This is because less energy is consumed in moving their light and thin bodies and because the heart of ectomorphs need not work as hard since there is less tissue calling for oxygen and nutrients and removal of carbon dioxide.

Mesomorphic somatotypes possess a number of advantages with respect to success in a variety of sports. The two major advantages are their strength and distribution of weight or mass over the body levers. Distribution of weight over the arms and legs is more uniform than that of endomorphs. Their large forearms, wrists, hands, and fingers increase the moment of inertia that can be generated when throwing implements. Their massive lower legs and large feet make possible a greater moment of inertia when kicking balls.

Mesomorphs require a large amount of physical activity for maintenance of cardiovascular fitness and prevention of obesity. During their middle years and beyond, they must learn to avoid engaging in reveries of their past athletic exploits and participate actively even though their ego may be slightly damaged in the process.

LEVERAGE APPLIED TO PROJECTILES

Many different projectiles are used in sports. These projectiles are of a great variety in shape, size, weight, density, and coefficient of restitution. They are thrown, pushed, or struck with the hand or foot. Some are projected with the aid of an implement. The projectiles include baseballs, softballs, the discus, the javelin, footballs, soccer balls, golf balls, arrows, handballs, basketballs, tennis balls, squash balls, volley balls, bowling balls, the shot put, badminton birds, horseshoes, the hammer, hockey pucks, lacrosse balls, darts, and the human body. The objects are projected with the hand, foot, or head or with implements such as golf clubs, bows, racquets, hockey sticks, bats, and lacrosse sticks.

Throwing and striking can be classified into overhand, underhand, diagonal, and sidearm patterns. Other projection patterns have been classified as pushing (shot put, one- and two-hand basketball push shots, and volleyball set-up). Certain principles must be applied for greatest efficiency regardless of the pattern. Furthermore, similar procedures are utilized in each of the patterns regardless of the projectile or implement.

The objectives with respect to projection in sports are distance, velocity, and accuracy. The following principles relate to direction and distance of projection:

1. The force must be of sufficient magnitude to overcome the projectile's inertia and all restraining forces such as friction with the supporting surface, resistance of wind or water, and the weight of the lever arm.

2. The force transmitted to the projectile as a result of muscular contractions requires an equal counterforce from the supporting surface. The coefficient of friction between the performer's feet and the supporting surface must be great enough to allow exertion of maximal thrust without slipping. The supporting surface must also be sufficiently firm that it will not absorb some of the thrust.

3. The sequential movements of body lev-

ers terminating in the object to be projected must each be timed to add to the peak velocity of the preceding movement. Each body lever receives the velocity of the movement of levers preceding and adds its own velocity to the sum of the velocities.

4. The linear velocity of the body resulting from a forward step, steps, or a run can be added to the velocity of the projectile.

5. Since velocity is greatest at the distal end of both internal and external levers, an object can be projected farthest from the end of the lever, all other factors being equal.

6. If the strength of muscles involved in moving the internal levers is inadequate, projectile speed, distance, and accuracy are diminished.

7. The projectile's direction is determined by the direction of the force applied at the moment of impact or release. When the force consists of two or more components, the projectile's flight will be in the direction of the resultant of the components according to a parallelogram of forces.

8. The point of application of force with respect to the projectile's center of gravity determines whether its motion will be linear or rotatory.

9. The greater the initial velocity of a moving projectile when it is impacted by a striking lever (internal or external), the greater the resultant velocity of the projectile in the opposite direction after it is struck.

10. The greater the mass of a struck ball, the greater its velocity after impact unless its mass is so great as to overcome the momentum of the striking lever.

11. The velocity that can be imparted to a struck ball is directly related to the mass of the striking implement. The heavier and longer the bat the baseball player can swing with accuracy and control, the greater the velocity and distance of the ball.

12. Greater distance can be secured in a discus or football throw or football kick by varying the angle of inclination of the plane of the projectile according to the direction and intensity of the wind.

13. The higher the coefficient of restitution or elasticity of the ball and of the striking implement, the greater the velocity of the struck ball.

14. The direction of rebound of a ball from a flat surface (such as a wall or a tennis racquet) is dependent upon the projectile's angle of approach as well as its direction of spin.

15. The further an object is projected and the longer the backswing, the greater the probability of accuracy.

16. The longer the backswing, the further an object can be projected.

17. Dense objects are less influenced by air resistance and wind than are less compact objects.

The student is referred to Chapter 6 for specific topics dealing with the production and application of force.

Overarm Patterns

The overarm pattern is used in throwing baseballs, footballs, and javelins, in the overarm serve in volleyball, and in the tennis serve. As in the underarm and sidearm patterns, a number of anatomic levers are used sequentially, giving a "whiplike" action to the distal end of the system of levers. A distinct feature of the overarm pattern is flexion of the elbow and medial rotation of the humerus during the forward or force-producing phase of the arm action. Next to wrist flexion, medial rotation of the humerus is the fastest joint action of the arm. Additionally, the length of this rapidly moving lever (forearm) is longer than most of the other involved levers; consequently, its contribution to linear velocity of the projectile is substantial. The moment or resistance arm of this lever is longest, and, therefore, its speed is greatest when the forearm is at a right angle to the humerus.

Other lever actions that are used in the overarm pattern (as well as in the underarm pattern) are pelvic rotation, spinal rotation, spinal flexion, and wrist flexion. A forward step of the leg opposite the throwing or striking arm adds linear velocity to the throw or strike. The foot on the side of the throwing or striking arm is pointed sideward (90 degrees) to the direction of the throw or strike on initiation of the movement. This increases the range of motion of the pelvic lever. During the movement, the projectile is "pulled" with the elbow leading.

Throwing a Baseball (Figure 7.10). The pitcher's wind-up and stretch does not contribute to the velocity of the ball or accuracy of the throw. These actions may relieve the pitcher's tension and confuse the batter. A backward step with the left foot (right-handed pitcher) will increase the distance of the stride of the left leg, which will increase the distance through which momentum can be generated (Figure 7.10a). A push off this foot follows. The right foot is pointing sideward as are the thorax and pelvis at this point. During the long forward step with the left leg, the pitcher pivots on his right foot, rotating his body toward the batter to bring the levers of the pelvis and thorax into motion (Figure 7.10b). At the same time, the arm is drawn back preparatory to its forward movement and the humerus is laterally rotated. The farther the arm is drawn backward, the greater will be the distance over which velocity can be increased. The right leg pushes hard as the left leg strides forward (Figure 7.10c).

During the forward step of the left leg, the motion of the throwing arm begins with hori-

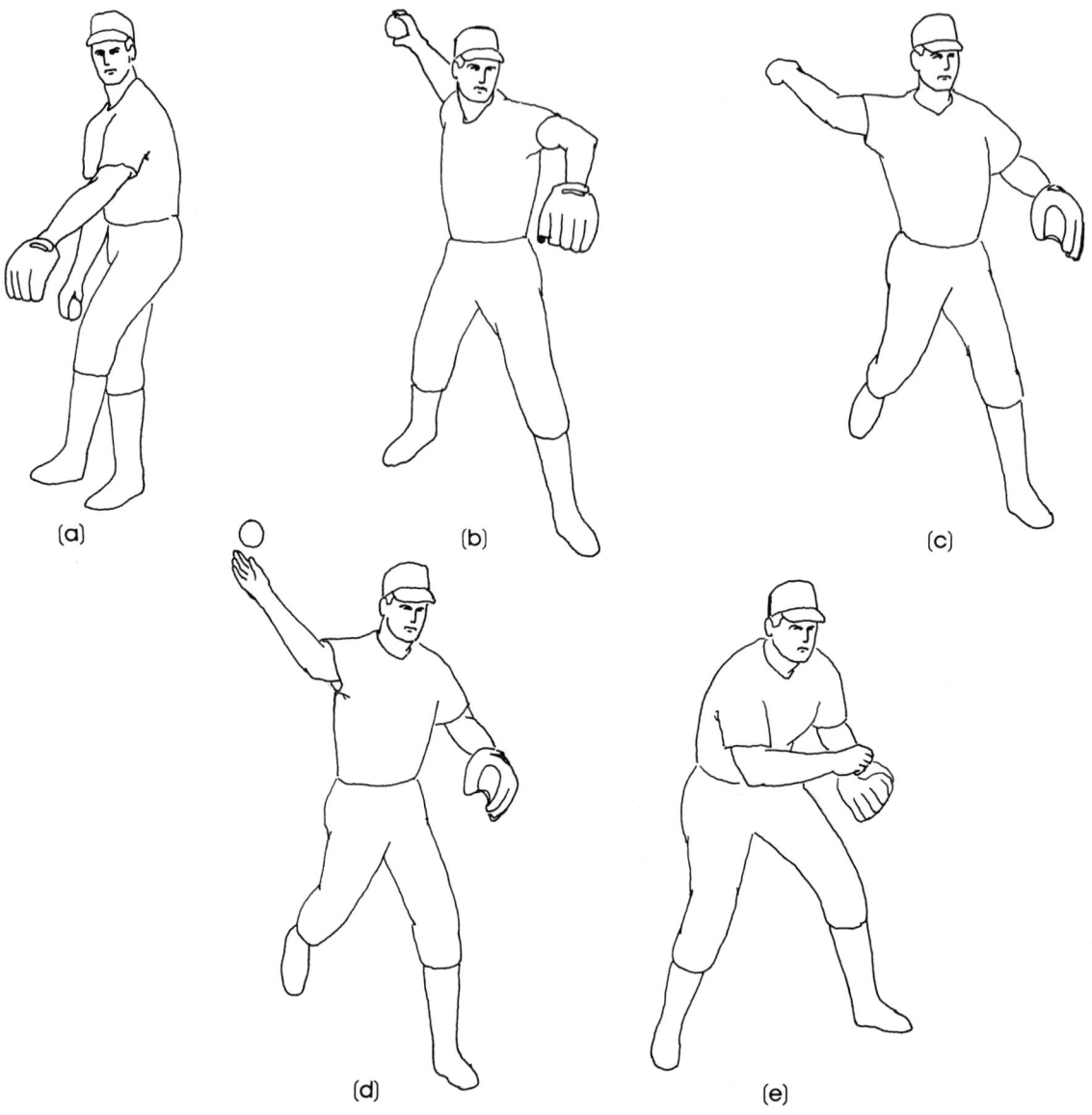

(a)

(b)

(c)

(d)

(e)

Figure 7.10 Baseball Pitch (a) Push-off from right leg initiated and body mass beginning to move forward. (b) Counterclockwise trunk rotation initiated (c) Humerus outward rotated and weight moving over left foot (d) Humerus rotating inward to accelerate rotational speed of the right hand and hips flexing to get mass of the trunk into the pitch. (e) Completion of pitch

zontal flexion of the humerus as it is brought in line with the plane of the thorax. This is followed by medial rotation of the humerus which brings the hand up over the elbow. The wrist is hyperextended. As the humerus approaches the frontal or lateral plane, the forearm begins to extend. This extension is quickly followed by flexion of the wrist as the ball is released. As these two movements occur, the trunk is brought forward to add the momentum of this large mass. The ball leaves the hand immediately after the forearm passes the vertical (Figure 7.10d). At this point, the sequential action of the stride and the levers of the pelvis, thorax, medial rotation of the humerus, extension of the elbow, hip flexion and wrist flexion have given the ball its greatest velocity (Figure 7.10e).

A recent study by Toyoshima et al.[4] utilizing electromyographic and electrogoniometric techniques showed that the greater the number of internal levers brought into play, the greater the final speed of the thrown ball. These researchers found that with five throwing patterns—(1) overhand with step, (2) overhand without step, (3) overhand with lower body immobilized, (4) overhand with upper body immobilized, and (5) overhand with the upper arm placed on the arm of a chair and immobilized—regardless of the weight of the ball (balls weighing 100, 200, 300, 400, and 500 grams were used), greatest velocity was achieved with pattern 1, that is, when the maximum number of body levers were used. With pattern 1, a 300-gram ball was thrown with the same velocity as a 100-gram ball with pattern 2. Contribution of body parts to the velocity of the ball was independent of the ball weight. They found that 50 percent of the velocity of the overhand throw resulted from the step and body rotation and the remainder from the shoulder, elbow, wrist, and finger action. They also found strongest action potentials from the gluteus maximus, adductor magnus, and pectoralis major in pattern 1, substantiating the contributions made by pelvic and shoulder rotation. Further, contribution of extension of the elbow joint to the velocity of the ball was greatest when the torque produced by rotation of the body was included.

Kunz studied the influence of the type of movement and mass of the ball on the speed of release.[5] He measured the path and velocity of the hand and hip with two rubber-band goniometers attached to the forefinger and the crest of the ilium. He found a linear relationship between the best performance (of three trials) and the velocity of the hand at the moment of release. The skilled throwers (group 1) achieved higher velocities than did the poor throwers (group 2). Effective throwers achieved greater velocities with a wind-up than without one. The distance over which force was applied decreased with increase in ball mass. Skilled throwers achieved higher maximal velocities of the hip. However, this movement was stopped earlier by the better throwers through intensive pressing of the left foot against the ground shortening the path of both the hand and the hip. This technique produced greater back arch tension because the posterior foot was able to maintain contact with the ground for a longer period. This provides a firm base for the sequential actions of the anatomic levers.

Throwing a Javelin (Figure 7.11). The mechanics of throwing a javelin are like those in throwing a ball except that the javelin thrower may execute a short run previous to release.

The thrower approaches the line at full speed (Figure 7.11a) and plants his left foot so that this foot points to the right (Figure 7.11b). Next, he crosses his right leg in front of the sideward turned left leg in the direction of the throw (Figure 7.11c). This action increases the distance through which the pelvic lever can move. As this is done, the javelin is brought into position for the throw to give greater distance through which to increase

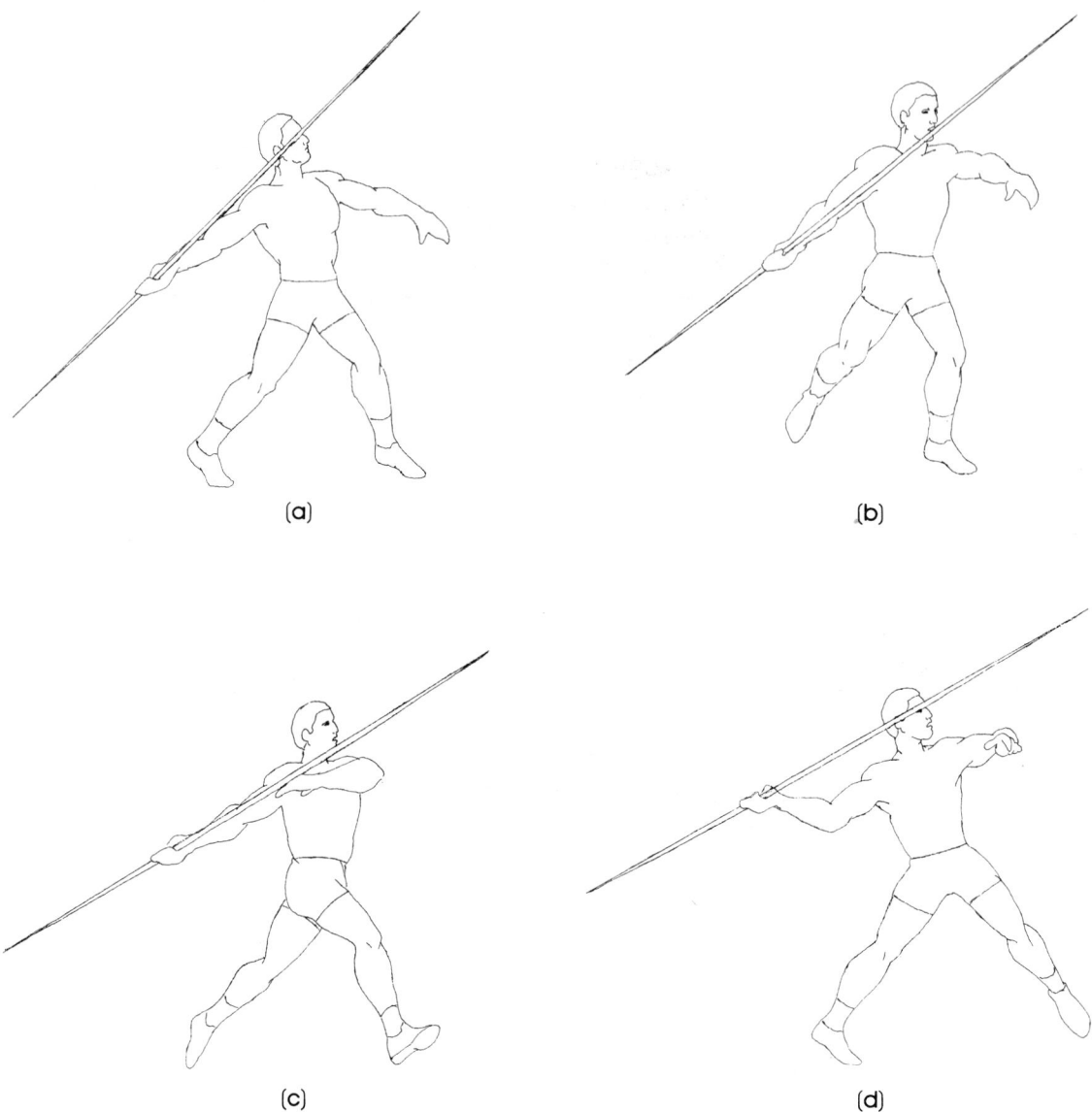

Figure 7.11 Javelin throw (a) Muscles of throwing arm placed on a stretch (b) Push off from right foot (c) Forward step with right foot to establish momentum in the body and the javelin. Note clockwise rotation of trunk and shoulder girdle (d) Weight on right foot moving forward to left foot. Humerus externally rotated and elbow flexing to secure greatest possible rotatory speed of hand during medial or inward rotation of humerus just prior to release (e) Back hyperextended to facilitate increase in the distance this large mass can accelerate to add its momentum to that imparted to the javelin (f) Elbow brought forward prior to extension. In pitching a baseball, the elbow remains to the side during its extension due to the object's lighter weight (g) Shoulders, trunk and hip levers undergoing clockwise rotation (h) Note follow through

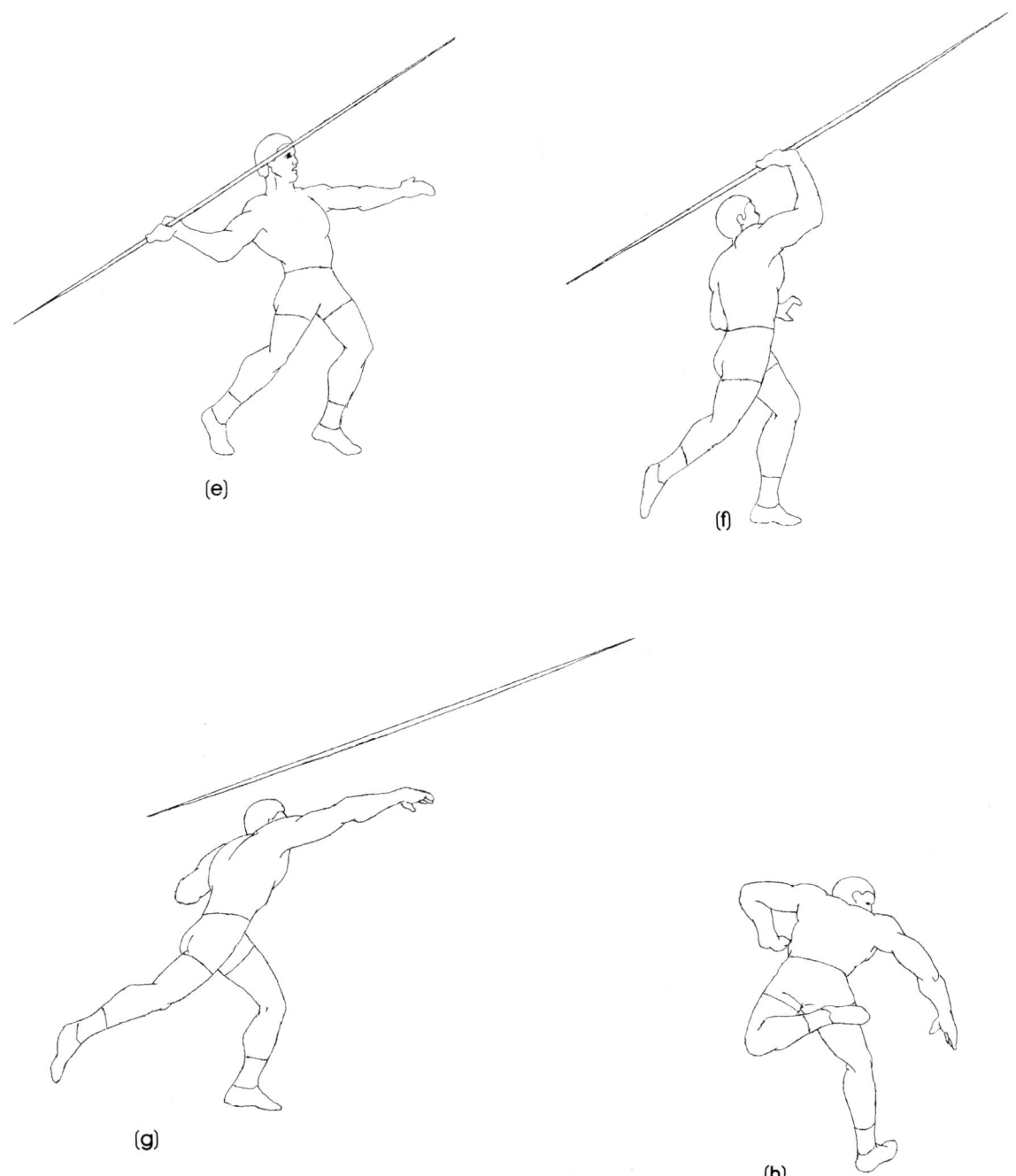

(e)

(f)

(g)

(h)

velocity (Figure 7.11d). At the same time, the body is tilted backward so that the center of gravity is behind this foot (Figure 7.11e). The backward tilt of the body provides this massive lever a greater distance through which to move when it is next thrust forward while the arm also moves forward in the same manner as the pitcher's arm (Figure 7.11f). The magnitude of arm and wrist snap cannot be as great as when pitching a baseball due to the greater mass of the javelin. The arm and hand follow through in the direction of the javelin's line of flight in order to insure that all the force is directed along the javelin's long axis (Figure 7.11g).

After the javelin has left the hand, the feet are reversed and the thrower lowers his center of gravity to better check his momentum in order to avoid stepping over the line (Figure 7.11h).

The humerus is rotated laterally as the arm is brought backward before the throw and then rotated medially during the throw. The most important muscles involved in this action are the pectoralis major and the latissimus dorsi.

Tennis Serve. Basically, the mechanics of the tennis serve are the same as in the baseball throw. The same overhand pattern used in the tennis serve is used in the tennis and badminton smash and the overhead clear in badminton.

The serve begins with a "toss," really a "push" of the ball vertically upward above the forward foot to a height of at least eight feet or as high overhead as the player can reach with the arms and legs extended and up on the toes. "Pushing" the ball upward insures a vertical flight path of the ball, making it easier to hit. The ball is thrown over the forward foot because it is at a point above this foot that the racquet head achieves its maximal speed. The body weight is shifted to the forward foot and the racquet is in the center of its arc at the moment the ball is contacted.

The ball is thrown to the height specified to insure use of the longest possible levers and to decrease the probability that the ball will travel into the net when struck horizontally or slightly below the horizontal.

Beginners should direct the ball horizontally until they can develop a ball velocity of at least 80 feet per second.[6] The ball is usually struck at a height of about eight feet. It must travel 39 feet before clearing the net and may not travel more than 60 feet before striking the ground without being beyond the service area. The force of gravity will pull the ball downward a distance of 16.1 feet per second. At a speed of 80 feet per second, 0.75 of a second will be required for the ball to travel the distance to the back line of the service area and 0.5 of a second will be required for it to travel the almost 40 feet to a point above the net. Gravity will cause the ball to drop

$$\tan 5° = \frac{8}{AC}$$

$$0.08749 = \frac{8}{AC}$$

$$0.8749\ AC = 8$$

$$AC = 91.4$$

$$DC = 91.4 - 39'$$

$$DC = 52.4'$$

$$\tan 5° = \frac{ED}{52.4}$$

$$0.08749 = \frac{ED}{52.4}$$

$$ED = 4.58'$$

by the time it crosses the net. It will cross the net at a height of 3.975 feet, adequate to clear the net by 11.5 inches (since the net is 3 feet high) if the ball is hit horizontally.

If the ball is hit downward at an angle as small as 5 degrees from the horizontal, it will strike the net. This is illustrated by the following trigonometric computations. Since at a speed of 80 feet per second the ball will drop 4.025 feet by the time it crosses the net, an angle of 5 degrees will drive the ball into the net (Figure 7.12). The purpose of the preceding exercise is to illustrate the importance of developing speed and striking the ball at maximal height, and the hazards involved in driving the ball downward. A downward angle of 2 to 3 degrees from the horizontal for accomplished tennis players is a more reasonable goal than the 5 to 8 degrees sometimes recommended.

Underarm Patterns

In the underarm pattern, the extended arm moves forward in the anterior-posterior or sagittal plane in striking or throwing. The action begins with the arm in a position of hyperextension being elevated rearward to approximately shoulder height at the height of the backswing. The arm is then moved rapidly downward and the object is struck or released when the arm is in line with the trunk or slightly beyond. As in the overarm patterns, the levers of the hips, trunk, and wrist are used to add their acceleration and speed to that of the arm. If an implement such as a racquet or club is used, it also acts as a lever and adds its acceleration and speed to that of the internal levers. The length of this external lever extends from the grip to the point of contact of the implement with the object being struck.

Several levers can be utilized in underarm patterns. The number used and the extent to which they are used depends upon the necessity for speed. Each successive lever used is brought into play at the point of greatest speed and least acceleration of the preceding lever. Several actions are utilized for the purpose of increasing the range of motion of levers. This will give the performer's movements greater time and distance to accelerate the motion.

The first lever brought into play is that of the pelvis. The distance of pelvic rotation is increased by a transfer of weight to the right foot (for right-handed throwers and batters), which is turned clockwise. At the same time, the left foot is lifted off the ground to facilitate as much as 90 degrees of pelvic rotation. As the pelvis is rotated counterclockwise and the left leg swings forward, the throwing arm is abducted and extended overhead and backward to increase the length of the arm lever. Some momentum is transferred to the implement as the body lunges forward onto the left foot as a result of the long and powerful forward stride of the left leg. Rotation of the spine acting through the sternoclavicular joint at the shoulders adds a second lever to the sequential actions. A third lever is that of the hand and phalanges acting at the wrist joint. If a striking implement is being used, wrist flexion, because of its speed and the length of the implement, can add greatly to the striking force. The moment arm of a badminton racquet or baseball bat, for example, is quite large.

Underarm Throw. The procedures just described for underarm patterns are those that should be followed in throwing or pitching underarm. Individual variations in form can be observed, but among skilled performers these differences are only superficial modifications.

Figure 7.12 Line of flight of tennis ball after service

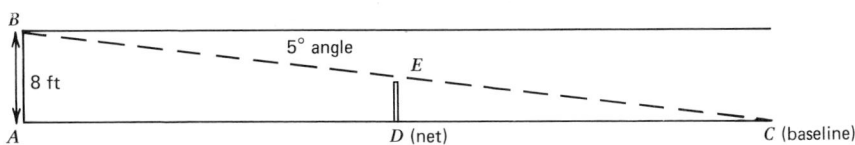

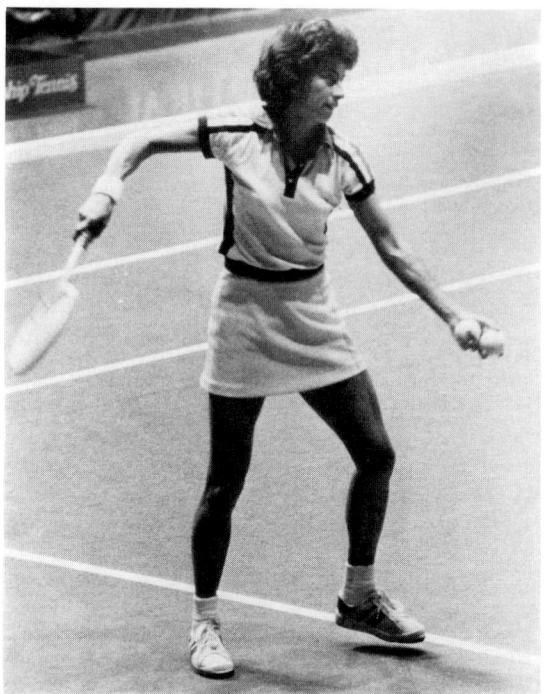

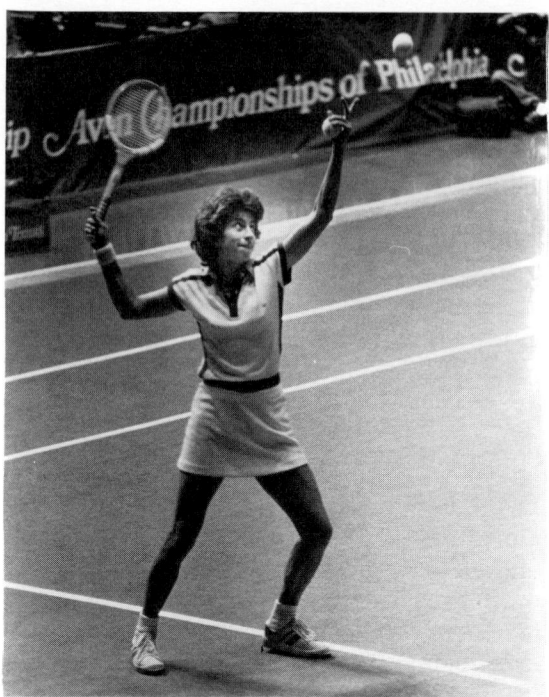

Figure 7.13 Sequence in Tennis Serve Note: Appreciation is expressed to Virginia Wade 1977 Wimbleton and U.S. Open Women's Champion and a member of the N.Y. Apples Tennis Team. Photographer Maria Garcias. (a) Body mass moving forward in order to produce greater momentum. Racquet arm moving upward is almost fully extended in order to generate greater velocity by lengthening lever. Left foot stepping forward and to the right to facilitate counterclockwise rotation of hip and shoulder levers during forward swing of racquet

Figure 7.13b Right elbow flexing to increase rotatory speed of racquet

During the underarm throw, the arm is kept in the sagittal plane as it swings forward through shoulder adduction and flexion. During the forward step with the left foot, the trunk should face to the right to secure maximum rotation of the pelvis and the trunk. Lack of skill in underarm pitching is often distinguishable by failure to turn the pelvis and trunk to the right. Extreme hyperextension of the wrist as the arm is swung downward, followed by very rapid flexion at release of the ball gives the ball great speed.

The ball is caused to rotate and curve to the left by medial rotation of the humerus and supination of the forearm. It will curve to the right when the humerus is rotated laterally and the forearm is pronated.

Cooper and Glassow[7] report velocities of 64 to 109 feet per second of balls pitched underarm by women physical education majors and male pitchers on softball teams, respectively. They also found that the shoulder joint contributed 45.3 percent; the wrists, 32.4 percent; the hip, 14.3 percent; and the spine, 7.9 percent to the total velocity of the ball.

Handball Underhand Stroke. The underarm pattern is followed in several strokes in handball. These include the power serve, the underhand stroke, and the "kill" shot. The movement pattern is basically that of the underhand softball pitch. However, adaptations are made to meet

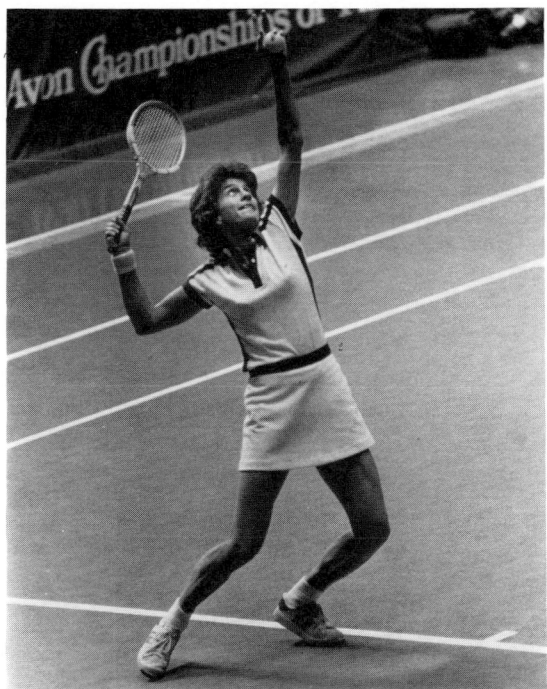

Figure 7.13c Note lateral flexion of the trunk to the right

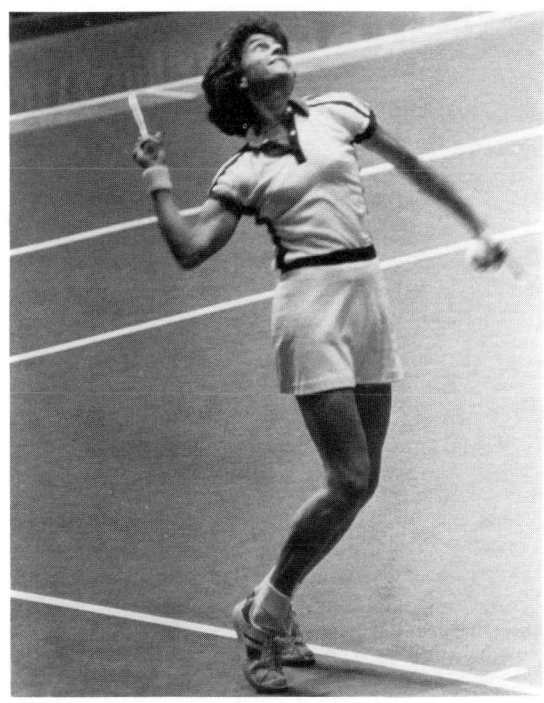

Figure 7.13d Humerus outward rotated to increase range of motion of forearm lever during later inward rotation of the humerus. Right foot has moved up to left foot

the peculiar requirements of the game of handball.

As in softball pitching, the forces generated by several body levers are summed, the force of each successive lever being added at the point of least acceleration and greatest speed of the preceding lever. The body unwinds with the rear foot thrusting against the floor as first the hips and then the shoulders rotate followed by the swing of the arm, flexion of the elbow, and, finally, flexion of the wrist to provide a whiplike action as the ball is flung against the wall. Additional momentum is transferred from the body to the ball as the body is moved forward throughout the swing by a shifting of the body weight from the rear to the forward foot.

Because of the necessity for quick action, since a moving ball must be struck at a relatively precise moment in its flight, there is inadequate time to step forward, to rotate the pelvis and trunk as far or to utilize as long a backswing as is used in softball pitching. In handball there is not as great a premium placed upon accuracy as there is in softball pitching or in bowling. Therefore, it is not essential in handball that the plane of the shoulders be at a right angle to the path of the ball. Additionally, it is more important for the handball player than for the softball pitcher to be in balance after releasing the ball since the handball player must be prepared to move quickly to retrieve the next ball.

The handball player will drop the shoulder of his striking arm and bend his knees and hips further than the softball pitcher because in handball the lower the ball strikes the wall, the more difficult it is to return. In pitching, the ball must be projected through a relatively prescribed area. In order to strike the ball as low as possible so that it will travel horizontally close to the floor and strike the wall low,

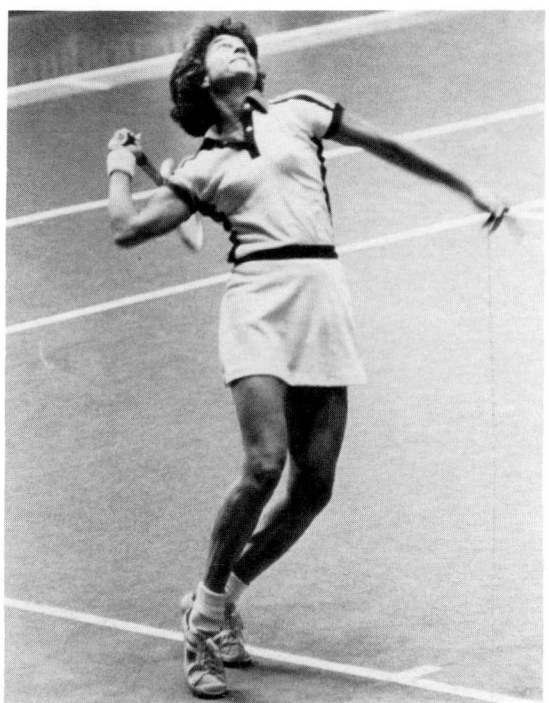

Figure 7.13e Note hyperextension of vertebral column to increase range of motion of trunk. Also note extreme clockwise rotation of shoulder and pelvic levers

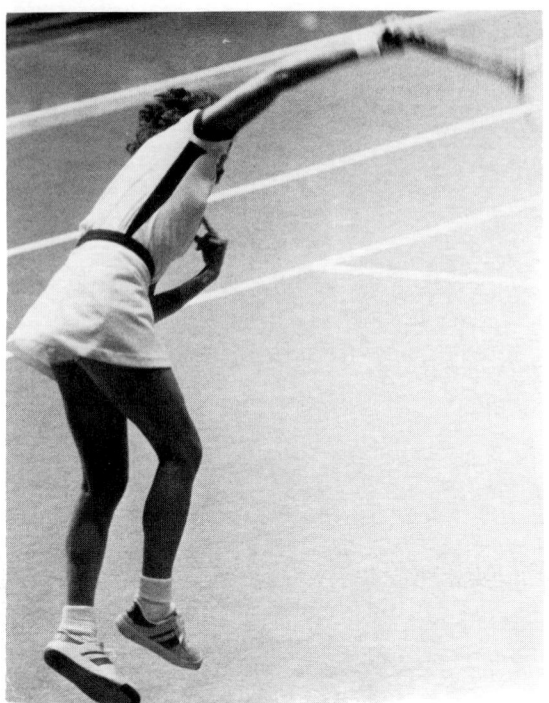

Figure 7.13f Hip and shoulder levers rotating counterclockwise. Humerus has completed inward rotation. Elbow has extended. Wrist flexing. Hips have flexed to add momentum of the trunk. Ball has been contacted

the handball player will often flex his elbow so that the forearm is almost parallel to the floor. This procedure requires considerable knee and hip flexion and lowering of the shoulder of the striking arm.

Notwithstanding these differences, the underhand stroke in handball utilizes the same principles of levers and mechanics as does the softball pitch. These include the principles of summation of forces; action and reaction; the laws of gravity influencing projectiles; the longer the lever, the greater the linear speed; shortening the radius of rotation accelerates the speed of rotation; backswing; and follow-through. In both movements, momentum is also transferred to the ball as a result of forward movement of the entire body.

Golf. The golf stroke is a reversed underarm pattern in that (for a right-handed person)

the left arm provides most of the force and the left shoulder is abducted rather than adducted.[8] In most other underhand patterns only one arm is used.

In the golf stroke, not only do the arms move in the sagittal plane as in other underhand patterns but there are other major similarities. Body weight is shifted from the rear to the forward foot during the stroke. The pelvis, vertebral column, and shoulder girdle are rotated clockwise during the backswing to facilitate a greater range of movement during the downswing, with consequent greater acceleration (Figure 7.16a). Greater rotation is made possible through flexion of the left knee and elevation of the left heel. As the downswing begins, body weight is shifted toward the left foot, the hips begin to un-

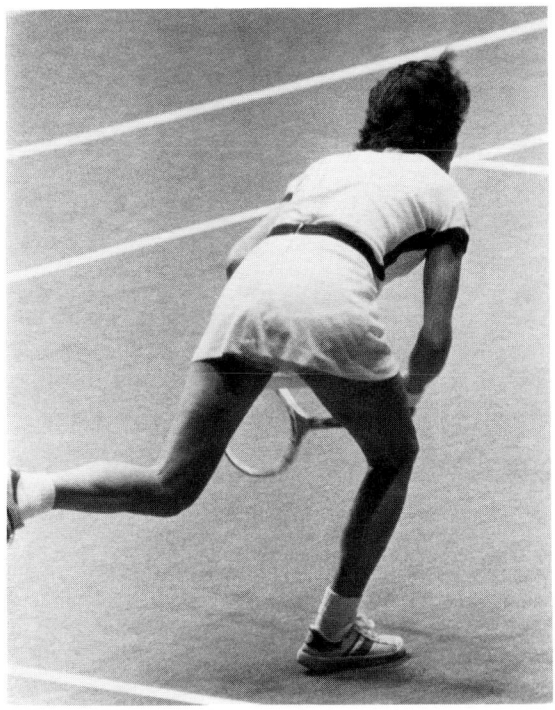

Figure 7.13g Follow-through. Momentum has carried the player over the base line and she is now facing the net. In 7.13e, she was facing almost to the rear

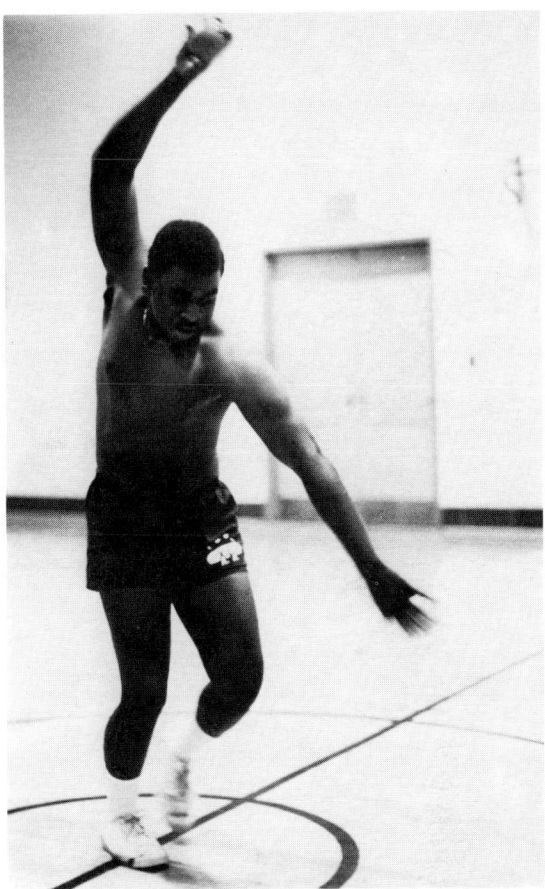

Figure 7.14 Underhand Pitch (a) Inadequate counterclockwise rotation of pelvis, trunk, and shoulder girdle.

wind, followed by an unwinding of the shoulders (Figure 7.16c). Pelvic rotation initiates the downward movement of the arms, while the shoulder action begins at about the time the arms are horizontal. The lever of the wrists adds tremendous rotary speed to the sum of the speeds generated by the other levers (Figure 7.16d). The wrist snap occurs as the arms approach the vertical. As in other underhand (and overhand) patterns, the forces generated by the several involved levers are summed, each being added at the point of greatest speed and least acceleration of the preceding movement.

The differences that exist between the underhand patterns of the golf stroke and the softball pitch arise out of the great need for accuracy during the golf swing. Both the ball and the striking surface of the club are very small, making a controlled swing a key factor in skillful play. Further, the great projection distances of golf drives magnifies an inaccuracy. For example, trigonometry will show that an error of 10 degrees in a 300 yard drive will place the ball 156.24 feet to the right or left of the center of the fairway. (Sine of 10 degrees = 0.1736×900 ft = 156.24 ft). Additionally, distortion of the golf ball at impact is considerable. As the ball regains its shape, the club head must follow through in the same direction it attained at impact or the ball will be hooked or sliced. If control and accuracy were not so necessary, greater speed could be generated in the club head if

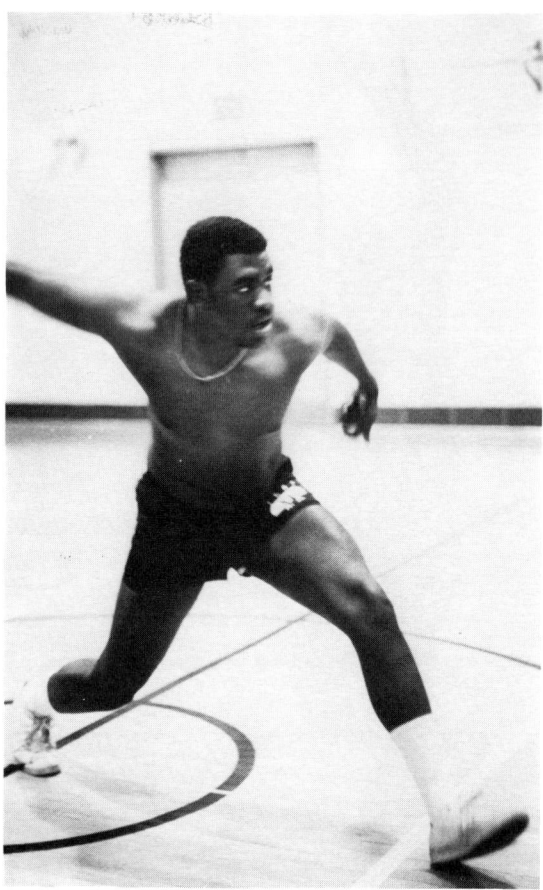

Figure 7.14b Note long, powerful stride of left leg

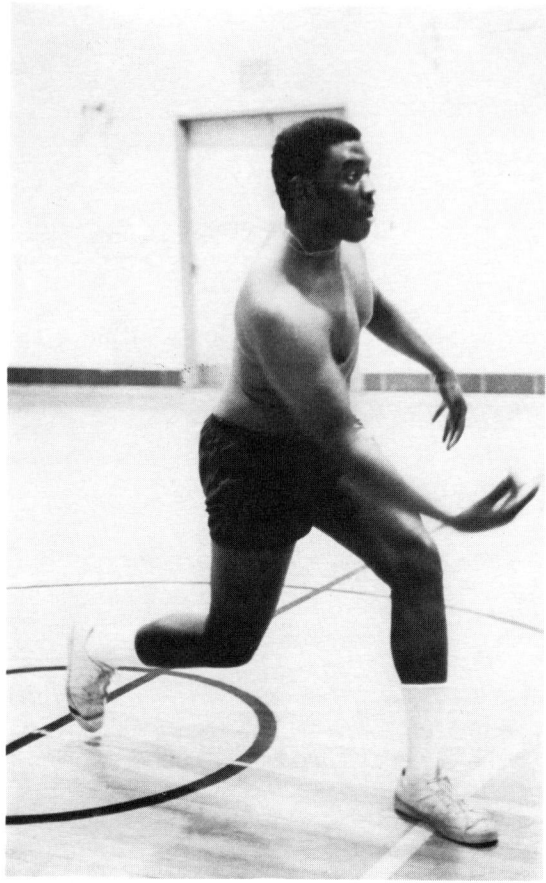

Figure 7.14c Note flexion of wrist and fingers

some of the procedures used in the softball pitch such as stepping forward and increasing pelvic rotation were utilized.

Because of the great need for control, it is necessary to develop a consistent swing. To facilitate development and use of a consistent or "grooved" swing, golf clubs are designed to control the distance and height the ball may be hit through different shaft lengths (differing lever lengths) and angle of pitch of the face of the club. In a matched set there is a 5 degree difference in the angle of pitch of successively numbered clubs. This means that the beginner in golf need learn only one swing, which can be used for all shots except putting. Regardless of the club used, the

arms and shaft should form a straight line at the moment of impact in order to provide the longest possible lever. In all swings with all clubs (except the putter) the backswing, downswing, club head trajectory, club head speed, and stance should be the same. Exceptions to this rule, which will not be discussed here, include chip shots and uphill, downhill, and sidehill lies. Bunn[9] advocates the following for increasing control:

1. The long axis of the body should be held stationary throughout the swing. To accomplish this, it is necessary to keep the eyes on the ball and to continue to focus on this point after impact. The body may rotate about its long axis but it should not

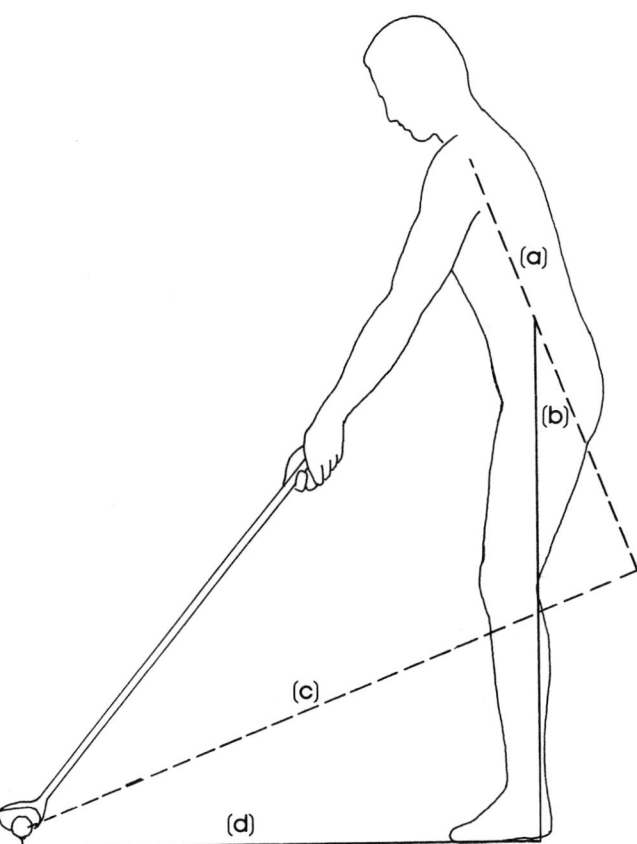

Figure 7.15 Moment arm lengths in golf swing: (a) axis of spinal rotation; (b) axis of hip rotation; (c) length of moment arm of spinal rotation; (d) length of moment arm of hip rotation; (adapted from J. M. Cooper and R. B. Glassow, **Kinesiology**, 4th ed., C. V. Mosby Co., St. Louis, 1976, p. 148)

move from right to left or forward or backward (Figure 7.16a).

2. The left arm should be fully extended, particularly through the center of the swing, in order to maintain a uniform radius of rotation.

3. As additional insurance that the club head will move through a consistent arc, the right elbow should be held against the side of the body until the ball is contacted.

4. Follow-through should continue until the hands are head high. This helps to insure that the club head will remain in its arc and plane before the ball is hit (Figure 7.16e).

5. Finally, the proper speed and sequence must be learned. Backswing should be slow. There should be a slight hesitation before the downswing is begun. The downswing should progressively increase in speed reaching its maximum speed as the ball is impacted.

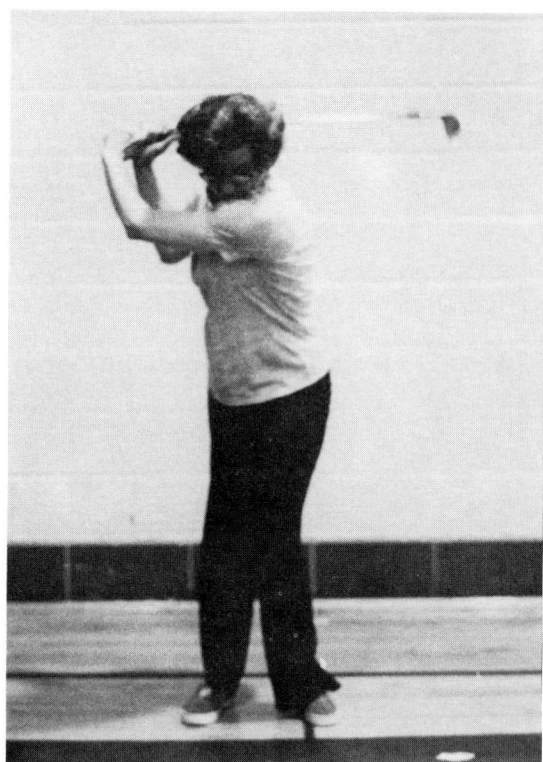

Figure 7.16 Golf Swing (a) Left arm should be extended. Note pelvic rotation, right leg extended and head down

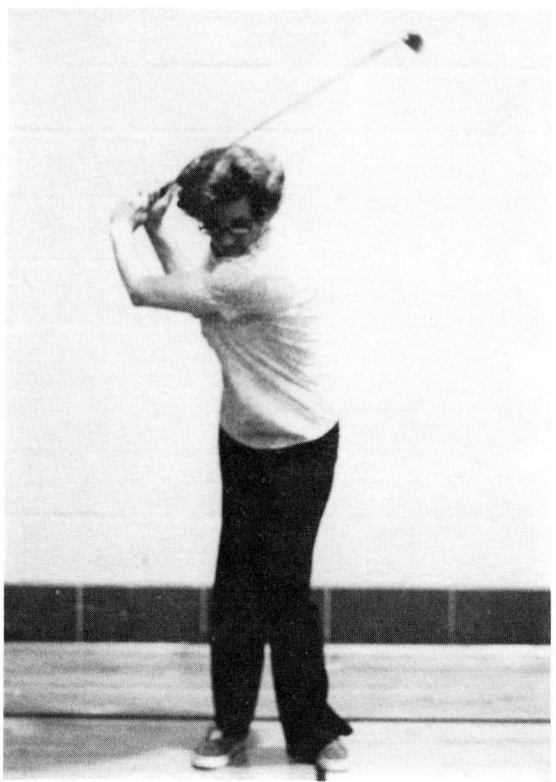

Figure 7.16b   Right elbow against trunk

Sidearm Patterns

The most easily distinguishing feature of the sidearm pattern is that the movement is made in the transverse plane. In this pattern, the force arises principally from pelvic rotation with the arm held almost immobile in an abducted position. The pelvic lever, which extends from the axis of the left hip to the point of applied force, is the longest lever that can be used in throwing and striking actions. When a tennis racquet or baseball bat is used, the length of the moment arm could be six feet or more. The internal levers used in this pattern include, in addition to the pelvic lever, the spine, the shoulders, and the wrist.

The Discus (Figure 7.17).   The discus thrower must confine his/her movements to a circle

with a diameter of 8 feet, 2.5 inches. This forces the performer to secure maximum linear motion of the discus through circular motions of the body and its parts. The body rotates one-and-a-half times while the discus itself may move through an arc 80 degrees greater or a total of 620 degrees. This highly complex skill requires precise timing and demonstrates the importance of a smooth and continuously accelerating flow of energy culminating in an explosive burst at the climax.

The thrower begins his/her movements facing the rear of the circle with feet apart and the throwing arm behind the body. (Figure 7.17a) He/she whirls around in a tight circle, accelerating as rapidly as possible by taking steps that resemble those of a sprinter. (Figure 7.17b) During the first full turn the

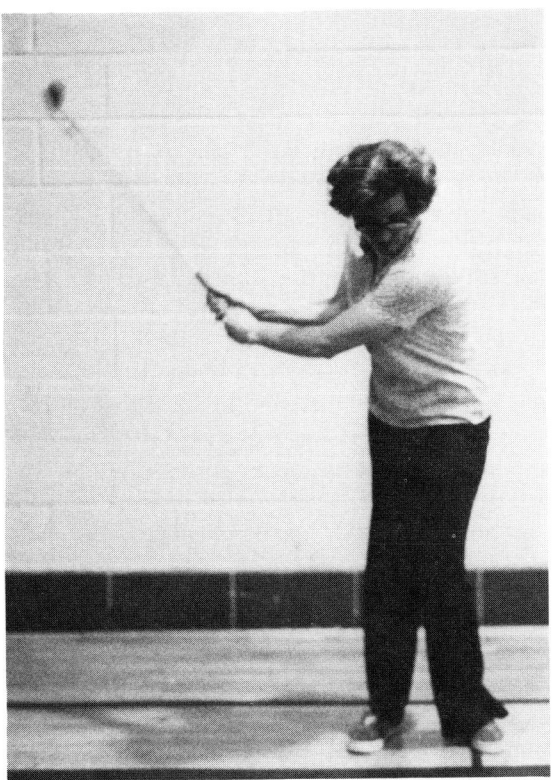

Figure 7.16c Wrists extending. Club head accelerating

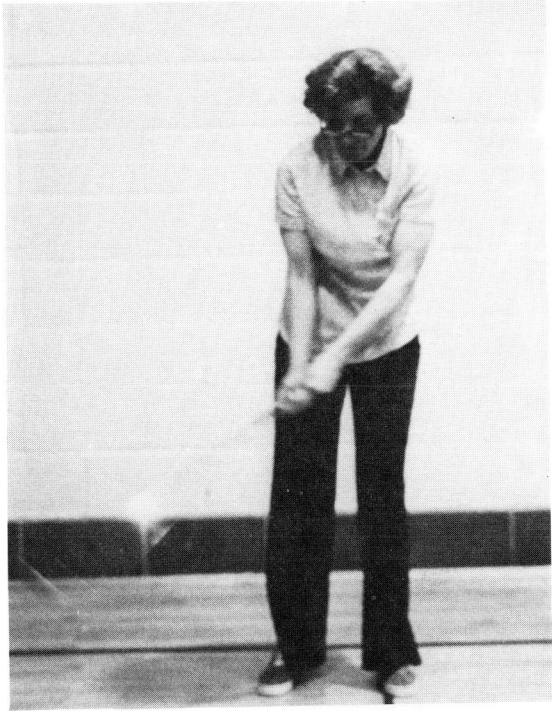

Figure 7.16d Weight has shifted toward left foot and trunk has rotated counterclockwise

throwing arm is held close to the body to reduce development of unbalancing centrifugal force and to facilitate acceleration in rotational speed (shortening the radius of rotation accelerates the speed of rotation). The knees are flexed to lower the center of gravity, increasing stability (Figure 7.17c). Greater stability will enable the thrower to rotate more rapidly without losing balance. The feet should maintain contact with the ground at all times in order that the force generated can act against a reacting surface.

The radius or moment arm of the lever should be as long as possible just prior to release. (Figure 7.17d) If the thrower is strong enough to retain grasp of the discus during the throw while its edge rests against the first joint of the fingers, the longest possible lever will be utilized. During the last half of the one-and-a-half turns, the arm is abducted to lengthen the moment arm. The discus should be behind the shoulder and the shoulder should pull the discus around. The final movements begin with a powerful push from the right leg followed in sequence by pelvic rotation, blocking action by the left leg, spinal and thoracic rotation, shoulder girdle rotation, abduction of the throwing arm followed by adduction, and a wrist snap to send the projectile on its way.

The optimum angle of inclination of the plane of the discus was found by Taylor,[10] as early as 1932, to be 35 degrees. When throwing into the wind, this angle should be less and when throwing with the wind, this angle should be greater in order to maximize the push of the wind.

Batting (Figure 7.18). Batting is a sidearm pattern in which an implement is used. On

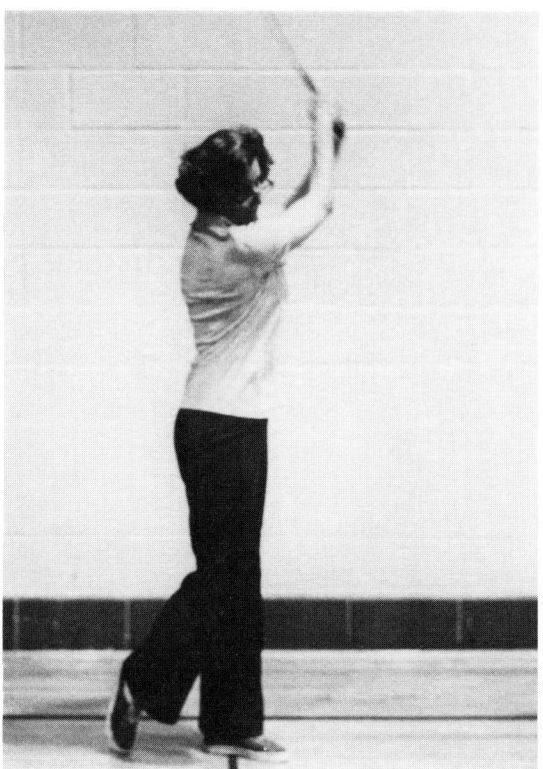

Figure 7.16e Note follow through and that golfer is still looking downward

the average, it takes 0.5 of a second for a pitched ball to travel from the pitcher's hand to the plate. According to Bunn,[11] a fast ball will travel two-thirds of the distance from the pitcher's mound to the plate by the time the batter begins the swing. A pitched ball travels between 55 and 80 mph. The preceding points out the importance of speed and quick reactions to successful batting. Adaptations of the basic sidearm pattern are made to facilitate a quick reaction with a minimum loss of force and control.

Since force is a function of the square of the velocity, maximum *controlled* velocity of the bat is essential. Although, when all other factors are equal, the ball can be batted farther with a heavier bat, velocity and control of the swing will be lost if the bat is too heavy for the batter's available strength.

To minimize recoil of the bat, it should be gripped firmly at the moment of impact, and the rear foot should maintain contact with the ground until after the ball has been hit. While awaiting the pitch, the batter should stand with feet spread shoulder width and with the bat resting on the shoulder. When the pitch is begun, the bat is drawn behind the shoulder with the long axis of the bat slightly above the horizontal plane. The hands should be at shoulder height (Figure 7.18a). During the early portion of the swing, the hands and arms should be close to the body to shorten the radius of rotation, which will make possible a more rapid swing. This is necessary in view of the speed of the ball and the short time to swing the bat. The linear velocity of the bat is then increased by extending the right elbow (right-handed batter) as the bat is swung toward the ball (Figure 7.18b).

As the ball is released, the batter takes a short step to establish linear momentum. This step is slightly to the left to facilitate greater hip rotation. At the same time, the shoulders are rotated slightly backward to increase the range of motion of the shoulder lever. Additionally, the hands are radially flexed to increase the range of motion of the bat (Figure 7.18c). Upon completion of the forward step, the shoulders and hips are rotated forward, pulling the arms around. The forearms are extended, as previously mentioned, and the hands are adducted (wrist snap) as the ball is contacted (Figure 7.18d).

The head should be turned in the direction of the ball at all times and the eyes should track the ball right up to the bat. The bat is swung in a horizontal plane (Figure 7.18e).

Tennis Drive (Figure 7.19). The forehand and backhand drives in tennis are sidearm patterns and, like other sidearm patterns, utilize the linear momentum generated by a forward step and forward movement of the body and the levers of the pelvis, spine, and shoulder

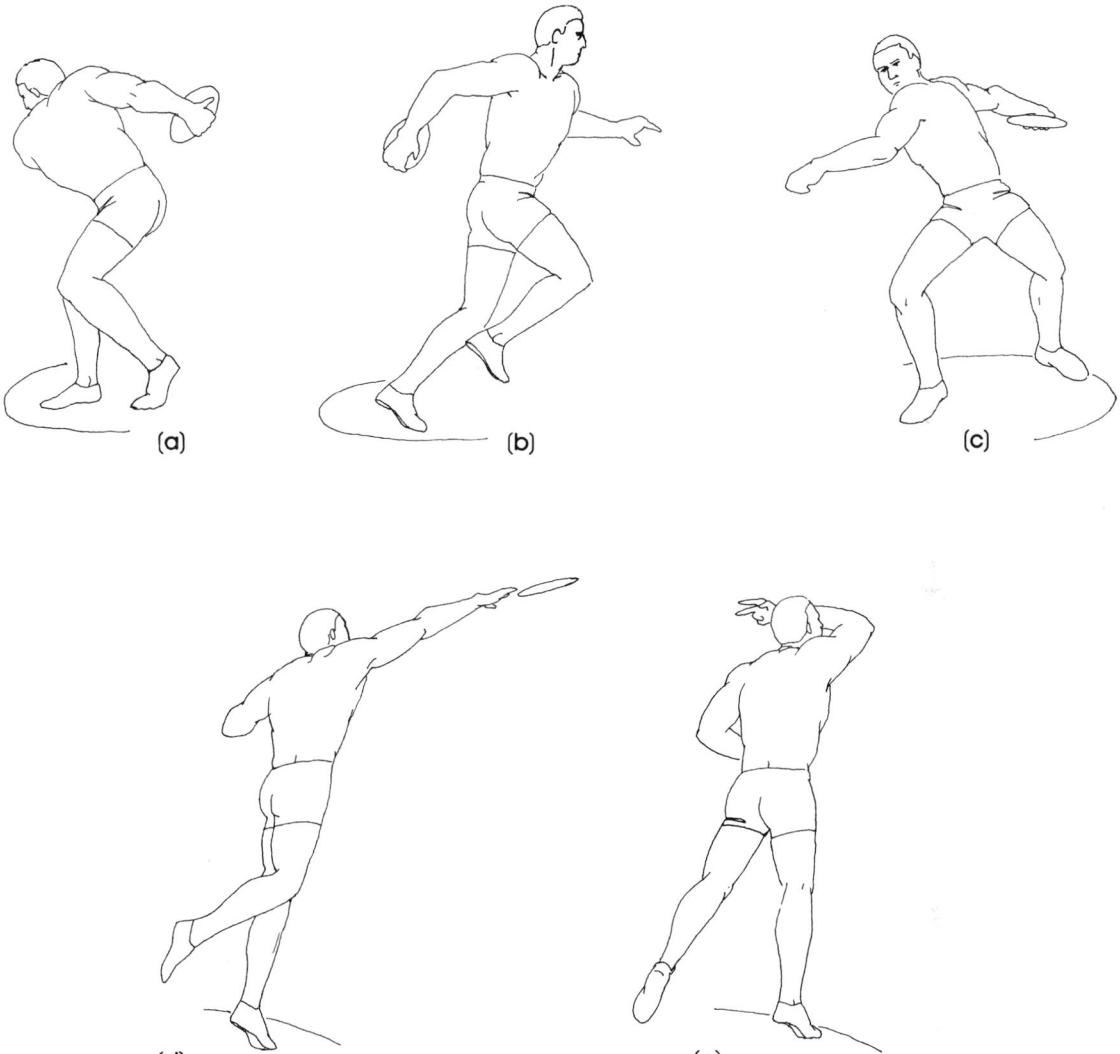

Figure 7.17 Discus Throw (**a**) Hips, trunk, add shoulders rotated clockwise. Weight principally on right leg (**b**) Spin around left leg (**c**) Right arm abducting for longest possible lever (**d**) Rotation has been counterclockwise and the body has come out of its low crouch (**e**) Follow through and hop to right leg

girdle. In the backhand drive, some players use both arms, making the movement almost identical to that of batting.

All tennis stroking begins with the "ready position," in which the player stands facing the net with the feet shoulder width apart, knees flexed, back inclined slightly forward, head up, weight on the toes, and eyes on the

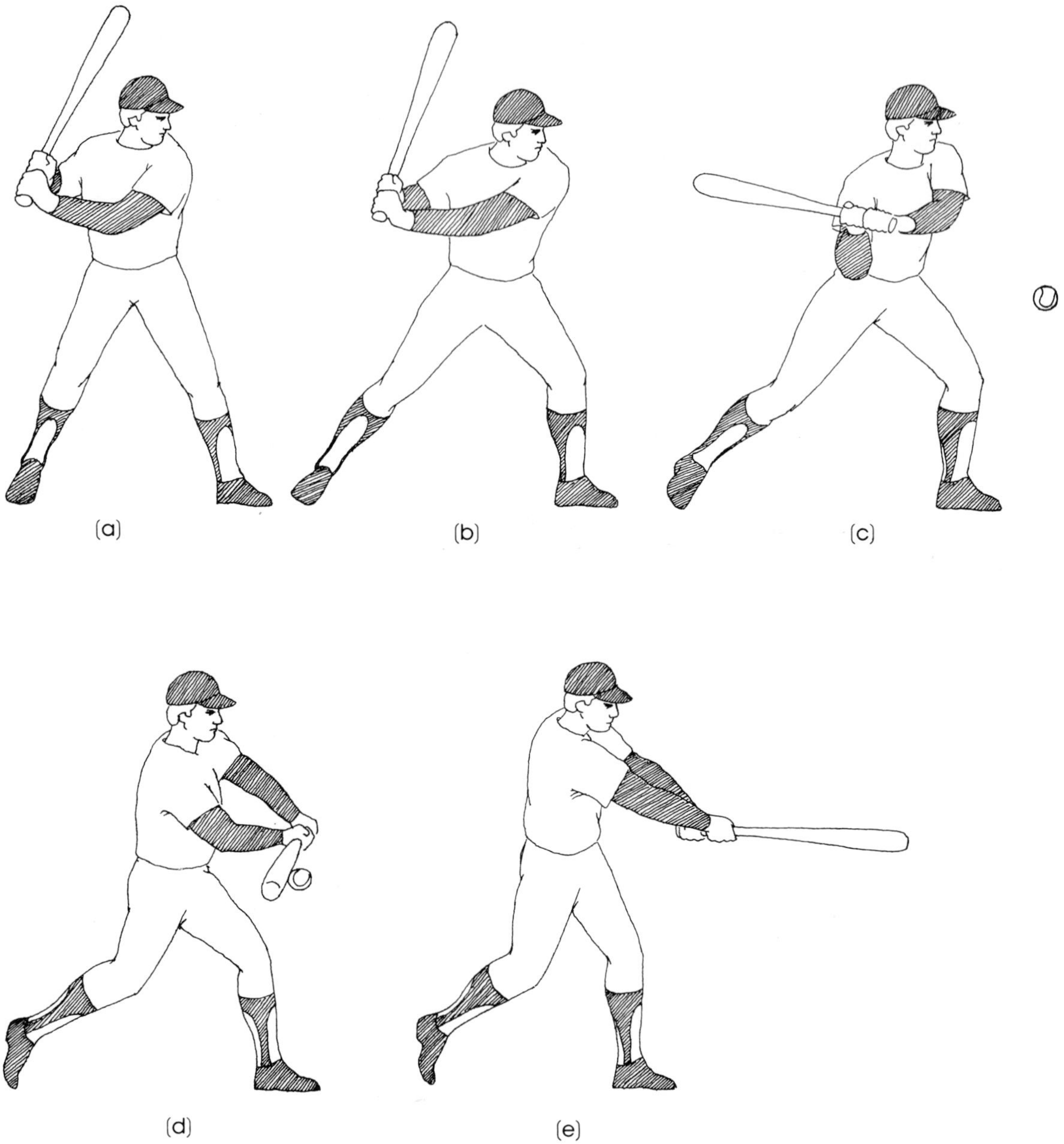

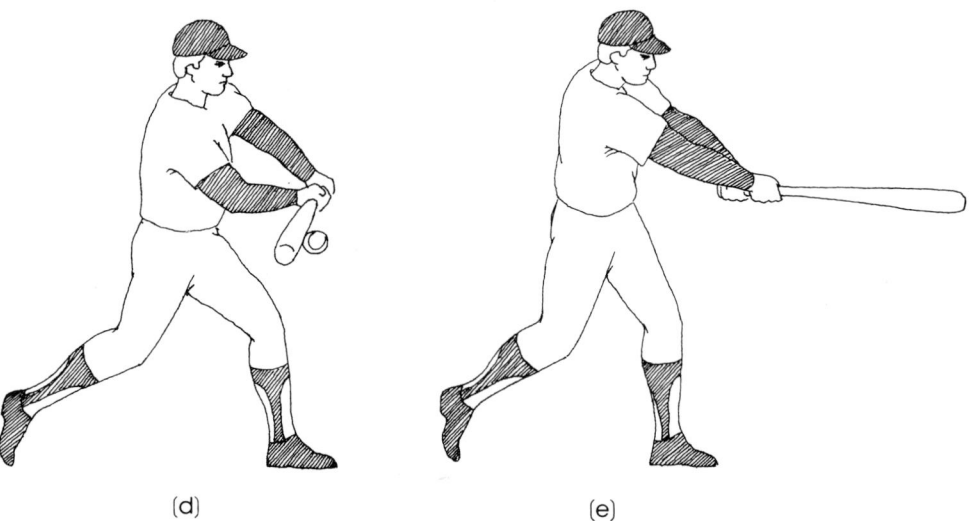

Figure 7.18 Batting **(a)** Bat slightly above horizontal plane and hands at shoulder when pitch is begun **(b)** Hands and arms close to the body to shorten radius of rotation and time of swing **(c)** Step slightly to left to facilitate hip rotation, wrists flexed **(d)** Hips and shoulders rotated counter-clockwise pulling the arms around **(e)** Elbows extended and wrists flexed, batter watches ball meet bat.

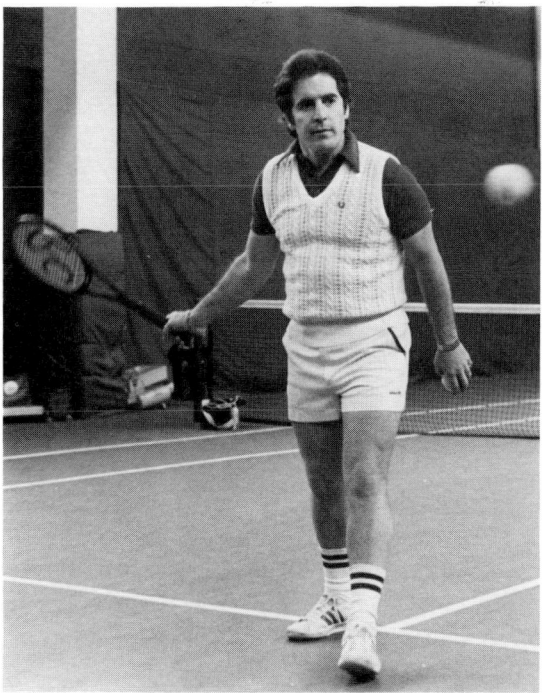

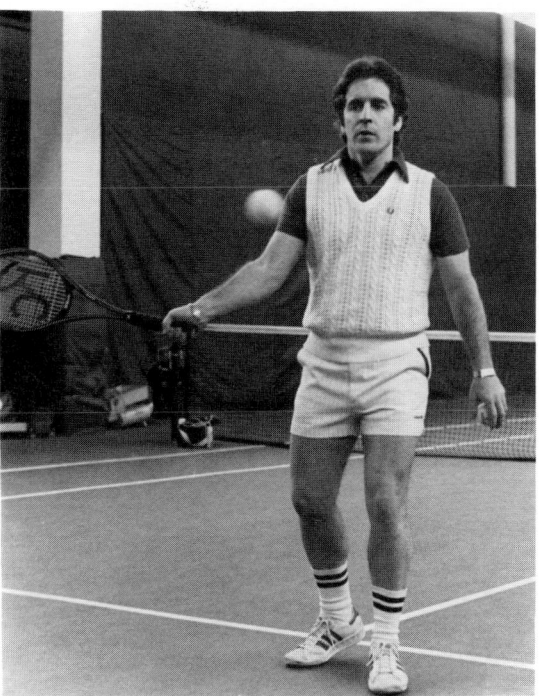

Figure 7.19 Forehand tennis drive (across width of court). The subject is Robert Coriat who represented Venezuela in the Davis Cup Tournament. (a) Left leg moving **diagonally** forward to increase distance through which hip and shoulder levers will be able to move and to initiate forward movement of body mass. Right arm brought backward to increase distance through which racquet head can be accelerated.

Figure 7.19b Eyes on the ball. Body weight shifting forward over left foot. Hip and shoulder levers rotating.

opponent. When the ball comes to the player's right side, a step is taken toward the net with the left foot and the weight is shifted onto this foot as the ball is hit (Figure 7.19a). The amount of the contribution of this action to the force imparted to the ball can be appreciated by trying to strike the ball with all the body weight on the rear foot. If the greatest force is desired, the rear foot must push against the ground at the moment of contact with the ball (Figure 7.19b). This is in conformity with Newton's third law. Boxers, baseball batters, and golfers all push off the rear foot to generate greatest possible momentum.

The backswing should be continued until the arm muscles are placed on a stretch, since they can then generate their greatest force. However, time available to complete the stroke and the force desired are limiting factors on the length of the backswing. At the end of the backswing, the weight should be on the rear foot. During the backswing, as well as during the forward swing up until the moment of contact with the ball, the upper arm and elbow should be close to the body. This will shorten the radius of rotation and accelerate the speed of rotation to conserve energy and to enable the player to get the racquet into position to meet the ball more quickly. As in batting and the discus throw, the striking arm is extended just prior to making contact with the ball (Figure 7.19c). This action increases the length of the mo-

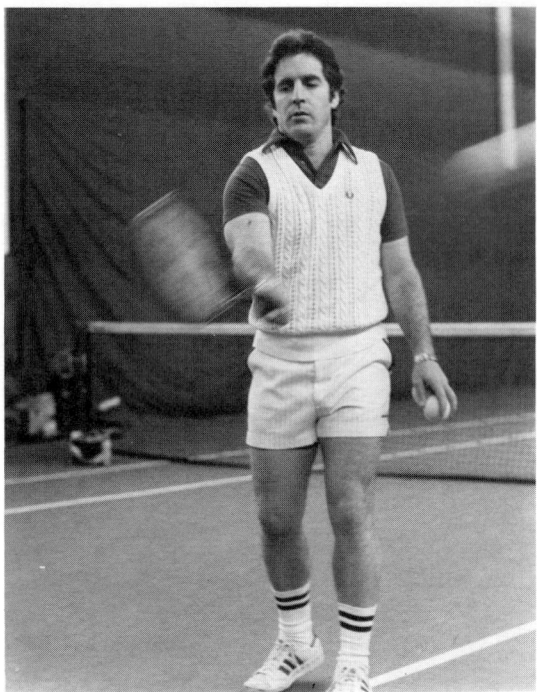

Figure 7.19c Ball has been struck. Hip and shoulder levers continuing to rotate. Right arm extended to increase linear speed of racquet head.

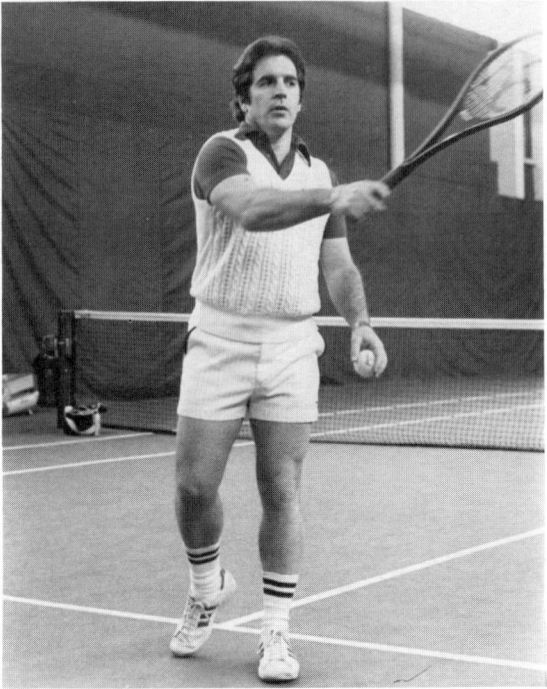

Figure 7.19d Follow through. Elbow flexing. Racquet face closed. Shoulder joint in horizontal flexion-adduction.

ment (lever) arm, which will increase the linear speed of the head of the racquet.

The forward step is taken just prior to the beginning of the forward swing. This forward step is immediately followed by pelvic and shoulder rotation toward the net, which pull the arm and racquet around. These long levers, extending in the forehand drive from the left side of the body to the point of contact of the racquet face with the ball, produce considerable linear velocity in the racquet face. When hip and shoulder rotation are at their greatest speed, shoulder action swings the arm and racquet forward. The elbow is almost fully extended at contact with the ball to secure the greatest lever length possible. Although many writers advocate that the wrist be locked at the moment of contact in order to avoid recoil, there is some question as to whether a locked wrist will prevent recoil better than one that is flexing and consequently imparting greater velocity to the racquet.

According to the law of rebound discussed earlier, the tennis ball will rebound in the direction the racquet face is moving at the moment of contact. Consequently, efforts should be made to keep the racquet head moving in the direction one wishes to hit the ball for as long as possible. This is facilitated by extending the arm and laying back the wrist at the moment of contact so that the ball is given somewhat of a push. The tennis ball, unlike most other balls used in games where they are struck, collapses by as much as one-half its diameter when it is struck. This means that it is in contact with the racquet face for a relatively long period of time. A follow-through in a horizontal arc would bring the ball to the left in a forehand drive.

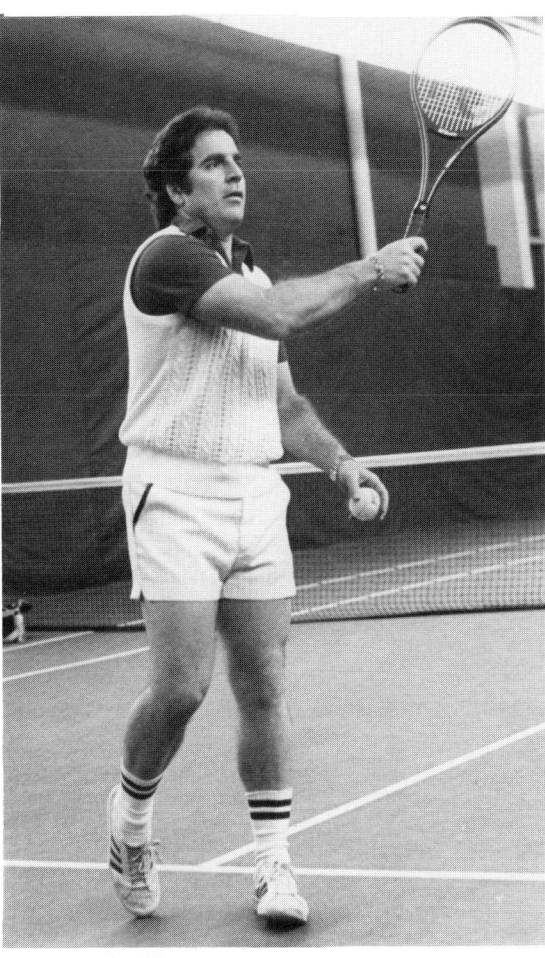

Figure 7.19e Follow through completed. Shoulders and hips have moved through 90 degrees of rotation between illustrations 7.19a and 7.19e.

The preceding procedures apply to the backhand drive except that the step forward is taken with the right foot rather than the left and the ball is impacted opposite the forward hip rather than opposite the center of the body.

Use of Body Levers in Thrusting or Jabbing

Examples of thrusting or jabbing activities are the basketball chest pass, shooting a basketball from the chest, the jab in boxing, and

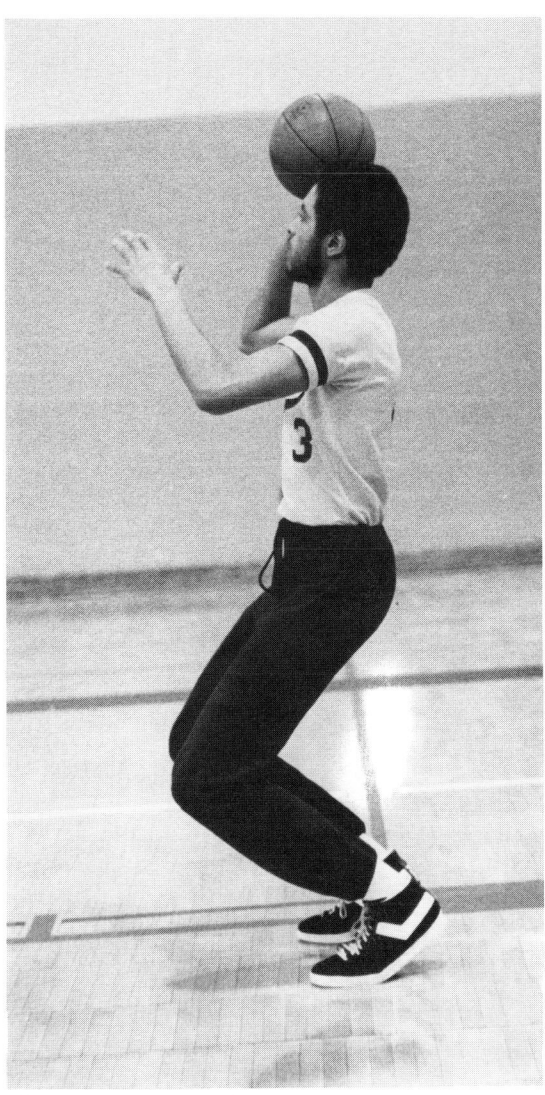

Figure 7.20 One-hand Push Shot (a) Right humerus horizontal, body in balance

shot putting. In these activities, there is horizontal flexion of the humerus and elbow extension, sometimes with body movement. The thrust is through the long axis of the bones of the forearm.

One-handed Push Shot (Figure 7.20). The one-handed set shot used in basketball pro-

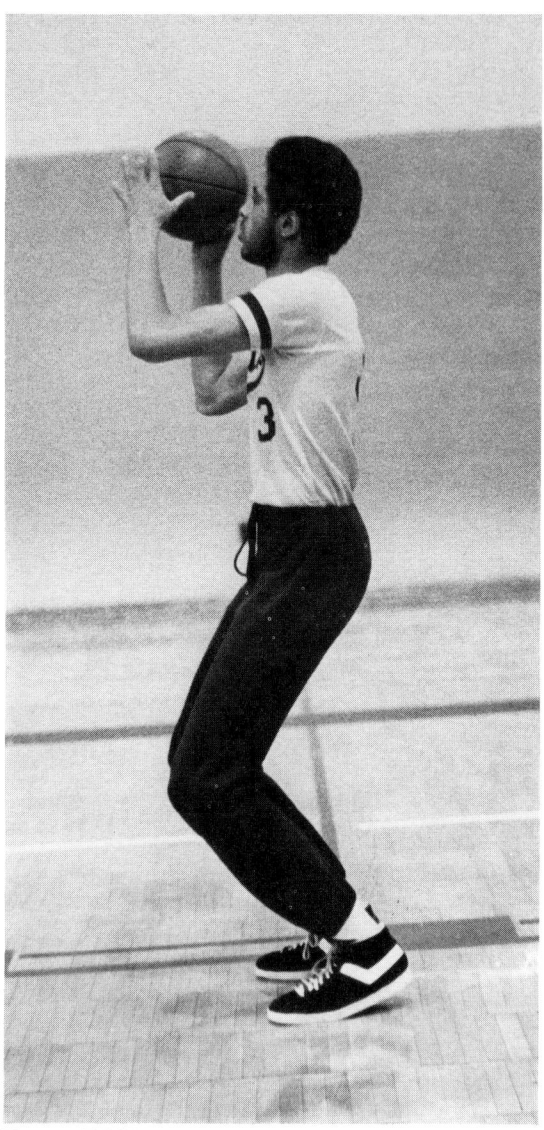

Figure 7.20b Knee and hip extension initiated, trunk vertical

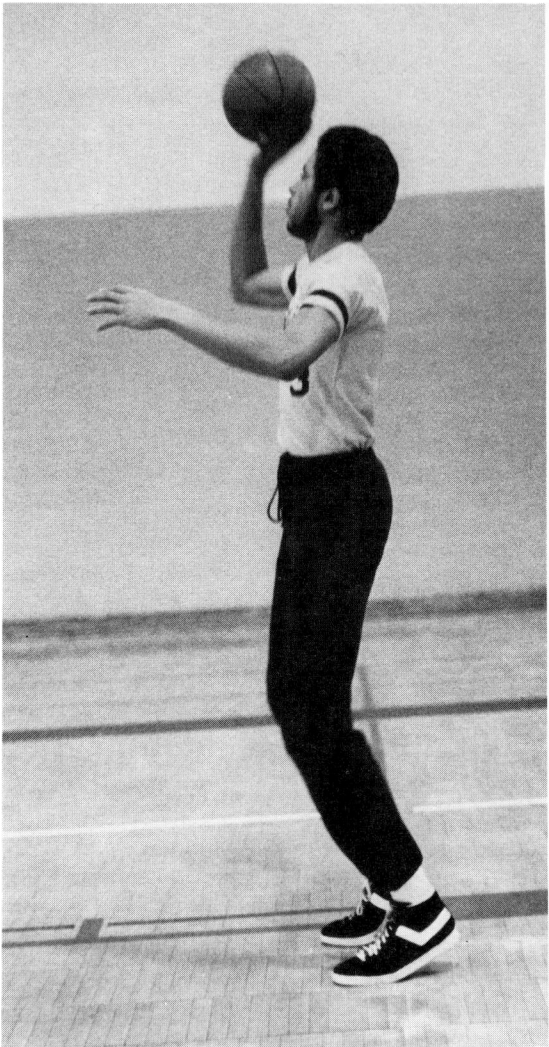

Figure 7.20c Elbow extension initiated

vides a relatively simple example of the use of body levers in a thrusting motion. Upon receipt of the ball, the elbows are flexed to bring the ball above the elbow. Elbow flexion continues to a 45 degree angle while the humerus is held in a nearly horizontal position. Since the pelvic lever is not utilized in this procedure and balance is a prime requisite

for accuracy in throwing, the foot on the side of the throwing arm is forward as the shot is made (Figure 7.20a). This enables the line of force generated through ankle, knee, and hip extension to pass in a straight line through the center of gravity of the ball. Simultaneously with ankle, hip, and knee extension (Figure 7.20b), the shoulder is flexed to move the humerus upward and the elbow is extended (Figure 7.20c). Near the completion

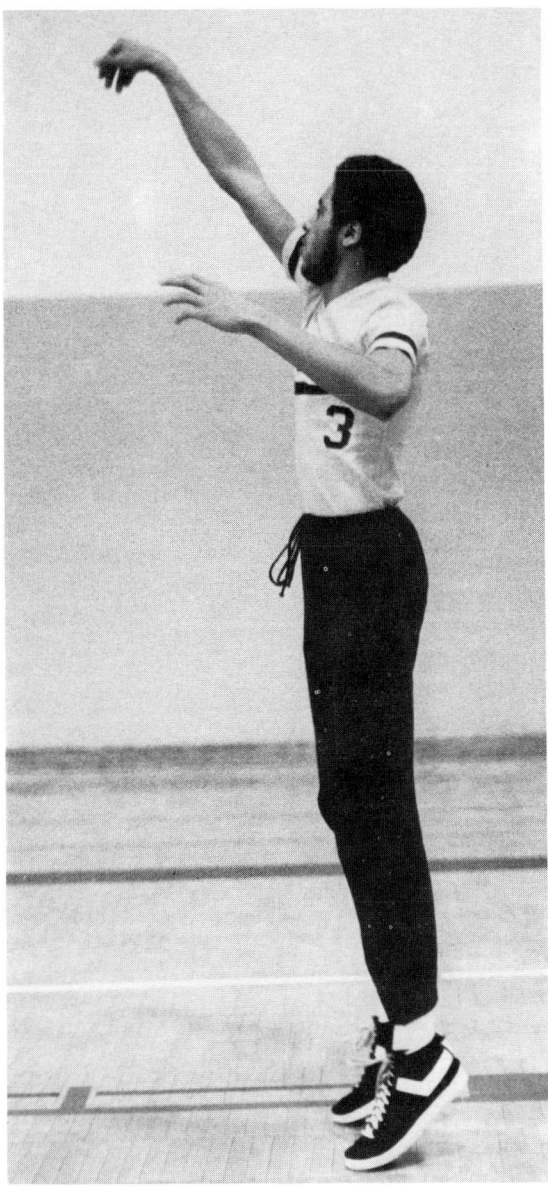

Figure 7.20d Plantar flexion of feet and wrist and finger flexion and final impetus to ball

of these movements, the wrist is flexed to impart additional impetus to the ball (Figure 7.20d). The internal levers involved are those of the feet, lower legs, thighs, and the humerus, forearm, and hand of the throwing arm. The rotary movements of all these levers

culminate in linear motion upward of the body, which is transferred to the ball. The amount of force generated and the angle of projection will be dependent upon the distance from the basket.

The one-hand set shot, or jump shot, has a higher probability of success because fewer muscles are used, decreasing the probability of error. It is necessary, however, that the player possess sufficient strength to propel the ball to the basket without having to strain. It is especially important that the player have a large hand and strong fingers, wrist, arm, and shoulder muscles. Weight training programs have proven helpful.

Shot Put (Figure 7.21). The shot put provides a more complex illustration of a thrusting action in the use of internal levers. While the one-hand set shot places a premium upon fine and delicate coordination, the shot put event places a premium upon explosive power. Power is a function of strength and quickness. However, unless the shot putter can execute the movements in proper sequence and with continuous acceleration, he will not secure maximum possible distance on his put.

The action starts with the shot putter facing the rear of a circle. The right toe is against the inside edge of the ring so that the maximal linear distance can be used. The diameter of the circle is only 7 feet in the women's event and 8 feet 2.5 inches in the men's event. The weight is on the right foot and the ball is cradled against the neck just below the jaw bone. The wrist is hyperextended. The elbow is under the ball. The putter crouches low to increase the distance over which force may be applied to the ball (Figure 7.21a). The left leg is next lifted behind the body and forcefully extended toward the front of the circle to initiate the generation of momentum toward the front of the circle (Figure 7.21b). As the weight is taken on the left foot (Figure 7.21c), the right foot slides forward to the center of the ring and as soon as it is planted,

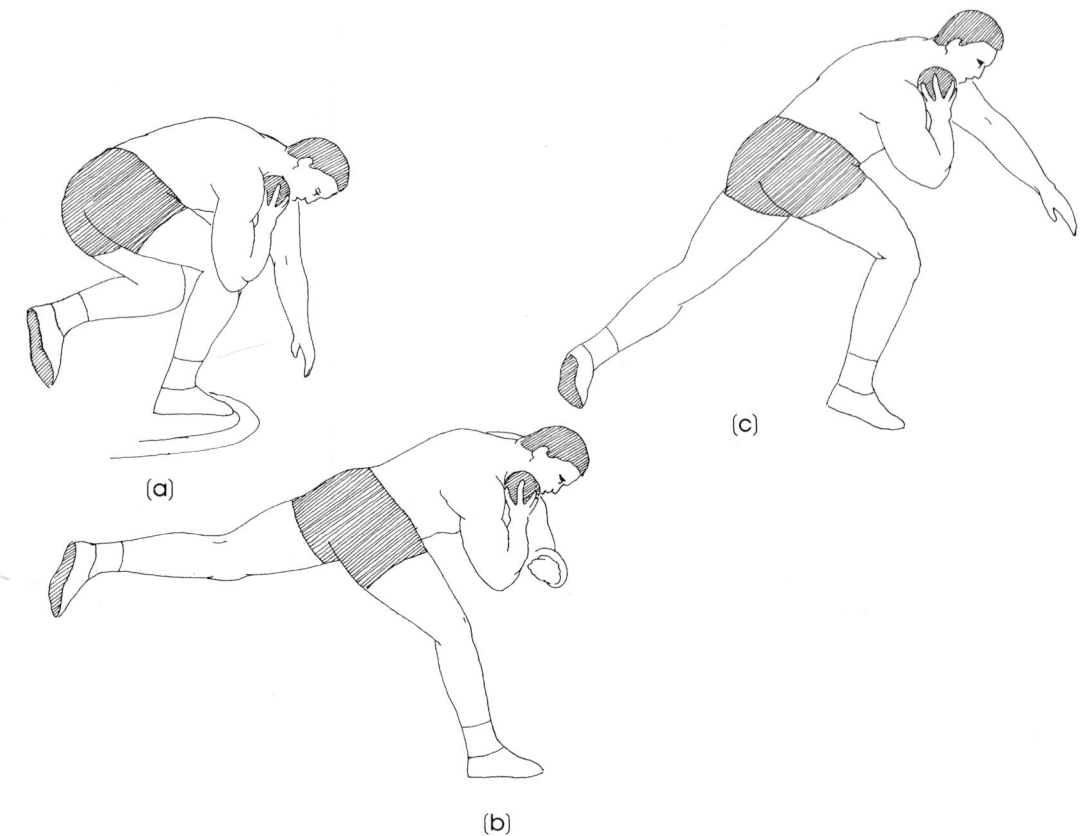

(a)

(b)

(c)

Figure 7.21 Shot Put (a) Facing rear of circle, weight on right foot, ball cradled at neck, elbow under the ball, putter crouched low. (b) Left leg lifted and extended to the front of the circle to initiate forward momentum. (c) Left foot on ground and body beginning to rotate. (d) Elbow lifting, right leg beginning to extend explosively. (e) Body rotating around left leg, wrist flexing, elbow extended. (f) Note extent of rotation between illustrations a and f.

the right leg is explosively extended while the body extends and rotates so that it faces forward at the moment of release (Figure 7.21d). During the rotation, the elbow is lifted to place the upper arm in a horizontal position (Figure 7.21e). This will increase the length of the pelvic lever, which provides the major force. This lever will extend from the left hip as the body rotates around the left leg to the tip of the elbow.

Near the end of the trunk rotation, the shoulder is adducted and flexed, thereby moving the upper arm forward and upward. At the same time, the elbow is extended. Finally, the wrist is flexed. The shot should be projected at an angle of about 41 degrees. Throughout the action, the movements should continuously increase in speed with no hesitations or stops so that maximal speed is achieved at the moment of release. The levers used are those of the feet in plantar flexion, the lower legs, thighs, and trunk in extension, the pelvis and shoulder girdle in rotation, the humerus in shoulder adduction and flexion, and the forearm and hand in elbow and wrist extension.

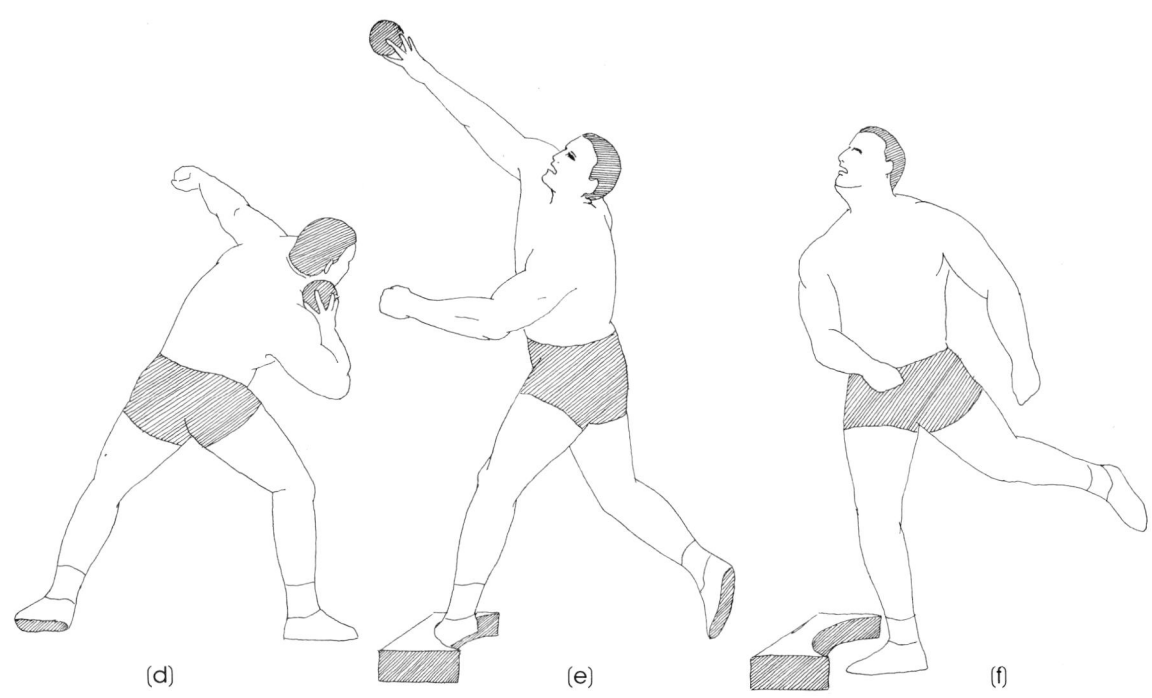

(d)   (e)   (f)

SUMMARY

Three of the six kinds of simple machines are found in the human body. These are the lever, pulley, and wheel and axle. External levers appear as bars. Levers are classed as first-, second-, or third-class depending upon whether the fulcrum or axis, the resistance, or the force is located between the other two. Levers perform the function of enabling a force to move a greater resistance a lesser distance than the force moves or to move a resistance a greater distance than the force moves at the cost of applying greater force. Whether the advantage lies with overcoming a greater resistance with less force or with moving the resistance a greater distance than the force moves is dependent upon the relationship between the length of the resistance arm and the length of the work arm. When the resistance arm is longer than the force arm, the resistance will move a greater linear distance than will the force but force must be greater than the resistance. When the force arm is longer, the force expended will be less than the resistance overcome but the force will move a greater linear distance than the resistance. This is known as the *principle of levers* and may be stated as an equation:

$$F \times FA = R \times RA$$

where F = force; FA = length of the force arm; R = resistance; and RA = length of the resistance arm.

A pulley is used to change the direction of force. Pulleys in the human body in the form of sesimoid bones, condyles, and trochanters change the angle of pull of muscles to enable them to function more efficiently in producing movement of the body levers. Since muscles must lie along bones, their line of pull upon contraction would be in the direction of the long axis of the bone if it were not for the protuberances over which their tendons must pass. With respect to production of movement, the most efficient angle of pull is at a right angle to the long axis of the lever. However, in addition to producing movement, it is the job of the muscles to supplement the work of the ligaments in holding adjacent bones in juxtaposition. This is known as the stabilizing component of force of muscles.

An accurate definition of the force arm is "the perpendicular distance between the fulcrum and the line of force," while the specific definition of resistance arm is "the perpendicular distance between the fulcrum and the line of resistance." These are called, respectively, the force moment arm (FMA) and the resistance moment arm (RMA).

The movements of all individual levers in the body are rotatory, but combinations of various rotatory movements may produce linear motions of body parts as in jabbing, pushing, or lifting. Also, rotatory movements of body levers may produce linear motion of the entire body or of implements such as balls or javelins.

Lengthening of anatomic levers produces greater linear velocity at the end of the lever but greater force is required to move this longer lever. Shortening of anatomic levers produces greater angular velocity and reduces the amount of force required to initiate and sustain rotation. Different combinations of lengthening and shortening of anatomic or internal levers are utilized to execute various sports skills. Where high angular velocity is desired, the movement is initiated with a long lever that is then shortened. This is illustrated in twists and somersaults. Where high linear velocity is desired, as in throwing or striking, the motion is begun with a small lever that is lengthened throughout the motion.

The third type of simple machine found in the body is the wheel and axle. When the force is applied to the rim of the wheel, the effect is that of a second-class lever with the fulcrum on one end, the force on the opposite end, and the resistance in the middle. When the force is applied to the axle, the effect is that of a third-class lever with the force being applied between the fulcrum and the resistance. The relationship between body type and levers has been discussed. Endomorphs, because weight is concentrated nearer the fulcrum of the legs and arms than it is in the other two types, will be unable to generate as much angular momentum. Angular momentum is the product of the moment of inertia times the angular velocity. The moment of inertia is computed by multiplying the mass of each particle by the square of its distance from the axis and then adding all these products. Particles nearer the fulcrum or axis will add less to the moment of inertia than will those further away. Consequently, endomorphs with their "hammy" upper arms and thighs with most of the mass near the axis are unable to generate the great momentum so necessary in throwing and kicking.

Seventeen principles respecting the direction and distance of projectiles set in motion by internal or external levers have been presented. Maximum success in kicking, throwing, and striking activities cannot be achieved unless these principles are observed.

The overarm, sidearm, and underarm patterns of throwing and striking have been discussed, Detailed analyses of several of each of the overarm, sidearm, and underarm patterns of throwing and striking have been made. A distinct feature of the overarm pattern is flexion of the elbow and medial rotation of the humerus during the force-producing phase of the arm action. In all three patterns, the pelvic lever is the greatest force contributor. Other internal levers used include those of the spine and thorax (wheel and axle), shoulder girdle, humerus, forearm, and hand. **The baseball pitch, javelin throw, and tennis serve were analyzed in detail.**

In the underarm pattern, the throwing or striking arm (or arms) move forward in the sagittal plane. As in the overarm pattern, great force is contributed by the pelvic lever. The spinal, thoracic, shoulder girdle, arm, and hand levers add their force to the movement. The lever actions in the softball pitch, the underhand stroke in handball, and the golf swing were analyzed.

The sidearm patterns followed in the discus throw, batting, and the tennis drive were described. In these patterns, the arm moves in the transverse plane.

Finally, the use of body levers in thrusting or jabbing as in the one-handed push shot in basketball and the shot put were described and analyzed. In these patterns horizontal flexion of the humerus combined with elbow extension produces thrust or linear, rather than rotatory, movement of the hand.

REFERENCES

1. Cates, H. A., and Basmajian, J. V., *Primary Anatomy*, 3rd ed. Baltimore: Williams and Wilkins, 1955, p. 108.

2. Karpovich, Peter V., "Mechanics of Rising on the Toes." Paper presented at the Spring Convention of Connecticut Association of Health, Physical Education, and Recreation, Storrs, Connecticut, April, 1968.

3. Roozbazar, A., "Biomechanics of Lifting," *Biomechanics IV*, edited by R. C. Nelson and C. A. Morehouse. Baltimore: University Park Press, 1974, pp. 37–43.

4. Toyoshima, S., Hoshikawa, T., Myoshita, M., and Oguri, T., "Contribution of Body Parts to Throwing Performance," *Biomechanics IV*, edited by R. C. Nelson and C. A. Morehouse. Baltimore: University Park Press, 1974, pp. 169–174.

5. Kunz, H., "Effects of Ball Mass and Movement Pattern on Release Velocity in Throwing," *Biomechanics IV*, edited by R. C. Nelson and C. A. Morehouse. Baltimore: University Park Press, 1974, pp. 163–168.

6. Cooper, John M., and Glassow, Ruth B., *Kinesiology*, 4th edition. St. Louis: C. V. Mosby, 1976, p. 148.

7. *Ibid.*, pp. 123–124.

8. *Ibid.*, p. 124.

9. Bunn, John W., *Scientific Principles of Coaching*, 2nd edition. Englewood Cliffs, N.J.: Prentice-Hall, 1972, pp. 264–266.

10. Taylor, James A., "Behavior of the Discus in Flight," *ICAAAA Bulletin*, February 27, 1932.

11. Bunn, *op. cit.*, p. 172.

8 BIOKINETICS OF BALANCE AND EQUILIBRIUM

CONCEPTS

1. Human balance control is derived from interrelated and interacting anatomical/physiological/mechanical sources.

2. Stationary and dynamic balance are uniquely different, each requiring specific skills.

3. The arrangement of body weight, center of gravity, and line of gravity is a vital condition in attaining and maintaining balance.

4. Upright and inverted balance classifications are not necessarily related skill variables.

5. Short stature is an advantage in maintenance of balance.

6. Muscular strength aids in balance control.

7. The predominant internal third-class lever system of the human physique does not favor balance and equilibrium.

8. When body weight is equally distributed, maintenance of balance over a narrow support base is enhanced.

9. Sensory mechanisms of vision, ears, proprioceptors, and kinesthesia are vitally affiliated with balance control.

10. Conductive deafness does not necessarily indicate poor balance. Individuals with middle-ear impairment often display superior balance ability.

11. Balance and equilibrium are integral components of kinesthesia.

12. Stationary and dynamic balance tests re-

veal clues to specific balance skills and are not absolute indicators of general balance ability.

13. Balance and buoyancy in water are directly related to the body density of the individual.

14. Orthopedic aberrations usually change the body center of gravity and generally make balance control more precarious.

GENERAL CONSIDERATIONS

Balance and equilibrium skills are paramount for efficient and effective movement. These qualities generally rate high priority among the specific objectives of physical education. Balance control enhances the "safety insurance" of individuals. Certain minimum levels of competence are essential in sitting, walking, running, and the myriad of physical activities surrounding man. It is not uncommon to hear the following remarks: "How did he fall on the trampoline?" or "How did she dislocate her elbow joint?" The frequent response stated is: "I lost my balance!" Equilibrium results from the integration of (1) *anatomical* (somatotype structure), (2) *physiological* (neuromuscular functioning, kinesthesia, acuity of senses), and (3) *mechanical*

286

(levers, forces, laws of motion) components, which are all interacting elements. Stability and balance can be improved significantly through games and appropriate physical activities.

Definitions and Classifications

Two general types of balance descriptions are entailed in human motion, (1) *stationary balance* and (2) *dynamic balance*. A subordinate division is further categorized as upright and inverted posture. Stationary balance, sometimes referred to as static balance, is defined as a hold position of the body in any given posture. Figures 8.1 and 8.2 illustrate upright and inverted stationary balance positions. Dynamic balance is identified as the ability of

Figure 8.1 Stationary upright balance

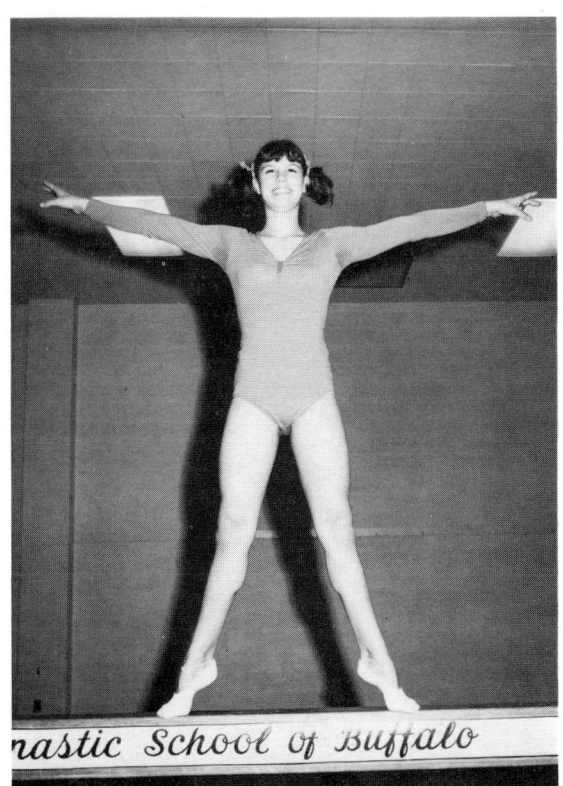

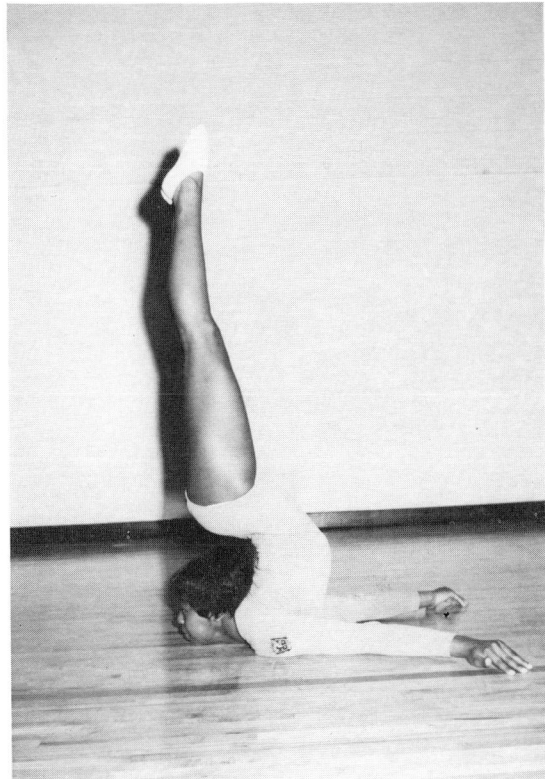

Figure 8.2 Stationary inverted balance. Observe the broad support base and low center of gravity permitted by extreme flexibility of the performer

the individual to maintain balance during a body movement. Figures 8.3 and 8.4 exemplify upright and inverted dynamic balance actions.

Elements of Equilibrium

Balance control is affected by the gravitational constant of 32.2 ft/sec/sec, which simply means that an object falls freely in the absence of air resistance by 32.2 ft/sec each second; its rate of speed is 32.2/sec². It should be noted that this rate applies to objects falling in a vacuum, not within the normal environment of the earth's atmosphere. Due to air resistance and variability of aerodynamics in structural forms, certain bodies

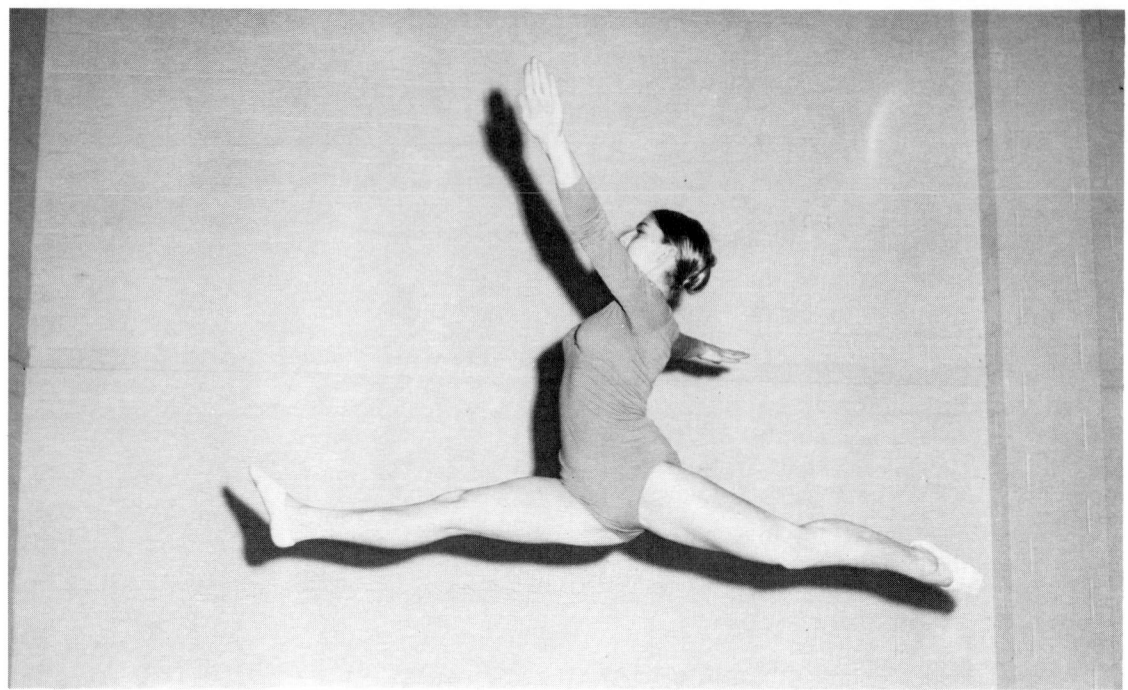

Figure 8.3 Running straddle leap—dynamic balance in upright position

tend to fall more quickly than others. Notwithstanding, in the maintenance of adequate stability and balance, this constant downward pull toward the earth must be considered as an important element in the understanding of equilibrium.

In addition to considering the constant force of gravity for correct balance, other factors affect equilibrium. These elements are (1) mass or weight of the object, (2) base of support, (3) center of gravity, and (4) line of gravity.

Mass or Weight of the Object

If mass or weight were the only factor affecting human equilibrium, the heavier the body, the more stable the object would be. This variable is obvious in inanimate items such as a brick. Theoretically, the density of such an object is uniform and the center of

the brick is also the center of its gravity. The heavier the brick, the greater its stability. More weight, evenly distributed over its supporting base, tends to give the object stability. For example, heavier individuals should be placed as base men in sports acrobatics with the lightest individuals utilized as "top men." Correct weight placement in concert with other elements is important in achieving stationary and dynamic balance control.

Base of Support

In stationary balance position, support bases that are wide, other factors being equal, possess greater stability. Narrow bases of support tend to make it difficult to keep the line of gravity over the supporting structure. For example, it is more difficult for the individual to balance on one foot than on two feet slightly separated since the gravity line must be

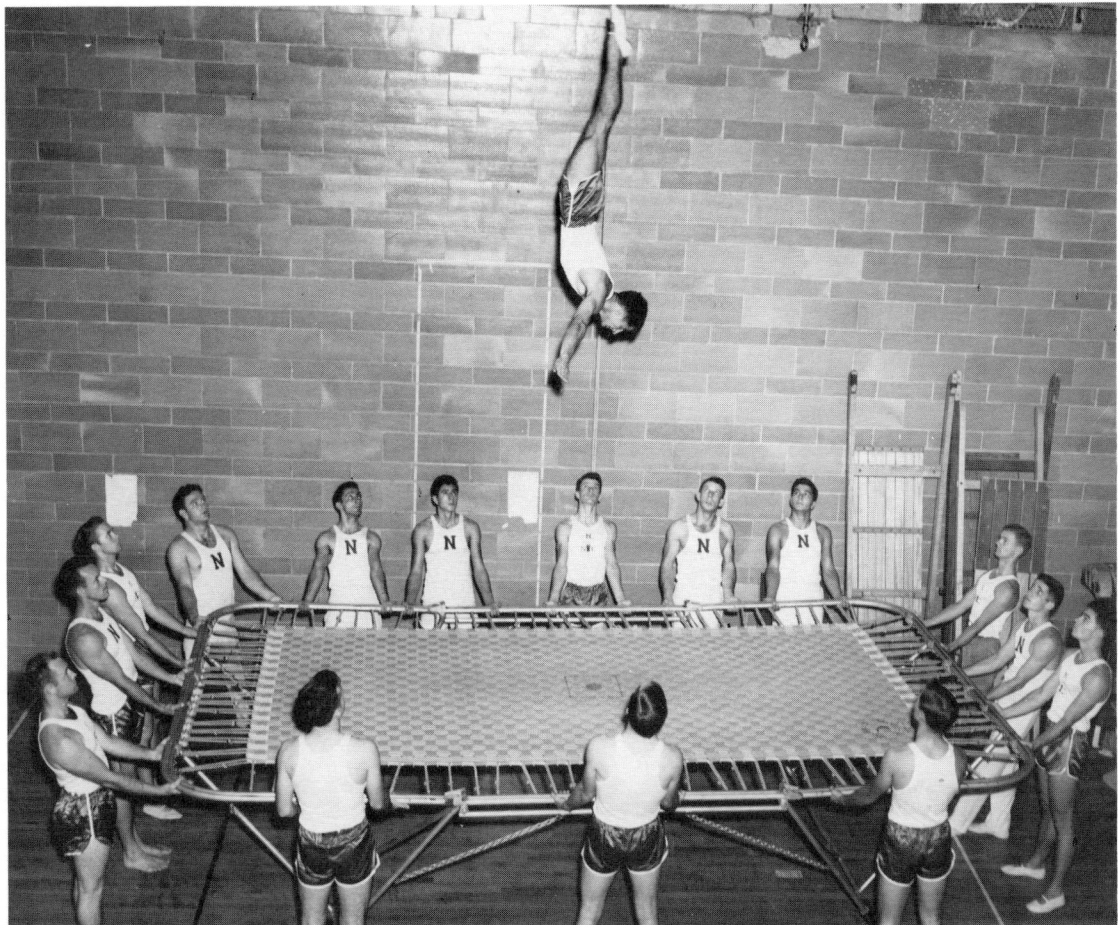

Figure 8.4 Inverted dynamic balance. Performer is actually in the middle of a backward somersault

concentrated directly over one foot. Jumping and landing movements are easier to perform when separating the feet shoulder width than with legs held close together. Narrowing the support base increases the difficulty of maintaining stationary balance positions. Figure 8.5 illustrates various support bases affecting stability.

Center of Gravity

The geometrical center of a uniform object is also its gravity center; however, the human body is dynamic, constantly moving from one position to another. Stationary balance appears to be static, but in reality small oscillating moves are being made by the individual to hold the center of gravity over its supporting base.[1]

The center of gravity in the normal standing position of the adult male, arms hanging at the sides, is at approximately 56 to 57 percent of the height. In women it is approximately at 55 percent of standing height, and in children the center of gravity is higher due to a proportionately larger thorax.[2]

The problems of human stability are quite different from those of a constant homoge-

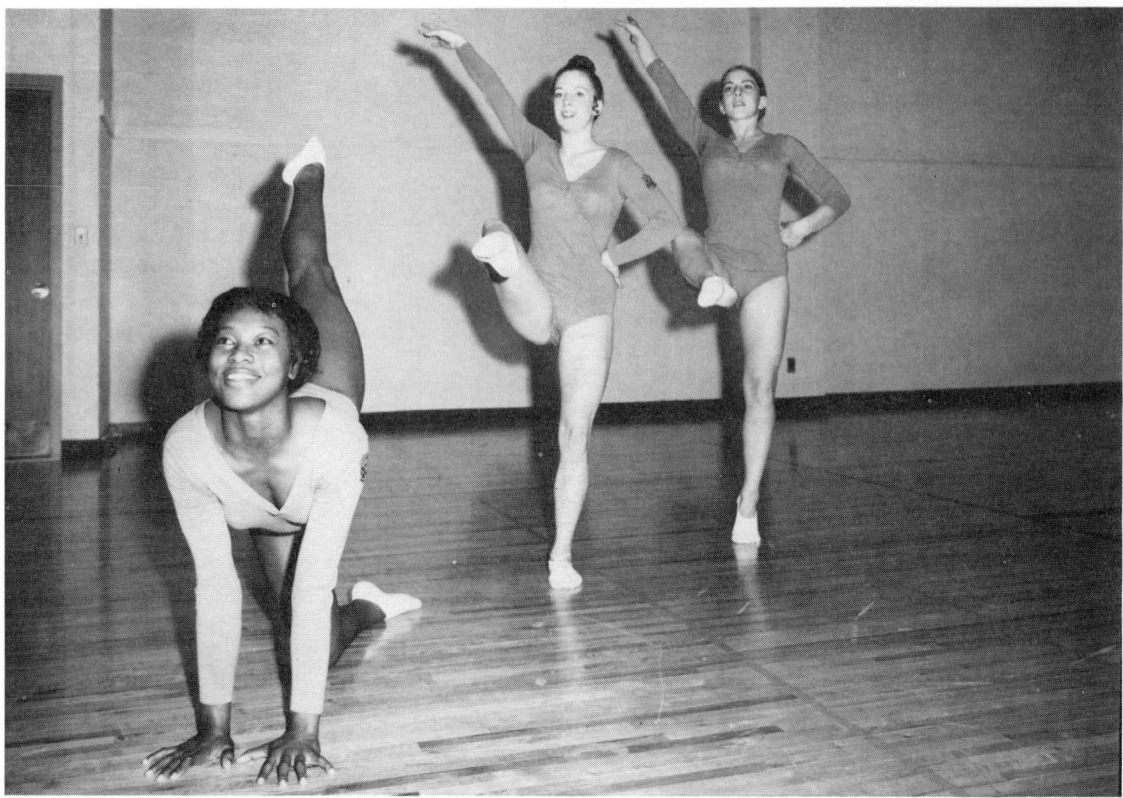

Figure 8.5 Upright stationary balance positions. Observe the gradual reduction of support base size to the half-toe standing posture

neous mass of uniform density such as a block of wood. The human body is not uniform but has varying densities of bone, muscle, liquid, and other living tissues, which, in effect, change its gravity center with each different movement.

Segmentally, each body area contains its own center of gravity. Each segment has a weight center, for example, arm, leg, head, trunk, which is subject to gravitational forces affecting equilibrium depending upon its relational location to the segment's supporting base. Segmental weight center information is particularly useful for therapists working with amputees and other orthopedically disabled individuals when balance and stability are important elements in the performance of

walking, running, turning, and general motor mobility. The student is referred to Table 3.5 in Chapter 3 for specific data on segmental weights and percentages of total weight.

Figure 8.6 illustrates changing lines of gravity to accommodate various support bases in upright stationary positions.

Line of Gravity

The line of gravity is defined as an imaginary line that passes through the object's center of gravity. In balanced positions, the line of gravity passes approximately through the geometrical center of the support base. Upright and inverted balance control postures

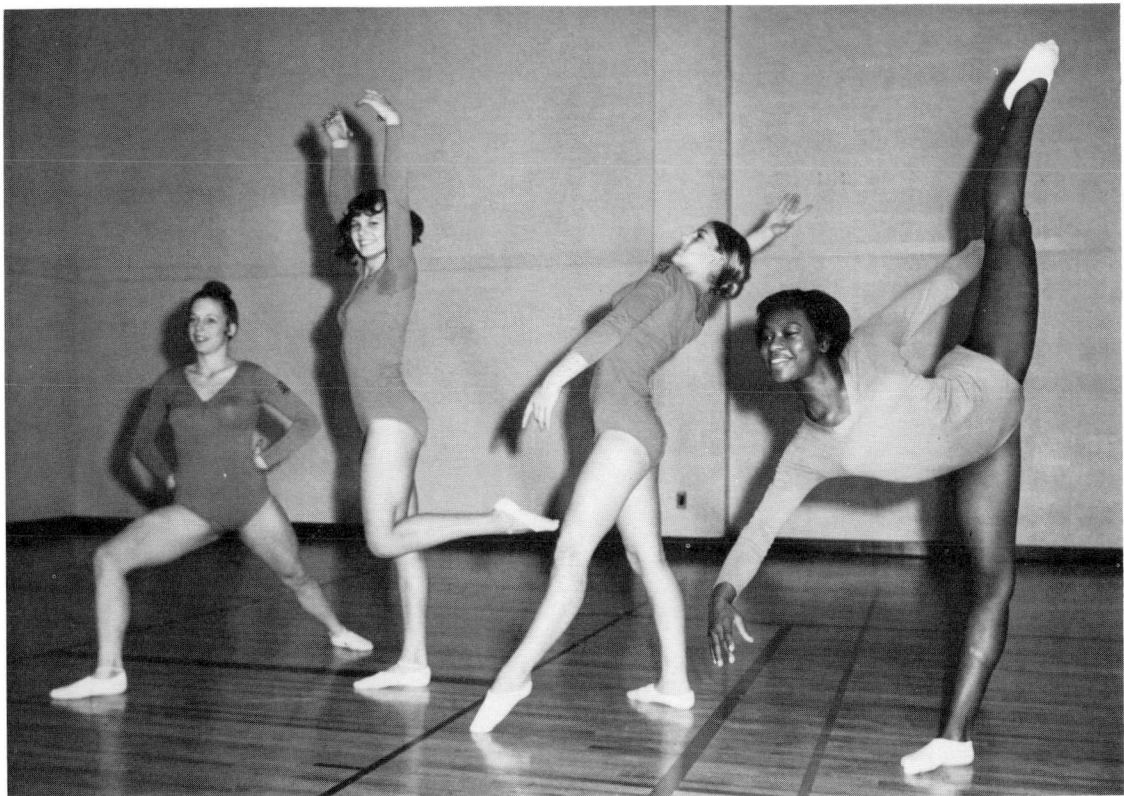

Figure 8.6 Various stationary upright balance positions with changing lines of gravity

demand that the line of gravity be over its supporting base; otherwise balance is lost. Figure 8.7 illustrates passage of the gravity line through the center of gravity inside the base of support.

ATTAINING AND MAINTAINING UPRIGHT AND INVERTED BALANCE

Why is it less difficult to walk on the balance beam with arms outstretched in a frontal plane? Is balance easier to maintain with feet apart or together in performing a handstand? Maintaining balance requires the proper positioning of the following factors: (1) base of support, (2) center of gravity, and (3) line of gravity.

In stationary balance positions, ease of stability is attained by broadening the support base, keeping the gravity center low with the line of gravity within its support base. A simple illustration of the triangular-shaped object exemplifies maximum ease of equilibrium and stability. Figure 8.8 clearly illustrates the easier form of attaining balance. The application of this principle may be utilized in physical activity classes with pyramid constructions as follows:

Each of these shapes reflect low gravity centers and broad support base profiles, which give a hold posture maximum mechanical stability.

Although stationary balance posture is easier to attain, as shown in Figure 8.8, the reverse order is true in the maintenance of

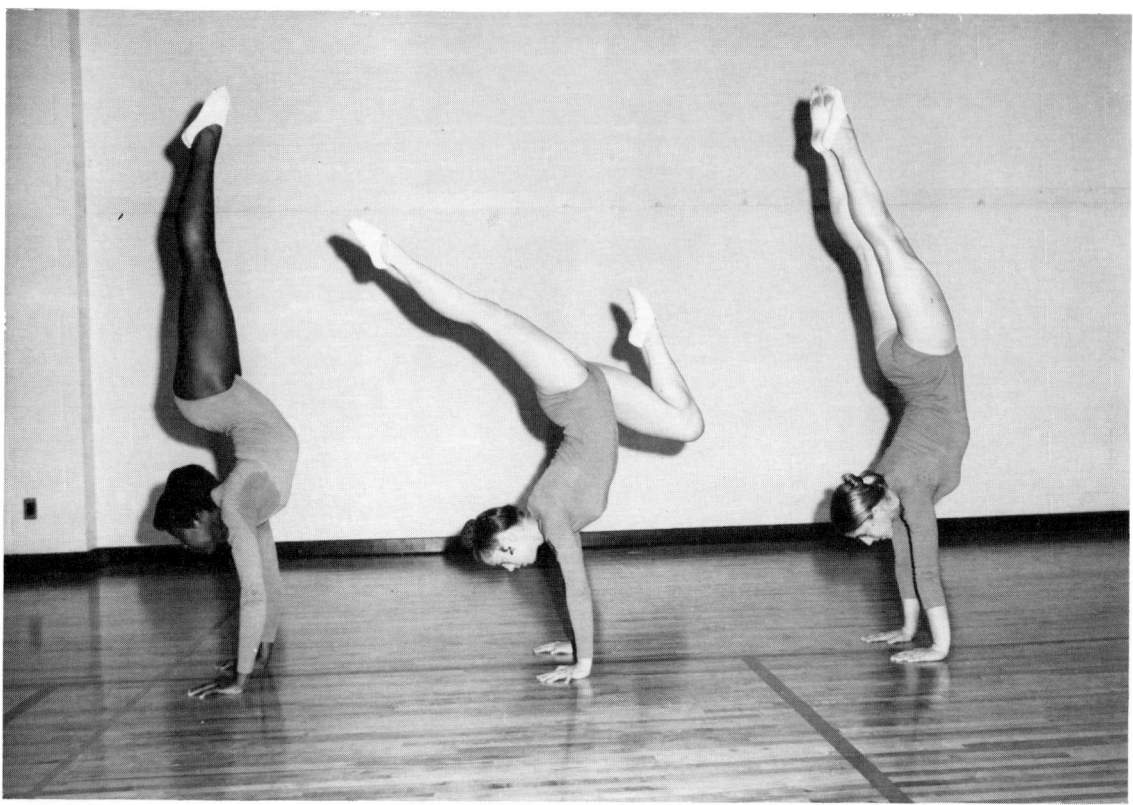

Figure 8.7 Various handstand styles. Observe the line of gravity between the hands irrespective of body form. Center of gravity is in front of hands (under head) in first performer

balance maneuvers. Regaining loss of balance of an object is easier with the weight center high, rather than low, as illustrated in Figure 8.9.

When the center of gravity is high, a balanced position is more difficult to *attain*. However, correction of balance is easier because the speed of the center of gravity decelerates as its distance above the base lengthens.[3] This mechanical principle explains in part, why it is possible for performers utilizing a "perch pole" described in Chapter 9 to balance the topmounter. In addition to the object's base area and gravity height, balance is also affected by the horizontal distance between the center of gravity and its pivoting edge. The handstander in Figure 8.10 is using her legs as a balance pole to maintain the line of gravity over its narrow support base of the hand. The inverted triangle-shape form is indicated when feats of balance must be executed over small or narrow bases such as a one-arm handstand, standing on toes, and other similar positions.

Although studies have been completed relevant to specific upright dynamic and static actions, it is interesting to note that research is meager showing the relationship, if any, between upright and inverted balance positions.

Balance activities are found in many human kinetic movements that accent upright

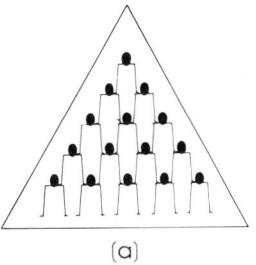 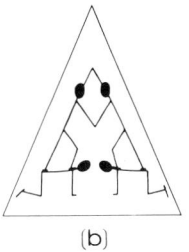 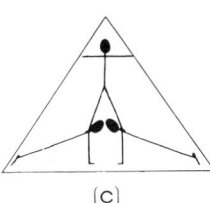

Figure 8.8 Broadening the base of support in pyramid building

dynamic position such as the shot put, basketball dribbling, high jumping, leaping, or gymnastic activities that inescapably involve inverted balance postures centering around the basic handstand. Indeed, it would be important to know whether or not developing inverted balance ability directly or indirectly improves upright balance. It does not necessarily follow that an individual who possesses expert balance precision with handstands will also have the keen balance ability in walking on a balance beam or standing on one foot in the upright position. Chapter 9 contains specific applications and examples of mechanical principles applied to gymnastics.

ROLE OF SOMATOTYPE IN HUMAN BALANCING

In previous discussions three important elements have been stressed for correct balance skill, namely, base of support, center of gravity, and line of gravity. The physique of an individual also plays an important role in balance performance. Somatotypes are indeed variable, and it is important to realize the concept that balance styles must conform to the shape and size of the individual's structure. Various methods of identifying and assessing physique are described in Chapter 3.

The height and length of the individual's limbs does have an affect on stationary and dynamic balance ability. Short, stocky individuals tend to have a lower center of gravity while a high center of gravity is possessed by

tall individuals. Applying the principle of gravity height, tall individuals find it more difficult to attain balance positions than shorter persons. It follows that tall individuals with long arms will find it difficult to maintain balance while swinging on the parallel bars or performing a handstand on this piece of apparatus, since the gravity center of each arm is considerably higher over its support base than in those appendages of the shorter individual. Tall individuals must

Figure 8.9 Effect of center of gravity height on a pivoting base: (a) low center of gravity accelerates tipping action; (b) high center of gravity (COG) decelerates tipping action

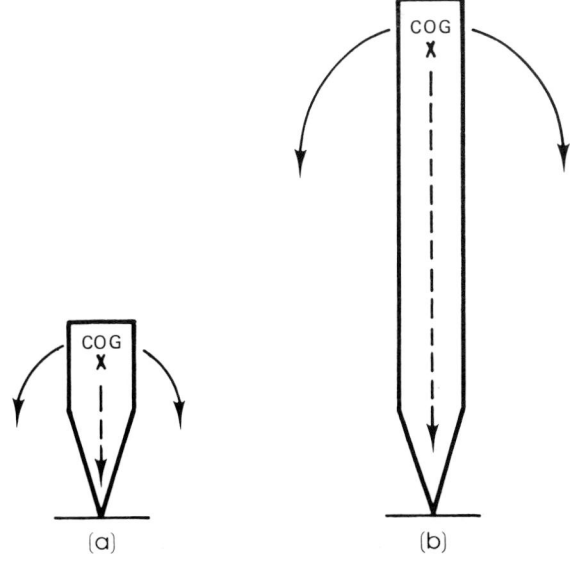

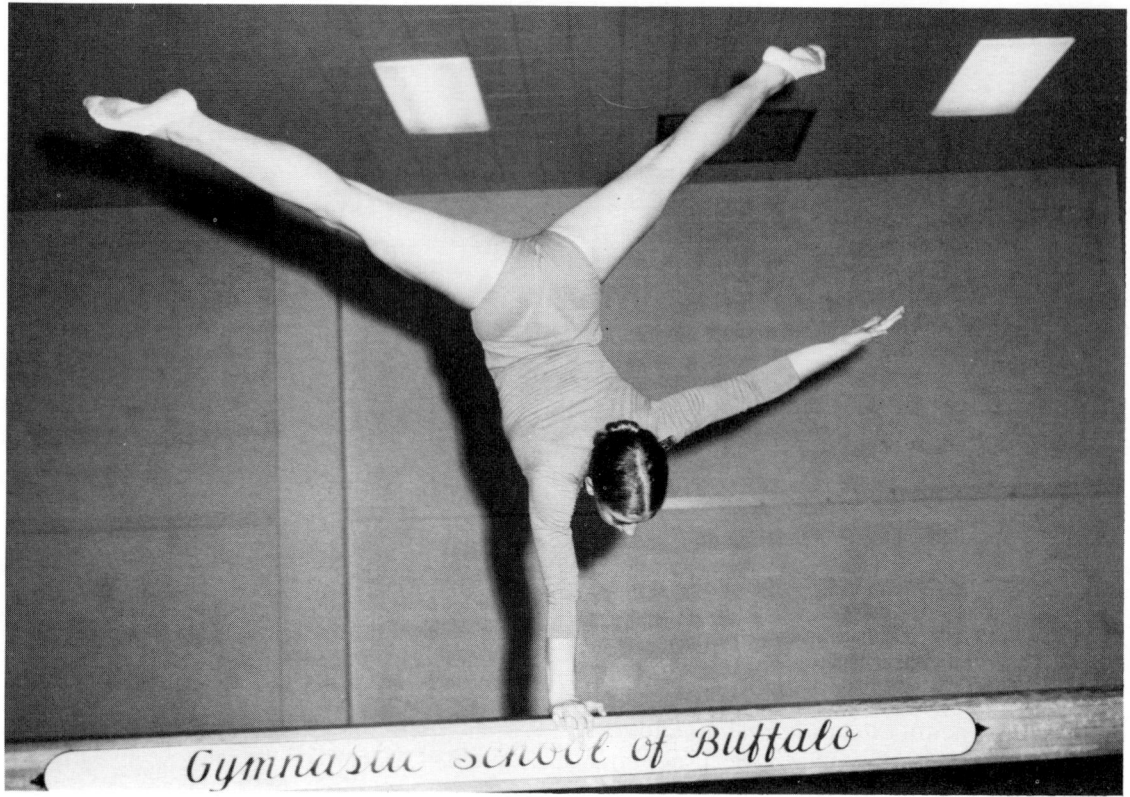

Figure 8.10 Advanced inverted stationary balance position. Observe the first-class lever effect of the legs assisting the performer to maintain the line of gravity directly over the hand.

compensate by developing greater strength and skill through practice.

Balance control can be enhanced with strength development. Force provided by muscular strength can correct errors in joint angles that are important for the proper alignment of the critical line of gravity. However, it should be noted that strength alone is not the most single important requirement for balance precision. Other aspects such as kinesthesia, motor ability, and skill ability must be considered in successful balance performance. Superior strength allows the individual reserve power to correct errors in attaining and maintaining the line of gravity within its base of support and as such assists the tall person in achieving good balance control.

ROLE OF LEVERS IN STATIONARY AND DYNAMIC POSITIONS

Maintaining stability and equilibrium also involves consideration of lever construction. The principles of internal and external levers apply to static and dynamic postures, as pointed out in Chapter 7. Internal levers are constructs of anatomical structure; for example, the extension of the elbow articulation is classified as an internal lever of the first class, which functionally does not favor balance.

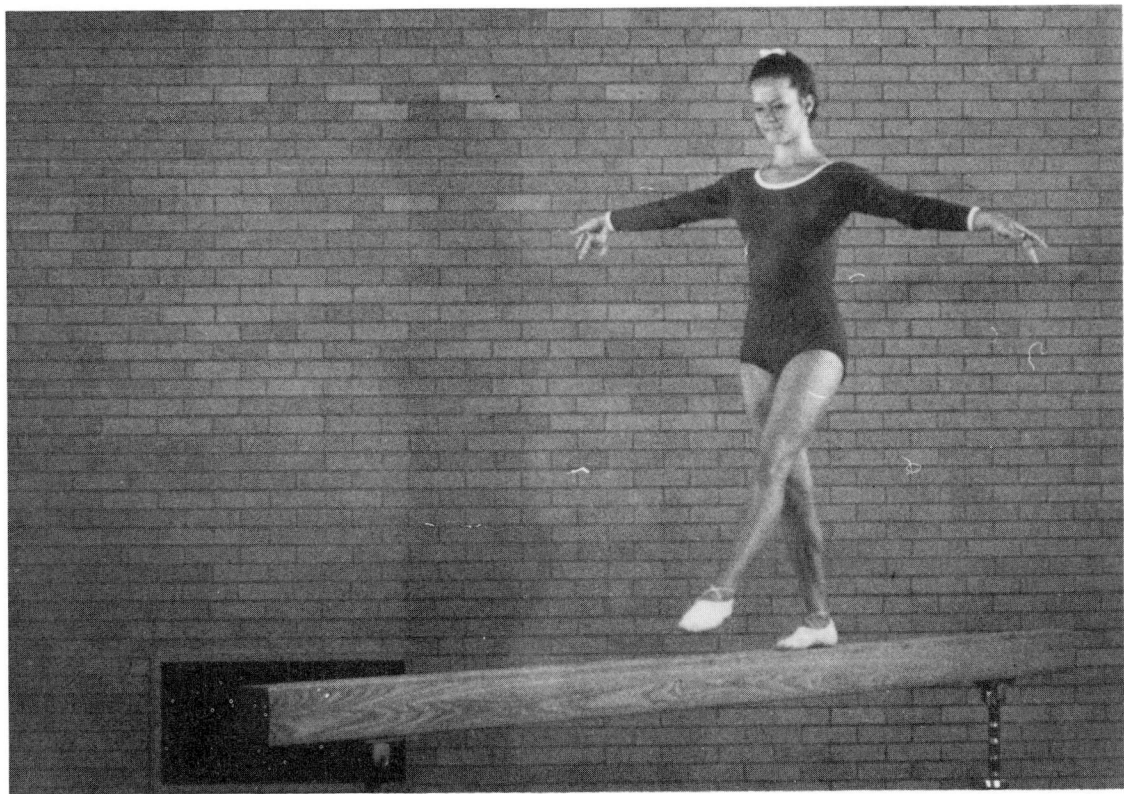

Figure 8.11 Lever effect of arms maintaining upright dynamic balance

Most muscle insertions, which represent force points, are located close to body joints that reflect long resistance and short force arms resulting in leverage instability. External levers involve the positioning of the body and/or external apparatus affecting change in the fulcrum position, favoring or unfavoring equilibrium. In stationary balance moves, perfect balance is attained when the fulcrum is exactly between the resistance point and the force point (first-class lever). Therefore, in posture manipulations or physical activity, the participant should strive to equalize rotatory movements, when equilibrium is the objective, by centering the fulcrum point. The Great Wallenda of high tight-wire walking fame utilized long poles to help maintain balance by creating long first-class levers, with the fulcrum located at the hands, and the ends of the pole representing force and resistance points. The ends of the poles help to maintain the line of gravity over its small supporting base, which in this case is the feet. Figure 8.11 illustrates a similar "lever effect" maintaining balance as the performer walks along the balance beam.

Most balance movements can be learned and improved with practice, provided the individual has intact anatomical and physiological attributes. However, simple balance control can be a problem for individuals with spinal cord lesions and/or other types of central nervous system impairments. The paraplegic patient must learn to master the delicate interplay or position between the pelvis and his head and shoulders. When one of these segments moves forward, the other must move backward to compensate. An understanding of segmental balance with reference to segment weights and location of centers of gravity, discussed in Chapter 3, can help the handicapped individual gain balance control in basic functional walking and turning movements.

SENSORY INVOLVEMENT IN HUMAN BALANCING

Balancing and equilibrium are psycho-neural-somatic phenomena of the total organism. The potential for development lies with heredity, and the improvement of that potential depends upon the degree of positive nurturement. Four sense factors have considerable influence upon an individual's balancing ability, namely, (1) eyes, (2) ears, (3) proprioception, and (4) kinesthesia.

Eyes

Pioneer studies by Bass[4] and McCloy[5] support the premise that a vast difference exists in any balance exercise when performing a task with eyes opened or closed. This reality can be clearly demonstrated by walking the balance beam with eyes open and then repeated without visual clues. The participant immediately realizes that it is much easier with eyes open. Another example showing the importance of the eyes can be demonstrated by standing on one foot with eyes open and then repeating the exercise with eyes closed. The difficulty of maintaining balance without vision is immediately apparent. Vision provides a point of reference and, therefore, is important in the maintenance of balance. A diver reinforces balance control by watching the end of the board during the initial forward running approach. Balance beam walking movements can be improved by looking at the far end of

the beam. Stressing eye focus at specific reference points can assist the student in the early learning stages before he attempts difficult balance maneuvers. However, a word of caution should be given about the avoidance of rigidity and overdependence upon visual clues. For example, gymnasts attempting a one-arm handstand by focusing vision on a particular point or area soon discover a rapid increase in oscillatory movements both in magnitude and amplitude, resulting in a loss of balance.

Elements of proprioception and kinesthesia are also important component elements in developing precision balance, especially in advanced and intricate exercise patterns. Rasch and Burke[6] point out that a skilled performer becomes very sensitive to proprioceptive sensations in the tendons and joints and semicircular canals of the inner ear, and too much visual information may inhibit a development of proprioceptive and labyrinthine mechanism. Conversely, overstimulation of the labyrinthine receptors, such as whirling or rapid tumbling, may produce dizziness and even nausea. A common practice of dancers and figure skaters, whose routines include rapid spins, is to fix the eyes on a distant point and to watch that point until the head has turned as far as is compatible with comfort. The eyes rest on a focus object until the limit of the turn is sighted. The exact specificity of vision contribution to balance and equilibrium probably cannot be stated in absolute terms; however, it is recognized that sight can assist the individual in the improvement of this motor constituent when utilized correctly as an integral adjunct with other sensory impressions arising from the nervous system.

Ears

The function of the ear is not only to receive sound but to serve as a sensory balance mechanism. The ear is divided into three major segments, external, middle, and internal or inner sections. The external and middle ear deal primarily with the conduction of vibrations via the ear drum and three ossicles: malleus, incus, and stapes.

The internal ear or labyrinth contains the structures and fluids that affect equilibrium, particularly head orientation. The power to coordinate the movements of the body and to maintain balance resides in the cerebellum. However, this power of coordination, which involves equilibrium, is shared with vestibular apparatus of the inner ear. Gardner[7] refers to "vestibular feedback," which is particularly responsible for the equilibrium aspect of skilled movements. Responses of the vestibular apparatus from angular and linear acceleration and changes in the head position in relation to gravity assist with other sensory mechanisms to produce the "righting reflex." Whenever these detectors signal a head position other than associated with normal posture, control centers intitiate movements of the head to correct the position of the head with the line of force of gravity. The understanding of this vestibular mechanism system can aid the learner to improve the balance component of motor skills and confirms the concept of the well-known axiom that the "body follows the head."

Poor balance has often been attributed to deaf students. This quality may or may not be true, depending upon the degree of vestibular inner ear damage. Deaf students at Gallaudet College, Washington, D.C., engage in dance, sports, and other recreational activities without problems.[8] Generally, if the conductive mechanism (ear drum and three ossicles) are impeded without damage to the inner sensorineural mechanism; balance may not be affected. Conditions such as meningitis, scarlet fever, and Meniere's disease, all of which are associated with sensorineural nerve loss, can result in poor balance ability if the vestibular apparatus is impaired. Few restrictions exist among the activities that may be offered to students with auditory handicaps in the regular physical education class.

Proprioception

An integral element of equilibrium involves proprioceptive receptors originating in the muscles, tendons, and joints. These receptors together with inner ear vestibular mechanisms are important components of skilled movements requiring precision balancing. Muscular contractions stimulate nerve endings in tendons and joints, sending neural messages to the cerebellum informing it of the actual state of contraction. This information, together with messages from the motor cortex of the brain, is integrated by the cerebellum, resulting in an adjustment of the rate and force of muscular contraction necessary for the balancing task at the moment. The anatomical structures of the Golgi tendon organs, Ruffini's corpuscles, and Pacini's corpuscles are the principal proprioceptive receivers found in muscular tissue and its nerve supply. Figure 8.12 illustrates the pathway of proprioceptive transmission to the brain. The pacinian corpuscles are found in the subcutaneous, submucous, and subserous connective tissue, especially in the palm of the hand, sole of the foot, and about the joints. The corpuscles of Golgi are found in the subcutaneous tissue of the pulp of the fingers. The corpuscles of Ruffini are a special variety of nerve endings in the subcutaneous tissue of the human fingers. The sensitive nerve structures can be developed to a point where ultimate kinesthetic efficacy is attained, as shown by the performance in Figures 8.13a and 8.13b.

Proprioceptive impressions are fed to the cortex and cerebellum with information on joint angulation and muscle tension; this information is eventually impressed upon mem-

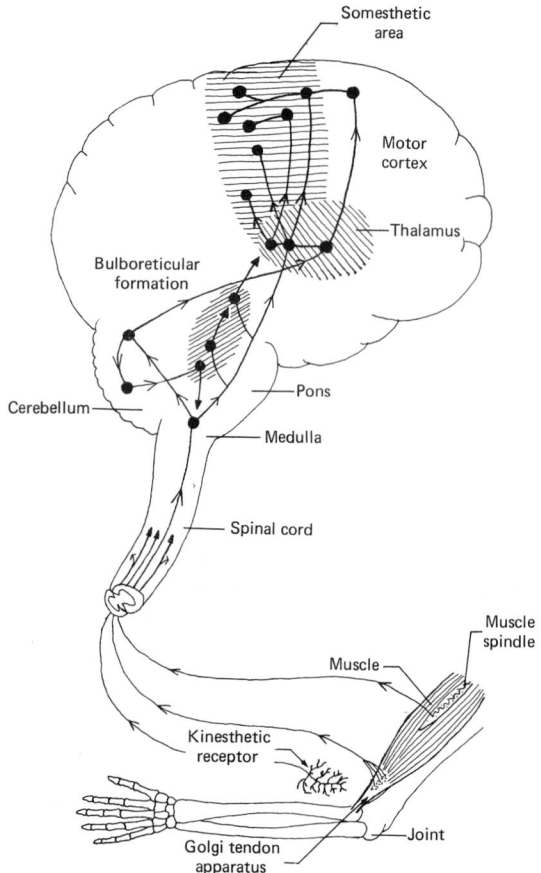

Figure 8.12 Proprioceptive transmission to the brain (from Arthur C. Guyton, **Basic Human Physiology**, W. B. Saunders Co., Philadelphia, Pa., 1977, with permission)

ory. As a result, repetitions of positions and movements at a later time without visual feedback can be effected.[9] Ultimately, refined motor skills reflect superb proprioceptive balance reflexes, which are intricately interwoven with kinesthesia. Balance control potential is determined by the individual's anatomical physiological proprioceptive circuit intactness. The positive development of the sensorimotor structures depend upon their stimulation and utilization. Active body exercise movements, dance, and gymnastics are excellent motor activities to cultivate pro-

prioceptive impressions and neural feedback circuits of the poorly skilled as well as the superior athlete.

Kinesthesia

Kinesthesia or kinesthesis is the mechanism by which one is aware of body position and/or its segmental parts. Often, this awareness is identified as "position sense." Specific analysis and discussion of this physiological mechanism is further explored in Chapter 4. Kinesthesia, only as it is related to balance, is examined in this chapter.

Balancing ability is a part of kinesthesia. In fact, visual clues, ears (vestibular mechanism), and proprioception are intricately related to the ability of the individual to initiate and maintain balance control.

An early study by Bass[10] points out the interrelationship of kinesthesia with balance. Scott[11] investigated 28 items as measures of kinesthesis among 100 college women, in which a balance leap test was utilized to measure dynamic balance. This researcher concluded that a balance test should be a part of any kinesthetic battery. Other static and dynamic balance tests have been utilized as integral elements in the assessment of kinesthesis.[12, 13, 14]

METHODS OF DETERMINING THE CENTER OF GRAVITY IN HUMAN BALANCE

The visualization of the center of gravity, line of gravity, and its supporting base is helpful in the understanding of human balance. Several methods of determining the center of gravity have been established. A common technique employed is the *reaction board method.* This procedure uses the principle of moments and relies on the fact that the sum of the moments acting on a body in equilibrium is zero.[15] The location of the gravitational line can be found in each plane, and

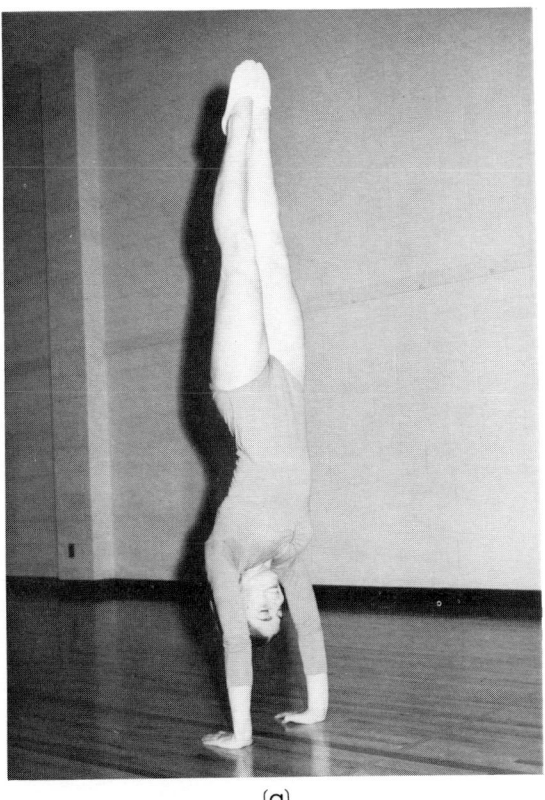

(a)

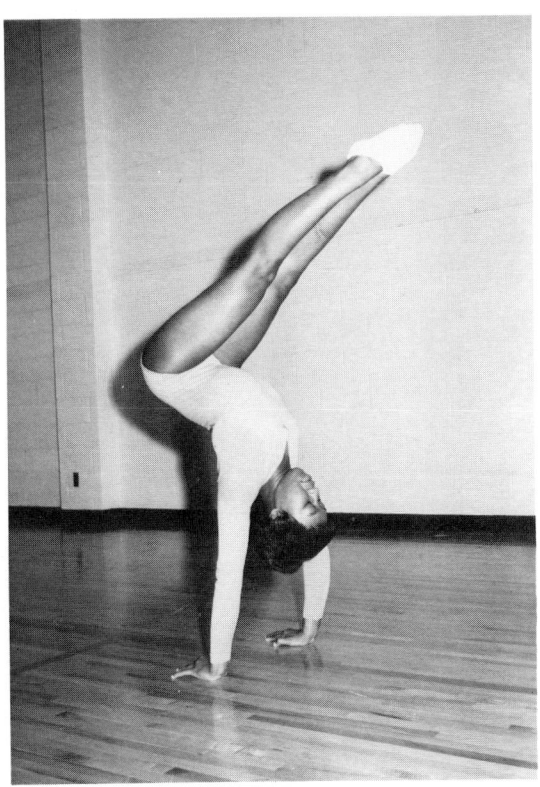

(b)

Figure 8.13 (a) "Needle" handstand; (b) "Yogi" handstand. Observe position held without visual clues. Inverted stationary balance positions cued to refined development of cutaneous proprioceptors and inner ear vestibular mechanisms in two handstand styles

the center of gravity becomes the intersection for each of these three planes. A scale, block and board about 40 cm wide and 200 cm long are necessary equipment items. The general position and equipment utilized for locating the line of gravity in the sagittal plane is shown in Figure 8.14. The student is referred to reference 15 for specific procedural details.

Rasch and Burke[16] describe the *photographic method* for locating the center of gravity whereby an individual is photographed from directly overhead. Detailed directions for locating the center of gravity in two planes simultaneously may be found in reference 16.

METHODS OF DETERMINING THE CENTER OF GRAVITY WITH INANIMATE OBJECTS

Weight centers of inorganic objects can be determined by a simple class of procedures of suspending small objects in air. Methany[17] describes the process of locating the weight center of a piece of cardboard utilizing a hairpin or paper clip, piece of string, and attached weight (Figure 8.15). This simple ex-

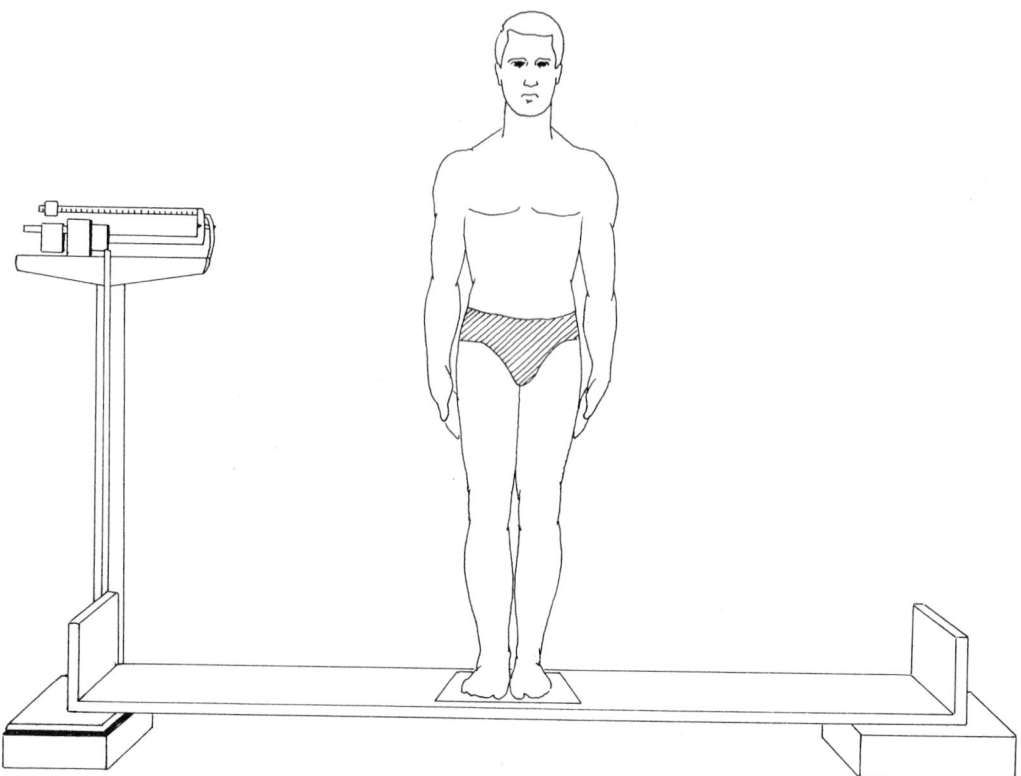

Figure 8.14 Method for locating the line of gravity in the sagittal plane (from Katharine F. Wells and Kathryn Luttgens, **Kinesiology**, W. B. Saunders Co., Philadelphia, Pa., 1976, with permission)

periment shows the center of gravity passing through that point at which half the weight of an object would be on either side of the object, an important concept in understanding principles of equilibrium.

A pattern for locating segmental centers of gravity has been devised.[18] A graphic triangulation schema called a "template" was constructed for the purpose of obtaining segmental gravity centers directly from a photograph of the subject. The template was drawn on a single sheet of transparent acrylic plastic arranged with eight triangles. The design utilized Dempster's proportions for locating segmental centers of gravity and the principle of similar triangles. The technique does have an advantage over the laborious method for ob-

taining the location of the center of gravity of the human body with photographs involved in finding the gravity centers of each major segment with respect to arbitrary X, Y axes. The calculations in obtaining the locations of each segmental center of gravity is often very arduous, if completed segment by segment. The "template method" offers a time-saving alternative for securing the data; its use is specifically described in reference 18.

STATIONARY AND DYNAMIC TESTS OF HUMAN BALANCING

Generally, tests for human balancing are specifically indicated for stationary and dynamic

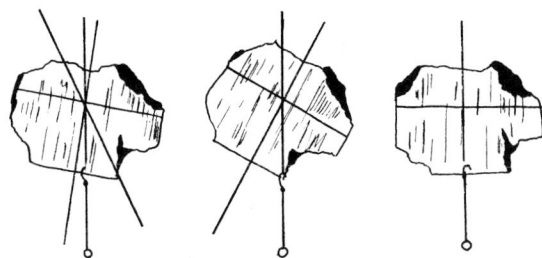

Figure 8.15 Method of determining the weight center of an object. (Note the irregularity of the model)

Directions for locating the center of gravity. The presence of the center of gravity may be illustrated by using a heavy irregularly shaped cardboard, bent hairpin or paper clip, and a piece of string with a weight attached to one end.

1. Make a hole at any point near the edge of the cardboard, large enough to insert the bent pin.

2. Slip the free ends of the string over bent pin, insert pin in hole.

3. Hold other ends of the pin easily between thumb and forefinger, allowing cardboard, string, and weight to hang freely.

4. Have someone mark with a pencil the line of the string through the center of the cardboard.

5. Now take another point on the edge of the cardboard, make a new hole, and repeat the entire process. The second pencil line should cross the first one at a point in the center of the cardboard. This point represents the center of gravity on the cardboard, the point through which the pull of gravity is pulling the cardboard down from its hook.

6. Make a third hole at another point near the edge of the cardboard and repeat the string-hanging process.

(From Eleanor Methany, **Body Dynamics**, Mc-Graw-Hill, New York, 1952, with permission)

balance postures. Certain tests attempt to measure stationary and dynamic balance variables in a single test. Other instruments attempt to measure balance ability in the inverted position.[19] It is important to remember that balance tests are specific in nature, but are broadly classified into stationary and dynamic categories in either the upright or inverted positions. Superior scores on upright dynamic tests do not necessarily transfer to high ability to inverted stationary balance performances. Research exploring the relationship, if any, between inverted and upright balance positions is sparse. Furthermore, research does not support the theory that a positive relationship exists between static and dynamic balance measurement criteria.[20]

Several tests are briefly described that are commonly utilized as instruments for the assessment of human balance.

Stationary Balance Tests

An upright static balance test called "gross body equilibrium factor" is advocated by Fleishman.[21] This test requires the individual to maintain his equilibrium without visual clues, standing on one foot upon a narrow rail. An exhibit of the test is shown in Figure 8.16.

Progressive Inverted Balance Test

Johnson and Nelson[22] developed a progressive inverted balance test that attempts to determine the subject's inverted stationary balance ability. The test consisted of five balance stunts: (1) tripod balance, (2) tip-up balance, (3) head balance, (4) forearm balance, and (5) handstand. Each balance may be held for a maximum of five points (one point for each second) with each balance from the tripod to handstand weighted one through five. Figure 8.17 illustrates several selected test items.

Piscopo* used a modified version of the inverted balance test for classification purposes

*Piscopo, John, "Gymnastic Classification Test" (unpublished data), Northwestern State University, Natchitoches, Louisiana, 1962.

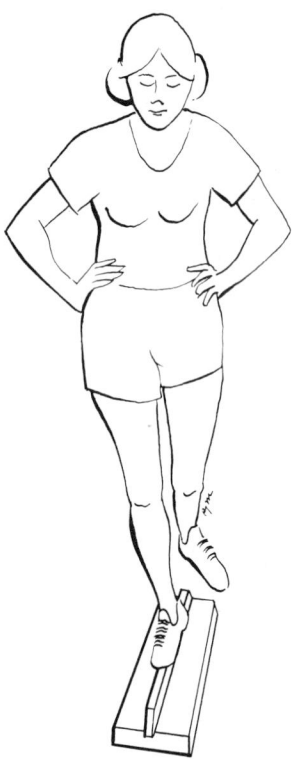

Figure 8.16 Gross body equilibrium test

in instructional gymnastics units. This test does give excellent clues about the subject's inverted balancing ability, as well as testing strength of the neck, arms, and shoulder girdle.

Stick Balance Tests

Bass[23] explored the reliability of tests for static and dynamic balance. This research resulted in the development of a stick balance test for stationary balance. Several variations of the test requiring different positions with eyes opened and closed were studied. Bass concluded that the eyes are important senses in maintaining equilibrium. The Bass stick test requires the subject to stand on a stick 1 inch wide, 1 inch high, and twelve inches long with one foot. This test can be completed with foot placement crosswise or lengthwise.

Dynamic Balance Test

The distinguishing variable between stationary and dynamic balance involves the moving pattern of the body. Dynamic balance requires constant gross changes in posture. These posture changes are in a stance and/or dynamic actions depending on the nature of motor skill required for successful performance. Walking, jumping, leaping, sitting, diving, putting the shot, twisting movements, and swimming are examples of motor movements that necessitate dynamic balance functions. Three tests commonly referred to in the literature as measures of dynamic balance are (1) *balance beam test*, (2) *stepping stone test*, and (3) *sideward leap test*.

Springfield Balance Beam-Walking Test. This test, developed by Harold Seashore,[24] consists of walking on nine beams of equal length and height but varying with widths from four to one-fourth inches. The objective is to walk ten steps on each of the progressively narrower beams in a heel-to-toe fashion with hands on hips. Variations of the Springfield Beam-Walking Test have been used by various investigators.[25,26] This test is reasonably reliable as one technique of assessing upright dynamic balance performance.

Stepping Stone Test. A classic dynamic balance test called the stepping stone test was developed by Bass.[27] Essentially, this test measures the ability to jump and maintain balance moving from a designated position to another. Figure 8.18 shows the jumping pattern. The subject stands on the right foot and leaps to the next circle on the left foot, holding a steady balance up to one but not exceeding five seconds. The individual jumps to the next succeeding circle (total of ten) alternating from right to left leg. Three practice trials are recommended with two attempts

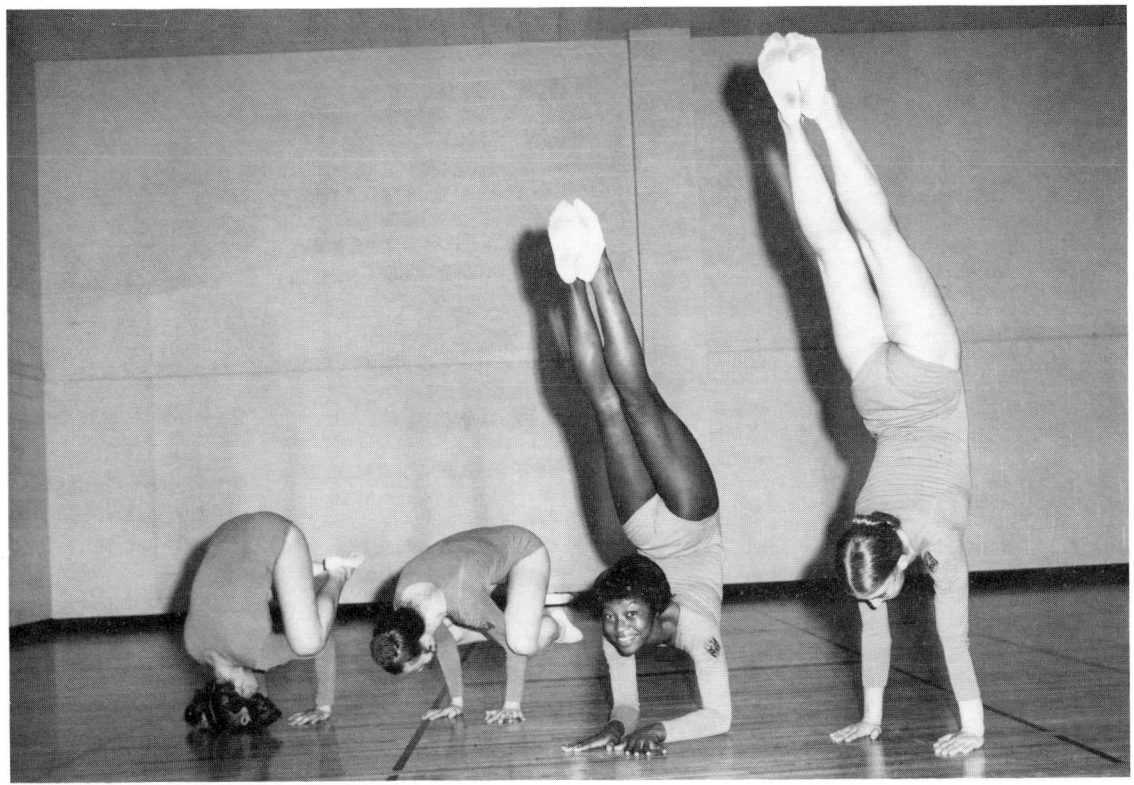

Figure 8.17 Progressive inverted balance positions: (a) tripod balance, (b) tip-up balance, (c) forearm balance, (d) handstand

used as official scoring. Specific test details may be found in reference 4.

It should be remembered that this technique attempts to assess upright dynamic balance and must not be interpreted to measure an individual's inverted or total balance ability in all dynamic movements.

Sideward Leap Test. This test attempts to measure the ability of the subject to jump and land accurately, perform a task, hold a balance position for five seconds, and return to a designated mark.

A similar balance leap was utilized as an integral element in the measurement of kinesthesis.[28] This test entailed a sideward leap,

forward bend, moving an object on the floor, and subsequently holding balance at least five seconds, with the score equal to the time balance is held. Essentially, this test is of the dynamic upright classification.

Other Balance Tests

Other dynamic balance tests have been devised utilizing various pieces of specialized apparatus. One of these, the *stabilometer*, consists of a platform mounted on a universal joint, which requires the subject to hold the platform as steady as possible, while standing with feet together and hands at the sides.[29] Blann[30] devised a *balance board machine*

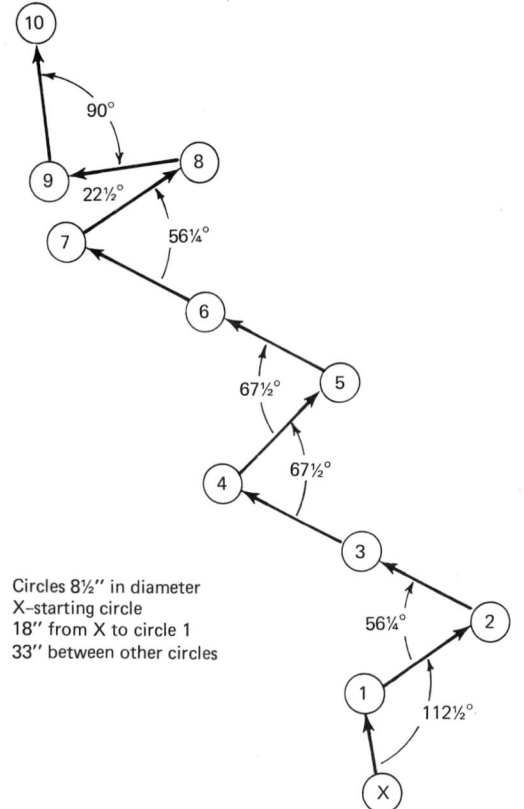

Figure 8.18 Stepping stone test (from Ruth Bass, "An Analysis of Components of Tests of Semicircular Canal Function and Static and Dynamic Balance," **Research Quarterly** X:33–51, May, 1939, with permission)

consisting of a wooden board measuring $36 \times 13 \times 1$ inches complete with an electrical microswitch attachment used as a timing device. Mitchem and Popp[31] constructed an *octagonal balance apparatus* similar to the balance board system using an eight-sided plane. Both systems graphically record the imbalance of the subject using microswitches.

Each of these devices, (1) *balance board*, (2) *stabilometer*, and (3) *octagonal balance sphere*, is chiefly operative in a laboratory setting. This sophisticated equipment requires a great deal of time to use and is of questionable value as a practical tool for measuring balance elements in school situations, especially where large classes are prevalent. However, the interested coach, working with small specialized groups concerned with balance assessment and skill development, may employ these research methods to secure fairly accurate balancing data.

SPECIAL BALANCE PROBLEMS

Balance in Water

Previous discussion of balance and equilibrium has been directed to man functioning on land and subject to the earth's gravitational pull of 32 ft/sec/sec. Man's land motor movements, including balance, are also governed by Newton's basic laws of motion. Under the first law, a body is in equilibrium if no free force is acting upon it. The determination of a weight with which a body is in equilibrium if a force applied to it is met by a counterforce of equal size and opposite direction supports Newton's second law. Under the third law, a body is in equilibrium if all forces acting upon it mutually neutralize each other so that the resulting force is zero. The application of Newton's laws affecting balance is significantly altered when man is submerged in an aquatic environment. These laws are affected by the individual's equilibrium in water. For most individuals, body position adjustments must be made in order for the swimmer to remain on the water surface. Insead of the normal constant pull of gravity toward the earth, as in land balancing activities, water can act as a *supporting* medium at varying levels depending upon the person's specific gravity and ability to control the rotating effect of his center of buoyancy. Generally, the movement posture in water is in the prone or supine position moving in a sagittal plane. Consequently, balance in water involves the control of a first-class lever system (total body). The lever components of man in water must accommodate the relative position of the center of gravity and center of buoyancy. The center of gravity and buoyancy loci is integrally interwoven with the individual's body density. As described in Chapter 3, heredity and ethnic backgrounds influence body density and directly affect buoyancy. Differences also exist between the sexes. Since women generally possess more adipose tissue than men, it is an accepted truism that females are superior to men in floating ability. Whiting[32,33] studied 875 females, ages 10 to 18 years of age and 1,040 males, ages 9 to 24 years and found that female floating ability is superior, compared with males from the age of 13 years and onward.

Center of Rotation in Water

Body density represents a somatotype component, which, as stated earlier, affects bouyancy. High body density enhances the "sinking ability" of the individual, whereas low body density promotes floating qualities. Additionally, bouyancy is affected by body positioning. Generally, an individual rotates around the fulcrum located in the *thoracic area*, since this part of the body is the most buoyant component when considering the body as a lever of the first class. Anthropometrically, the center of gravity is in the hip (slightly lower in females), which displaces a greater proportion of weight from the center of buoyancy located in the chest area. Consequently, the rotatory lever effect of body weight loci creates a downward pull of the leg, resulting in angular floating for most individuals. Persons with heavy legs and high specific gravity manifest sharper body angulation to the point where a few individuals are unable to float at any angle. This rotatory leverage force can be regulated, provided natural body density of weight per unit volume is less than that of water (specific gravity). Flexing hips and knees, and extending arms over head, raises the center of gravity (hips) closer to the center of buoyancy (fulcrum) or the point at which

the body rotates. The equalization of weight at each end of the fulcrum allows the body to balance and float in a horizontal supine position. Figure 8.19 shows the various body positions and its rotatory lever effects.

As the center of gravity moves closer to the center of buoyancy (fulcrum), the subject is able to float horizontally due to minimizing of the downward rotatory force of the legs.

In certain individuals, specific gravity is so low, because of adipose tissue, that they displace a volume of water that weighs more than their body. This results in a lowering of the center of buoyancy downward in the body to a point where the center of gravity and center of buoyancy coincide, and the individual floats easily in a horizontal position.

Figure 8.19 Lever affect on various floating positions. O = center of buoyancy; X = center of gravity

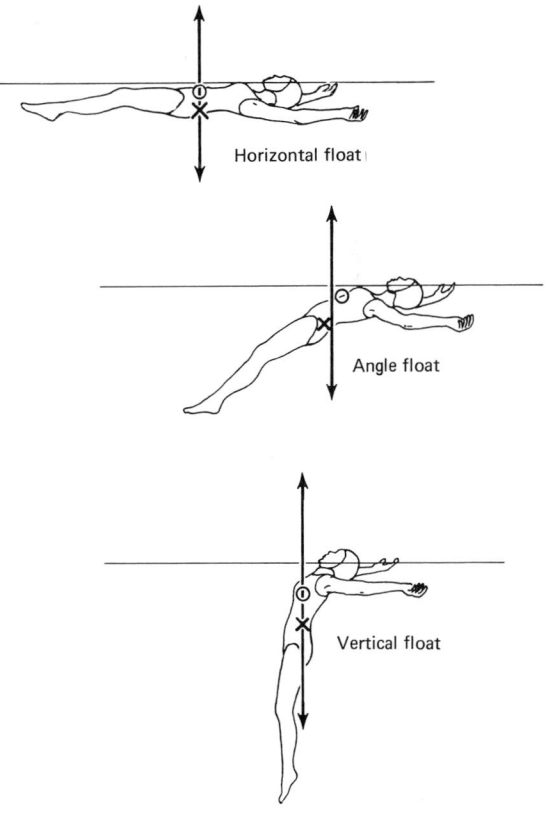

Horizontal float

Angle float

Vertical float

The general age trend of fat in man reflects the peaks of fatness being in early childhood and in late maturity.[34] These fat variations appear to give credence to Whiting's findings of poor floating ability among males between 13 and 18 years of age.[35] High body density generally characterizes male physiques during adolescence and early maturity and may explain why it takes longer periods of instruction to teach swimming skills to senior high school and college-age students. Balanced floating skills are simply more difficult among individuals with lean body mass and high specific gravity.

BALANCE AND ORTHOPEDIC ABERRATIONS

Balance and equilibrium among individuals with anatomical deviations such as loss of limbs, gross muscular deficiency, and extreme aberrations in somatotype can pose special balance problems. For example, it is more difficult for a person with one leg to hold a balanced starting position in swimming simply because the center of gravity is no longer located approximately between the pubic bones of the hips and equally distributed over both feet. The center of gravity has shifted to one side at a point directly over one foot, which represents a smaller base of support. Further instability is added by the center of gravity moving upward toward the chest, due to the loss of body weight by the absence of a leg. Prosthetic devices help to normalize the location of the gravity center by replacing the mass or weight loss.

Although prosthetic appliances aid the individual, these devices never seem to be equal substitutes, and the individual must relearn the kinetics and mechanics of controlling balance. Although changes in centers of gravity occur, stability follows the basic principle that the line of gravity and weight center must remain over the support base. Muscular strength development is an important part of

a corrective program for individuals with orthopedic problems since muscles provide the force in attaining and maintaining balance for everyday functioning activities. Moving from one position to another, whether inverted or upright, involves the loss and gain of body equilibrium. Muscular strength provides the force for correcting errors as the individual strives to maintain the line of gravity within its supporting base.

Inverted balance activities favor individuals with light hips and legs. Persons with paralytic limbs or other somatotype deviations, which result in centering the weight mass toward the chest area, possess greater stability in a hand-balance or inverted position. It is not uncommon for athletes with lower body orthopedic aberrations to become superior in gymnastic balancing activities. Muscular development of the upper body coupled with a lowered gravity center in the inverted position provides a natural equilibrium arrangement of the body.

CEREBRAL PALSY AND MOTOR DYSFUNCTIONS

Balancing, upright or inverted, for persons with brain injuries and other conditions such as cerebral palsy affecting the central nervous system can be exceedingly difficult (see Figure 8.20). These individuals must volitionally learn to keep the center of gravity within the base of support, in spite of impairment of the neural impulses from sensory perception to motor effectors. Balance in the walking process is usually laborious, since the alignment of the trunk over the pelvis is disturbed; the rhythmic shortening and lengthening of the leg is handicapped by the rigidity of the muscles, and for the same reason, the free forward and backward swing of the limb is impeded. Balance mechanisms, including proprioception and vestibular apparatus, may be intact among cerebral palsied individuals; however, the problem lies with the

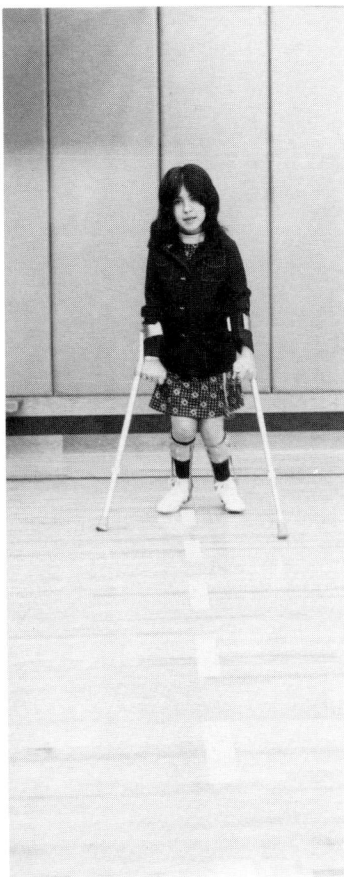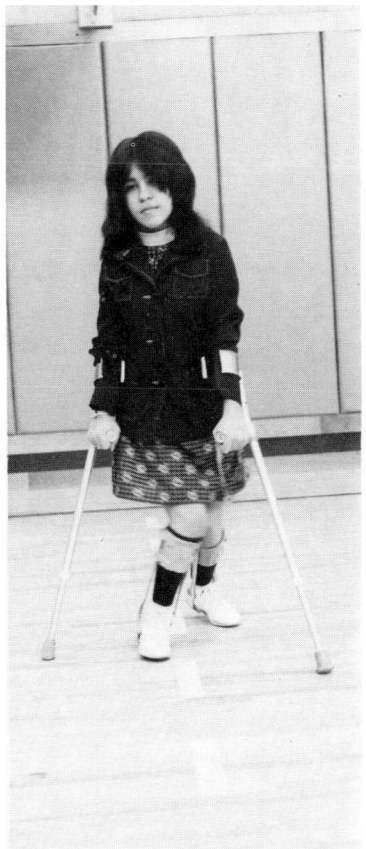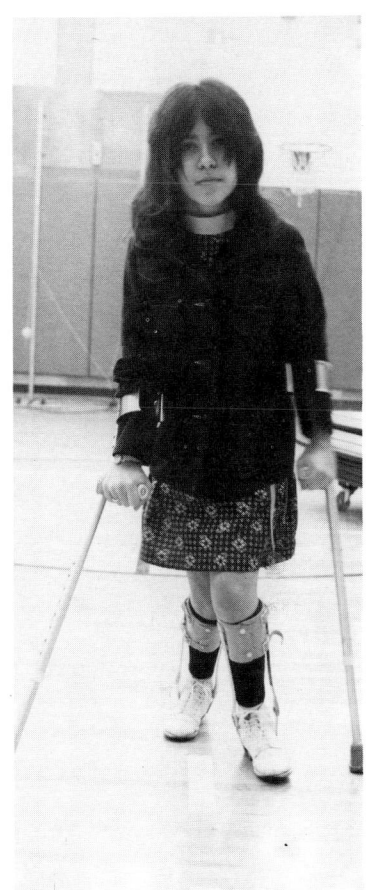

Figure 8.20 Student using floor vertical line as visual clue in maintaining crutch walking balance and stability

neuromuscular dysfunction and the inability of the individual to control muscular motor movements. Topographically, various parts of the body, depending upon the extent of brain damage, are affected. These conditions range from monoplegic (one limb involved) to quadriplegic (four limbs involved). It is not uncommon to observe spastic individuals moving swiftly. The maintenance of equilibrium is easier when the patient with precarious balance is moving hurriedly in order to decrease the requirements for lateral stability.

Other Specific Activities

Physical activities that reinforce dynamic fitness components of balance, strength, neuromuscular skills, and relaxation are suggested for individuals with conditions affecting motor performance. The concept of self-improvement rather than competition with others should be accented.

Upright dynamic balance skills can be enhanced through exercises utilizing the wide balance beam shown in Figure 8.21. Visual clues of eye focus at one end of the beam as-

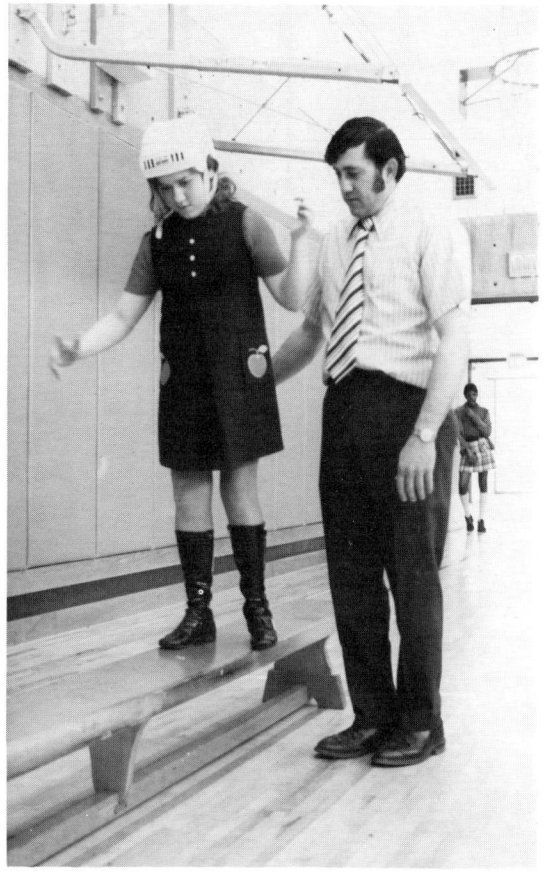
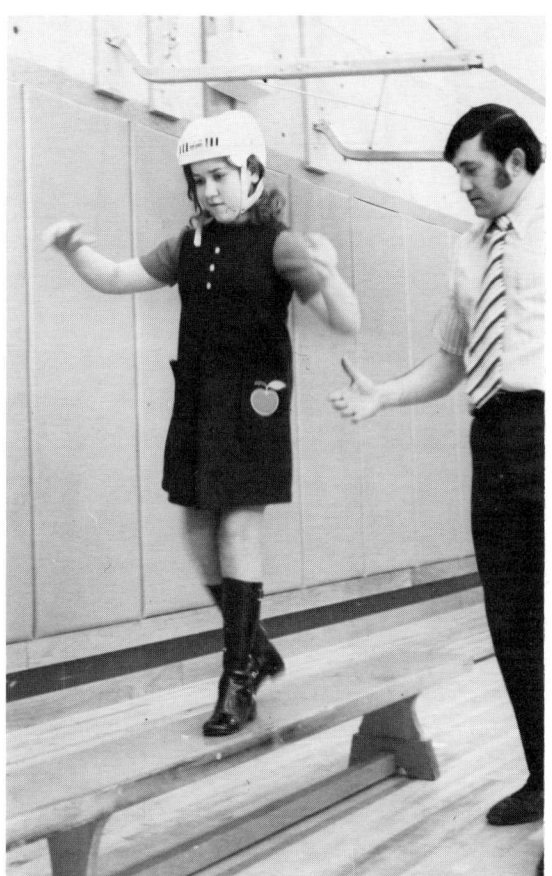

Figure 8.21 Improving upright dynamic balance using wide balance beam apparatus

sist the student in the maintenance of balance during the walking exercise.

Muscular strength provides the power and force affecting motor movements and is especially important as an antidote to fatigue. Muscular strength also aids in developing balance control. This element is particularly important in the correction of balance errors as the brain damaged youngster performs functional tasks of walking, running, turning, jumping, etc.

Learning how to shift the body center of gravity without loss of balance and stability in walking entails the reciprocal action of the agonistic and antagonistic muscles. Figure 8.22 illustrates a student with cerebral palsy (mixed type) using the low parallel bars and horizontal gait ladder apparatus.

An improvised strap shoulder harness (Figure 8.23), when equipment is not available, may also be utilized to assist the student in balance and neuromuscular coordination walking exercises.

Floating and swimming activities augment relaxation and balance elements of the cerebral palsied. The limited motor performance level of the spastic individual is made more relaxing and comfortable, since water buoy-

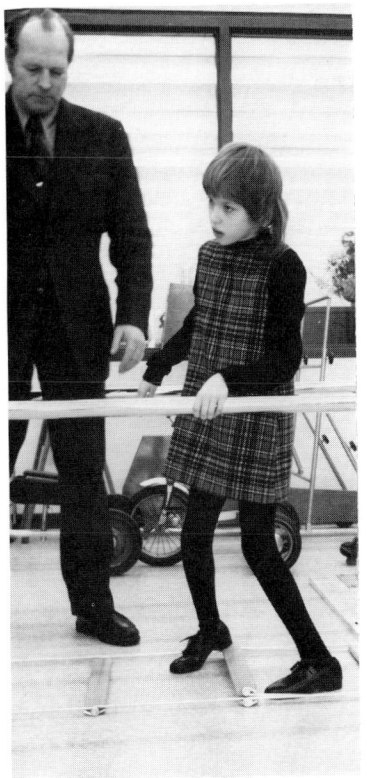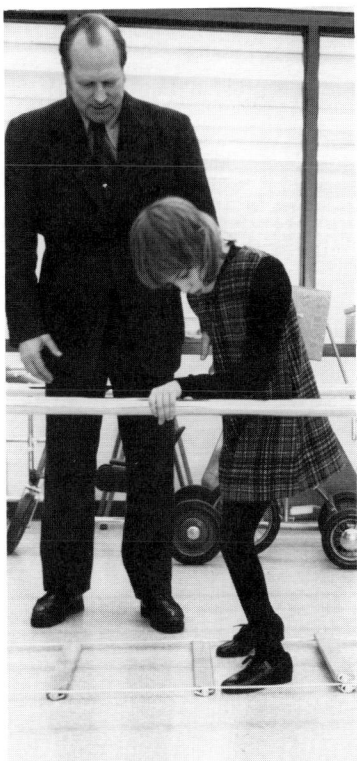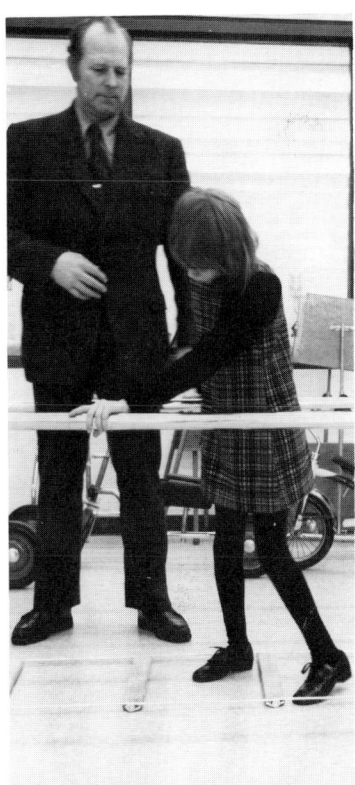

Figure 8.22 Parallel bars and walking gait ladder
utilized to improve balance in walking

ancy allows free movement of the youngster's limbs. Prone and back floating positions shown in Figure 8.24 also stimulate the balance sensory mechanisms of the ear vestibule and proprioceptors.

Youngsters with mild to moderate brain damage impairment, who can ambulate without instructor assistance, should be encouraged to use the hand-rail attachment as a progressive step to walking unassisted.

Activities designed to further develop neuromuscular control conducted at a slower than normal pace are recommended. Calisthenic exercises such as the jumping-jack and simple push-ups help to educate the antagonistic or stretch muscles as well as the overall balance ability of the individual.

SUMMARY

Balance and equilibrium are essential fundamental component elements for everyday efficient and safe living. Anatomical, physiological, and kinesthestic aspects dynamically interact to produce deficient or sufficient performance. Balance ability can be improved through physical activity. Balance classifications encompass two broad types, *stationary* and *dynamic* categories.

Balance control is affected by the following external and internal factors: (1) gravitational constancy, (2) mass, (3) base of support, (4) center of gravity, and (5) line of gravity.

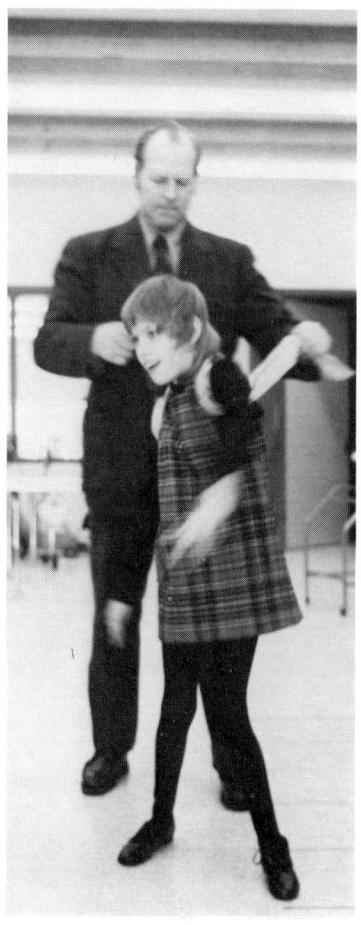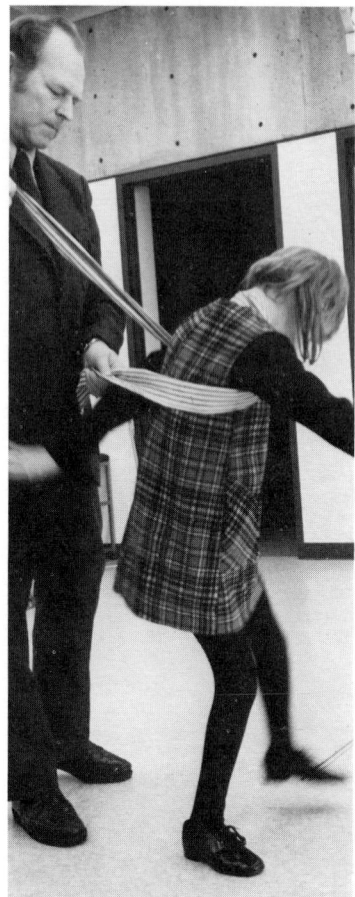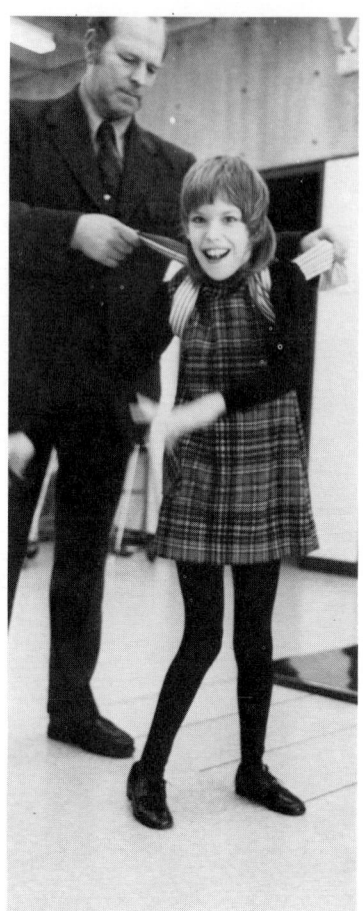

Figure 8.23 Instructor utilizing hand/shoulder harness to assist student in maintaining walking balance and stability

Attaining upright stationary balance is easier with a pyramid-shaped object than when the pyramid is inverted. Positive correlations do not necessarily exist between inverted and upright balance skills.

The height and length of the individual's limbs does affect balance ability. Inverted and upright balance positions are more precarious for tall individuals than for short persons with low centers of gravity. Inverted balance positions favor persons with light hips and legs.

Balance is also affected by *internal* and *external* leverage. Generally, internal body leverages are "out-of-balance," with short force and long resistance arms. Precise balance is attained externally, when the fulcrum is exactly between the resistance point and the force point (first-class lever).

Balance becomes more precarious when nervous system lesions interfere with the delicate interplay of the pelvis, head, and shoulders.

The human sensory apparatus of visual clues, ears, proprioceptors, and kinesthesis have considerable impact on the individual's balance ability. *Visual acuity and perception* serve as a physiological point of reference.

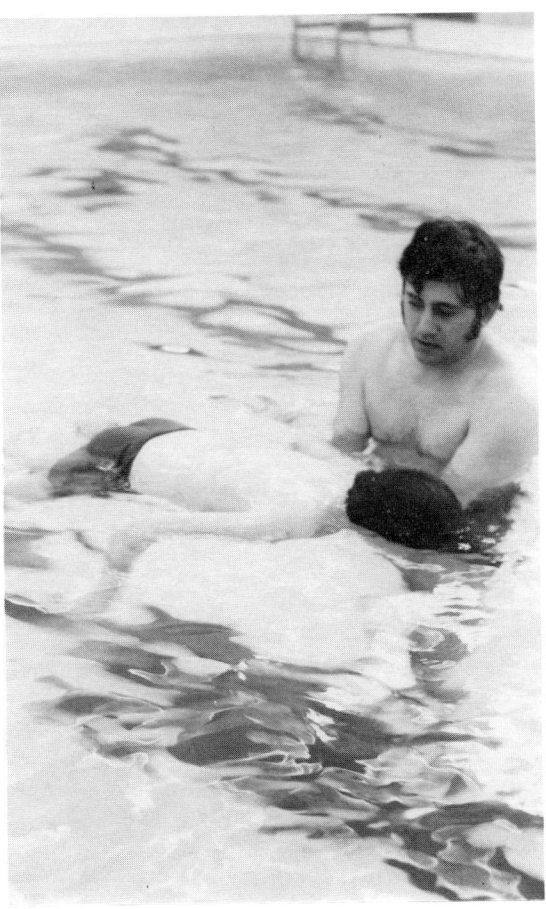

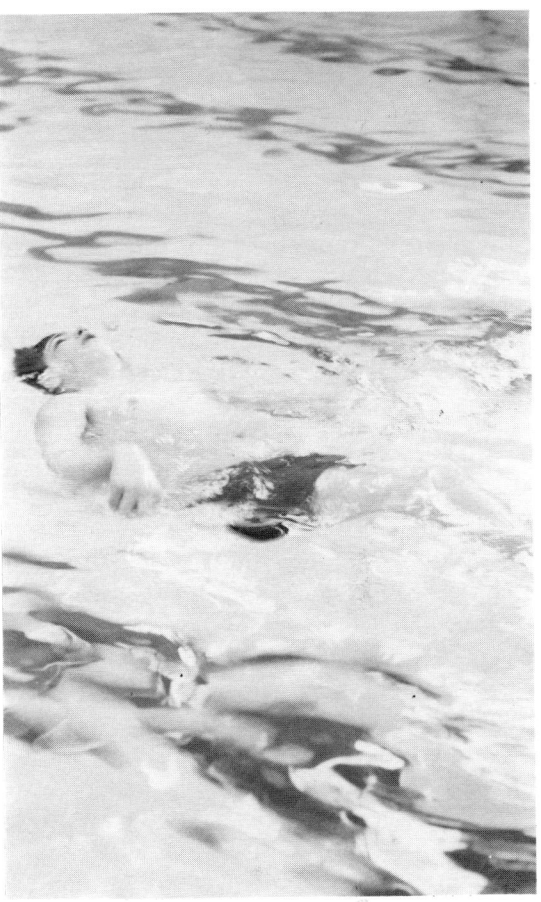

Figure 8.24 Improving balance in water through floating skills—cerebral palsy (spastic)

Ears contain the important vestibular apparatus essential for body position sense, particularly head movements. Deaf students do not necessarily have poor balance, unless the inner vestibule is impaired. *Proprioception* aids the individual's balance sensitivity by providing sensory perception originating in the muscles, tendons, and joints.

Balancing ability is an integral part of kinesthesia or "position sense."

The scale and photographic methods are utilized to determine the center of gravity in human balance.

Other methods of determining the center of gravity with inanimate objects have been devised. These methods include *cardboard and paper clip procedure* and *template method*.

A number of tests have been developed to assess human ability. The following stationary balance tests have been utilized by various investigators: (1) *gross body equilibrium test*, (2) *progressive inverted balance test*, and (3) *stick balance test*. The balance beam, stepping stone, and sideward leap tests have been utilized to measure dynamic ability. Other tests requiring laboratory procedures, such as (1) balance board, (2) stabilometer, and (3) octagonal balance sphere, have been used to measure balance in humans.

Special balance problems encompass the following areas: (1) balance in water, (2) orthopedic aberrations, and (3) other motor dysfunctions.

Low specific gravity and *low body density* favor high floating of the individual. When the center of buoyancy and the center of gravity are at the same point (hip area), the individual will float in a horizontal position. The center of gravity and center of buoyancy can be brought closer together by hip/leg flexion and arm extension, which helps to reduce the downward rotatory force of the legs in the horizontal float position.

Individuals with orthopedic aberrations possess different centers of gravity. Leg amputees generally have high gravity centers due to the loss of lower limb weight. In addition, a shift of gravity locus to one side of the body results when a single limb amputation exists. Prosthetic devices help to normalize the location of the gravity center by replacing the mass or weight loss.

Strength development is especially important for balance control among orthopedically handicapped individuals.

Individuals with spasticity and other motor dysfunctions have difficulty maintaining the line of gravity within its support base. Persons with impaired neuromuscular control often move more swiftly for the maintenance of balance in order to reduce the requirements of lateral stability.

Exercises that educate the stretching or antagonistic muscles, as well as the kinesthetic interplay of changing body positions, aid in the improvement of functional body balance.

REFERENCES

1. Rasch, Philip J., and Burke, Roger K., *Kinesiology and Applied Anatomy*, 6th ed. Philadelphia: Lea and Febiger, 1978, p. 100.
2. Rasch and Burke, *op. cit.*, p. 95.
3. Dyson, Geoffrey H. O., *The Mechanics of Athletics*, 6th ed. Warwick Square, London E.C4: University of London Press Ltd., 1973, p. 61.
4. Bass, Ruth I., "An Analysis of the Components of Tests of Semicircular Canal Function and Static and Dynamic Balance," *Research Quarterly*, X:33–51, May, 1939.
5. McCloy, C. H., "A Preliminary Study of Factors in Motor Educability," *Research Quarterly*, XI:28–39, May, 1940.
6. Rasch and Burke, *op. cit.*, p. 101.
7. Gardner, Elizabeth B., "Proprioceptive Reflexes and Their Participation in Motor Skills," *Quest*, XII:1–25, Spring, 1969.
8. Wisher, Peter R., "Dance and the Deaf," *Journal of Health, Physical Education and Recreation*, 40:81–84, March, 1969.
9. Gardner, Elizabeth B., "The Neuromuscular Base of Human Movement: Feedback Mechanics," *Journal of Health, Physical Education and Recreation*, 36:61–62, October, 1965.
10. Bass, *op. cit.*, p. 38.
11. Scott, Gladys, M., "Measurement of Kinesthesis," *Research Quarterly*, 26:324–341, October, 1955.
12. Johnson, Barry L., and Nelson, Jack K., *Practical Measurements for Evaluation in Physical Education*, 3rd ed. Minneapolis, Minn: Burgess Publishing Co., 1979, Chapter 18.
13. Wiebe, Vernon, "A Study of Tests of Kinesthesis," *Research Quarterly*, 25:222–227, May, 1954.
14. Mumby, H. Hugh, "Kinesthetic Acuity and Balance Related to Wrestling Ability," *Research Quarterly*, 24:327–334, October, 1953.
15. Wells, Katharine, and Luttgens, Kathryn, *Kinesiology: Scientific Basis of Human Motion*, 6th ed. Philadelphia: W. B. Saunders, 1976, p. 369.
16. Rasch and Burke, *op. cit.*, p. 94.
17. Methany, Eleanor, *Body Dynamics*. New York: McGraw-Hill, 1952, pp. 98–99.
18. Walton, James S., "A Template for Locating Segmental Centers of Gravity," *Research Quarterly*, 41:615–617, December, 1970.
19. Johnson and Nelson, *op. cit.*, pp. 239–240.
20. Walton, *op. cit.*, p. 615.
21. Fleishman, Edwin A., *Examiner's Manual for the Basic Fitness Tests*. Englewood Cliffs, N.J.: Prentice-Hall, 1964, p. 4.
22. Johnson and Nelson, *op. cit.*, pp. 230–232.

23. Bass, *op. cit.*, pp. 31–51.
24. Seashore, Harold G., "The Development of a Beam Walking Test and Its Use in Measuring Development of Balance in Children," *Research Quarterly*, 18:246-259, December, 1947.
25. Scott, *op. cit.*, pp. 324-341.
26. Espenschade, Anna, Dable, Robert R., Schoendube, Robert, "Dynamic Balance in Adolescent Boys," *Research Quarterly*, 24:270-275, October, 1953.
27. Bass, *op. cit.*, p. 36.
28. Scott, *op. cit.*, pp. 324-341.
29. Travis, Roland C., "A New Stabilometer for Measuring Dynamic Equilibrium," *Journal of Experimental Psychology*, 24:418-423, October, 1944.
30. Blann, Mary E., "An Investigation of Dynamic Balance Ability Among School Children," Unpublished Master's Project, State University of New York at Buffalo, 1967.
31. Mitchem, John C., and Popp, H. J., "A Modification of the Gilmore Octagonal Balance Apparatus," *Research Quarterly*, 40:246, March, 1969.
32. Whiting, H. T. A., "Variations in Floating Ability with Age in the Female," *Research Quarterly*, 36:216-218, March, 1965.
33. Whiting, H. T. A., "Variations in Floating Ability with Age in the Male," *Research Quarterly*, 34:84-90, March, 1963.
34. Keys, Ancel, and Brozek, Josef, "Body Fat in Adult Man," *Physiological Reviews*, 33:245-325, July, 1953.
35. Whiting, 1963, *op. cit.*, p. 90.

PART **3** APPLIED ASPECTS OF KINESIOLOGY

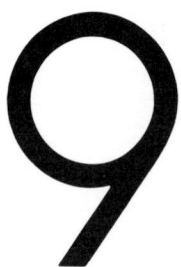

ANALYSIS OF SELECTED TUMBLING AND GYMNASTIC SKILLS

CONCEPTS

1. Gymnastics demands a high degree of both static and dynamic balance; therefore, gymnasts should learn the principles of balance.

2. The physical educator should present a large number of skills and permit students to select moves to be learned.

3. Physical educators teaching gymnastic classes and coaches of gymnastics should familiarize students with principles of spotting, absorption of impact, and other safety procedures and skills.

4. The execution of gymnastic and tumbling moves requires utilization of both kinesthetic and visual perception.

5. Many gymnastic and tumbling moves are the result of the summation of forces.

6. Gymnasts and tumblers need to understand the principles of centrifugal force in order to know when to effect releases or other movements during circling moves.

7. In many gymnastic moves momentum is transferred from a part of the body to the entire body and can be increased or decreased by changing velocity rather than mass.

8. The end of the body (or a body part) farthest from the center of rotation is moving faster than that part of the body nearest the

center of rotation and consequently possesses greater momentum, as is demonstrated in the giant swing.

9. The height reached and the trajectory of the center of gravity of the gymnast's body is determined at the instant of release from the apparatus or spring from the Reuther board, trampoline, mat, or balance beam.

10. The critical point in initiating a movement during circling moves around a fixed support is usually just as the center of gravity passes a point directly under the hands.

11. To initiate rotation around any of the three axes, force must be applied at an angle to the axis. The greater this force and the longer the force arm, the greater will be the speed of rotation.

12. There are three ways in which twisting movements are accomplished: (1) the "direct" method, (2) the "action–reaction twist," and (3) "twisting from a pike or arch."

13. Practice makes for consistency but not necessarily for perfection.

GENERAL CONSIDERATIONS

The major objective in the teaching of motor skills is to facilitate learning of motor skills. If the teaching is effective and efficient, the other more important objectives such as enhanced self-image, improved total fitness, enhanced social behaviors, and lifelong interest in the activity are more likely to follow. Physical educators should possess a reasonably thorough knowledge of human anatomy, particularly of muscles and joints, in order to prescribe exercises to facilitate student success in learning sports skills and to provide clues for first aid and athletic training procedures. However, a detailed analysis of the many muscle and joint actions involved in execution of even the simplest of movements serves research purposes but may be a deterrent to learning.

Gymnastics calls for an almost unlimited variety of movements and positions; consequently, this sport calls into use a greater number of the kinesiologic principles than does any other sport. For this reason, teachers and coaches of gymnastics should possess a thorough knowledge and understanding of kinesiology. This knowledge will enable them to analyze movements, body positions, and timing necessary for execution of any gymnastic movement even though they have never executed the movement themselves. If teachers of gymnastics teach some of these principles to their students, they will find that their students will learn more rapidly.

Doubles Balancing Skills

The front swan on feet shown in Figure 9.1 can teach students several important principles of balance. In the initiation of this move, efforts must be made to eliminate introduction of a rotary force upon the understander's legs as the topmounter moves into the final position. This is done by having the topmounter stand as close to the buttocks of the understander as possible. This enables the understander (who begins lying on his back with his feet on the topmounter's hips at his

center of gravity) to move his feet directly upward in a line perpendicular to the base of support—his own hip bones. At the same time, the understander must maintain his lower legs in as nearly a perpendicular position as possible. To attain this position, he must bend his knees and move his thighs downward against his torso as the topmounter lies down on his feet. After the topmounter is in position on his feet, the understander extends his knees so that the center of weight of the topmounter is directly over the vertical columns of the understander's legs. If the understander's legs are angled to either direction of the vertical, he will find it quite difficult to support his partner. Understanders have supported three people in a three-high stand in this position. As long as the weight is centered directly over the vertically aligned bones of the legs there is little strain. This stunt is a demonstration of the concept that states: *"The center of gravity should be as nearly as possible between the points of support."*

It will be noted that the entire back, as well as the hips and arms of the understander, are against the mat. This is in conformity with the concept that states: *"The larger the base of support, the greater the stability,"* as pointed out in Chapter 8.

MANIPULATION OF THE CENTER OF GRAVITY IN GYMNASTICS

Changes in the Location of the Center of Gravity

The location of the center of gravity of the body changes as the body or its parts are placed in different positions. The truth of this statement can be readily illustrated in the front swan on feet shown in Figure 9.1. If the topmounter bends her knees while in the final

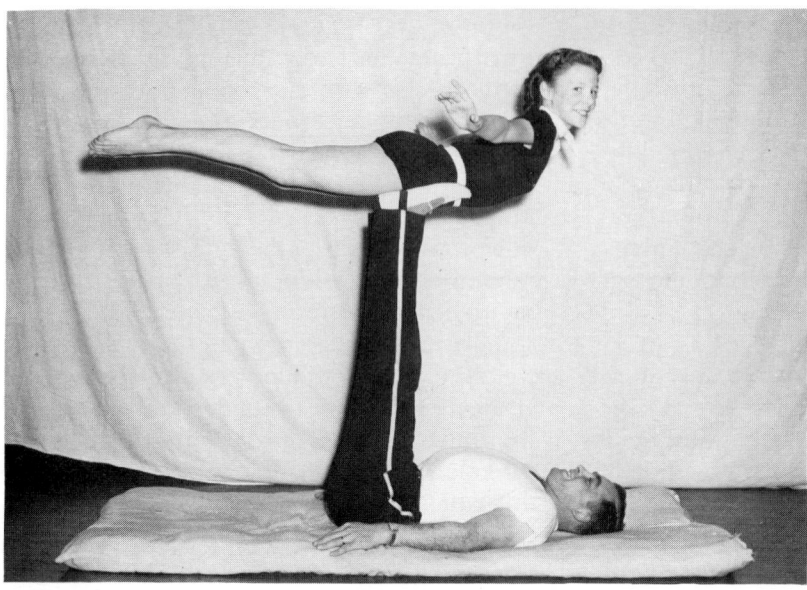

Figure 9.1 Front swan

balanced position, her trunk and head will drop downward. Also, by moving her extended arms forward or backward her center of balance will be moved forward or backward.

If the understander will attempt this skill first with a person who has heavy thick legs and relatively small trunk, shoulders, and arms and then with a person who has thin legs and buttocks and heavily muscled thorax, shoulders, and arms, he will be convinced that: "*The location of the center of gravity is different in different people.*" With the first person, the understander will find it necessary to place the feet on the lower part of the partner's hips while with the second he will have to place them higher—perhaps even on the partner's abdomen.

Center of Gravity and Base of Support

In the illustrations of the one-hand balance, the one-hand to one-arm half lever, the stand on knees, the fulcrum, the quadruple thigh stand, and the high father time (Figures 9.2 to 9.7), if a perpendicular line is drawn from the center of the base of support, it will be noted that half the weight of each ensemble is on each side of the line. Obviously, the center of weight must be over the center of support.

Visual Clues in Gymnastic Events

One of the authors received a lesson on the importance of keeping the center of support under the center of gravity when he decided to learn to do the 30-foot belt perch pole number outside for the first time. In the gymnasium, the pole was lined up with the ceiling girders. Outdoors (Figure 9.8), without realizing he was doing so, the understander lined up the pole visually on a cloud, which was moving. The understander ran the length of the field trying to keep the center of support under the forward moving center of gravity while the topmounter hung on for his life. Visual clues are important in balance activity whether the activity is static or dynamic. This is why beginners are instructed to focus on the center of the end of the frame when bouncing on the trampoline and on the end of the balance beam when performing in this event (see Chapter 8).

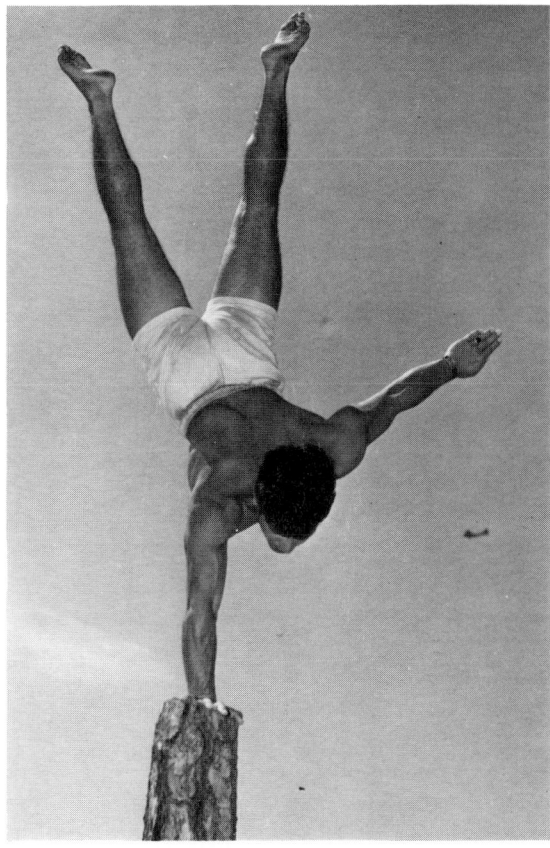

Figure 9.2 One-hand balance

Rotary Force in Lifts to a Balancing Position

When performing the clean and jerk or the snatch in weight lifting, or when lifting a partner overhead, the trajectory should be directly upward. This movement is illustrated in the jump into a high front swan on hands (Figure 9.9). In the jump into a high front swan on the hands, the understander places his hands on his partner's hips at her center of gravity. She grasps his shoulders while standing as close to him as possible. She leaps directly upward and, as she does, the understander bends his knees and hips to drop under her rising center of gravity, keeping his back and forearms vertical. While she still has upward momentum, he extends his knees, hips, and arms. If these movements

are properly timed, there will be a minimum of effort (summation of forces). It may be necessary for the understander to step forward in order to move the base of support directly under his topmounter's center of gravity. If the understander were to keep his arms extended during the lift, it is unlikely that he would have sufficient strength to lift his partner, and it is extremely unlikely that he would possess sufficient strength to prevent her from continuing to move beyond his head after she had reached the top. The straight-arm lift fails to keep the center of support at all times under the center of weight. This method also introduces a rotary force, which will force the understander's arms beyond the vertical position overhead, causing failure.

Figure 9.3 One-hand to one-arm half lever

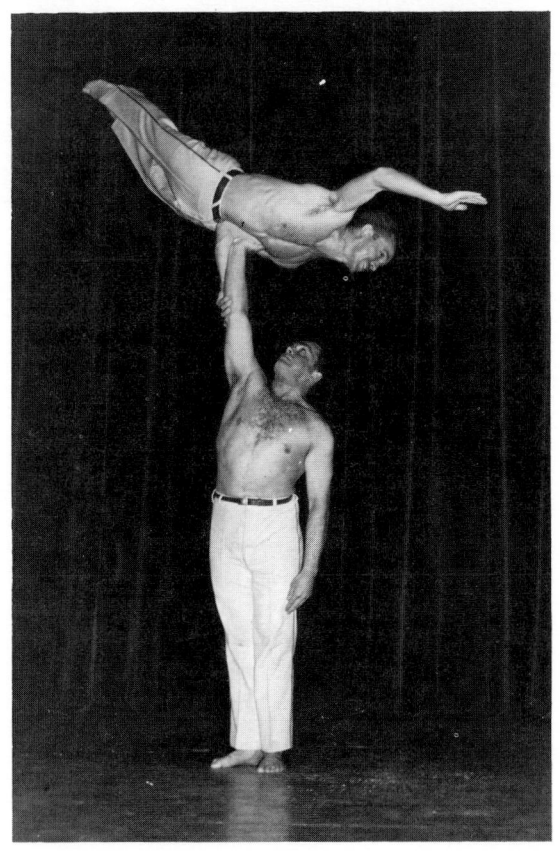

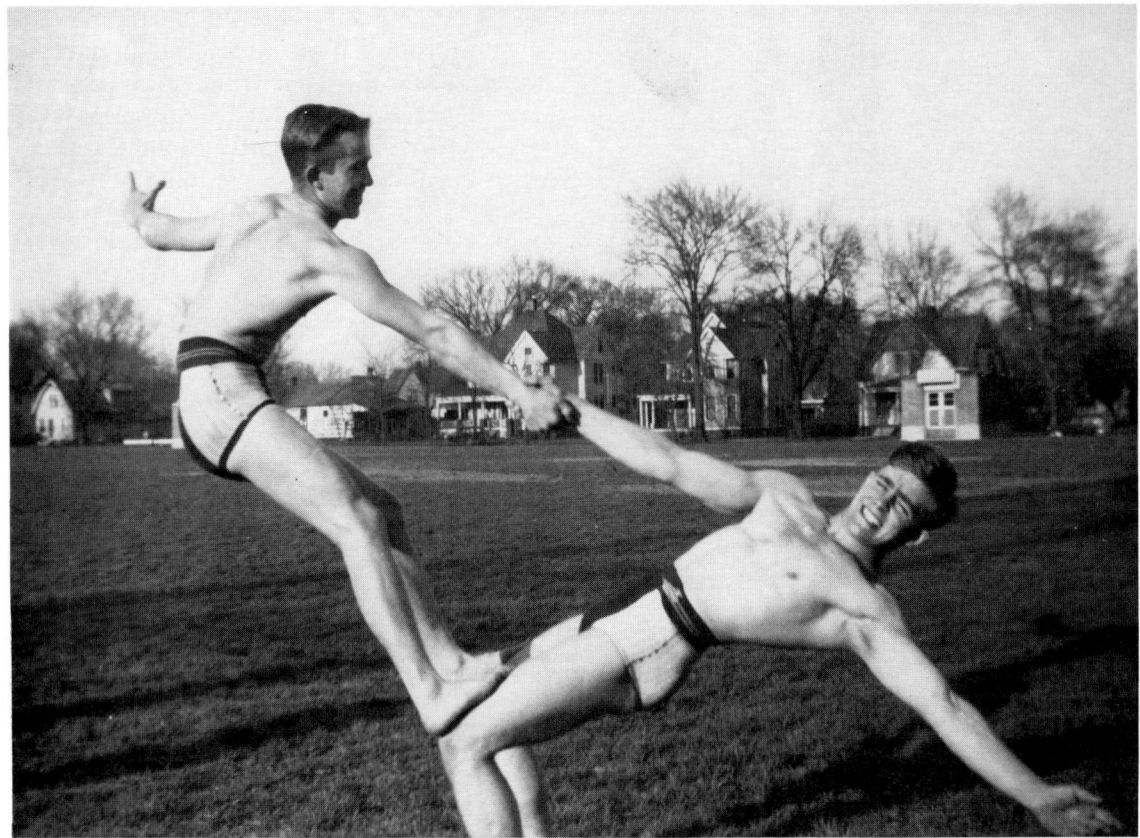

Figure 9.4 Stand on knees

FUNDAMENTAL GYMNASTIC SKILLS AND UTILIZATION OF KINESIOLOGIC PRINCIPLES

Most people enjoy those things that they do reasonably well. All persons participate most frequently in those leisure activities that they most enjoy. Obese or large-boned individuals will experience little success in gymnastics and tumbling. These people should be taught activities in which there is a higher probability of success. Participants of medial or ectomorphic-mesomorphic body type are most likely to succeed in gymnastics and tumbling. Mesomorphs have a higher center of gravity relative to their height, which is a decided advantage when executing handstands, circling moves, or twisting. Mesomorphs generally possess greater strength per unit of weight.

This quality, when combined with the leanness and light bones of the ectomorph, provides a great advantage in learning gymnastic skills. This is true because in gymnastics the participant is not required to manipulate an implement such as a ball, racquet, shot, discus, bat, javelin, nor to manipulate an opponent. He must manipulate his own body. This is why, in gymnastics, strength relative to body weight rather than raw strength makes for proficiency. The number of chin-ups a student can perform is a good single measure of gymnastic potential.

The Handstand

The strength of muscle groups involved in a particular move must be adequate for execu-

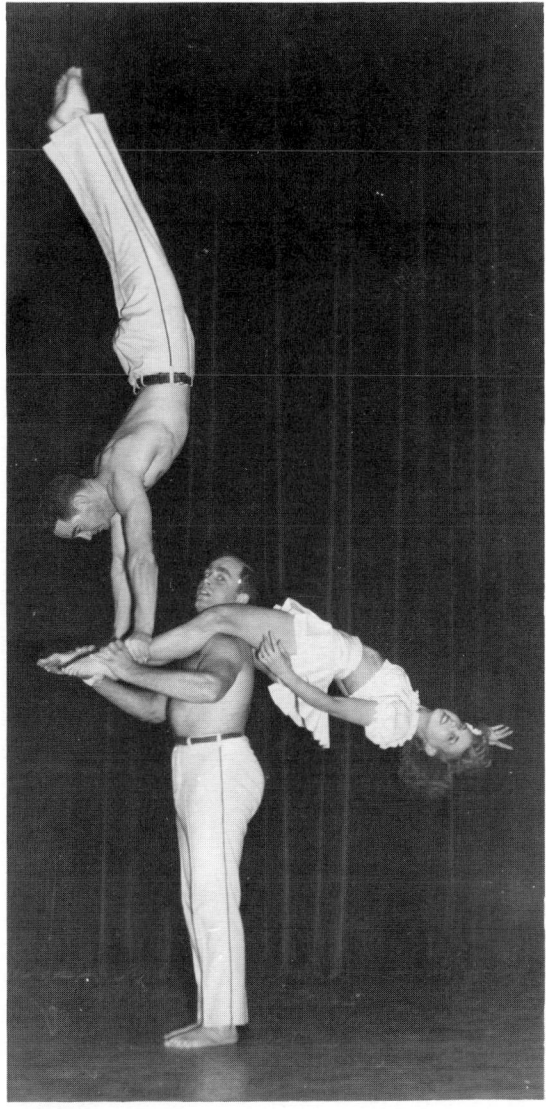

Figure 9.5 Fulcrum

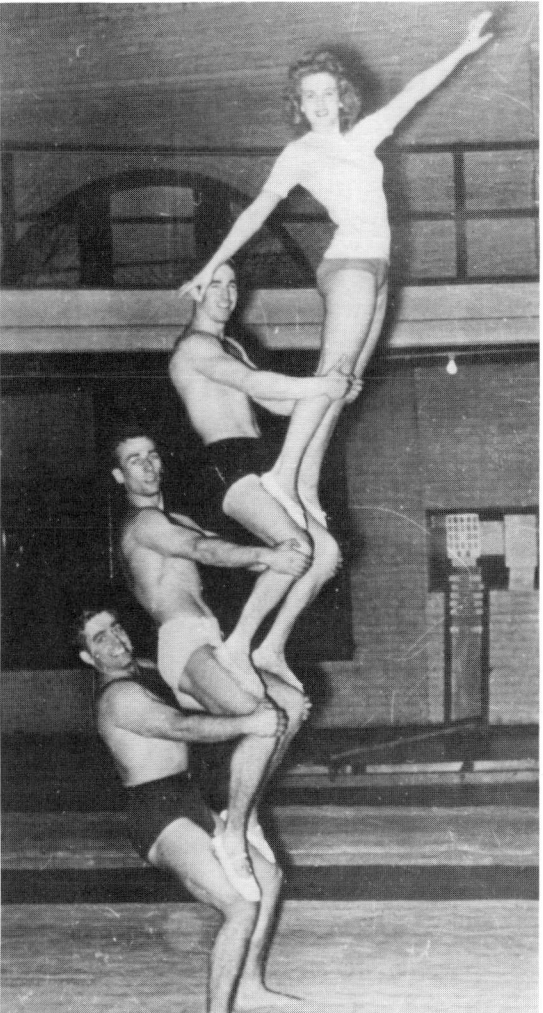

Figure 9.6 Quadruple thigh stand

tion of the move. Many boys and girls in physical education classes are unable to perform the handstand simply because the strength of their arm and shoulder muscles is inadequate to support their weight.

The most efficient method for moving into the handstand position on the floor is as follows: Place the hands on the floor at shoulder width with the fingers pointing forward (Figure 9.10). The head should be elevated with the eyes focused at a point on the floor between the hands and about eight inches in front of them. The left leg should be flexed and drawn under the body while the right leg is extended. The student upends by springing off the left leg while swinging (hyperextending the right hip joint) the right leg upward (Figure 9.10b). The arms are angled forward about 20 degrees beyond the horizontal at the start but as the legs move upward over the head, the shoulders move backward until, at

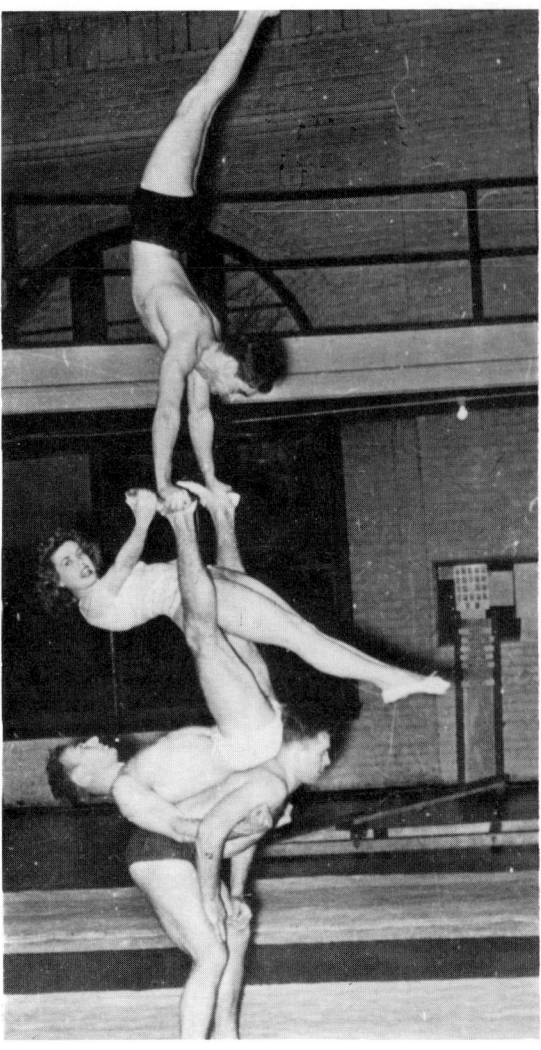

Figure 9.7 High father time

the time when the legs are over the head, the arms are vertical (Figure 9.10c). This angling of the arms keeps the center of gravity of the body more nearly over the center of support throughout the movement into the handstand. Without this forward inclination of the arms, the spring and swing of the legs must be so much more forceful that the probability the gymnast will overbalance is very great or he/she might correct for this excessive force by angling the arms backward to

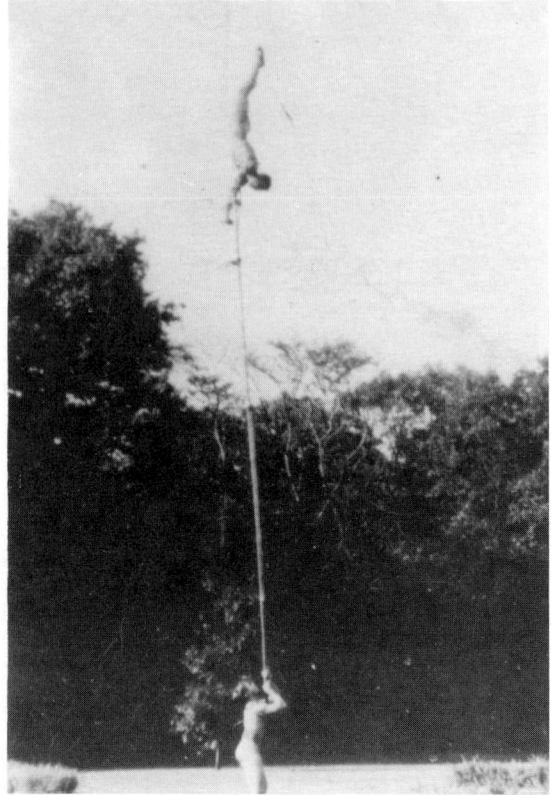

Figure 9.8 Perch pole

check the force. This latter action also often results in failure. Teaching beginners to kick up into a handstand from a standing position is a poor and ineffective teaching procedure because of the excessive amount of rotary force introduced which beginners and even advanced gymnasts find difficult to control (Figures 9.11a–9.11d). In the first method, the forward inclination and return to the vertical position is of great importance. However, the student with inadequate shoulder strength will be unable to hold the forward inclination sufficiently long. If he is to learn the handstand, adequate shoulder strength must first be developed through progressive resistance, isometric, or other exercise modalities.

The forward inclination of the arms is an application of the concept that states: *"The*

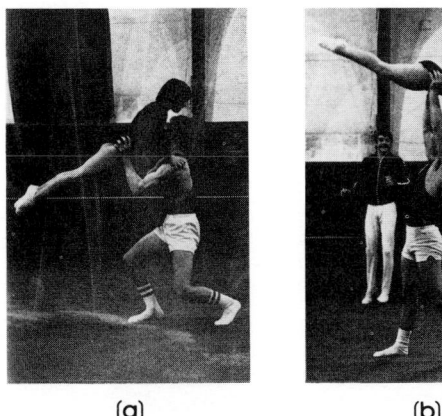

(a)	(b)

Figure 9.9 Sequences of jump into high front swan

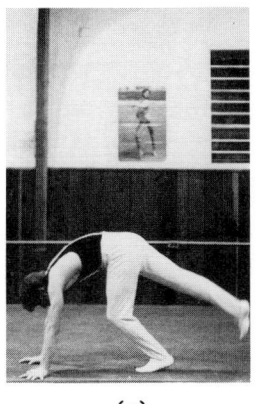
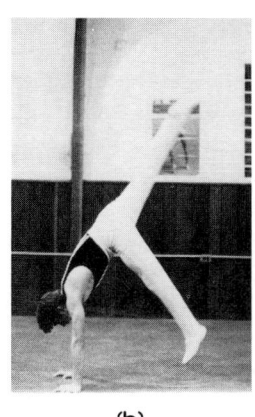

(a)	(b)

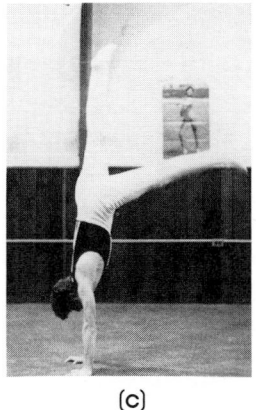
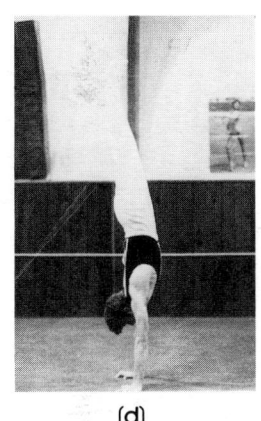

(c)	(d)

Figure 9.10 Kickup into Handstand (a) Hands on floor at shoulder width (b) Springing off left leg while swinging right leg upward (c) Center of gravity above hands (except left leg) (d) Handstand position

location of the center of gravity of the body changes as the body or its parts are placed in different positions." It is also an illustration of the concept that states: *"The center of weight should be as nearly as possible between the points of support."* At the beginning of the movement upward into the handstand position, a large portion of the body is behind the hands; therefore, the shoulders must be forward of the hands in order to move the center of gravity closer to a point between the hands. However, as the body and legs move upward, the center of gravity moves forward through an arc of 90 degrees. To retain the balanced position of the body, the arms must be brought back to the vertical position, where the body weight will be transferred downward through the vertically aligned bones of the arms. If the arms are inclined forward at this point, the center of gravity will fall forward of the hands.

Swinging and Pressing on the Parallel Bars

The same forward inclination of the arms followed by a return to the vertical occurs when swinging up into a handstand on the horizontal bar in preparation for a giant swing, in swinging into a handstand on the parallel bars, or in moving into a handstand on the balance beam. This action is illustrated in Figures 9.12 and 9.13.

The importance of the arm inclination is especially manifest in the straight-arm-straight-leg press into a handstand. The gymnast begins from a stand, then flexes his hips to place his hands on the floor as close to his feet as possible while keeping his legs extended. He angles his arms forward as he moves his hips upward until they are over his

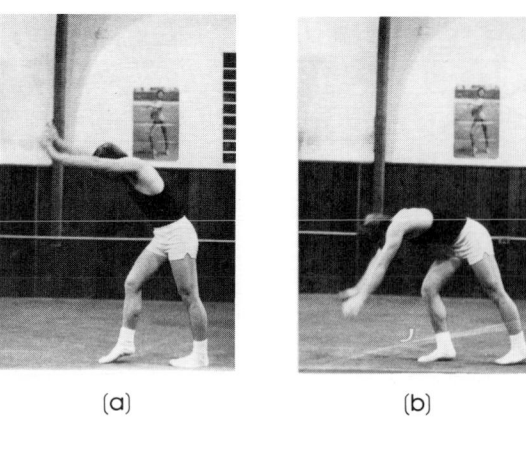

(a)   (b)

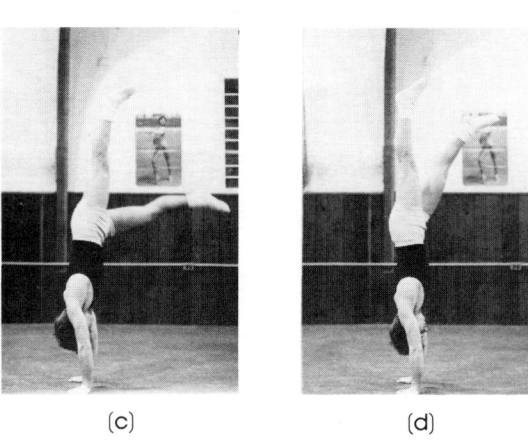

(c)   (d)

Figure 9.11   Hip Flexion into Handstand (a) Hip flexion initiated and rotatory momentum established (b) Weight principally on right foot (c) Left leg in final position, right leg moving into position (d) Slightly overbalanced position—note that arms are incorrectly angled forward of the vertical

head while keeping his feet low, legs extended, and hips fully flexed. After he is in a balanced position, he extends his hips, moving his arms backward in proportion to the displacement of the center of gravity as his extended legs move upward. Students who fail at this move do so because they do not keep their center of gravity over the points of

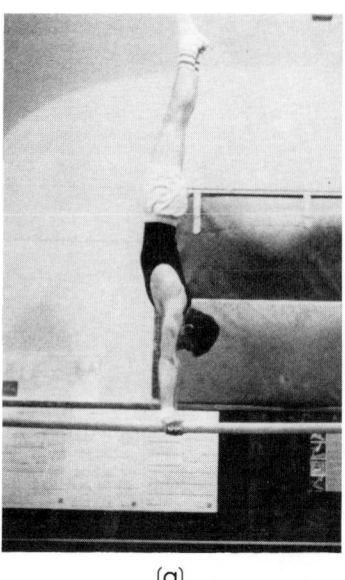

(a)

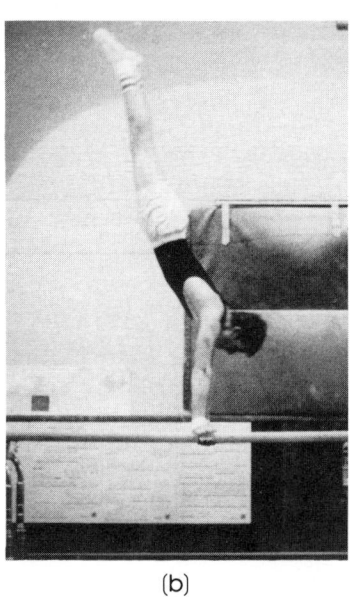

(b)

Figure 9.12   Swing in a Support Position on the Parallel Bars (a) Handstand. Note stretched position (b) Initiation of downward swing, arms beginning to angle forward of the vertical

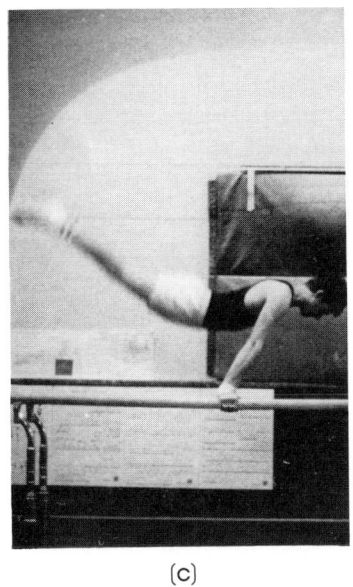
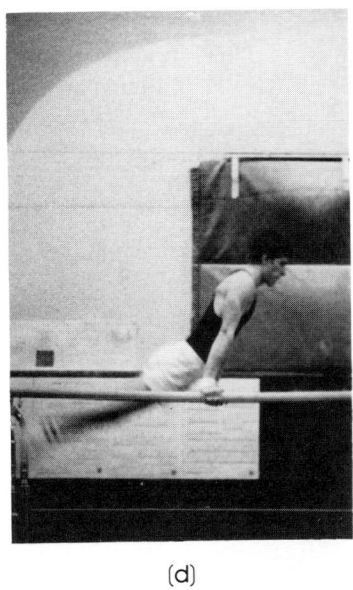
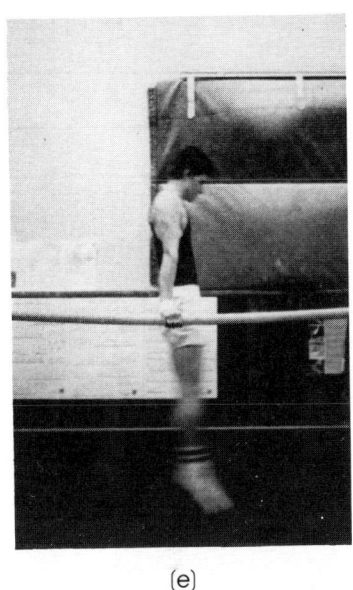

(c)　　　　　　　　　　(d)　　　　　　　　　　(e)

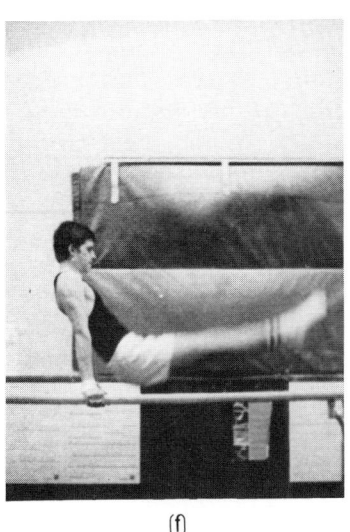
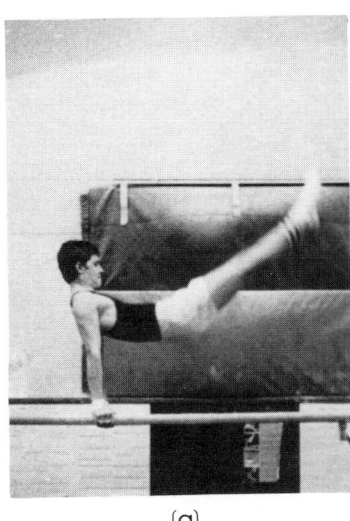
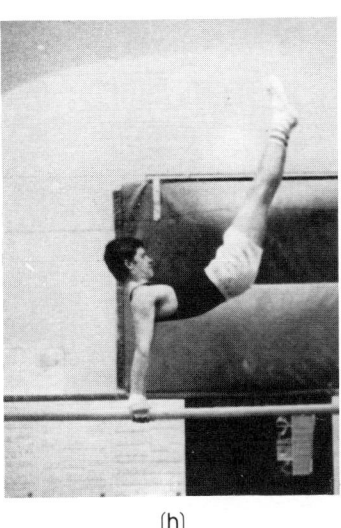

(f)　　　　　　　　　　(g)　　　　　　　　　　(h)

Figure 9.12 (c) Arms angled further forward. If this swing were to be into a back somersault, the body would be straight and the arms more nearly vertical to accelerate speed of swing (d) Arms moving backward toward the vertical position. Center of rotation at the shoulder joint—not the hip joint (e) Arms vertical and hip flexion being initiated (f) Hips flexed to accelerate speed of rotation and arms angled backward to maintain center of gravity of body nearer the hands (g) Hips extending to lengthen lever for backward swing at highest point in swing (h) Beginning of rearward swing

ANALYSIS OF TUMBLING AND GYMNASTIC SKILLS　　**325**

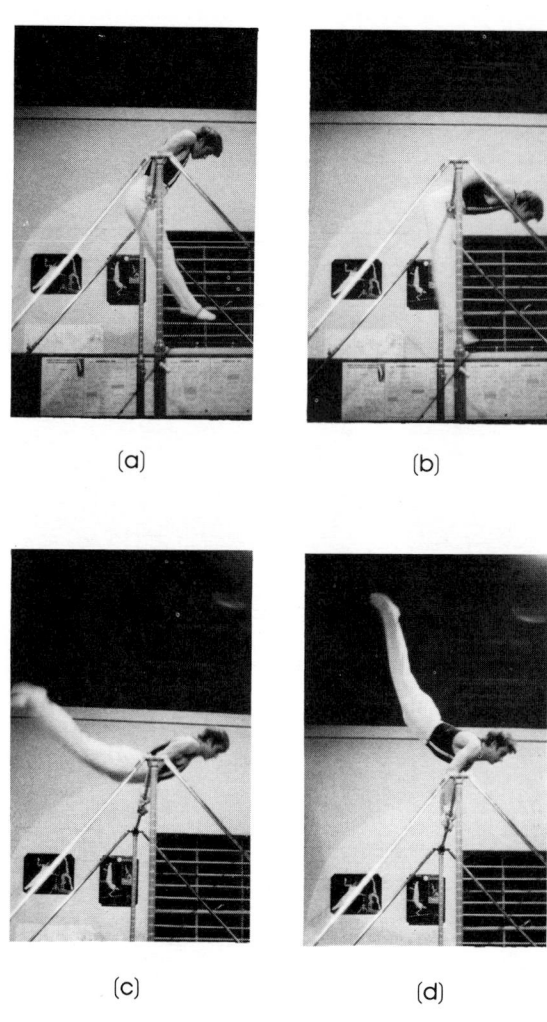

(a)

(b)

(c)

(d)

Figure 9.13 Cast into Handstand on the Horizontal bar (a) Hips flexing to bring legs forward in order to provide a greater distance through which to accelerate and to develop momentum during backward swing of legs (b) Legs swinging backward. Note forward position of shoulders, to maintain center of gravity over the bar. Arms should not be flexed (c) Arms moving toward the vertical. Legs and trunk moving upward toward the handstand position. Insufficient leg swing indicated by slightly flexed arms (d) Almost in the handstand. Elbows extending, feet moving above bar

support. However, often the reason they are unable to maintain the balanced position is because they lack adequate shoulder strength or adequate flexibility to assume the tightly jackknifed position necessary.

FLEXIBILITY NEEDS IN GYMNASTICS

An unusual degree of flexibility is required for skillful performance of gymnastic activity. Gymnasts should be familiar with a large number of both static and dynamic stretching procedures. In order to execute dislocates, inlocates, back bends, front and back walkovers (Figures 9.14 and 9.15), and handsprings (Figure 9.16), gymnasts need flexibility in the shoulder region. In order to tuck or jackknife tightly to perform somersaults and double somersaults in tumbling; straddle supports on the rings (Figure 9.17); stoop vaults on the long horse; stoop and rear vaults on the side horse vault; seat circles and back straddles on the uneven bars; and needle scales (Figure 9.18) and presses into handstands on the balance beam, the gymnast needs excellent hip flexibility. In order to execute backbends and yogi handstands in floor exercise, back handsprings in tumbling, codys on the trampoline, walkovers on the balance beam and other moves in other events, gymnasts need to be able to hyperextend the hips and spine. They also need to perform splits both forward and sideward. Static and dynamic stretching exercises are discussed in Chapter 14. These exercises will increase the range of motion in body joints. Chapter 14 also discusses exercises designed to increase muscular strength, power, and endurance. Additional references are provided. At this time, it should be pointed out that gymnasts and their coaches should select those exercises that most effectively develop the specific qualities needed in gymnastics. Gymnasts should perform stretching exercises of the hip flexors and extensors, spinal flex-

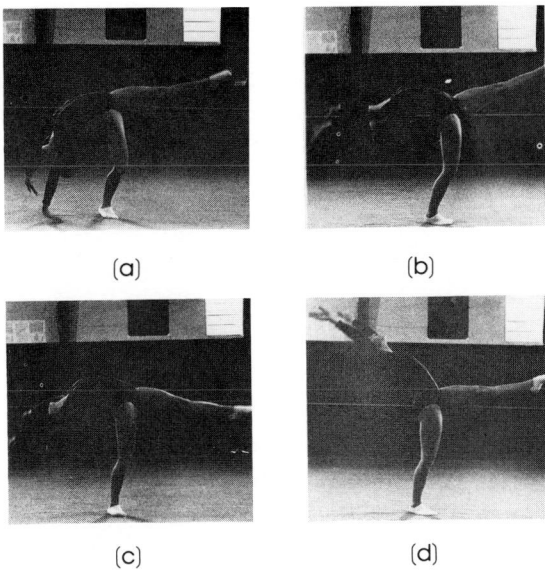

(a)   (b)

(c)   (d)

Figure 9.14   Front Walkover (a) The gymnast has come through the handstand position, her right foot has contacted the mat, and her hands are beginning to leave the mat (b) Note that the hips have moved forward and the left leg is extended horizontally to counterbalance the weight of the trunk (c) Note the left leg has moved downward. The momentum of the left leg is being transferred to the trunk (d) Move will be completed when the trunk and supporting leg are in a vertical line from the right foot and the left leg is lowered to the floor

ors, extensors, hyperextensors, and rotators, leg adductors and shoulder hyperflexors, hyperextensors, rotators, and horizontal flexor-adductors. Static stretching exercises are more effective than ballistic stretching exercises, for reasons pointed out in Chapter 14.

STRENGTH NEEDS IN GYMNASTICS

Gymnasts and their coaches should select strength and power exercises according to the demands of gymnastic activities. Heavily

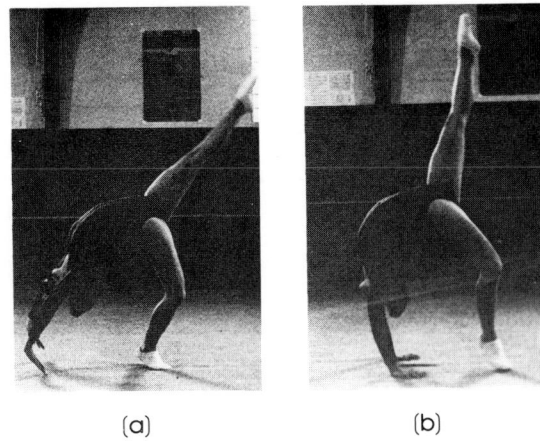

(a)   (b)

Figure 9.15   Back Walkover (a) The move has been initiated. Arms are reaching backward toward the mat. Hands are beginning to contact the mat. Left leg is moving upward (b) Note that shoulders have moved beyond a vertical line from the hands. Push-off from right foot has been initiated. Hips are moving above hands, led by the upward moving left leg

muscled legs and buttocks are a detriment to gymnasts, yet gymnasts need relatively powerful legs for long horse vaulting, mounts on the parallel bars, and tumbling moves in the floor exercise event. Gymnasts need both power and muscular endurance in the muscles of the arms, shoulder girdle, back, trunk, and abdomen. However, even in these muscle groups, great bulk can be a detriment rather than an advantage. Lean muscles have greater muscular endurance than bulky muscles. All-around gymnasts need muscular endurance as well as power. Consequently, a balance between muscular power and leanness must be achieved.

Exercise Prescriptions for Gymnasts

Fifteen to 20 repetitions in three sets using 60 to 70 percent of maximum is generally the correct prescription for gymnasts doing weight training exercises. Isometric exercises are of great value to gymnasts since bulk is not added to as great a degree as in weight training. Further, the energy cost of isometric exercises is smaller. Gymnastics calls for all three types of muscular contraction — concentric, eccentric, and static or isometric. In most skills, concentric contractions are used. Examples are provided in gymnastics and tumbling in springing upward in saltos, in a pull-up on the horizontal bar or uneven parallel bars, and flexing the hips during a straddle or stoop vault in the long or side horse vaulting event.

Examples in gymnastics of eccentric contractions are when landing after a dismount from the apparatus or after a salto, after the rear vault catch on the horizontal bar while lowering downward (Figure 9.19), lowering from a handstand to a shoulder stand on the parallel bars or rings, and absorbing impact on the balance beam after an aerial walkover. The most highly skilled gymnasts, however, minimize the force necessary in eccentric contractions by executing moves in such a manner that they need not lower themselves, but rather extend the body to secure swing for the succeeding move. An example is the rear vault catch on the horizontal bar.

Beginners barely clear the bar and, after catching, drop straight downward. Highly skilled gymnasts clear the bar with sufficient height and control that they can unwind their hips and extend in time to swing downward with body extended and generate momentum for the next move.

A static or isometric contraction is one in which the length of the muscle remains unchanged, the bone on which the muscle inserts and the one on which it originates remain at the same distance from one another, and no work is being done; i.e., physiologic work is being generated but foot-pounds of work are not since nothing is being moved although force is being exerted. Examples of isometric contractions in gymnastics are the

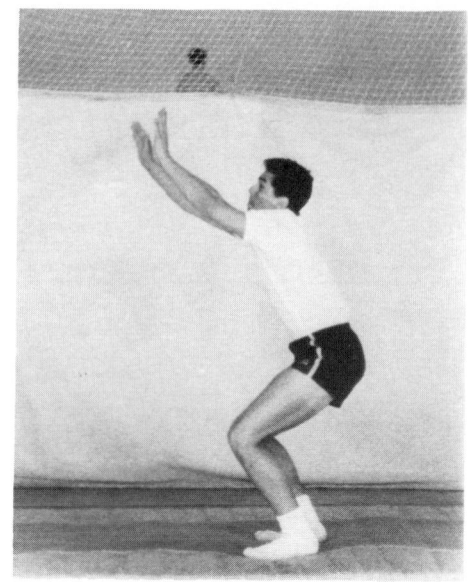

(a)

Figure 9.16 Back Handspring into Back Somersault (a) Arms swinging upward-backward to establish rotatory momentum

Figure 9.16b Center of gravity is behind the feet, neck hyperextending

(b)

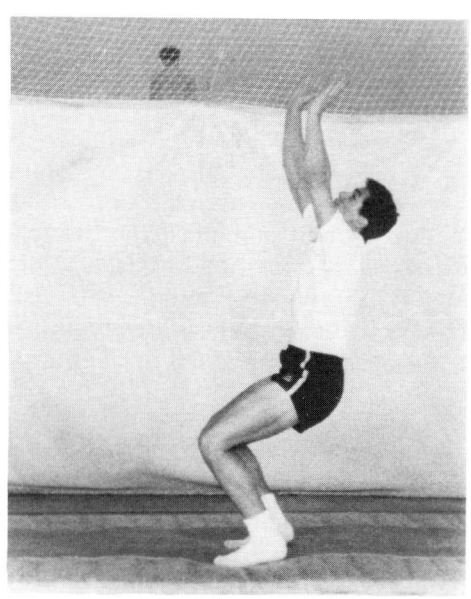

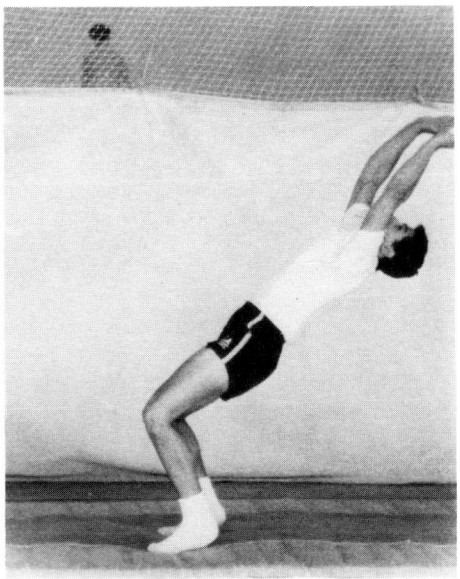

(c)

Figure 9.16c Hips and knees extending

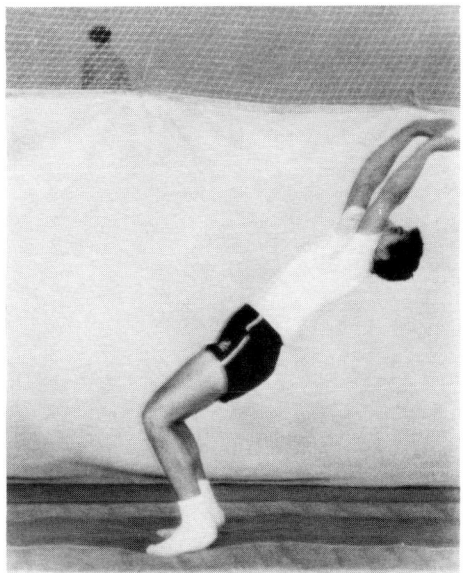

(d)

Figure 9.16d Hips hyperextended and lifting body vertically

Figure 9.16e Arms reaching for mat

Figure 9.16f Hands on mat, momentum carrying arms toward the vertical

(e)

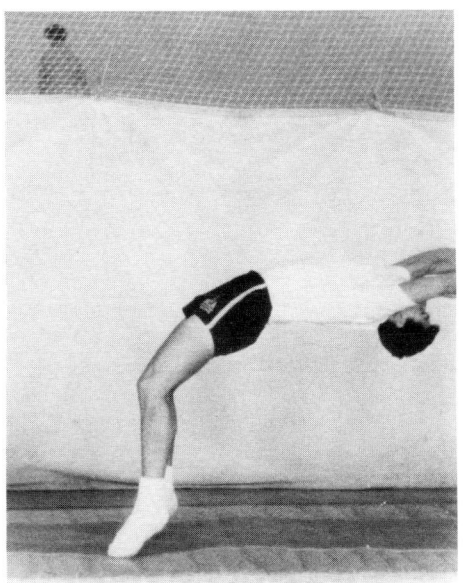

(f)

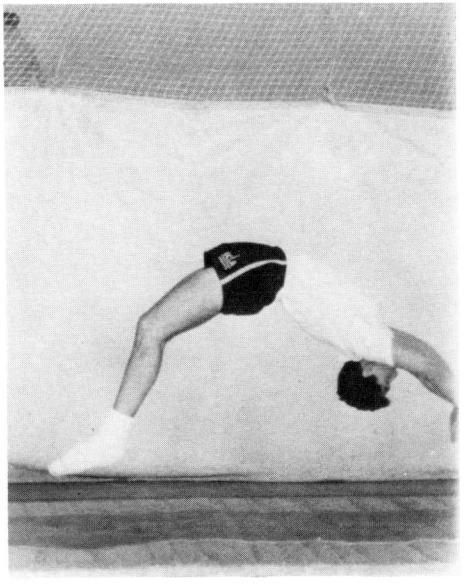

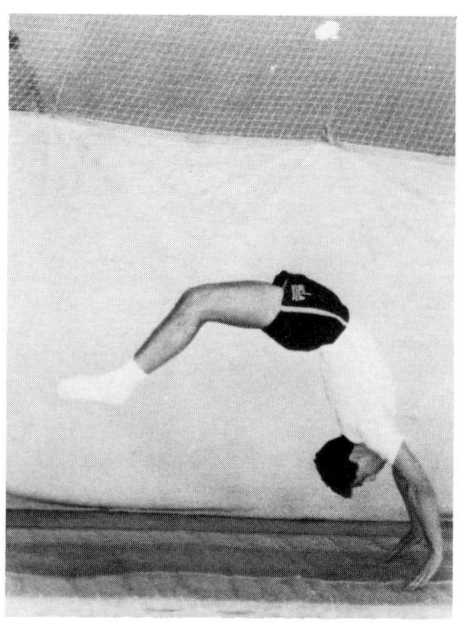

(g)

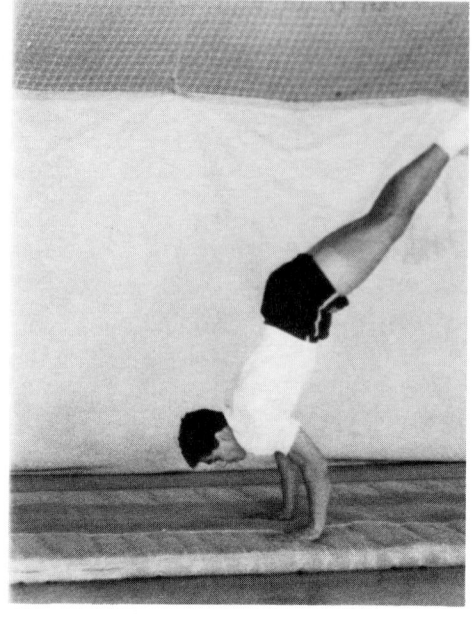

(h)

Figure 9.16g **to 9.16**i Hips flexing for vigorous snapdown, elbows extending and shoulder girdle being elevated to move trunk upward

Figure 9.16j Note angle of legs relative to the floor: this "blocking action" insures maximum lift

(i)

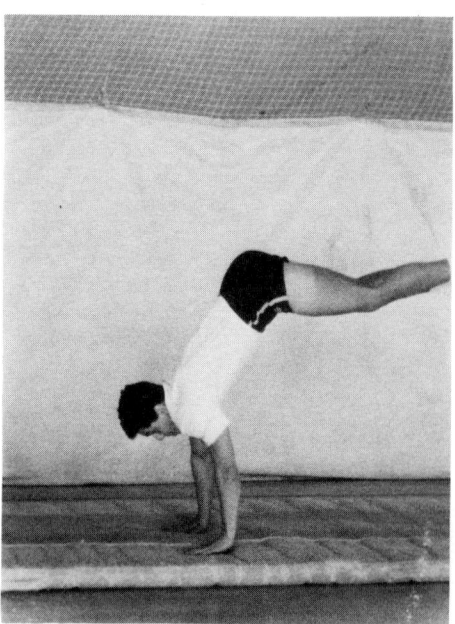

(j)

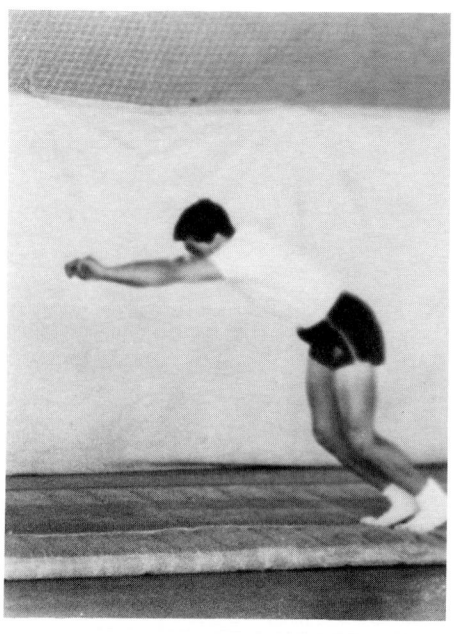

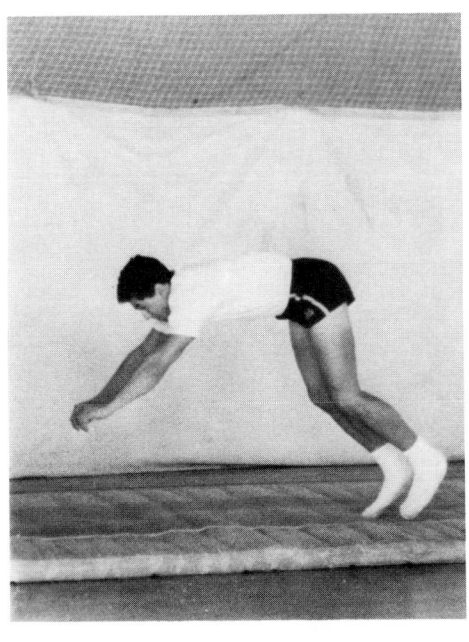

(k)

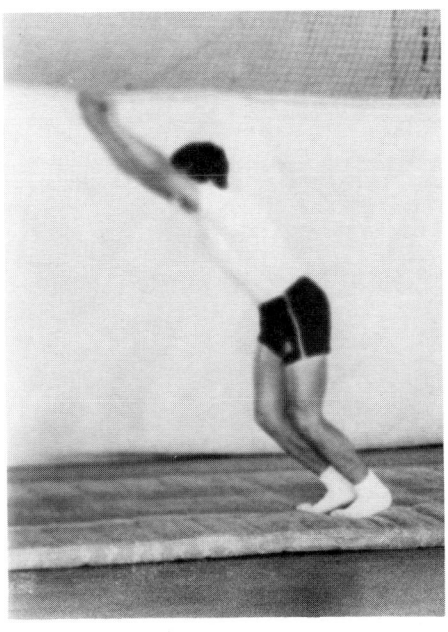

(l)

Figure 9.16k to 9.16n Hips and knees extending.
Note vertical lift (tumbler's body does not move beyond right edge of window)

(m)

(n)

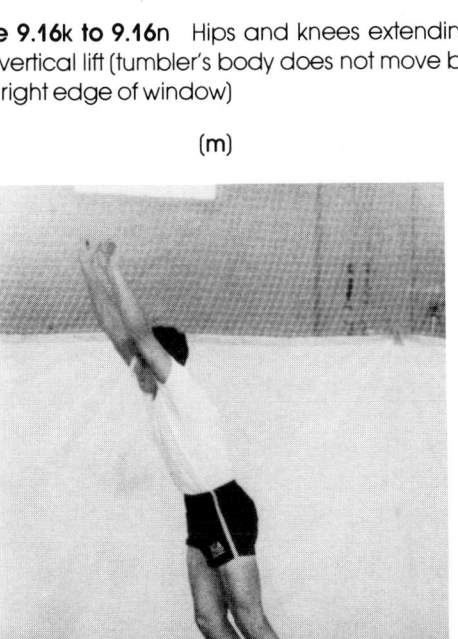
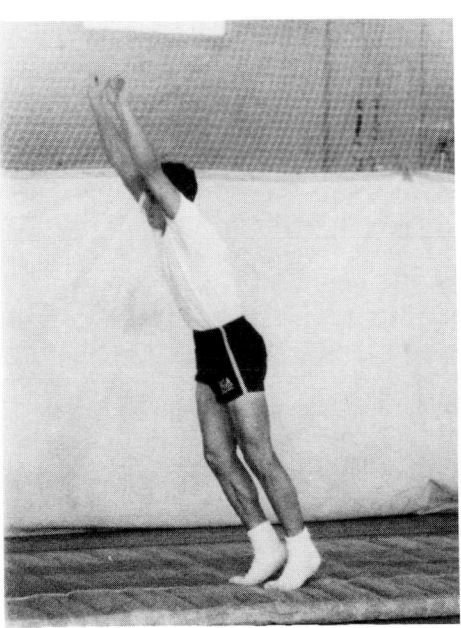

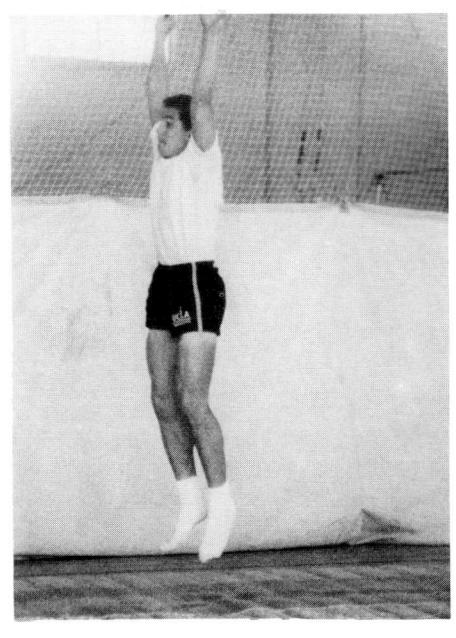

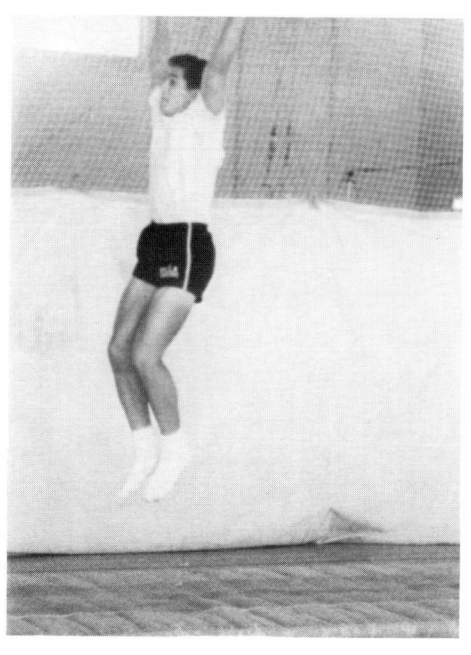

(o)

(p)

Figure 9.16o to 9.16s Knees and hips flexing to shorten radius of rotation

(q)

(r)

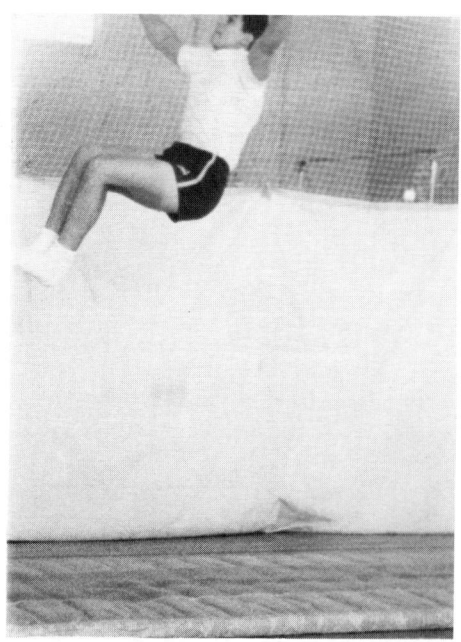

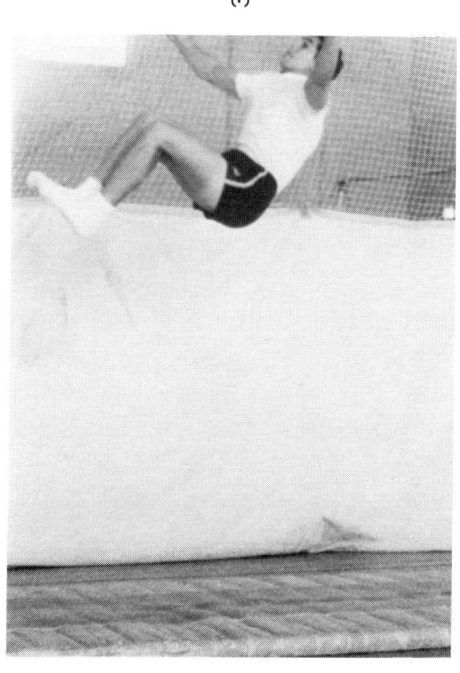

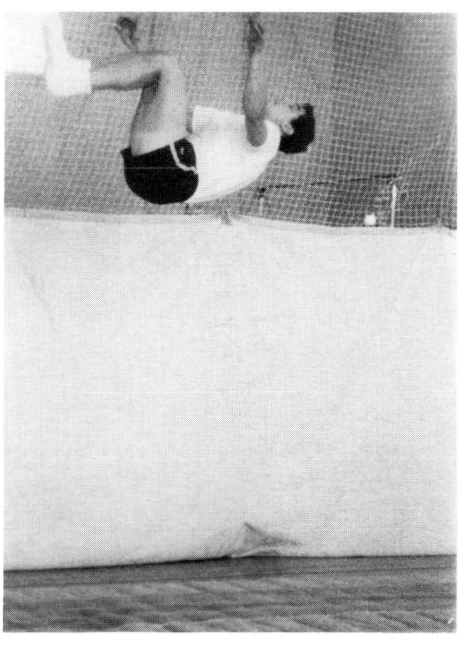

(s)

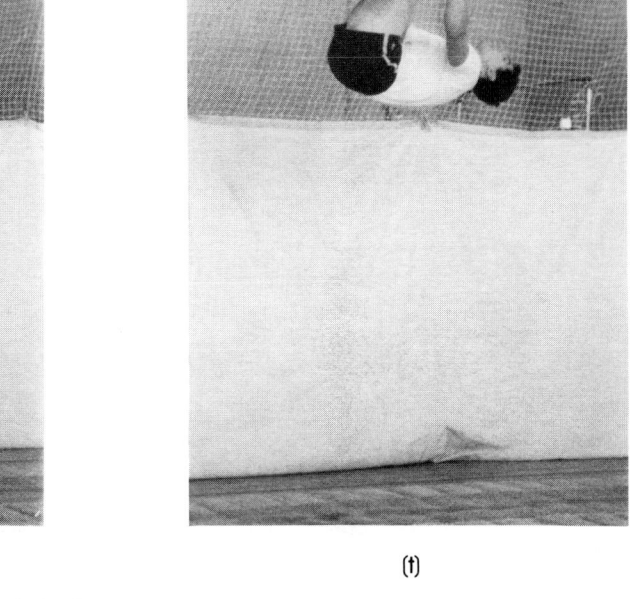

(t)

Figure 9.16t **to 9.16**v   Neck hyperextending to look
for mat, tuck tightening

(u)

(v)

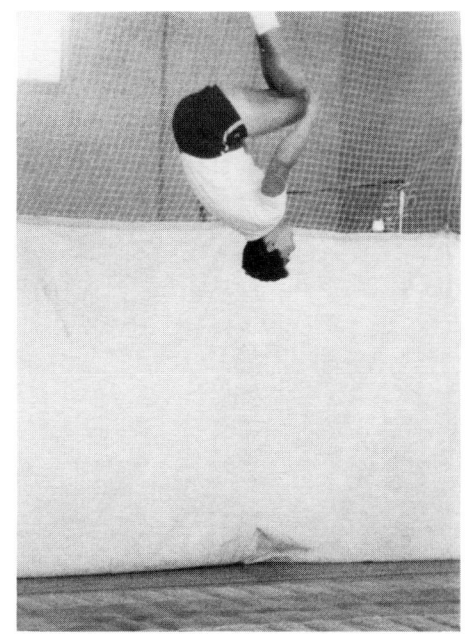

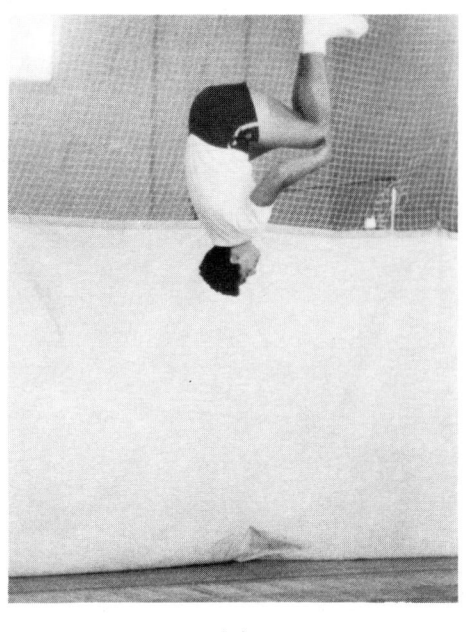

(w)

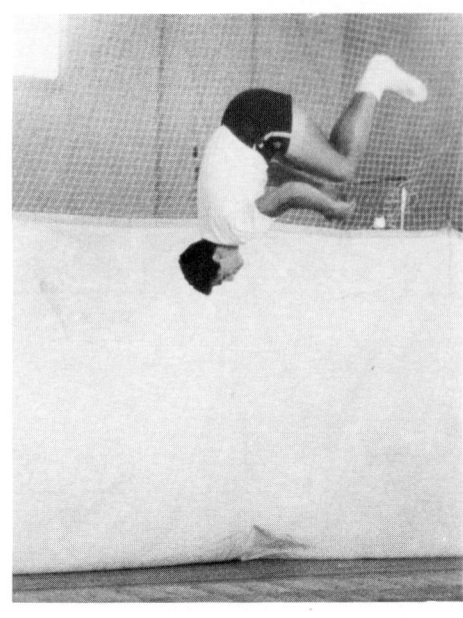

(x)

Figure 9.16w to 9.16z Hips and knees extending and head moving into straight line relationships with trunk to slow rotation

(y)

(z)

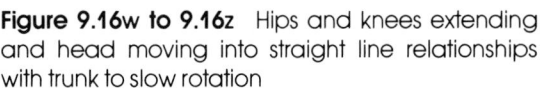

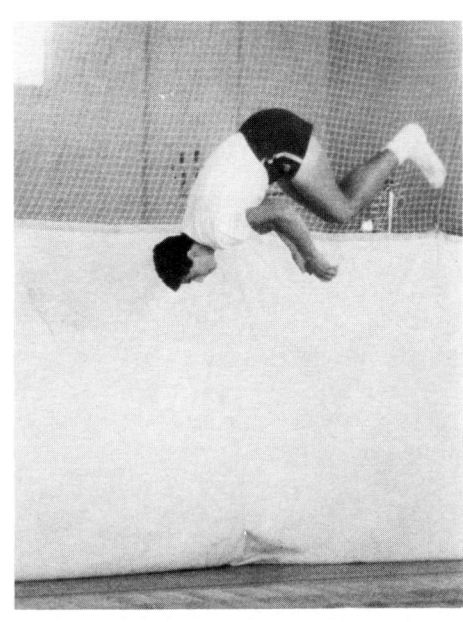

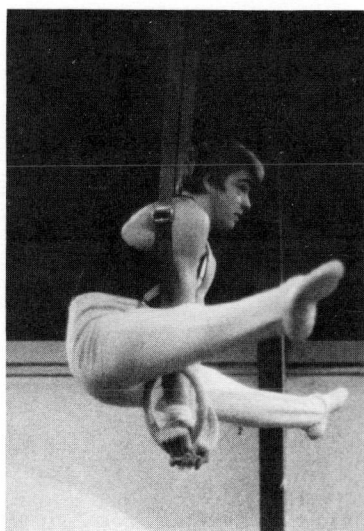

Figure 9.17 Straddle support on rings. Note vertical and extended position of the arms, depressed shoulders, elevated head position, and center of support as nearly as possible under center of gravity

crucifix, front and back levers, L-sits, straddle seats, handstands, and other held positions.

Strength and Prevention of Injury

Strength over and above that required for execution of a specific move is desirable in order to prevent injury or to "save" the move. This concept mandates that gymnasts practice strength-building exercises. If a gymnast executes an activity such as a kip on the horizontal bar, giant swing, stoop vault, leg circles, walkover on the beam, or any other move, only enough strength will be developed to perform that skill. To increase strength, the overload principle must be applied; that is, the resistance or the number of repetitions or both must be constantly increased.

If a gymnast in attempting a stutzkehre on the parallel bars (a move in which at the highest point in the forward swing in a cross-arm support, a half turn and catch to a support position is executed, Figure 9.20) re-

grasps with his body low and his arms bent, he can, if he has more than adequate strength, "save" the move. If his strength is inadequate, his arms will "fold" and he will fall below the bars. If in executing a handstand pirouette on the parallel bars, the gymnast finds his body in a levered position, he can, if he has more than the strength necessary to execute the move, "muscle" back up into the correct handstand position. In casts into giant swings on the rings, if the gymnast's timing is faulty or his momentum is insufficient to cause him to rise all the way into the handstand position, he can utilize his strength to push himself up by extending his arms.

SPOTTING

General Spotting Procedures

The spotter must stand close to the person being spotted so that the spotter can lift the per-

Figure 9.18 Needle scale. Note degree of both flexion of right hip and hyperextension of left hip. Unusual sense of balance is required due to small base of support and paucity of visual clues

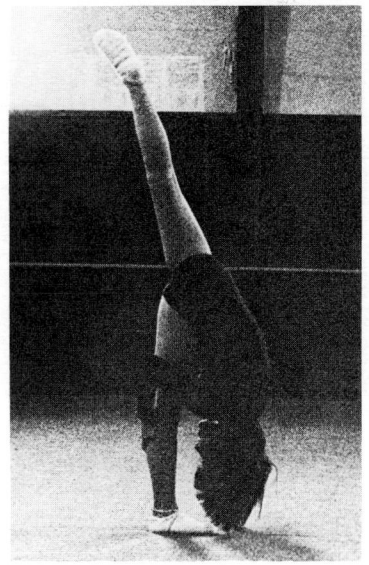

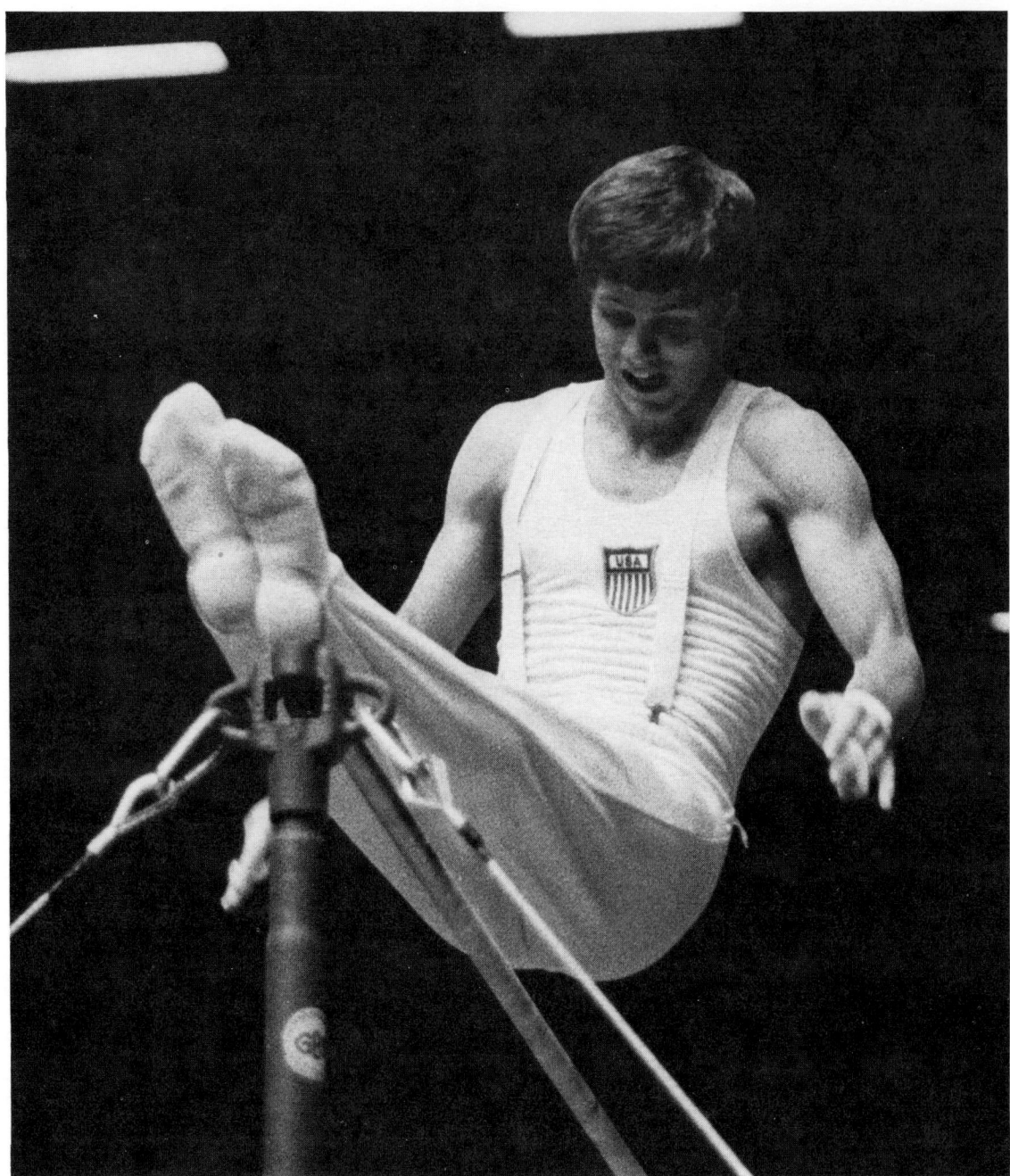

Figure 9.19 Rear vault catch. Gymnast will turn to catch the bar while extending the hips (Wayne Young). Photo courtesy of **International Gymnast**, Santa Monica, California

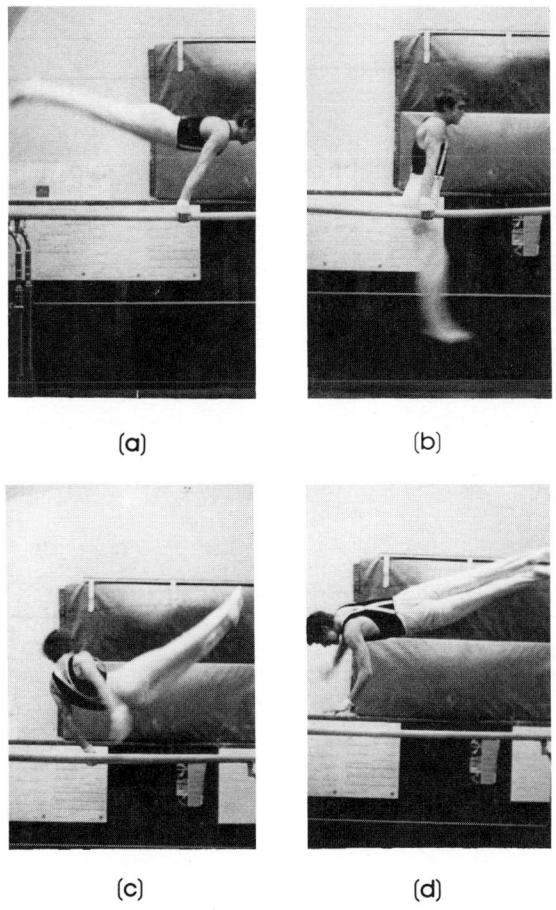

(a)   (b)

(c)   (d)

Figure 9.20 Stutzkehre (a) Note straight line relationship of legs and trunk to lengthen lever and thereby to increase momentum (b) Hip flexion being initiated (c) Rotation around vertical axis of the body initiated by rotation of head to the left and push-off by right hand. Note angle of supporting arm (d) Rotation almost completed, hands reaching for bars

former with the forearm held in a vertical position. If he/she is standing at arm's length from the gymnast, it will be necessary to support the gymnast with the arm extended hori-

zontally. This position greatly increases the length of the resistance arm. Very little weight can be supported on the horizontally extended arm. When a fall is imminent, the spotter must have the courage to move close to the gymnast in order to shorten the resistance arm of the arm lever.

Spotting Back Saltos and Back Handsprings

When spotting moves in which the gymnast is rotating around the frontal horizontal or lateral axis as in flyaways, salto dismounts, and front and back somersaults on the mats, the spotter's principal responsibility is to prevent under- or overrotation (Figure 9.21). To achieve this in the case of the back salto, if the spotter is standing to the gymnast's left, the right hand is placed on the gymnast's lower back or buttocks and the left hand is placed against the back of the gymnast's thigh. The right hand can lift the gymnast, and on completion of the somersault, if the gymnast is overrotating, this hand is moved up toward the gymnast's neck to prevent overrotation. With the left hand, assistance in rotation can be given. The procedure for spotting the back handspring is similar except that, since the gymnast's center of gravity is closer to the floor than it is in the back salto, the spotter must kneel alongside the gymnast in order to be able to lift effectively. The spotter must also be slightly behind the student because the performer's center of gravity will move backward. The spotter must position himself so that at the moment the performer is most likely to need support, the spotter will be able to provide support under the center of gravity.

In spotting almost all moves, the spotter must be so positioned as to be able to provide both lift and rotation at the crucial point in the move. When spotting the neck-, head-, and handspring, the spotter should kneel alongside the performer's left side, slightly

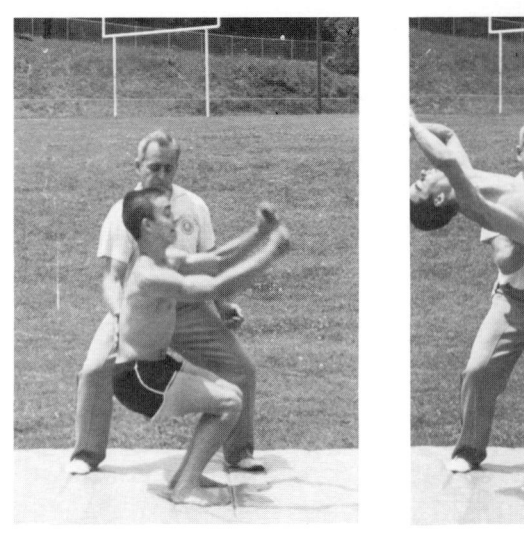
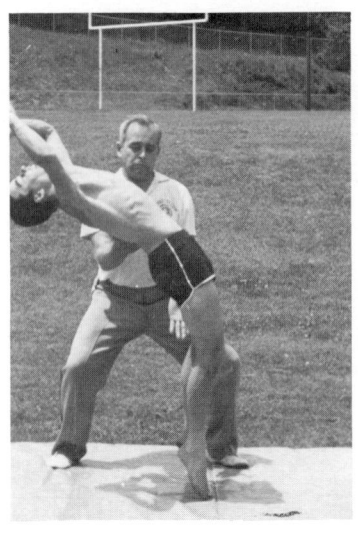
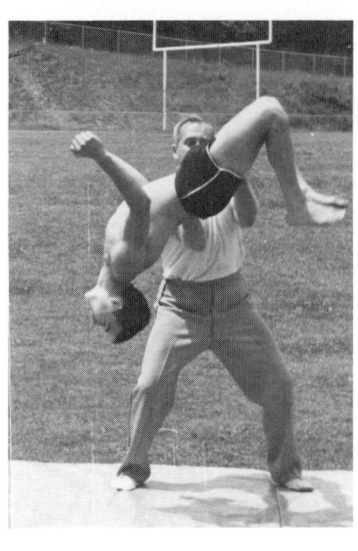

(a)　　　　　　　　(b)　　　　　　　　(c)

Figure 9.21 (a) Note that spotter is standing as close as possible to the tumbler (b) Note spotter's wide stance to increase stability (c) Note position of spotter's hands to facilitate providing both lift and rotation. Also note that the spotter's back is vertical (enhances stability and power) and his knees are flexed to assist in providing lift upon knee extension (d) Note spotter's left hand assisting in rotation (e) Spotter's legs have extended due to legs assisting in the lift (f) Move completed

(d)　　　　　　　　(e)　　　　　　　　(f)

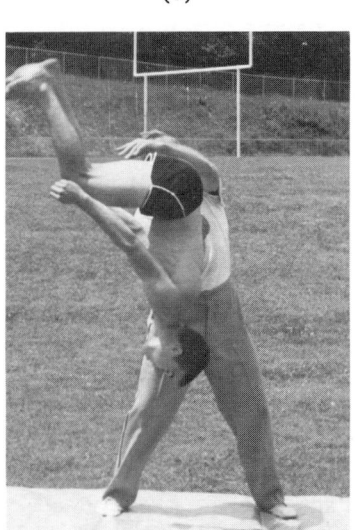
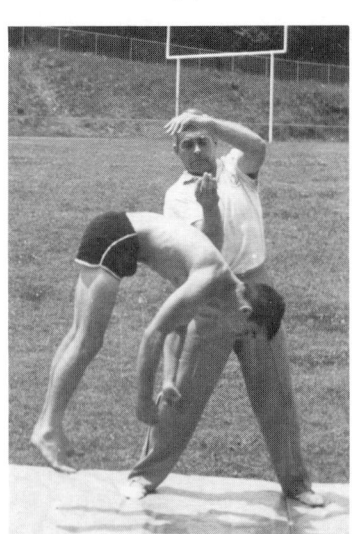
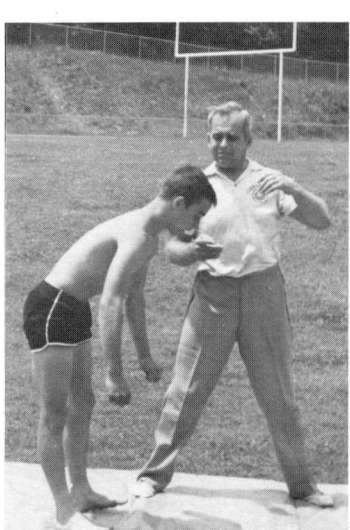

forward of the head and hands. The left hand (assuming he/she is on the gymnast's left) should be on the gymnast's lower back and the right hand should be under the performer's left shoulder. If the spotter rests the center of his right forearm against his own right thigh, better leverage will be provided for lifting the gymnast. These positions will facilitate assisting with rotation, if needed, as well as with lift or support in the event the gymnast extends directly upward.

SUMMATION OF FORCES

Many gymnastic and tumbling moves are the result of the summation of forces. A number of forces may be added to one another to propel the gymnast. These forces are provided by muscles acting upon bones. If the forces are applied simultaneously, the force generated will be limited by the weakest of the several forces. For maximal effectiveness, *succeeding forces should be added at the point of greatest speed but least acceleration of the preceding forces.* If this is accomplished, the resulting forces will be added to one another. Obviously, application of the succeeding force should not be delayed until speed is beginning to decrease. This principle points up the importance of good timing and explains why fluidity is an important criterion when judging competitive gymnastics. Application of the principle is illustrated in the take-off from the Reuther board. First, the gymnast drives the arms and shoulders upward; second, the back is "uncorked" (extension of the slightly rounded upper back); third, the hips are extended; fourth, the knees are extended; fifth, the feet are plantar flexed; and finally, the Reuther board imparts its lift.

Application of other kinesiologic principles will enhance performance in this skill to a great extent. We will present and discuss application of these principles in the order in which they affect the skill.

MOMENTUM AND VELOCITY

Use of the Reuther Board

Momentum is most often increased by increasing velocity rather than mass. The gymnast cannot increase momentum by changing body mass during the approach to the Reuther board (modified springboard type of equipment). Momentum can be increased, however, by increasing the velocity of the run. The gymnast should, therefore, accelerate rapidly during the run so that the Reuther board is reached at maximum controlled speed. The greater the momentum, the more force with which the gymnast can strike the Reuther board and the higher will be the vault. This is true because of the concept that *"For every action, there is an equal and opposite reaction."* The more forcefully the board is pushed downward, the more forcefully it will push upward against the gymnast. Because the gymnast lands on the board with legs angled backward at the moment of impact, it may appear that it is not true that the reaction is in the opposite direction. However, this conclusion is reached without allowing for the force represented by the forward momentum of the gymnast. As the gymnast is depressing the board, the forward movement of the body continues and the body begins to rotate around the horizontal axis. The body rotates between 90 and 180 degrees according to the move being executed. The reason for this rotation is stated in the concept that states: *"Rotation may be induced by slowing linear velocity at an extremity."* The gymnast is moving in a linear path as he approaches the long horse. One end of his body is suddenly stopped. This causes his body to rotate. This phenomenon is observed when we stub a toe and stumble. However, in the case of the gymnast, the spring (aided by the Reuther board) carries the legs upward over the head.

PARALLELOGRAM OF FORCES APPLIED TO GYMNASTICS

When several forces are applied simultaneously, the resulting direction and force is determined by the relative directions and amounts of the several forces according to a parallelogram of forces (as explained in Chapter 5). There are two principal forces propelling the gymnast off the board. These are forward momentum and rebound off the board. Assuming that the forces of the rebound and forward momentum are equal and that the forward momentum is 90 degrees forward of the vertical and the rebound off the Reuther board is 45 degrees behind the vertical, the gymnast would move upward 22.5 degrees forward of the vertical, which is halfway between the two forces. In moves such as the front handspring into a front somersault, in which the gymnast must get the legs up quickly and to a great height, slow-motion movies of champion gymnasts show that the gymnast uses more blocking action (greater angling of the legs backward on striking the Reuther board) than when executing moves such as the far tap stoop vault, which does not require that the legs move as high or as quickly above the head and shoulders.

HEIGHT AND TRAJECTORY OF CENTER OF GRAVITY

The preceding illustrates the concept that states: "*The height reached and the trajectory of the center of gravity of the gymnast's body is determined at the instant of release from the apparatus or spring from the Reu-*

ther board, trampoline, mat, or balance beam." Nothing the gymnast can do after he is airborne will alter the trajectory nor the height reached by the center of gravity.

Rebound Tumbling—the Spring

The trajectory of the gymnast's center of gravity is determined at the instant of release from the apparatus, spring from the Reuther board, trampoline, mat, or balance beam. This explains why it is so important to learn to bounce correctly and in control on the trampoline and to learn moves first with a low bounce. If the trampolinist does not strike the bed properly and lift off vertically, nothing can be done to change the trajectory or to prevent flight beyond the end or side of the trampoline. When the trampolinist notes on landing on the bed that the lift-off might be at too great an angle, the spring can be "killed" by flexing the hips and knees as the trampoline bed begins to lift the performer. This action will absorb the lift. This skill should be taught first on the trampoline.

Time of Release in Flyaways and Somersault Dismounts

Novice gymnasts trying to learn the cast or peach basket wonder why they land on the floor instead of in an upper arm hang on the bars. Other gymnasts wonder why, when they attempt a flyaway from the horizontal bar, they are forced to complete the somersault only 12 inches above the mat. *Gymnasts and tumblers need to understand the principles of centrifugal force in order to know when to effect releases or other movements during circling movements.* If gymnasts understood these principles, the probability that they would succeed in executing the above moves would be greatly enhanced. Gymnasts and their coaches should understand that *after releasing during circling movements, the gymnast will move at a tangent to the circle,* which is at a right angle to the radius at the moment of the release. The cast, peach basket, and flyaway are examples of circling movements in which this principle must be observed.

In Chapter 5 the reader was asked to imagine a key tied to the end of a string that was being swung in a circle in a vertical plane around a horizontal axis. If the key comes loose when the string is at the bottom of the arc, it will fly away horizontally. If it comes loose when the string is horizontal, it will fly vertically or directly upward. The human body follows the laws of physics just as do keys and other objects. The gymnast can gain maximal height in the front flyaway from the horizontal bar if he releases when his body is horizontal during the forward swing. However, although he would gain maximal height, the performer must compromise by releasing slightly before this point since his feet or legs would strike the bar if he held his body fully extended or arched (as he should) in order to maintain good form.

TRANSFER OF MOMENTUM

Momentum may be transferred from a part of the body to the entire body. This principle is applied in a great many gymnastic moves. We will illustrate its application in two beginning tumbling moves—the neckspring and the headspring.

Mechanics of the Neckspring

In the neckspring the gymnast begins in a supine position, hands under the shoulders, palms on the mat, and fingers pointing toward the feet. He/she lifts the extended legs up over the head until the toes touch the mat beyond the head (Figure 9.22a). He/she then rolls forward on the shoulder blades keeping the feet near the mat until the back is at about a 55 to 60 degree angle to the floor

(Figure 9.22b). At this point, the hips are extended, the arms push, and the head is moved forward so that the gymnast lands on the feet (Figures 9.22c to 9.22e). The gymnast must hold the legs in an extended position until just before the feet strike the mat and must fully hyperextend the hips while the back is maintained at a 55 to 60 degree angle to the floor. When the legs are extended, the lever is lengthened and consequently more momentum is generated since the velocity of the feet at the end of the lever will be greater when the legs are extended than it would be when they are flexed. When the hips reach the fully hyperextended position, the momentum generated in the legs will be transferred to the trunk, head, and arms and they will rotate upward (Figures 9.22f to 9.22h). The entire body rotates around the hips. Momentum of a part has been transferred to the whole.

Mechanics of the Headspring

The principle under discussion is illustrated through essentially the same movements of the body parts in the headspring. In the headspring (Figure 9.23), the student crouches to place her hands on the mat, shoulder width apart. Her head is placed on the mat in front of the hands at such a position that if a line were drawn connecting the three points of support (head and hands), an equilateral triangle would be formed. This provides a base of support of maximal area while allowing the elbows to be flexed so that they can later be extended to provide lift. The hips are then brought over the head, with toes on the mat, and with legs extended (Figure 9.23a). The trunk is tilted forward until the back is at a 55 to 60 degree angle to the floor with toes remaining near the floor (Figure 9.23e). When the gymnast is about to lose balance, the hips are vigorously extended into hyperextension, and the arms are extended to complete the move (Figures 9.23f

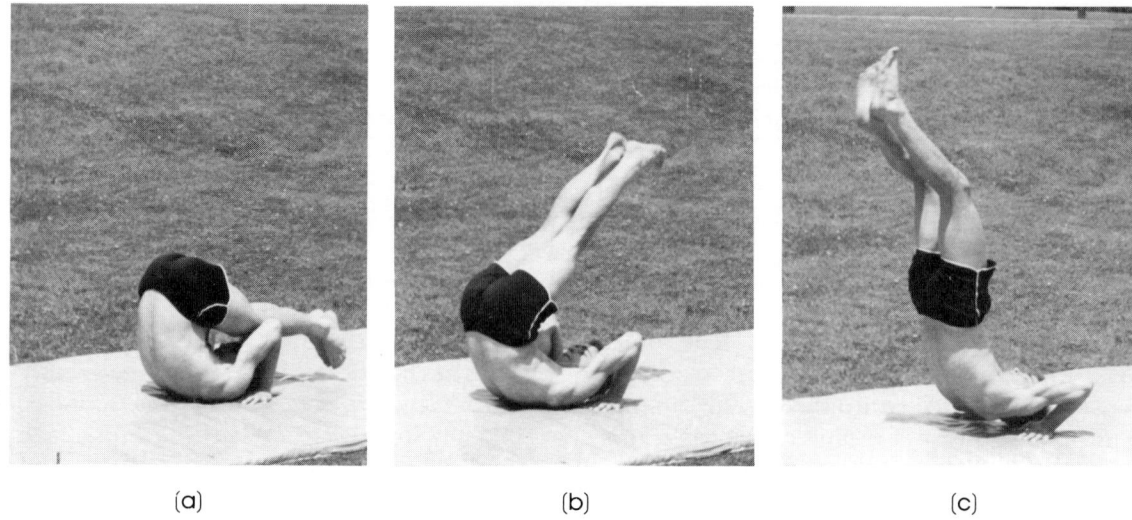

(a)   (b)   (c)

Figure 9.22 (a) Note direction of fingers. Weight is on the hands, shoulders, and head. Feet near the mat to provide maximum distance through which to accelerate movement of the legs (b) Hips extending. Note extended position of legs to maintain long lever and consequent greater linear speed of feet. Also note the angle of the back to the floor to maintain center of gravity as high as possible (c) Arms beginning to extend, hips ex-tended and moving toward hyperextension. Note angle of back to floor (d) Hips have reached hyper-extension and momentum is being transferred from the legs to the trunk; center of gravity has moved upward (e) Momentum is carrying trunk upward. Note forward position of head to move weight closer to vertical line from the feet (f) Arms sweep-ing forward to move center of gravity over the base of support

(d)   (e)   (f)

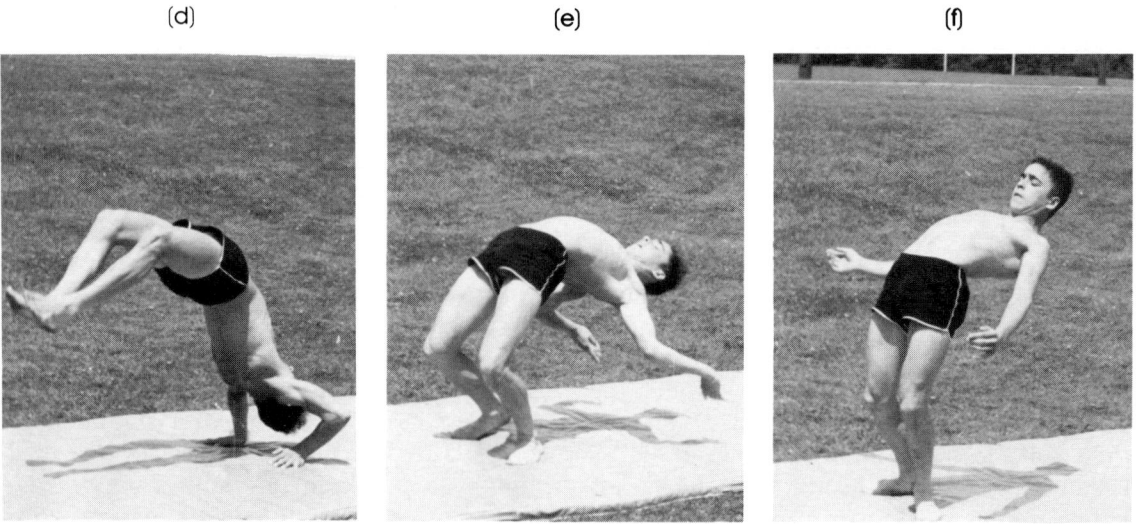

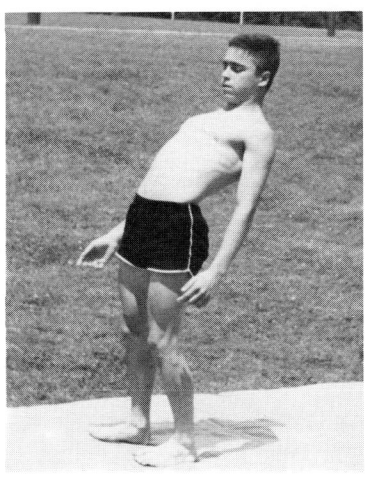

(g)

Figure 9.22g Head is forward to move center of gravity over base of support

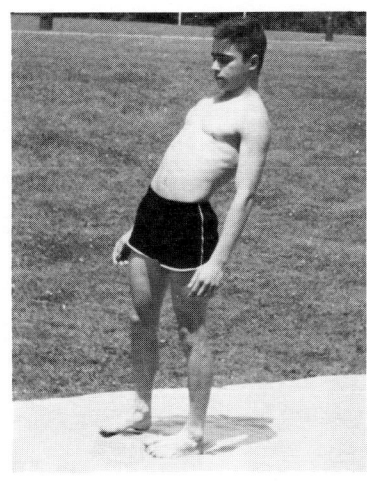

(h)

Figure 9.22h Move is almost completed

to 9.23*q*). The legs should be fully extended until just before the feet strike the mat in order to utilize a longer lever with consequent greater velocity, and therefore momentum, being generated (Figures 9.23*m* and 9.23*s*). By keeping the feet on the mat until the moment the vigorous hip extension is begun rather than extending the hips as the hips are brought over and beyond the head, a greater distance is provided through which the legs can accelerate to generate greater momentum. This serves the same purpose as the backswing in drives in tennis and badminton, in batting, and in throwing. When the hips reach the end of the movement in hyperextension, momentum of the part (the legs) is transferred to the trunk and head, and the arms and trunk rotate upward to complete the move (Figures 9.23*t* to 9.23*z*).

LENGTH OF LEVER AND MOMENTUM

Uneven Parallel Bars

One of the concepts states: "*The end of the body (or a body part) farthest from the center of rotation is moving faster than that part of the body nearest the center of rotation and consequently possesses greater momentum*." This concept is applied on the uneven parallel bars in the swing on the high bar into the back hip circle on the low bar. During the forward swing on the high bar, the legs are traveling at a greater speed than the trunk since they are closer to the end of the lever (extended arms and body) whose axis is at the hands. When the abdomen strikes the low bar and the gymnast begins to do the backward hip circle, the center of rotation is moved to the low bar, which is across her abdomen. Since the feet were moving faster than the head at the moment the abdomen struck the low bar, they will move rapidly around the bar and their momentum will be transferred to the trunk and head so that they will circle around the low bar. This is the same action that will occur when a weight attached to a string is swinging around in a circle and a finger or stick is interjected in front of the circling string. The weight will circle very rapidly around the new axis.

A greater velocity exists at the distal end of a longer lever than at the end of a shorter lever when both levers are rotating at the

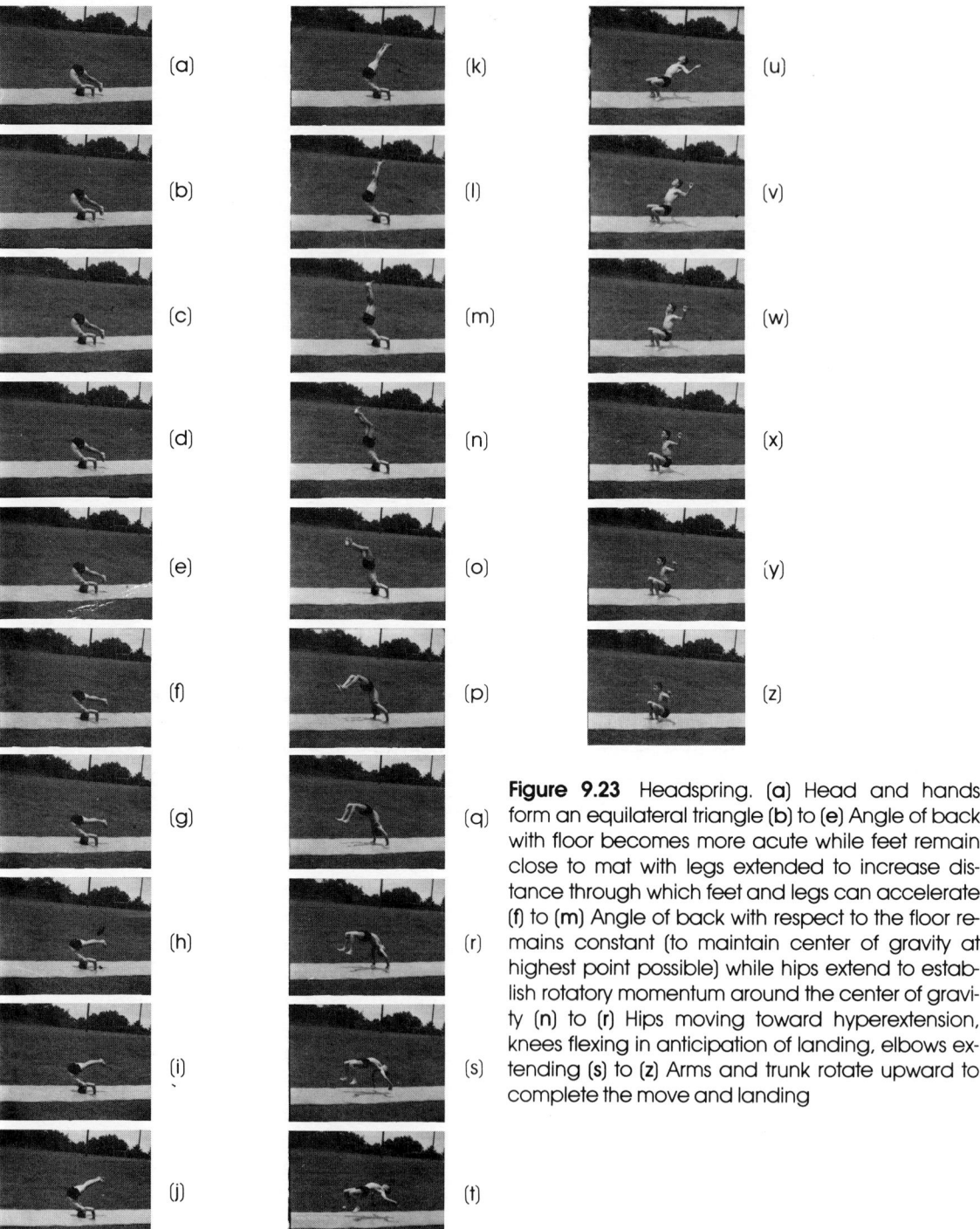

Figure 9.23 Headspring. **(a)** Head and hands form an equilateral triangle **(b)** to **(e)** Angle of back with floor becomes more acute while feet remain close to mat with legs extended to increase distance through which feet and legs can accelerate **(f)** to **(m)** Angle of back with respect to the floor remains constant (to maintain center of gravity at highest point possible) while hips extend to establish rotatory momentum around the center of gravity **(n)** to **(r)** Hips moving toward hyperextension, knees flexing in anticipation of landing, elbows extending **(s)** to **(z)** Arms and trunk rotate upward to complete the move and landing

same speed. The shoulder roll on the parallel bars is one of many moves that could be used to illustrate this concept.

Parallel Bars—Shoulder Roll

The gymnast starts in an upper-arm hang. He is grasping the bars with his forearms forming a right angle to his upper arms. The swing is initiated. On the forward swing, as the body passes the vertical position with feet directly under the head, hips and knees are flexed (shortens the radius of rotation and thereby accelerates the speed of rotation) and the gymnast flexes the arms to pull his body over his head. As the body reaches the shoulder stand position, the gymnast releases his grip and extends the arms sideward, pressing them downward against the bar while rolling around the upper arms. The bars are regrasped as soon as possible to finish the move in an upper arm hang. As skill is gained, the gymnast will avoid flexing his knees, will flex at the hips only minimally, and will pass through the shoulder balance position upon completion of the roll. It is obvious that as part of the same lever, the feet and hips will complete the same number of revolutions in a unit of time. However, since the feet are traveling through a circle with a longer radius and, consequently, a greater circumference than are the hips, they must be traveling faster or have greater velocity. Since momentum equals mass times velocity, greater momentum adequate to complete the roll in an extended position will be secured if the hips and knees are held extended to lengthen the lever during the downward swing.

ACCELERATION AND DECELERATION

The greater the mass of an object, the greater the force required for acceleration and also the greater the force required for deceleration. Possession of large mass is an advantage in sports such as football, heavyweight wrestling, or boxing, but it is a decided disadvantage in gymnastics and tumbling. Individuals with large, thick, heavy bones will find it difficult to become outstanding gymnasts or tumblers because a great force is required to secure the velocity of movement necessary to accomplish most moves. These body types find it more difficult to slow or stop their movement in the event they are slightly off balance during or after many moves because inertia is also directly related to mass.

INERTIA AND CHANGE IN DIRECTION OR VELOCITY

An object in motion possesses inertia and will remain in motion until some force causes it to change velocity, to change direction, or to stop. In the case of the gymnast, the force that causes the body to change its velocity or its direction of motion or to stop may be gravity, a spotter, eccentric muscular contractions, the floor, or the apparatus. In certain cases, the gymnast uses the apparatus to decrease velocity or to change the direction of motion. A tumbler running forward to do a front salto possesses inertia in a forward direction. The direction of this inertia from forward to upward is changed when skips are taken and landing is made on two feet with the legs angled backward (blocking action).

BASE OF SUPPORT AND STABILITY

The larger the base of support, the greater the stability. In the head balance, the forward part of the top of the head (*not* the forehead) and the hands should form an equilateral triangle to provide both lateral and forward–backward stability. This base should be as large as possible consistent with muscular efficiency of anatomic angles. If the arms are fully extended, the base is larger but

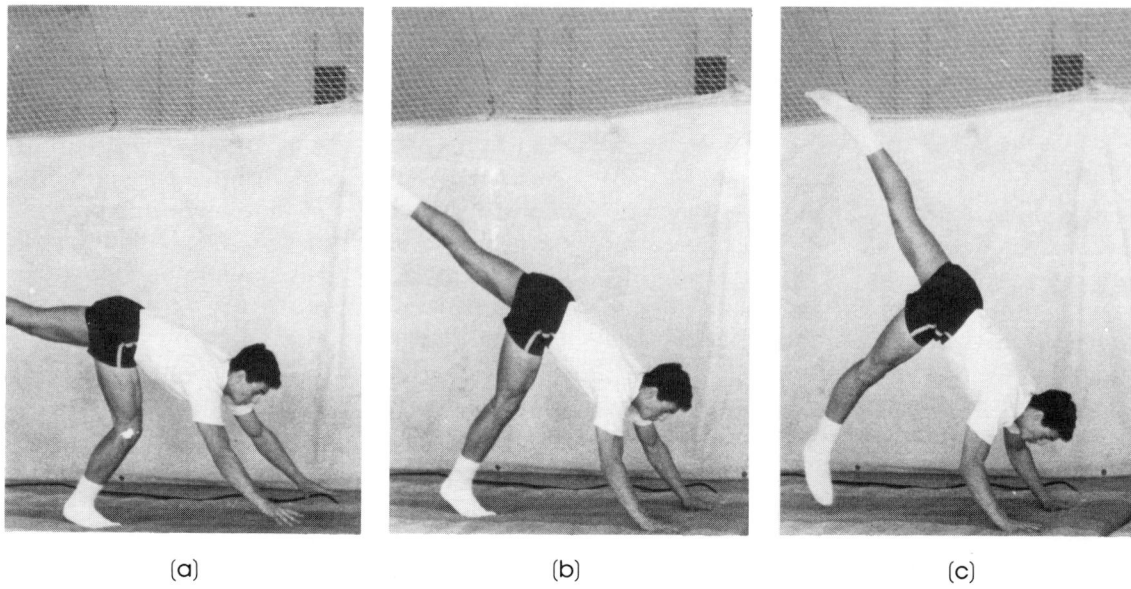

(a)   (b)   (c)

Figure 9.24 Front Handspring into Front Salto Piked Position (a) Note arms reaching forward for blocking action (b) to (e) Head is pulled backward; left leg is swinging upward; right leg extends for spring (f) to (h) Right leg moving closer to left leg, arms extending to elevate center of gravity (the hips) (i)

Note hyperextension of hips. Head moving forward, hands leaving mat, legs together (j) Note upward thrust of hips. Tumbler is completely off the mat (k) Contact of feet with mat. Arms moving toward the vertical axis of the body to provide lift. Note blocking action (l) Knees extending for lift-off

(d)   (e)   (f)

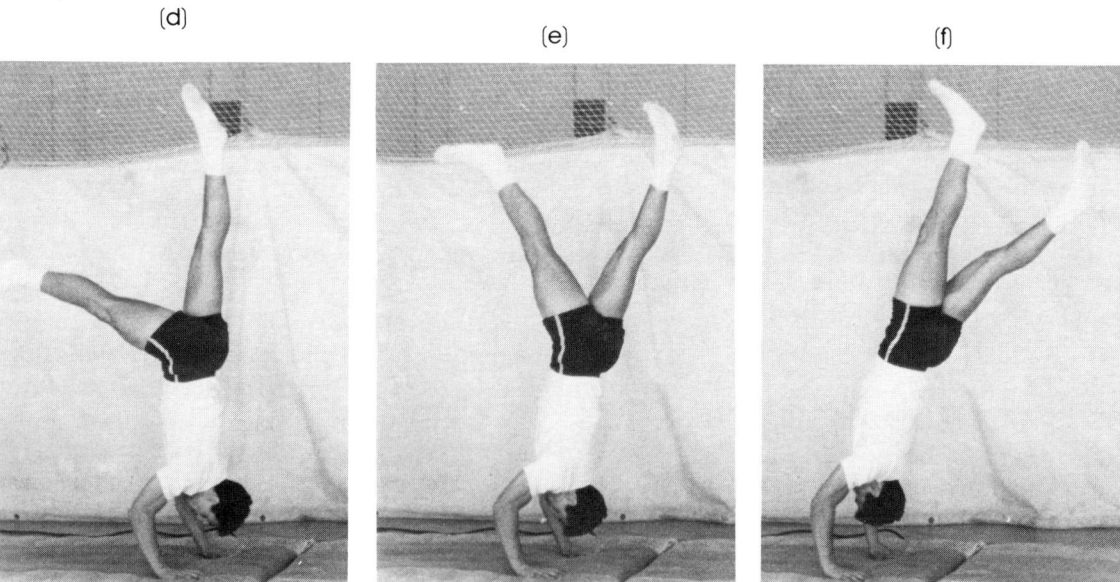

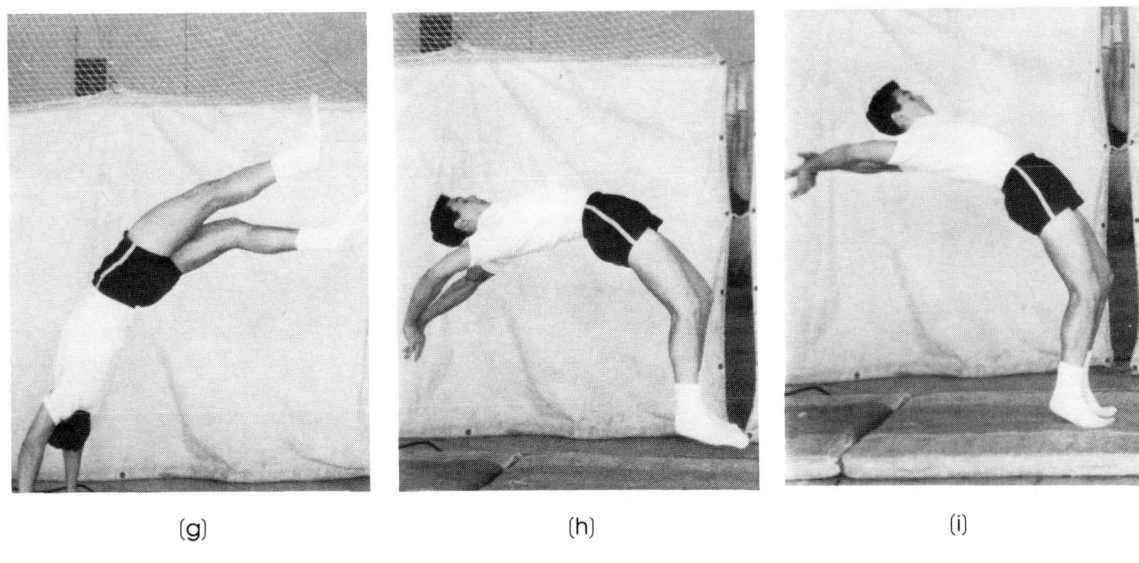

(g)   (h)   (i)

(j)   (k)   (l)

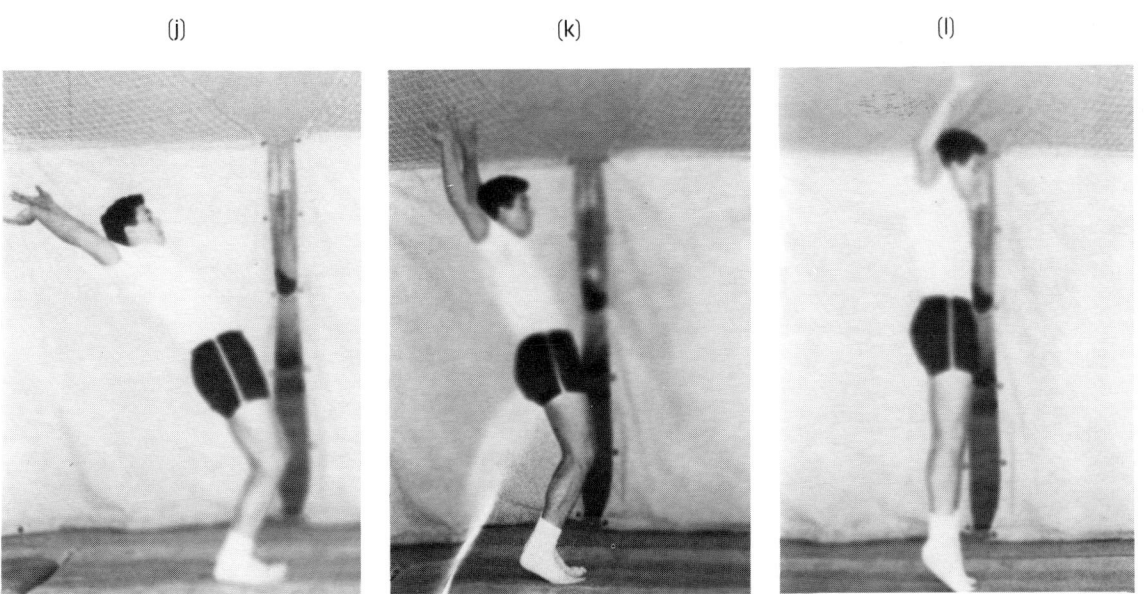

ANALYSIS OF TUMBLING AND GYMNASTIC SKILLS   **347**

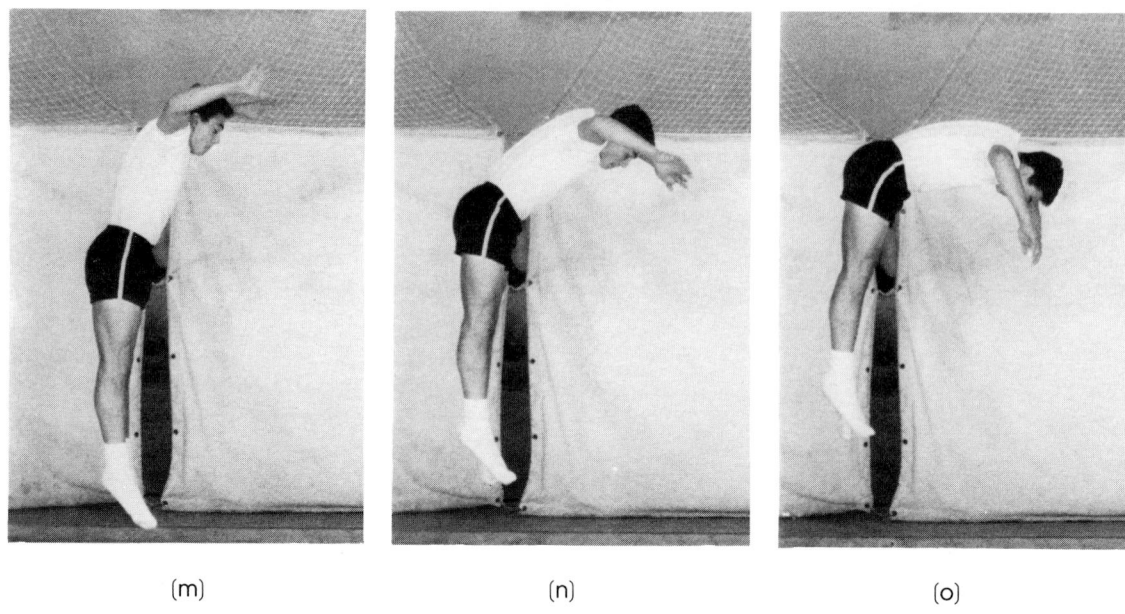

(m)   (n)   (o)

Figure 9.24 (m) to (o) Note that lift-off is vertical. Hips flex and head is brought forward initiating salto (rotation around lateral horizontal axis) (p) to (r) Arms moving downward to provide additional rotatory force (s) to (u) Highest point of center of gravity dur- ing the move. Hips maximally flexed to shorten radius of rotation (v) Hips beginning to extend (w) Arms elevating and hips extending to lengthen lever to slow rotation (x) Knees bending in anticipation of landing

(p)   (q)   (r)

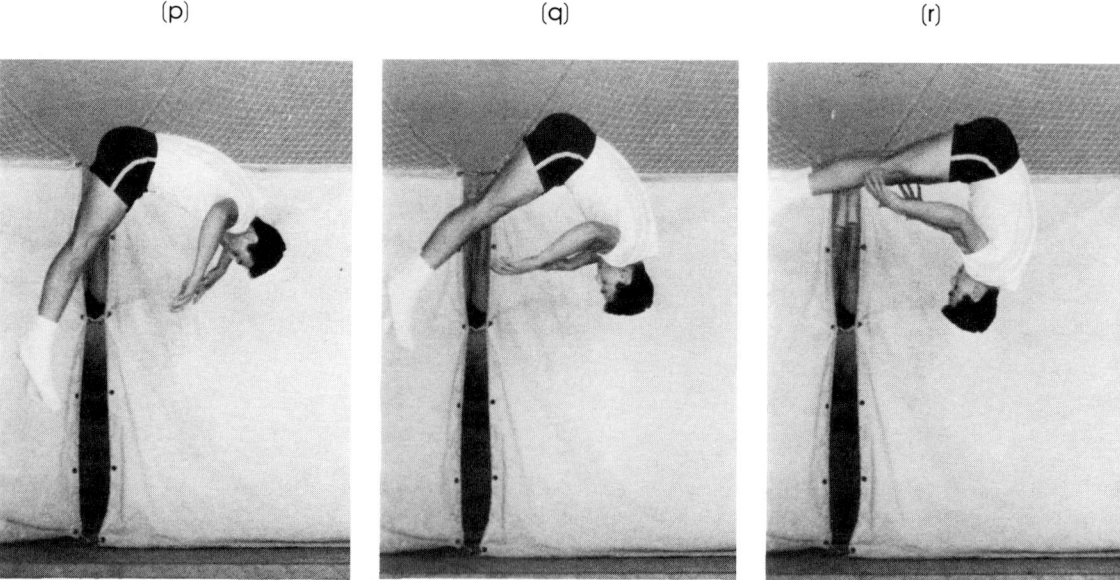

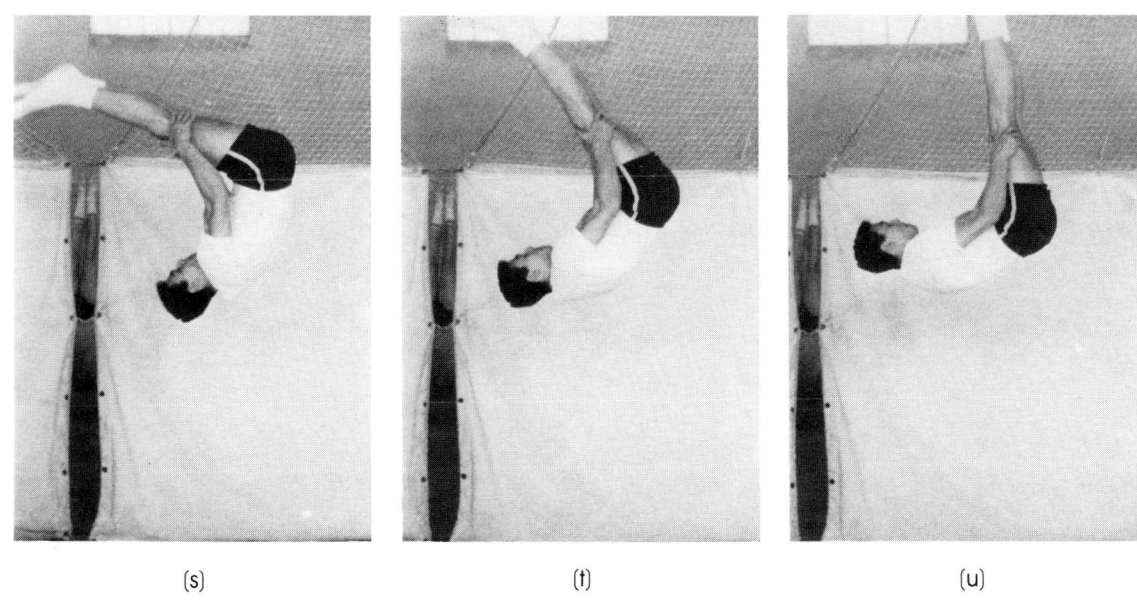

(s)	(t)	(u)

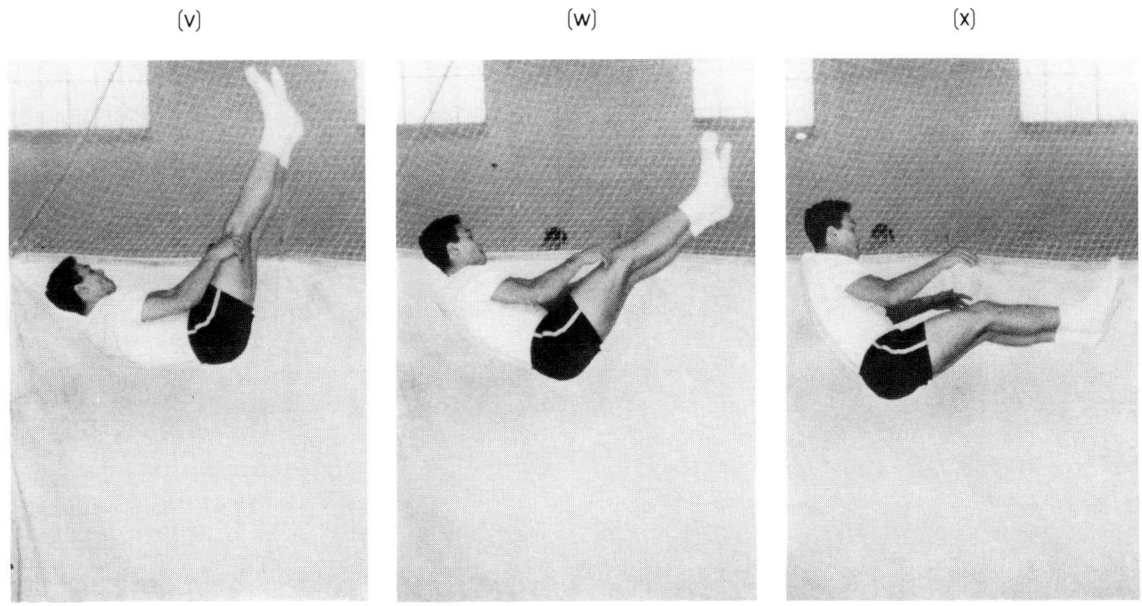

(v)	(w)	(x)

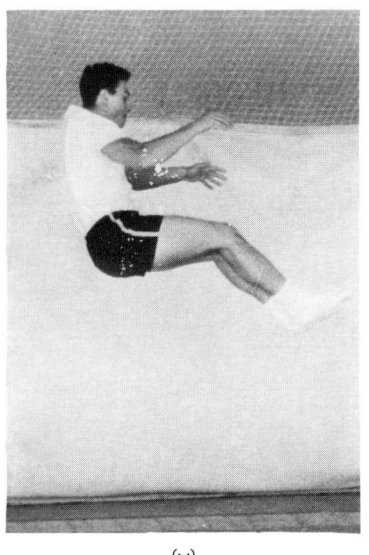
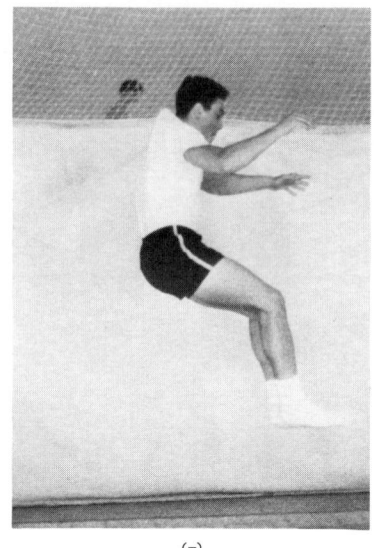

(y)   (z)

Figure 9.24y to 9.24z Landing

muscular efficiency would be very low; that is, the force that could be generated to correct balance would be insufficient.

The free head balance is more difficult than the regular head balance. The one-hand balance is more difficult than a regular handstand. The balance on one foot on the balance beam is more difficult than a balance on two feet. In all of these moves, the base of support is larger in the easier variation of the move. The reader is referred to Chapter 8 for further explanation of balance and equilibrium principles.

HEIGHT OF CENTER OF GRAVITY AND STABILITY

Raising or lowering the center of gravity affects stability. Execution of a 180 degree turn on the balance beam in a full crouch position is less difficult than it is in an erect position. This is true because in the crouched position, the center of gravity is lower. When gymnasts

land after a vault or dismount with the feet an insufficient distance in front of the body to allow for the body's excessive forward momentum, they lower their center of gravity by bending the knees and hips. This action lowers the center of gravity and facilitates maintenance of balance.

ENLARGEMENT OF BASE OF SUPPORT TOWARD ANTICIPATED FORCE

Enlarging the base of support in the direction of an anticipated force will increase stability. When gymnasts land after vaults over the horse, dismounts from the apparatus, or saltos, they move the feet in front of the forward-moving center of gravity. If they are unable to do this, they step forward to control balance. When skilled gymnasts anticipate landing in this off-balance position, they will often have one foot moving forward even before they land.

LEVER LENGTH AND ROTATORY FORCE

The longer the lever, the greater the force required to initiate rotation, but the greater the momentum at the end of the lever after the rotation has been established. In the neckspring, headspring, handspring, round-off, and back handspring, the legs should be extended throughout the move in order for the tumbler to be able to generate sufficient rotatory force to move into the succeeding skill easily.

Maintaining the extended position of the legs increases the length of the lever. Although greater force is required to initiate rotation with the legs extended, the moves cannot be executed properly from a mechanical as well as esthetic point of view if the legs are not maintained in the extended position. Most beginners flex the knees during these moves with the result that they fail to establish adequate rotatory force and consequently execute a low and ineffectual spring. Tall gymnasts must exert greater force to initiate rotation, but after rotation has been initiated, they perform giant swings and other circling moves with greater ease.

UTILIZATION OF MOMENTUM

Gymnasts and tumblers often utilize the momentum generated in a previous move (or moves) to successfully accomplish certain moves. The round-off is used not only to change the direction of movement from forward to backward but also to generate momentum for energetic back handsprings, which in turn are used to gain momentum for saltos, saltos with twists, and double saltos. In all moves on the side horse and horizontal bar in competitive exercises, the momentum of preceding moves is used to facilitate execution of succeeding moves throughout the ex-

ercise. Examples are provided in front giant swings into a rear vault catch, a hip circle into back giant swings, back giant swings into a front flyaway on the horizontal bar, and in double leg circles into a dismount on the side horse. Utilization of momentum generated in a previous move is not only mechanically efficient but also makes for more fluid and effortless movement. Momentum generated in a front handspring can be used to help in execution of a front salto (Figure 9.24). Fluidity and ease are earmarks of an esthetically pleasing exercise.

CENTER OF ROTATION AND POINTS OF SUPPORT

The center of rotation should be as nearly as possible between the points of support. The backward hip circle on the horizontal bar with the hips against the bar is considerably less difficult than is a backward free hip circle, which is done with the hips free of the bar, because in the latter move the center of rotation is not as near the points of support — the hands. Double leg circles on the side horse demonstrate application of this principle perhaps better than any other move in gymnastics.

Side Horse—Double Leg Circles

The gymnast initiates the double leg circle (Figure 9.25) in a front support. He swings the right leg over the right side of the horse until it meets the right arm. At the same time, he shifts his weight to the right arm. He raises the right leg upward until it is at a right angle to the trunk to increase distance through which momentum can be gained in this leg as he swings it clockwise over the right side of the horse. This move is utilized to gain momentum for the double leg circle, which is

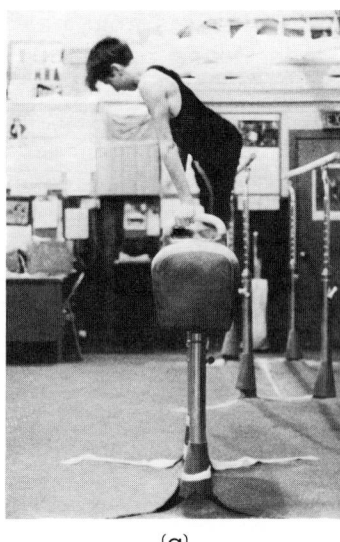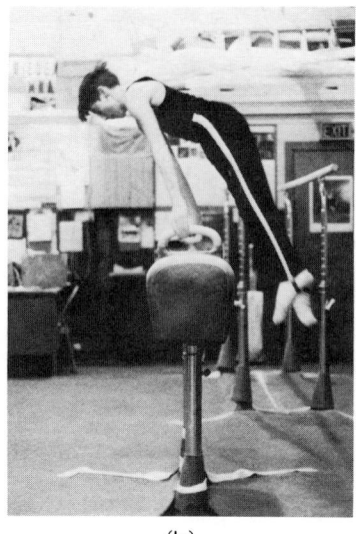

(a)   (b)

Figure 9.25 Double leg circles on the side horse. In (b) Legs beginning to clear left side of horse, left hand releasing pommel. Note greater forward inclination of arms. Center of gravity over pommels

executed out of this move. The right leg moves over the right side of the horse and continues over the left side, joined by the left leg. The gymnast has moved through the front support and at this point is moving through the rear support. He continues circling the horse with both legs. As the gymnast's legs move to the left, his shoulders move toward the right. As his legs move forward, his shoulders move backward. As his legs move to the right, his shoulders move to the left. As his legs move to the rear, his shoulders move forward. The continually changing angle of his arms with respect to the surface of the horse is always sufficient to just balance the weight and momentum of his legs as they circle around the horse. The movements of the body in this skill are similar to those of a pen if the center of the pen is held motionless while moving the lower end in a circle. The upper end of the pen will also move in a circle but always in the opposite direction. This action not only helps to maintain the center of gravity as nearly as possible

between the points of support but also places the center of rotation as nearly as possible between the points of support

CRITICAL POINT IN INITIATING MOVES

The critical point in initiating a movement during circling moves around a fixed support is usually just as the center of gravity passes a point directly under the hands or, when circling around a vertical axis such as the side horse, when the "uphill" movement begins. Another critical point occurs at the highest point in the swing, just before the body begins to swing downward, when the body is weightless. When executing circling movements around a fixed support such as the horizontal bar or parallel bars, velocity at the end of the lever (the body) is increased to gain momentum by lengthening the lever or extending the body on the downward swing. Speed of rotation is accelerated by shortening the radius of rotation by shortening the lever (the body) through flexion at the knees, hips, shoulders, or elbows (all these joints or various combinations of them are flexed in different moves). This flexion is usually initiated as the upward movement begins, just after the center of gravity passes a point directly under the hands (or shoulders if the axis of rotation is at the shoulders as in shoulder rolls on the parallel bars).

Back Giant Swings

An example is presented in back giant swings on the horizontal bar. In this move the gymnast starts in a front support with a front grip. He casts into a handstand, and as he begins to circle downward with his abdomen leading, he extends his body so that his legs, trunk, head, and arms are in a straight-line relationship (longest possible lever). As his body passes the uprights or as the center of gravity passes a point directly under his hands, he flexes the hips and shoulders slightly to shorten the radius of rotation and thereby accelerate the speed of rotation. These actions bring his body above the bar to complete the move.

Swinging Moves

Another example is provided in the swing on the parallel bars whether in an upper-arm hang or in a cross-arm support. As the gymnast's body passes the vertical position, at which time his center of gravity is directly under his shoulders when he is swinging in an upper-arm hang and between his hands when he is swinging in a cross-arm support, he flexes the hips to shorten the radius of rotation. When the body reaches the highest point in the forward swing, he extends the hips to lengthen the radius of rotation.

In double leg circles and many other moves on the side horse, the gymnast is circling around a vertical axis. The feet circle somewhat in a horizontal plane although the action is basically pendular. As the gymnast's body circles around to the front of the horse, he extends his body. As it circles over the left side (if he is circling clockwise), he flexes his hips slightly. He extends his hips again as his body swings over the right side of the horse.

APPLICATION OF FORCE AND SPEED OF ROTATION

To initiate rotation around any of the four axes, force must be applied at an angle to the axis. The greater the force, the greater will be the speed of rotation. The longer the force arm, the greater will be the speed of rotation. In the back handspring, the force to initiate rotation around the transverse horizontal axis is provided by the backward swing of the arms, the thrust of the head backward, and the movement of the trunk toward hyperextension. All of these forces are applied at an angle to the axis that is located at the center of gravity in the hip area. The more vigorously the arms are thrown backward or the greater the force, the greater will be the speed of rotation. If the arms are held extended as they are swung backward—in other words, if the force arm is lengthened—the handspring will be faster or the speed of rotation will be greater.

Cartwheel

In the cartwheel, rotation is around the anterior-posterior horizontal axis. The force initiating rotation arises out of the forward-sideward flexing of the trunk, the swing of the right arm overhead or across the body and to the mat alongside the legs, and the swing of the right leg sideward and overhead. All of these forces are at an angle to the anterior-posterior horizontal axis. For most effective execution, the right arm and the right leg should be held fully extended as they are swung in order to provide a longer force arm.

The more vigorously the trunk, arm, and leg are moved, the faster the cartwheel will be executed or the greater will be the speed of rotation.

THREE TYPES OF TWISTING MOVEMENTS

The three ways in which twisting movements are accomplished are (1) the direct method, (2) the action–reaction twist, and (3) twisting from a pike or arch.

Direct Method

In the direct method the twist is initiated from the mat, bed of the trampoline, or the piece of gymnastic equipment. The feet or hands push laterally as well as downward against the supporting surface to initiate the twist, and the action is against the supporting surface. As the feet leave the supporting surface or the hands release the equipment, the head and shoulders turn to the left and the right arm, which is extended (longer force arm) as it starts its movement, is swept in the direction of the turn. After the twist has been initiated, the arms are held as close to the body as possible, or are moved parallel to the body's long axis (shortens radius of rotation to accelerate speed of rotation). Since the twisting action is initiated while the feet or hands are still in contact with the bed, mat, or equipment, the reaction to the push from the feet or hands is against the mat, bed, or equipment and the lower body cannot move in a direction opposite to that of the arms, head, and trunk. The momentum generated by the head, shoulders, and arms is transferred to the body and legs to bring them around for the twist.

Action-Reaction Method

In the action–reaction twist, the twist is initiated after the feet have left the supporting surface. The action of the arms in one direction causes a reaction of the body in the opposite direction, causing it to twist to the left when the horizontally forward-extended arms are swung to the right to initiate the twist and slightly upward to help initiate somersaulting action. When the left arm runs into the chest, no more force or torque can be applied. In order that a twist of the body will not occur in the opposite direction when the arms are brought back into position, they are either dropped to the side or brought overhead in line with the body to shorten the radius of rotation, thereby increasing the speed of rotation.

Twisting from a Pike

In twisting from the pike or arch (Figure 9.26a), the twist is initiated after the feet have left the mat, bed, or board, or the hands the equipment. In this respect, the procedure is like that of the action–reaction method. In twisting from the pike, the twist is initiated when the body is in a tightly jackknifed position by throwing the right arm to the left in the direction of the twist. The body is then extended and the twist follows. The twisting action is made possible by the successive use of several laws of motion. With the body piked, when the arm is thrown across the chest in a plane that is at about a 45 degree angle to that of the chest, there can be little reaction to this movement because the arm movement is parallel to the vertical axis, which in the piked position is forward of the hips. To produce rotation, the force must be at an angle to the axis. Sometimes there will be a slight side somersaulting action, but this would be small because of the considerably greater mass of the body than that of the arm. This makes it possible to build up considerable momentum without producing a reactive twist in the opposite direction. When the hips are extended, the vertical axis moves behind the arm (through the center of the

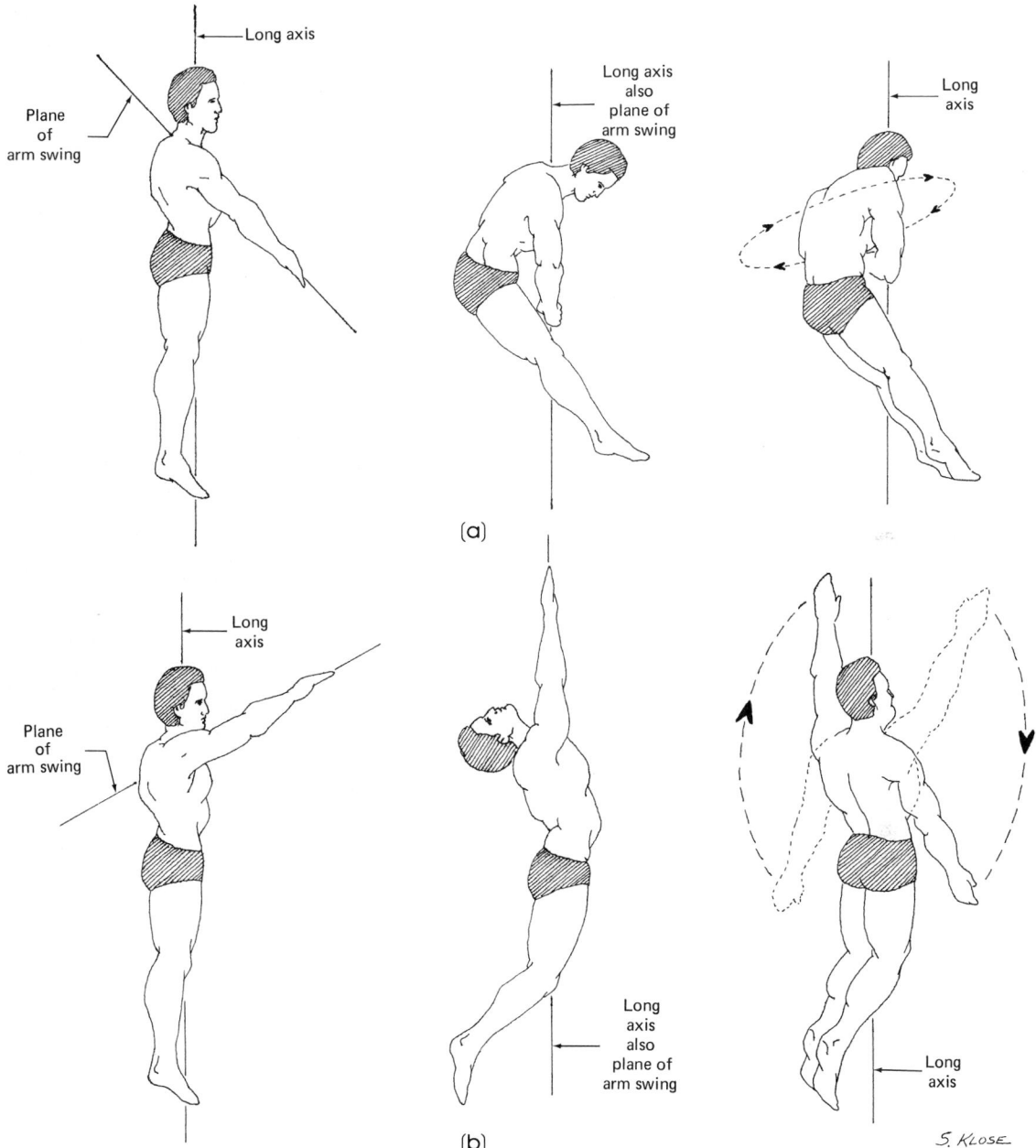

Figure 9.26 (a) Twisting from a pike—arm swing while in jackknifed position cannot produce rotation since action is in the plane of the long axis. Rotation occurs after hips have extended when arm action will be at an angle to the long axis (b) Twisting from an arch—diagonal swing of arms in oppo-site directions is in the plane of the long axis when the body is arched. However, when the body extends, the long axis moves forward relative to the body and the arm swing is then at an angle to the long axis and produces rotation

ANALYSIS OF TUMBLING AND GYMNASTIC SKILLS   **355**

body) and the momentum of the arm can now provide a force to act at an angle to the vertical axis, and the body twists.

Twisting from an Arch

The same mechanical principles are utilized in twisting from an arch in the back salto as are utilized in twisting from a pike in the front salto. During the jump after the arms have reached a position in line with the body's vertical axis in their upward swing, they are swung sideward in the plane containing the body's vertical axis. Consequently, no twisting reaction occurs. Only a slight sideward somersaulting reaction is produced. However, momentum has been generated in the arms. This momentum acts to produce torque upon the vertical axis when the body moves from its arched or hyperextended position to a straight position because the arms are now at an angle to the body's vertical axis, which now passes through the center of the body rather than behind the hips and forward of the shoulders and feet (Figure 9.26*b*). After the momentum of the arms acts upon the straight body, the arms are wrapped around the body to shorten the radius of rotation, and the twisting salto has been completed.

INCREASING MOMENTUM BY INCREASING DISTANCE

The greater the distance, and therefore time, over which momentum is developed, the greater the momentum possible. Momentum equals mass times velocity. Mass cannot be altered; however, velocity can be changed. Velocity is the product of acceleration times the time of acceleration. Therefore, momentum can be increased by increasing the time of acceleration. This is achieved in racquet sports, throwing of balls and implements, and in batting by increasing the backswing. In tum-

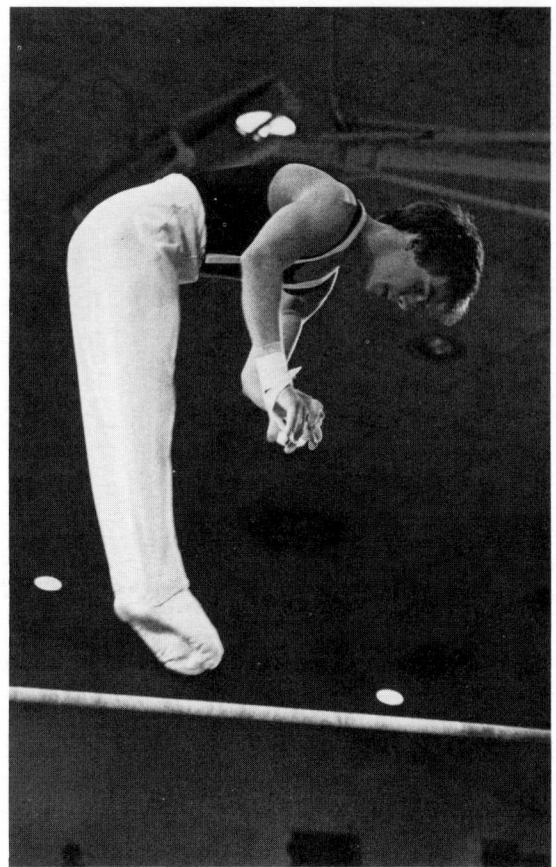

Figure 9.27 U.S. Olympian Kurt Thomas executing a Veronin. Photo courtesy of **International Gymnast**, Santa Monica, California

bling and gymnastics, it is achieved in a variety of ways. For example, in the back handspring, the tumbler swings the arms backward in the extended position during the sitback preparatory to swinging the arms forward-upward and backward above the head to move into the back handspring. The backward arm swing during the sit-back increases distance and, therefore, the time during which the speed of the forward arm swing can be accelerated. For this reason also, a high and long forward swing is advised in a back uprise or stem on the parallel bars or in the back uprise on the horizontal bar. In side horse moves, the higher the pendular swing

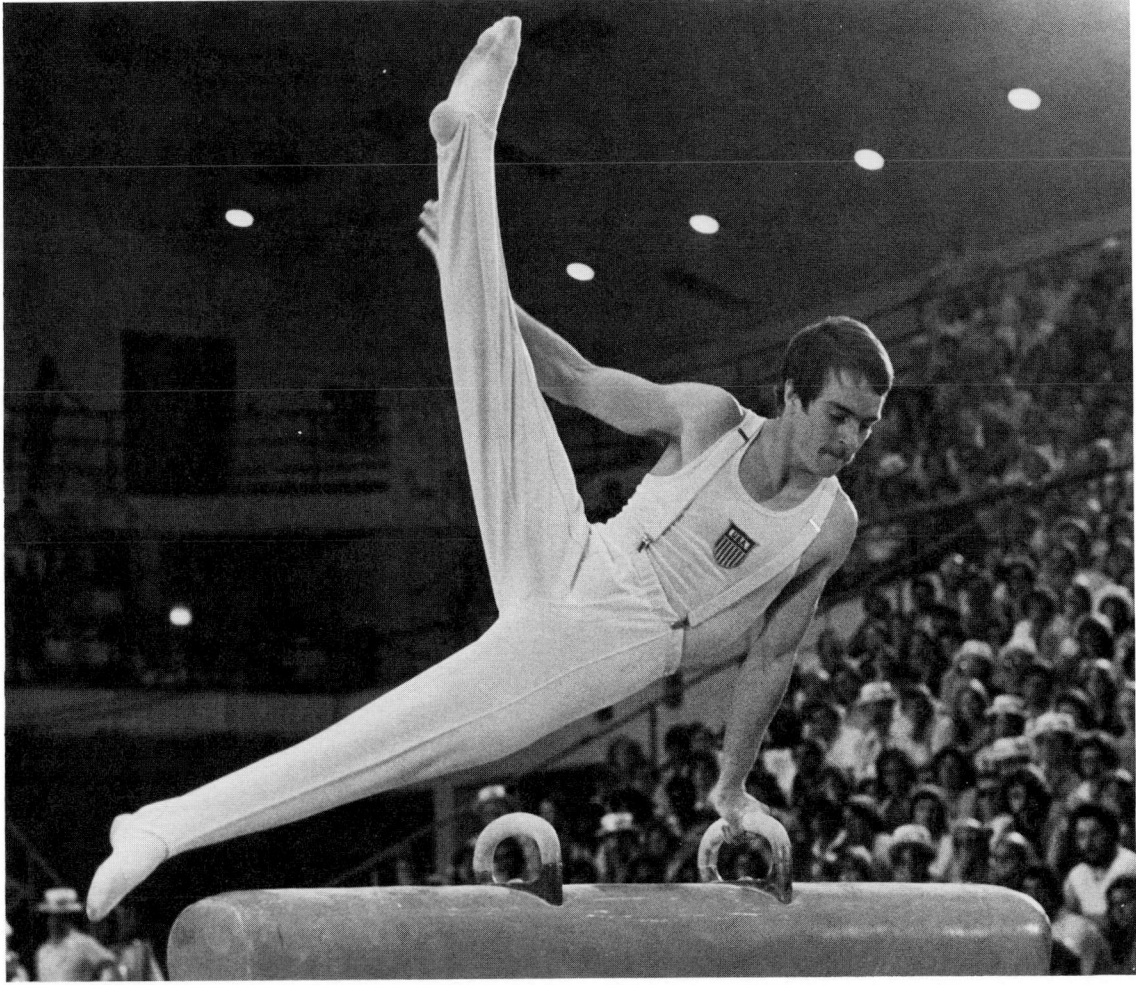

Figure 9.28 Tom Beach performing a scissors. Photo courtesy of **International Gymnast**, Santa Monica, California

on one side, the more momentum can be generated to make possible a high position as the body clears the opposite side of the horse, since the high position will increase the time of acceleration. These positioning or preparatory movements not only increase the time of acceleration but also place the muscles on a stretch. It is well known that muscles on a stretch can generate a greater pull than when they are already shortened.

DESIGN OF A GYMNASTIC EXERCISE OR ROUTINE

During a routine or exercise, the preparatory movements discussed above are incorporated into the design of the exercise so that there are no intermediate or extra swings or unnecessary hesitations. This is accomplished by utilizing the follow-through or momentum

ANALYSIS OF TUMBLING AND GYMNASTIC SKILLS | **357**

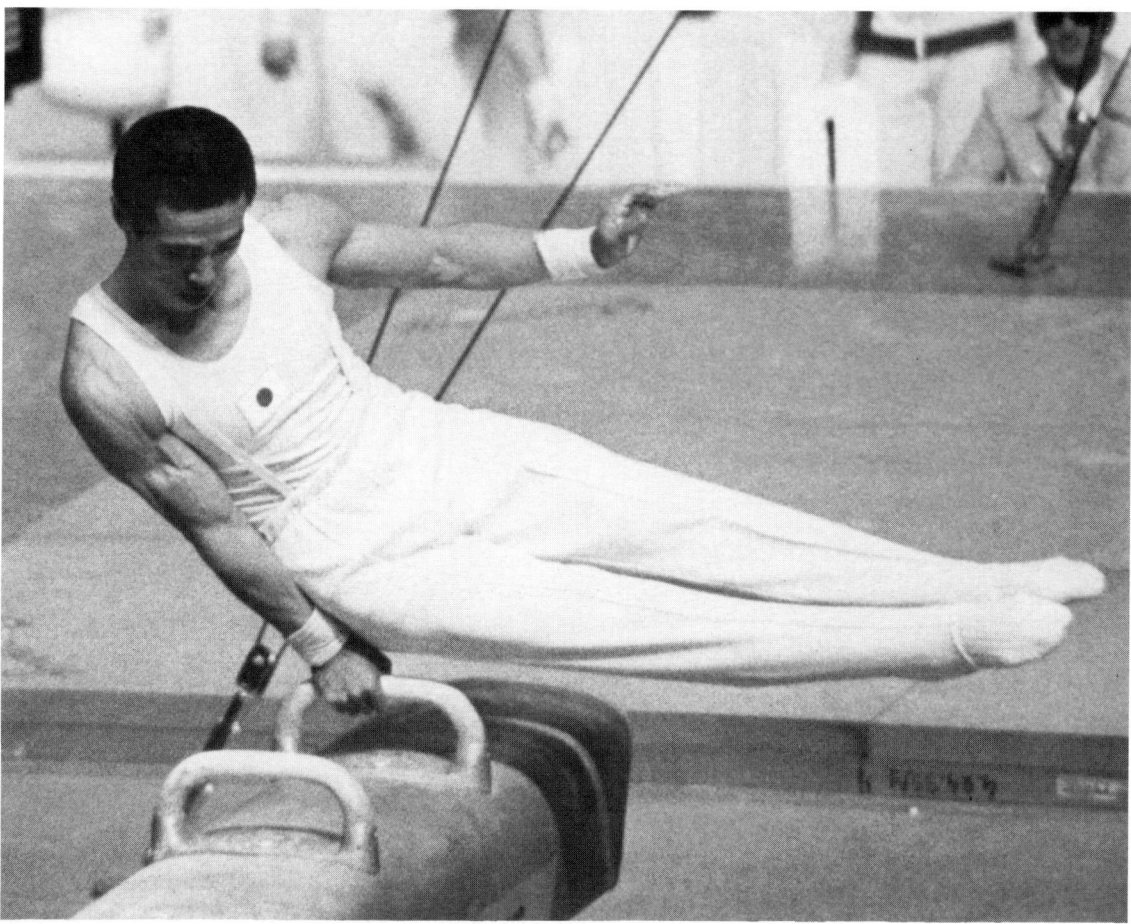

Figure 9.29 Sawao Kato, Olympian, doing a double-in. Photo courtesy of **International Gymnast**, Santa Monica, California

remaining from the previous move to initiate the move. The position of the body and its parts is also considered when determining, during the design of an exercise or routine, what the next move should be. This makes possible a continuous flow of movement with a minimum of stops. When the gymnast and his coach are planning a routine, moves and their sequences are selected so that the follow-through is used to generate momentum, to place the muscles on a stretch, and to establish the direction of application of force for the next move in the exercise. The follow-

through also facilitates relaxation and conservation of energy.

SUMMARY

Throughout this chapter we have shown how execution of gymnastic movements is facilitated by application of kinesiologic principles. Procedures for execution and spotting of a number of tumbling, trampoline, balancing, uneven parallel bars, horizontal bar, parallel bars, vaulting, floor exercise, and

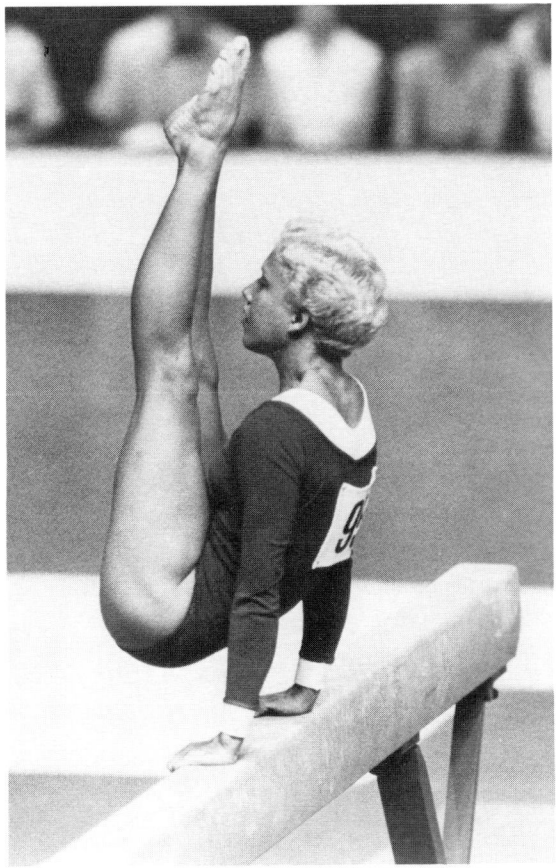

Figure 9.30 Kim Chase, U.S. Olympian, holding a V-sit. Photo courtesy of **International Gymnast**, Santa Monica, California

the location of the center of gravity; (3) the utilization of visual clues in maintenance of balance; (4) the relationship of the height of the center of gravity to stability; and (5) enlargement of the base of support in the direction of an anticipated force. In the area of momentum, the relationship between velocity, distance through which a movement may be accelerated, length of the lever and momentum were discussed. Efficient utilization of force was presented from the point of view of gymnastics in discussions of summation of forces, point of application of forces, parallelogram of force, and the point of application of force on a human lever that is at an angle to an axis around which the gymnast wishes to rotate. Transfer of momentum from one body part to another as illustrated in skills such as the neck- and headspring were discussed. Procedures for accelerating and decelerating rotatory velocity were illustrated.

Figure 9.31 "Aristocrats of Balance." Photo courtesy of Dr. David A. Field

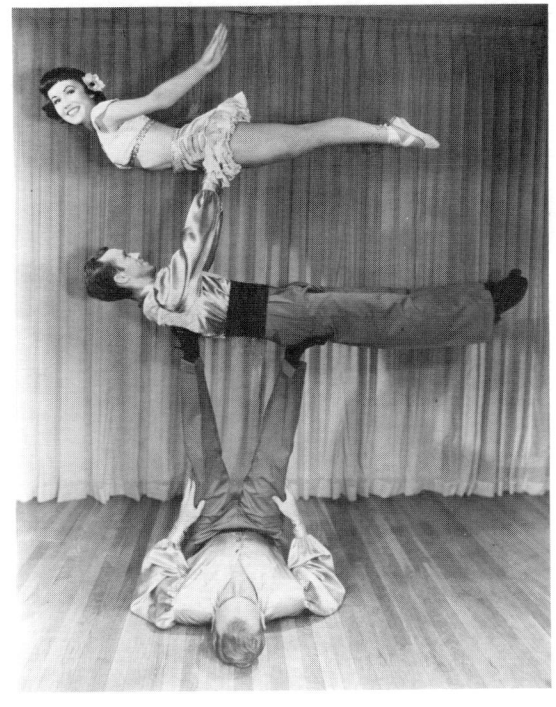

balance beam skills were presented. Procedures for most efficient execution and spotting of these skills was presented from the point of view of utilization of mechanical principles. The utilization of several mechanical principles in each skill described was explained.

Principles of stability, momentum, velocity, force, levers, and inertia as they apply to gymnastics were discussed. More specifically, in the area of balance these have included: (1) the relationship of the center of gravity to the base of support in skills of static and dynamic balance; (2) procedures for changing

ANALYSIS OF TUMBLING AND GYMNASTIC SKILLS **359**

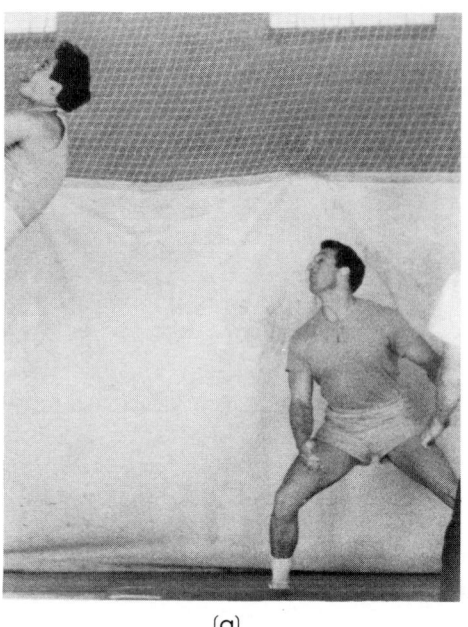

(a)

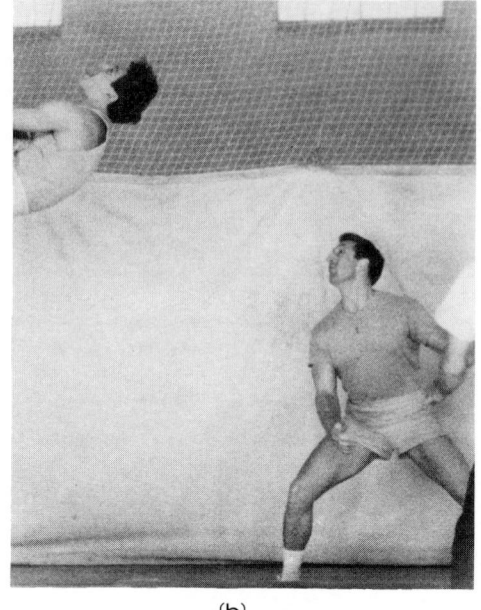

(b)

Figure 9.32 Double back somersault. (**a**) First somersault one-quarter completed (**b**) to (**d**) Center of
gravity rising. Note spotter's position (**e**) Center of
gravity at highest point (**h**) First somersault completed. Note amount of rotation between frames (**i**)
to (**p**) Completion of second somersault.

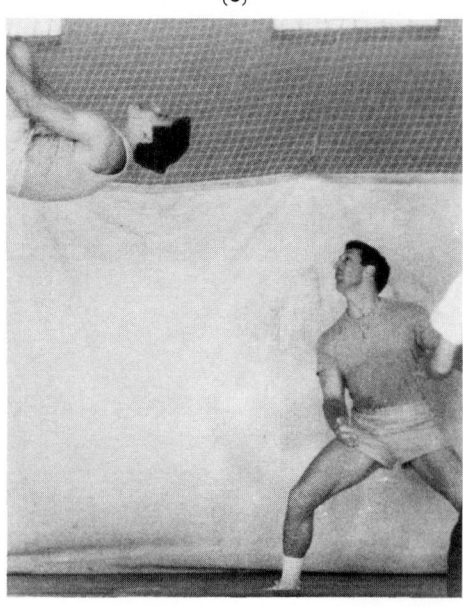

(c)

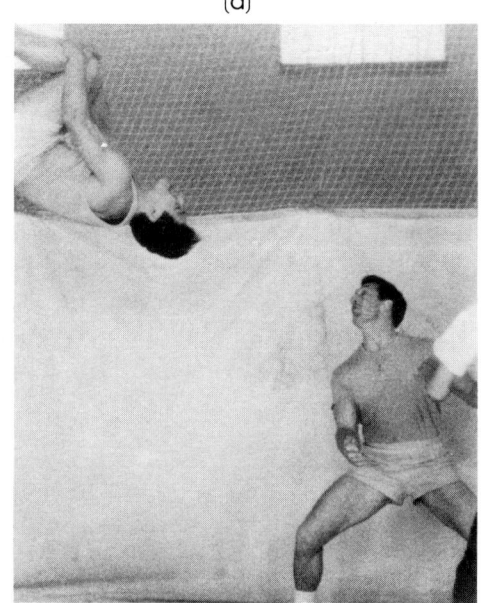

(d)

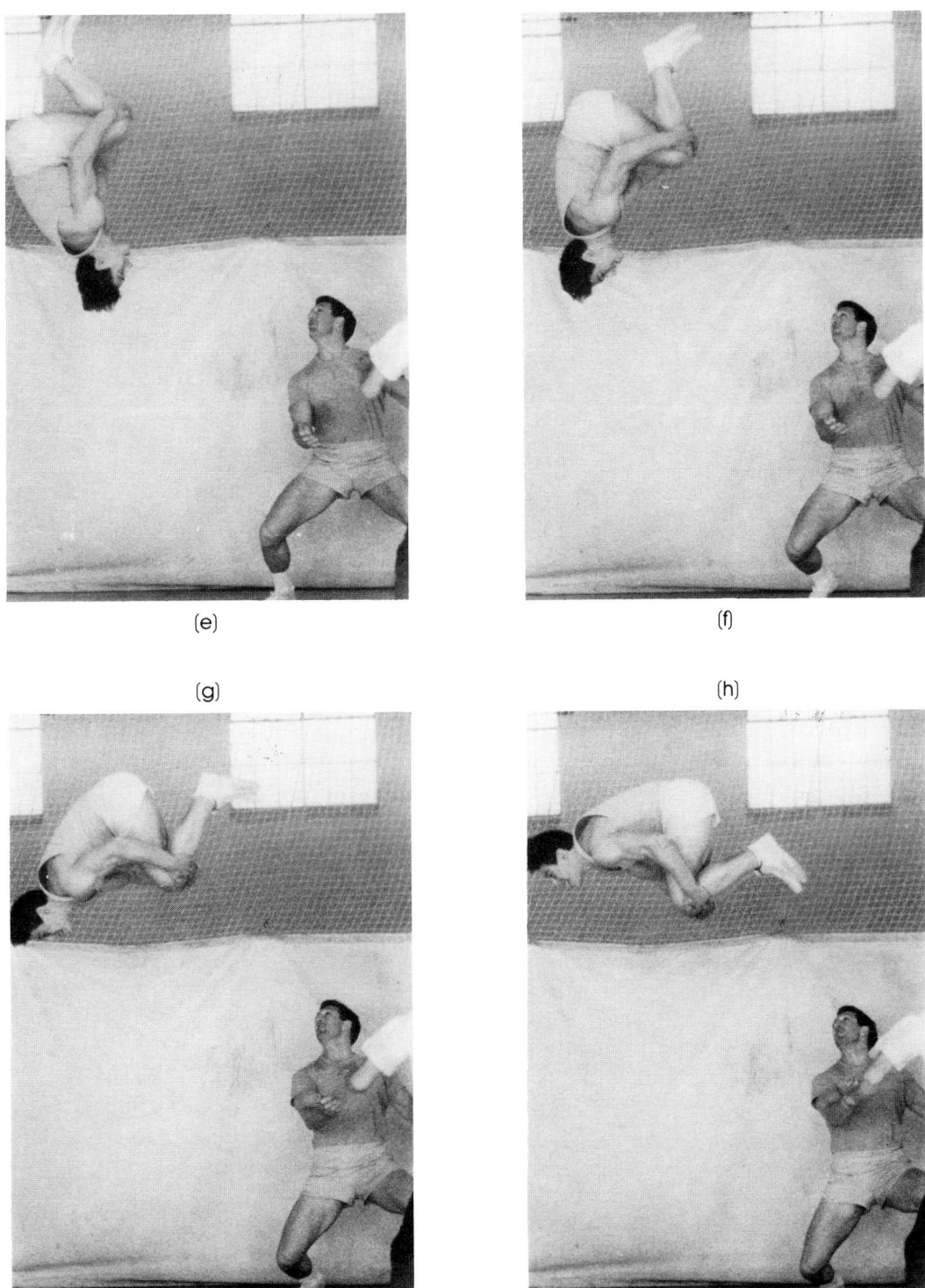

(e)

(f)

(g)

(h)

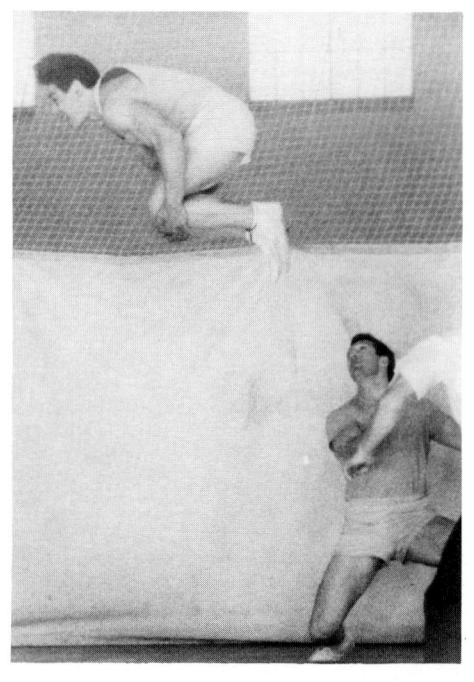

(i)

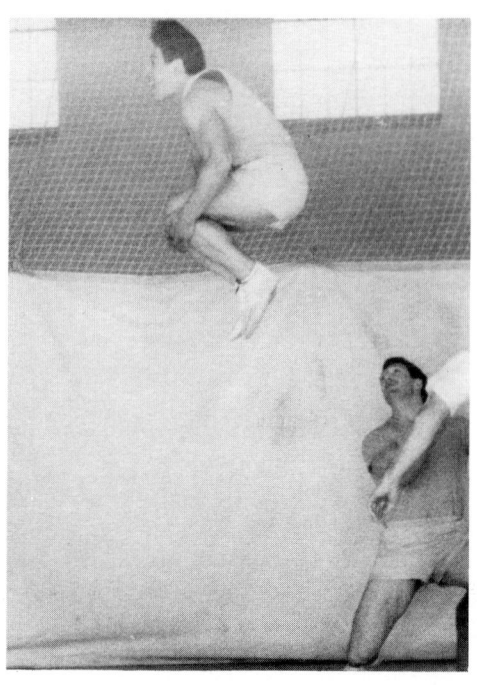

(j)

(k)

(l)

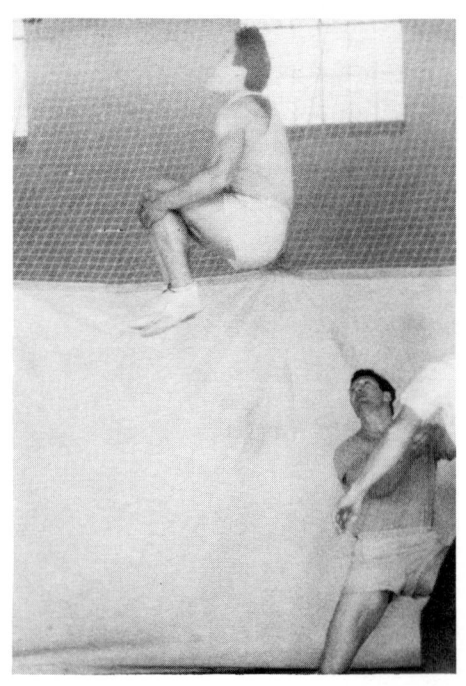

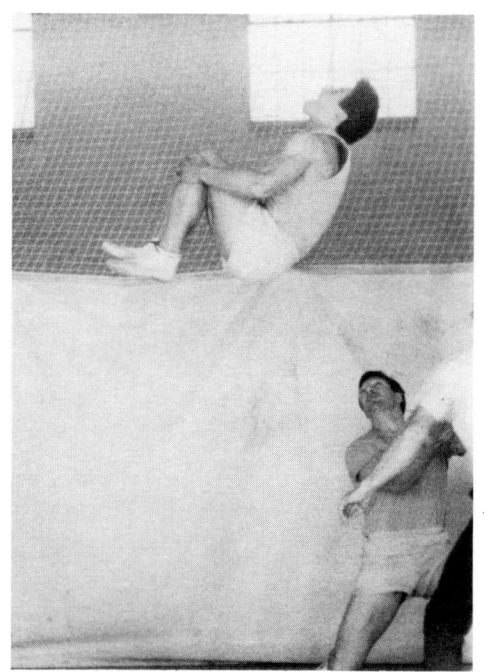

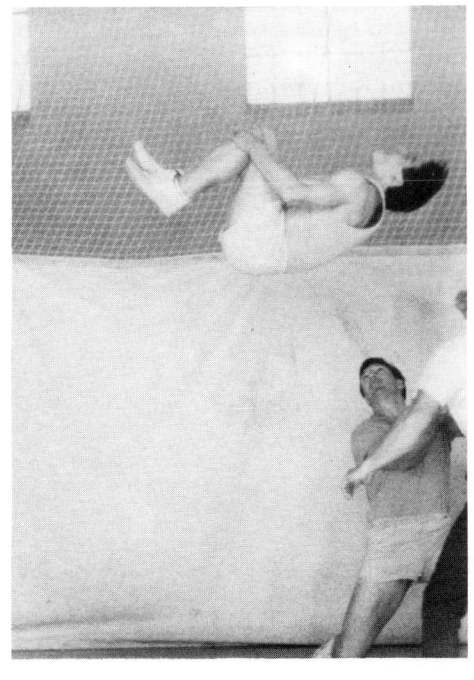

(m)

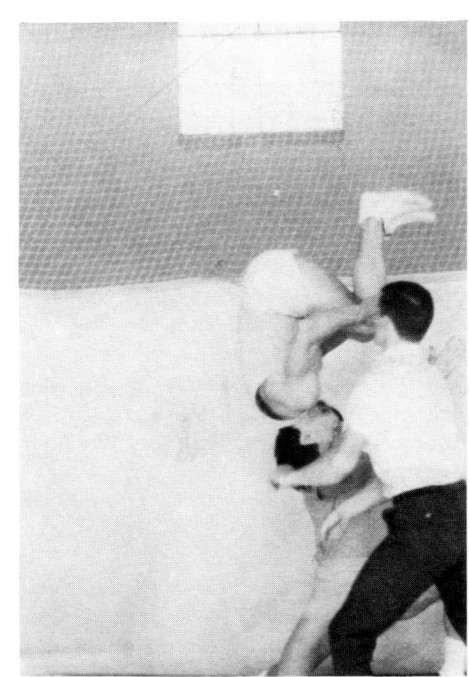

(n)

(o)

(p)

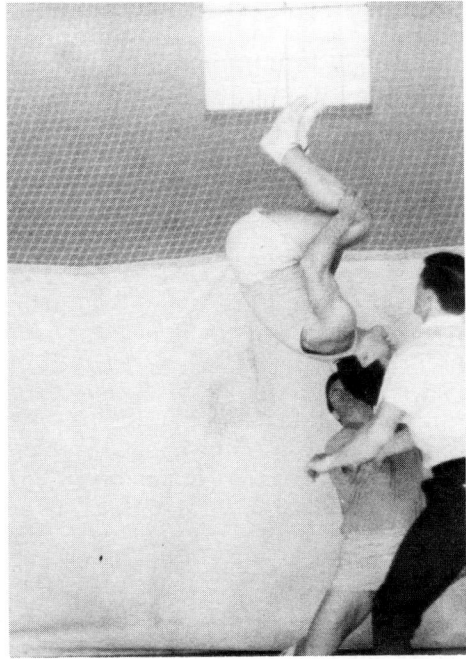

The discussion has included application of kinesiology principles in prevention of injury through developing understanding of how to absorb impact, spot, and fall with least probability of injury. Several methods of twisting during salto movements, instructions for execution of beginning skills such as headstands, handstands, cartwheels, front swan on feet, neck- and headsprings, shoulder rolls, cast to hip circles on the uneven bars, and use of the Reuther board, and instructions for such intermediate skills as giant swings, saltos, back handsprings, and stutzkehres were presented. Finally, suggestions were given for designing routines or exercises that possess continuity and fluidity.

SUPPLEMENTARY READINGS

Books

Allison, June, *Advanced Gymnastics for Women*. London: Stanley Paul and Co., Ltd., 1963.

Babbitt, Diane, and Haas, Werner, *Gymnastic Apparatus Exercises for Girls*. New York: Ronald Press, 1964.

Baley, James A., *Handbook of Gymnastics in the Schools*. Boston: Allyn & Bacon, 1974.

Baley, James A., *An Illustrated Guide to Tumbling*. Boston: Allyn & Bacon, 1967.

Baley, James A., *Illustrated Guide to Developing Athletic Strength, Power and Agility*. West Nyack, N.Y.: Parker Publishing Company, 1977.

Cochrane, Tuovi Sapinen, *International Gymnastics for Girls and Women*. Reading, Mass.: Addison-Wesley, 1969.

Cooper, Phyllis, *Feminine Gymnastics*, 2nd ed. Minneapolis: Burgess Publishing Co., 1973.

Edwards, Vannie M., *Tumbling*. Philadelphia: W. B. Saunders, 1969.

Farkas, Jim, *Age-Group Gymnastics Workbook*. Tuscon: The United States Gymnastic Federation Press.

Hughes, Eric, *Gymnastics for Girls*. New York: Ronald Press, 1963.

Hughes, Eric, *Gymnastics for Men*. New York: Ronald Press, 1966.

Johnson, Barry L., *Beginning Book of Gymnastics*. New York: Appleton-Century-Crofts, 1966.

Kjeldsen, Kitty, *Women's Gymnastics*. Boston: Allyn & Bacon, 1969.

Loken, Newton C., and Willoughby, Robert J., *The Complete Book of Gymnastics*. Englewood Cliffs, N.J.: Prentice-Hall, 1959.

Maddux, Gordon, *Men's Gymnastics*. Pacific Palisades: Goodyear Publishing Company, 1970.

Ryser, Otto E., *A Manual for Tumbling and Apparatus Stunts*, 5th ed. Dubuque, Iowa: William C. Brown, 1968.

Schmidt, A. B., and Drury, B. J., *Gymnastics for Women*. Palo Alto: Mayfield Publishing Co., 1977.

Articles

Baley, James A., "Beginning Triples Balancing," *Athletic Journal*, February, 1952.

Baley, James A., "Beginning Singles Balancing," *Athletic Journal*, January, 1954.

Baley, James A., "Vaulting Stunts over the Side Horse," *Scholastic Coach*, December, 1959.

Baley, James A., "Advanced Doubles Balancing Stunts," *Scholastic Coach*, December, 1959.

Baley, James A., "Advanced Parallel Bar Stunts," *Coach and Athlete*, January, 1964.

Baley, James A., "Advanced Tumbling Stunts," *Athletic Journal*, March, 1964.

Kerr, Beth, "Vision, Kinesthesis, Consciousness, and Skills," *Journal of Health, Physical Education and Recreation*, November–December, 1976, pp. 46–49.

Piscopo, John, "Assessment of Forearm Positions upon Upper Arm and Shoulder Girdle Strength Performance," *Kinesiology IV*. American Alliance for Health, Physical Education and Recreation, Washington, D.C., pp. 53–57, 1974.

Piscopo, John, and Hennessy, Jeff, "Trampoline Safety," *Journal of Physical Education and Recreation*, April, 1976, pp. 33–36.

Schvartz, Esar, "Effect of Impulse on Momentum in Performing on the Trampoline," *Research Quarterly*, Vol. 38, No. 2, May, 1967, pp. 300–304.

Sinning, Wayne E., and Lindbert, George D., "Physical Characteristics of College Age Women Gymnasts," *Research Quarterly*, Vol. 43, No. 2, May, 1972, pp. 226–234.

10 ANALYSIS OF SELECTED AQUATIC SKILLS

CONCEPTS

1. Forward propulsion in water is generated by a coordinated pattern of fixed and rotary joint actions.

2. Body drag in water is significantly less in females than males.

3. Magnitude of hydroplaning is dependent upon the swimmer's buoyancy and velocity.

4. Arm and hand movements generate the major source of force in front crawl swimming, whereas legs serve as the primary source of propulsion in the breast stroke event.

5. Newton's third law is operative during swimming strokes, since reaction forward is equal to the force of the backward thrust against the water.

6. The efficiency of the flight in starts depends upon the magnitude of force generated by the legs, as well as the direction of that force off the starting platform.

7. The forward flip turn entails the application of Newton's first law, principles of rotary velocity, and reduction of body drag resistance.

8. The one-arm glide turn is faster than the two-arm glide method of turning in the forward and backward crawl strokes.

9. The quality of forward running dives is governed by the approach, hurdle, takeoff, execution, and entry and depends upon an uninterrupted sequential chain of movements.

10. A slight lean on the forward approach lessens the resting inertia of the body.

11. "Pushing" the board rather than "lifting" the feet is essential for maximizing the effects of Newton's third law of motion.

12. Increasing body lean on the takeoff augments the speed of dive rotation.

13. Twisting dives can be initiated directly from the board or free-in-air after the takeoff.

14. Twisting free-in-air resembles the action of a cat falling from a designated height and exhibits the action–reaction principle of Newton's third law.

GENERAL CONSIDERATIONS

Locomotion in an aquatic medium is profoundly different from movement on land from a kinesiological perspective. Anthropometrical factors, such as body shape, size, and composition, as well as flexibility and skill elements, affect progression through water. Whenever the human body is immersed in water, Archimedes' principle is operative. This principle states that the upward force of the water is equal to the product of the density of the liquid and the volume of the object or the volume of liquid displaced. Therefore, body composition, as a biomechanical parameter, affects the swimmer's position. Simply stated, a person with high density usually swims with the legs lower than the chest. An individual who possesses low density normally floats in a horizontal position without difficulty. Since efficient forward propulsion in water requires that the body be parallel to the water surface, buoyant individuals possess a biomechanical advantage over nonbuoyant, heavy boned, and muscular persons.

The relative locations of the center of gravity and of buoyancy, as described in Chapter 8, govern body floating positions. These elements of physical buoyancy should be considered in analyzing flotation and/or propulsive skills. For example, in males certain age periods are characterized by different body density characteristics due to growth and developmental patterns. Basic swimming strokes require a horizontal position, which can be held with less difficulty during prepubescence.[1] This buoyancy variable may partially explain why it is more difficult to teach beginning swimming skills to college-age students than to elementary-school pupils. The buoyancy factor also represents a natural biological differential between males and females, which favors the female, who possesses approximately 10 percent more adipose tissue than males. This buoyancy advantage may also be a significant factor in superior performance of women in long-distance swimming.

Two important elements in generating forward propulsion entail (1) decreasing water resistance and (2) maximizing the production of force by applying correct biomechanical principles. The body moves most efficiently when it is in the horizontal position, prone or supine, as compared with vertical positions such as treading water. The production of force is a coordinated pattern of fixed and rotary joint characteristics. A physique that contains high buoyancy qualities, together with the utilization of a faultless mechanical

style, can reduce water resistance and generate maximum propulsion from beginner to championship caliber swimming levels.

RESISTIVE FORCES AND FORWARD PROPULSION

Body Alignment

A streamlined body position, as opposed to angular postures of the hips and head, significantly reduces body drag. It is interesting to note that body drag is significantly less in women than in men swiming the front crawl stroke.[2] Since hip and leg segments of men are heavier and have higher density values than those of women, streamlining or keeping the legs in line with the center of buoyancy is more difficult for men. The tendency for the male feet to sink is much greater than it is in women. Increased angulation of the hips/ legs creates greater resistance to forward propulsion. Figure 10.1 exhibits the mathematical relationship of resistive surface size with angulation of the feet that illustrates this principle.

Exaggerated angles or extreme flexion and extension postures should be avoided. These positions create vertical deviations from the supine or prone body form and increase drag, impeding forward propulsion of the swimmer. In speed swimming, the concept of *hydroplaning* assumes greater importance. Hydroplaning tends to lift the head, shoulders, and upper trunk, thereby reducing the area of body surface in contact with the water, decreasing the drag coefficient. Certain sprint swimmers performing at high velocities commonly "plane" with the resultant diminishment of body drag.

Hydroplaning is directly related to the lifting force generated at right angles to the drag force of the swimmer. Since water is of considerable density, body lift can be great, depending upon the buoyance and velocity of the swimmer. Lift is proportional to velocity,

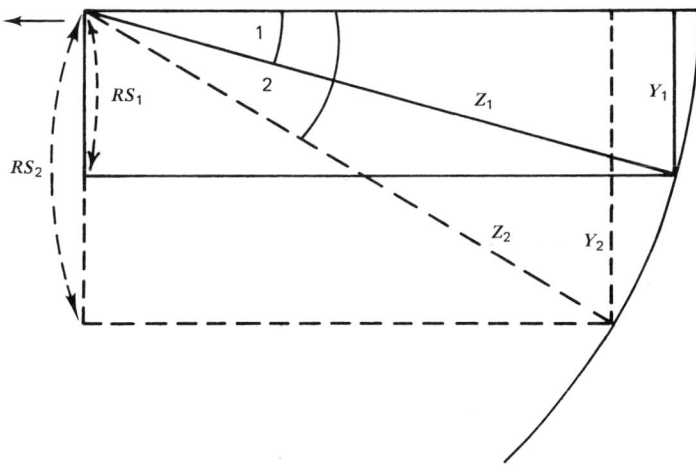

Figure 10.1 Relationship of resistive surface to sine of angle

$$\sin \text{angle}_1 = \frac{Y_1}{Z_1}$$

$$\sin \text{angle}_2 = \frac{Y_2}{Z_2}$$

$$Z_1 = Z_2$$

$$\frac{\sin \text{angle}_1}{\sin \text{angle}_2} = \frac{\dfrac{Y_1}{Z}}{\dfrac{Y_2}{Z}} = \frac{Y_1}{Y_2}$$

Y_1 = resistive surface (RS_1) caused by angle$_1$

Y_2 = resistive surface (RS_2) caused by angle$_2$

$$\frac{\sin \text{angle}_1}{\sin \text{angle}_2} = \frac{RS_1}{RS_2}$$

Resistance varies with the sine of the angle of inclination (from Marion R. Broer and Ronald F. Zernicke, **Efficiency of Human Movement**, W. B. Saunders Co., Philadelphia, Pa., 1979, with permission)

and hydroplaning of swimmers with favorable specific gravity qualities is desirable for drag reduction when speed is the primary objective. The assumption that swimmers should swim low because there is less resistance under water than on the surface is without scientific support. When considering water resistance alone it is preferable to swim on the surface instead of under the water. Swimmers developing more or less resistance performing various strokes at different velocities evidence mixed resistant values. The retarding effect is dependent upon a combination of variables including anthropometric dimensions, body position, and speed during swimming performance. The principle of hydroplaning is sound for buoyant individuals when seeking efficiency at high velocities; however, it is important to consider the swimmer's position and style. If an elevated posture of the upper trunk and shoulders conflicts with the natural head, shoulder, and arm movements, then this particular principle may create a retarding effect rather than an increase in speed. Every person has a unique structural physique and functional style; the concept of limiting a swimmer to one or two specific patterns, ignoring anthropometrical and psychomotor differences, may not be the most efficient technique for teaching swimming. The principle of hydroplaning for certain individuals with low body

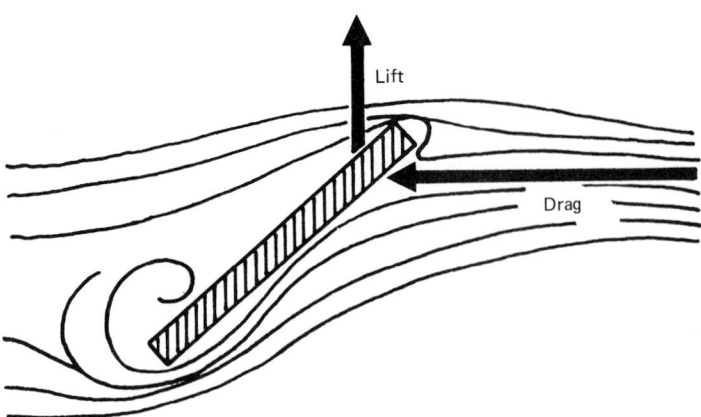

Lift

Drag

Figure 10.2 Drag and lift forces (from Marilyn M. Hinson, **Kinesiology,** Wm. C. Brown Co., Publishers, Dubuque, Iowa, 1977)

density is valid, provided excessive up and down body movements are avoided and a streamlined style is maintained.

Turbulent water drag is related to smoothness of the surface. Calm water presents less drag on the swimmer than choppy waves. A lone swimmer moving through a smooth surface, before other persons enter the pool, feels the ease of forward propulsion due to a significant reduction of turbulent drag. As the swimmer moves through the water, drag and lift forces are generated as shown in Figure 10.2. The component force acting at right angles to the drag component is known as the lift.

Forward Propulsion

An integral component of generating movement through water entails the propelling forces stemming from coordinated actions of torso, arms, and legs. The goal of swimmers is to minimize resistance forces and maximize propulsive thrusts. Arms and legs rotate in an angular fashion around joints as the entire body moves linearly in an extended supine, prone, or sideward posture.

Observation of fish and aquatic mammals illustrates the profound advantages of joint flexibility and extensive range of motions natural to sea creatures. Humans are limited to constricted movements and ranges, which impede forward propulsion, when compared with the suppleness and rubberlike characteristics of fish. Propulsion is clearly illustrated in Figure 10.3 by the dolphin kick, which resembles the motion of a fish tail with the legs moving in the vertical plane.

Perhaps one of the most important anatomical characteristics of excellent swimmers is reflected by their superb flexibility pattern, particularly of the knee and ankle articulations. Coaches generally agree that individuals lacking full plantar and dorsiflexion ranges of the ankle joint seldom achieve high kicking efficiency. Sheeran[3] compared electrogoniometric movements of competitive and noncompetitive swimmers and found that the kicking action at the knee of varsity swimmers exhibited a greater degree of movement in the front flutter, back flutter, and dolphin kicks than in nonvarsity performers. The range of movement at the ankle in these three types of kick was also greater with the varsity group. This evidence supports the concept of leg flexibility as an important element in efficient performance of the leg kick.

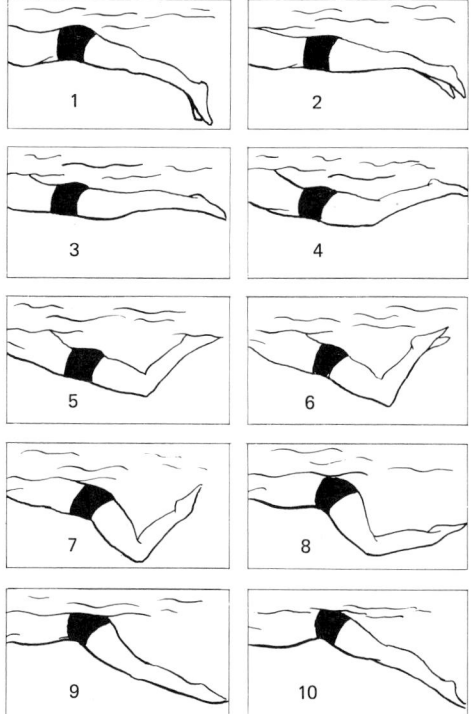

Figure 10.3 Underwater leg action of the dolphin kick (from James E. Counsilman, **The Science of Swimming,** Prentice-Hall, Englewood Cliffs, N.J., 1968, pp. 27–72, with permission)

Arm and Leg Forces

Most swimming authorities agree that the prime propulsive force for moving a body through water in crawl stroke swimming emanates from the arms and shoulder girdle, rather than from leg power. An early study by Karpovich[4] indicated that 70 percent of the propelling force in the crawl stroke is derived from the arms. Recent data support Karpovich's contention that the major contribution to propulsion in front crawl swimming is obtained from the arms.[5]

Most swimmers use the kick as a balance mechanism and to lift the legs, thereby reducing body drag. However, the work of the legs makes a much larger contribution to the total propulsive force in the breaststroke than in the crawl stroke. In butterfly swimming, Magel[6] found that the arms and legs deliver approximately the same propelling forces. In analyzing propulsive force values of the arms and legs, attention should also be directed to the anatomical and physiological attributes of the individual, which significantly affect the overall performance in all swimming strokes and events.

SWIMMING STROKES

Front Crawl

The front crawl continues to predominate as a popular stroke and is commonly taught in most units of swimming instruction at all age levels. This style is the fastest known human stroke.

Several variations in leg beat and the arm action exist; however, all techniques employ an alternating flutter kick and an overarm recovery with the face underwater. The technique described in this discussion is known as the "American crawl," employing a six-beat kick characterized by six leg kicks to one complete cycle of the arms. Three components of the crawl stroke entail (1) arm action, (2) leg kick, and (3) rhythmic breathing. These elements must be mechanically and neuromuscularly coordinated for achievement of maximum efficiency. Figure 10.4 illustrates a basic position of coordinating arms, kick, and breathing elements.

Timing of arms and legs is central to learning an efficient front crawl stroke. Proper rhythm is similar to a waltz tempo of three kicks — one-two-three, one-two-three — to each arm pull; a complete revolution of both arms has six kicks, three with each leg. The breathing mechanism should also be integrated with stroke action; inhaling on the preferred side at the end of the arm press.

An effective forward propulsion results when arm strokes and leg kicks are used in such a way that the movement is executed in

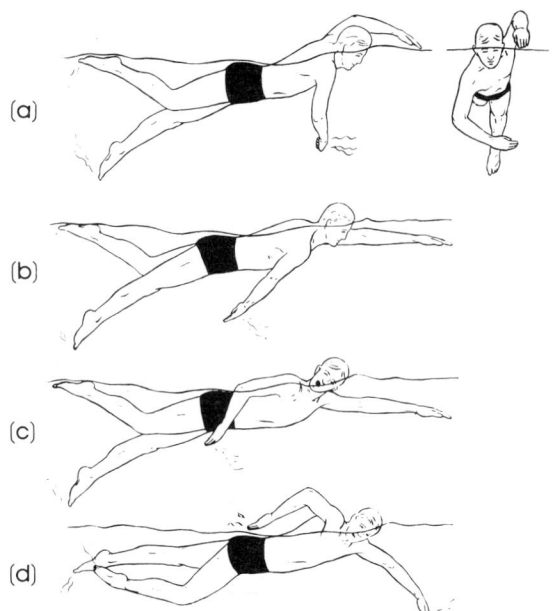

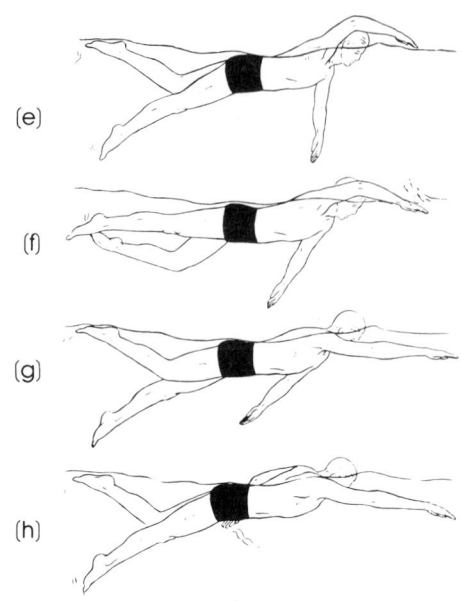

Figure 10.4 Coordination of the front crawl (from David Armbruster, Robert H. Allen, and Hobert S. Billingsley, **Swimming and Diving,** 6th ed., The C. V. Mosby Co., Saint Louis, Mo., 1973 with permission)

a continuous ballistic fashion. The force backward against the water employing Newton's third law of motion where the reaction forward is equal to the backward push is applied. As indicated previously, linear motion of the body moving in a horizontal position requires rotary movements in the kinetic chain of human levers. As the right arm is pulling down and backward during the armstroke, the left leg is thrusting up and backward as shown in Figure 10.4a. The same coordinating motion is reversed using the left arm and right leg (Figure 10.4e). This basic pattern is integrated with a six beat action of the American crawl. Specific mechanics of the arm action, leg kick, and breathing mechanism are described in the following section.

Arm Action. The arms provide the main source of propulsion in the front crawl stroke.

Earlier techniques favored a longer gliding action for distance swimming and no-glide for sprints. Modern speed swimmers employ the no-glide technique with the arms moving continuously with minimum changes in velocity and direction. Some rolling action of the body is allowed, since a side position of the body places the pulling arm in a better mechanical position by permitting greater rotation of the glenohumeral articulation. The arm stroke is comprised of three important segments: (1) catch, (2) pull, and (3) recovery.

Catch

The catch begins when the swimmer contacts the water and begins the push backwards. The actual "catch" should be made with the arm flexed. The bent arm position allows greater backward force and minimizes upward and downward body movement that may dissipate the arm thrust.

Pull

The pull applies to the actual propelling phase of the arm stroke. The arm stroke force is generated by the contraction of arm and shoulder muscles. Since pulling power provides approximately three-fourths of crawl propulsion, it seems logical to develop specific muscles of the arms and upper torso as a foundation for achieving high-speed performance. Underwater films reveal that as the skilled swimmer pulls, the hand does not follow a straight path, but the path of the hand resembles an inverted question mark.[7] The arms pull in a flexed position. The bent elbow allows for greater forward propulsion by exerting a better straight-line action of the body and increases the mechanical advantage of the third-class lever arrangement of force. Bending the elbow increases the mechanical advantage by (1) minimizing the zig-zag motion of the body as the swimmer surges forward and (2) allowing the upper arm to exert a greater force by reducing the distance between the fulcrum and resistance point. Figure 10.5 illustrates the pulling pattern utilizing three bent arm techniques. The bent arm pull is universally accepted by swimming authorities as a sound technique for maximizing arm propulsion in the front crawl stroke.

Recovery

This phase of the arm action begins after the pull–push of the arm and hand, as the elbow is lifted out of the water. The shoulder joint is rotated with the arm circumducting. The elbow is raised higher than the hand as the entire arm moves forward. The recovery phase of the arm action allows a brief pause for relaxation. Maximum roll should be avoided since excessive lateral deviation of the body can increase resistance to forward propulsion. However, some roll is desirable to permit greater shoulder mobility, although the exact quantitative roll deviation is difficult to specify because of interrelatedness of the swimmer's anthropometrical, physiological, and individualistic style of propulsion.

Leg Kick. The leg action used in the front crawl is called the "flutter kick." The kick is characterized by an undulating movement emanating from the hips, in a wavelike fa-

Figure 10.5 Pulling pattern of three bent arm techniques in the front crawl (from James E. Counsilman, **Science of Swimming,** Prentice-Hall, Englewood Cliffs, N.J., 1968, p. 58, with permission)

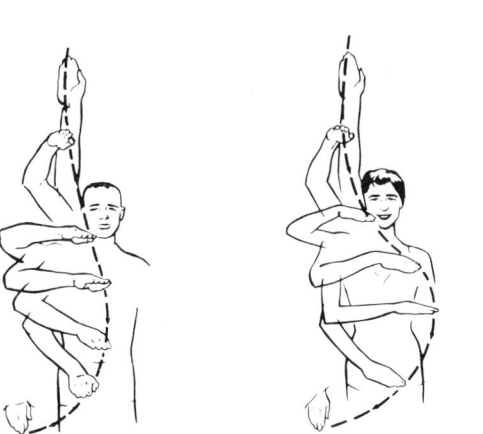
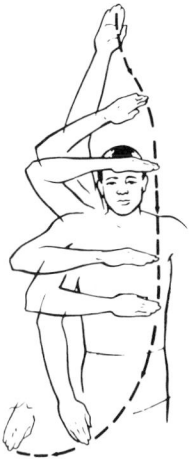

shion, and moving toward the knees and feet. An efficent kick resembles the sinuous motion of a fish's tail, except that the movement is in the vertical (up and down), instead of the lateral (side-to-side) plane. Flexibility of the hips, knees, and ankles, in addition to large feet, is a functional advantage in the flutter kick. Swimming experts attribute less than 50 percent of forward propulsion to the leg kick in the front crawl stroke; however, the kick does have a major role in preventing excessive lateral roll and maintenance of proper body balance. Backward force can be produced by the upward and downward beats of the kick. The effectiveness of both phases of the kick depends largely upon the flexibility of the talocrural joint (ankle joint) in the foot. Highly skilled swimmers consistently exhibit a greater range of ankle joint motion. Motions that favor restricted movements of the ankle as opposed to the "rubberlike" action of swim fins can actually hinder forward propulsion. Movements with the emphasis on the down-

beat, with extreme dorsiflexion, can in certain instances cause the swimmer to travel backward. The backward force of the legs is dependent upon the flexibility of the ankle joint and it is unlikely that persons with poor talo-crural ranges will attain maximum flutter kick velocity. Disagreement does exist since some experts believe upbeat is merely a "recovery phase" of the kick, while others maintain that considerable force can be generated by the sole of the foot, since a greater body surface is exposed in the upward thrust action. Figure 10.6 illustrates the up and down movements of the flutter kick with a resultant force thrusting the body forward.

Breathing. Rhythmic breathing, coordinated with the arm pull, is important for economical oxygen consumption and the maintenance of proper body position of the swimmer. Sprinters attempt to minimize the number of breaths taken because of the loss of time and change in body position. Skilled

Figure 10.6 Up and down phases of flutter kick pattern in the front crawl; **EU** = Effective upward force component. **ED** = Effective downward force component. **TFU** = Total force of up-kick swirls. **TFD** = Total force of down-kick swirls. (from T. K. Cureton, Jr., "Mechanics and Kinesiology of Swimming (The Crawl Flutter Kick)" **Research Quarterly**, 1:101, 1930, with permission)

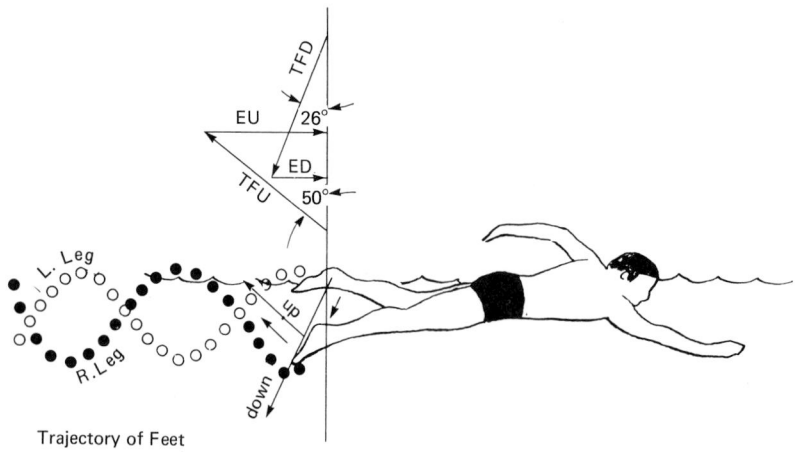

Trajectory of Feet

swimmers inhale rapidly by rotating the head sideward and returning to the prone posture with minimum changes from the elongated horizontal position. The mechanics of head turning vary with style and swimming proficiency. Swimmers usually breathe on a preferred side, which is often the side of the strongest arm pull. They inhale at the end of the push phase of the arm stroke. The head is quickly returned to the prone position independently of the arm stroke. The objective is to keep any lateral movement of the body at a minimum since such movement may interfere with forward propulsion. Proficient speed swimmers learn to breathe on both sides. This technique is desirable because it is less fatiguing and allows the swimmer a choice of sides at each turn as either arm approaches the end-wall before executing a somersault turn. The objective in rhythmic breathing, at least over long distances, is to maintain correct horizontal body posture, which helps reduce body drag, and to execute head turning movements in coordination with the arm stroke so that less oxygen is consumed.

Back Crawl

The back crawl is the third fastest stroke known to humans, exceeded in speed capabilities only by the front crawl and butterfly. Mechanically, two basic differences occur in this stroke as compared with the front crawl: (1) breathing mechanism is in the face-up posture, and (2) the flutter kick is the inverted position. Slight variations from the front crawl occur in arm and leg action. However, it is not unusual for the front crawl swimmers to perform outstandingly as backstrokers. These two strokes are related, employing flexors and extensors of the torso and appendages in identical planes. Underwater film observations of world class back crawl competitors reveal that the bent-arm pull is the most frequently used method. Mechanically, the bent-arm pull allows the arm to move overhead more rapidly. The faster the

hand moves through the water, the greater propelling resistance it creates; since propulsive resistance increases with the square of the speed, i.e., doubling the speed increases the resistance approximately four times, the faster the arm moves, the greater the resistance created at the hand, and the more efficient the propulsion.[8] Figure 10.7 illustrates the competitive six-beat back crawl stroke using the bent-arm pull and recovery.

The major components of the back crawl are (1) arm action, (2) leg action and (3) breathing. These elements and their interrelatedness to the total stroke are described in the following section.

Arm Action. The arm action consists of (1) recovery, (2) entry and catch, and (3) pull and push elements. A rhythmic counterbalance of arms and legs is necessary to propel the body forward in a continuous motion. The bent-arm pull is described in this analysis because of its shortened lever arm advantage, which consequently strengthens the moment of force by decreasing the distance of force application (hand pressing the water) from the fulcrum (shoulder joint). The underwater pulling action of the bent-arm technique is shown in Figure 10.7c, d, g.

Recovery Phase
The arms begin the recovery phase when the hand and arm are extended alongside of the thigh as shown in Figure 10.7a. The arms are flexed slightly at the elbow joint and move out of the water vertically around a horizontal axis. A slight lifting of the shoulder of the recovery arm and hip rolling occur, which serve to counterbalance the opposite side. The recovery phase ends when the arm is fully extended overhead, slightly lateral to the shoulder.

Entry and Catch Phase
A smooth ballistic movement of the arm follows the recovery with the shoulder and elbow

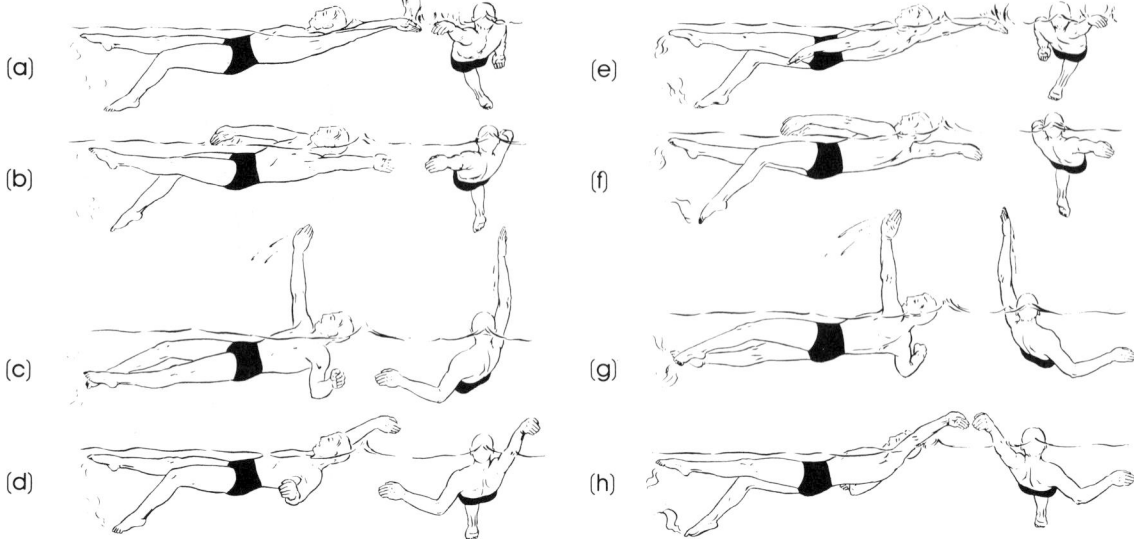

Figure 10.7 Coordination of the back crawl (from David A. Armbruster, Robert H. Allen, and Hobert S. Billingsley, **Swimming and Diving**, 6th ed., The C. V. Mosby Co., Saint Louis, Mo., 1973, with permission)

joints contacting the water before hand entry (Figure 10.7d). The entry phase should emphasize proper hand placement with the hand parallel to (facing) the water and slightly flexed. The hand and arm are now in correct position for the catch phase of the arm stroke, as shown in Figure 10.7e, f. The catch begins with an initial press of the fingers and the hand slightly below the water surface. The catch usually pulls at a shallow depth, which becomes deeper as the arm stroke moves into the pull phase.

Pull and Push Phase

A powerful thrusting motion is initiated with the pull phase of the arm stroke. This action resembles the letter "S" as the arm is adducted to the side of the body toward the feet. The "S" pattern reduces the length of the lever and makes it easier for the arm pull. Additionally, this action facilitates the application of Bernouli's principle of fluid dynamics by allowing the swimmer to alter the pitch of the hand, creating increased velocity of the

arm moving in the water and thereby maximizing forward propulsion. The large depressor muscles of the lattissimus dorsi and trapezius come into play, as the swimmer proceeds pulling in a bent-arm position. The backward thrust movement is completed with the "push" action of the forearm and hand, terminating at the side of the body in an extended position as shown in Figure 10.7g, h.

Leg Action. As in the front crawl, the flutter kick is used in back crawl, but it is inverted. Refer to the section above on leg kick.

Breathing. The face-up position of the head allows for easier breathing in the back crawl than swimming in prone postures. Exhalation is usually executed through the nose and inhalation is taken through the mouth.

Breaststroke

The breaststroke is the most seaworthy of all strokes from a stability perspective. The head position allows the swimmer a forward view, which, coupled with the lateral simultaneous double arm pull and recovery of the arms, favors this stroke for balance and equilibrium, especially in choppy water. The breathing mechanics are not difficult to coordinate, since the pulling phase allows a natural extension of the head out of water for a quick inhalation through the mouth; and the glide phase of the stroke places the head in the water for exhalation through the nose. The breaststroke is the slowest of all strokes. The timing mechanism of the breaststroke in sequential order is (1) *pull*, (2) *kick*, and (3) *glide*. The glide phase should be performed with the body in elongated position and with the arms extended overhead. Legs should also assume the position of full extension (Figure 10.8*a*). Emphasis should be placed on assuming a streamlined body position, which facilitates minimum body drag, as the swimmer glides with face in the water while receiving the resultant propulsive thrusts created by the coordinated arm and leg actions.

Females may have a decided advantage by possessing a lower specific gravity than males and, thus, a greater potential for reducing body drag through the "hydroplaning" effect of body position. It should be noted that swimmers accenting long glides will lower their speed. Prolonged glide duration alters the rhythm of the stroke cycle, and the relationship between propulsive and drag phases of the stroke. A continuous action of arms, legs and breathing to maintain forward propulsion should be sought in the breaststroke. Figure 10.8 illustrates the various phases of breaststroke. As the arm pull is initiated, the legs sequentially adduct. Inhalation is taken during the arm pull (Figure 10.8*b*). Recovery precedes the forward thrust and glide.

The breaststroke analysis entails three major components: (1) arm action, (2) leg action, and (3) breathing. The body position is similar to the crawl stroke and can be adjusted by positioning the head and/or varying

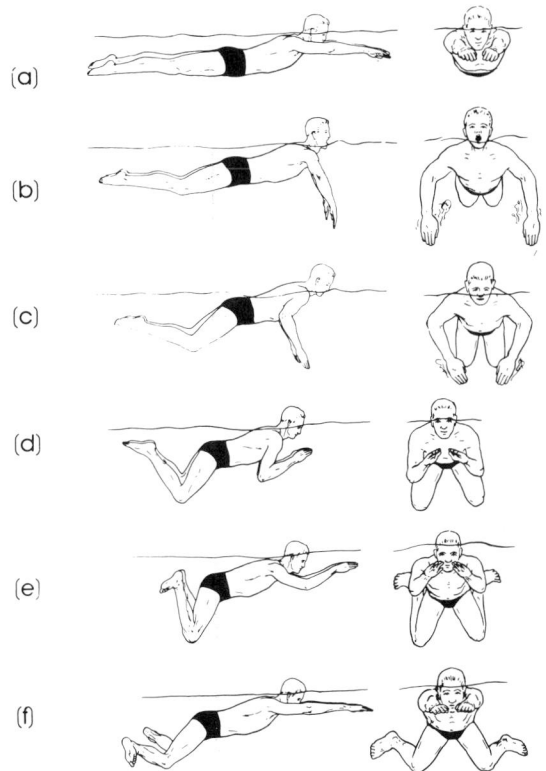

Figure 10.8 Breaststroke coordinated arm/leg stroke pattern (from David Armbruster, Robert H. Allen, and Hobert S. Billingsley, **Swimming and Diving**, 6th ed., The C. V. Mosby Co., Saint Louis, Mo., 1973, with permission)

the arm pull. High head extension and quick shallow arm pulls tend to accent the planing effect by elevating the shoulders while lowering the hips. A streamlined posture should be maintained throughout the whole stroke with the head elevated slightly higher than other body segments throughout each phase.

Arm Action. The pulling action of the arms appears to be a simultaneous lateral, onward, and backward motion. However, cinematographic data indicate efficient breaststroke pulling is a "sculling" action.[9] Hand motion is predominantly sideways—an out and in scull with only a slight motion backwards. The resting phase of the arm action is the glide. The glide position is held when swimming at a slow pace; however, this pause is reduced in sprint breaststroke swimming since considerable forward propulsion is lost without the continuous thrusts of the arms and legs. The bent-arm pull is employed, similar to the arm action of the crawl stroke; however, a circular pattern of motion is used, which differs from the "S" path of the front crawl arm pull.

Leg Action.   Two types of kick are generally utilized that satisfy competitive rule protocol: (1) orthodox kick and (2) whip kick. The orthodox kick is usually taught in noncompetitive instructional classes, while the whip kick is advanced by most coaches for maximum speed. Although it has an overall low efficiency rating in terms of speed performance, the propulsive phase of the breaststroke is powerful and is considered more efficient than the crawl stroke. Homer[10] found that the propelling force of the breaststroke leg kick was higher than the crawl and butterfly strokes and suggested that the increase in propulsive force seems to be better in the breaststroke kick. Detailed electromyograms also indicate that the kick (adducting) phase increases the speed and the leg recovery decelerates velocity.[11] It should be noted that the greatest resistance during the breaststroke occurs with the recovery of the legs.[12] Research supports the importance of the leg thrust in the breaststroke, and it is perhaps the most important single element creating forward propulsion. The orthodox kick is characterized by a wide abducting action of the thighs on the recovery, and a true adducting motion of the thighs on the thrust. The whip kick is executed with a narrower knee spread, followed by circumducting motion of the hip joint creating a circular "whiplike" squeezing action of the legs. Swimming authorities agree that the whip kick is faster than the orthodox fashion. However, the older orthodox kick, commonly called the

"frog" kick, is easier to coordinate and has some merit when teaching beginners for whom recreation is a primary objective. Figure 10.9 illustrates the general pattern of action in the whip kick.

Breathing.   Patterns of breathing vary with the physiological needs of the swimmer and the distance swum. Breathing with every stroke is usually employed in long-distance

Figure 10.9   Breaststroke whip kick (from James E. Counsilman, **Science of Swimming**, Prentice-Hall, Englewood Cliffs, N.J., 1968, pp. 120–121, with permission)

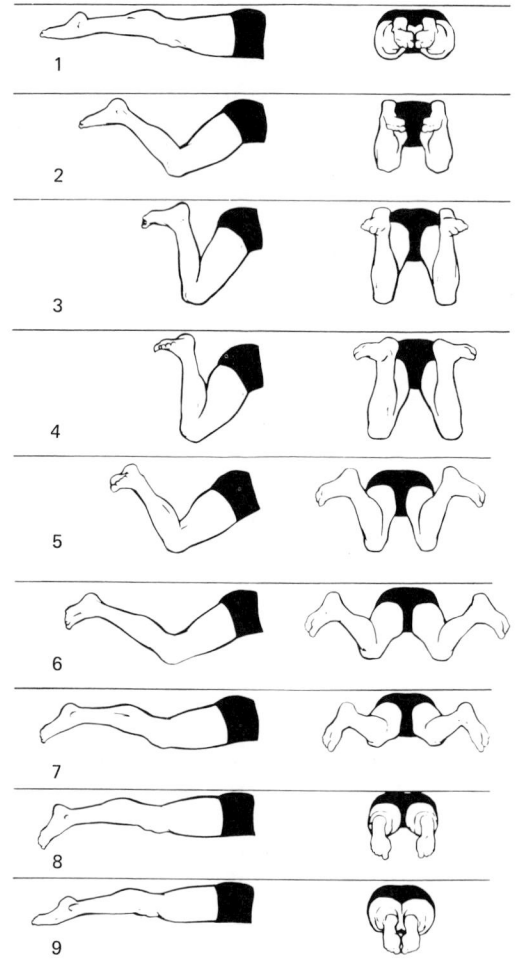

events. Breathing on every second or third stroke is preferred for sprinting. Raising the head does create some body drag by lowering the legs. This movement has a tendency to decelerate the swimmer and should be held to a minimum, particularly in sprint events. The head is extended up and forward in line with the swimmer's forward thrust, and inhalation is performed quickly through the mouth on the arm pull. At this time, the head and shoulders are at their highest point and provide an optimum position of inspiration. As the arms and hands extend forward, the face is placed in the water, and expiration through the nose occurs. Figure 10.8 illustrates the timing sequence in a complete breathing cycle of the breaststroke.

SWIMMING STARTS

Forward Start

Starts utilized in the front crawl, breaststroke, and butterfly events are made from a starting platform not over 30 inches above the water surface.

Any analysis of start mechanics should conform to rules governing competitive starts. Swimmers employ two forward start methods known as the *grab start* and the *conventional start*. Highly skilled swimmers prefer the grab start over the conventional style, and research studies support the speed superiority of the former technique. Figures 10.10*a* and 10.10*b* illustrate the grab and conventional types.

Figure 10.10 (a) Grab start and (b) conventional start

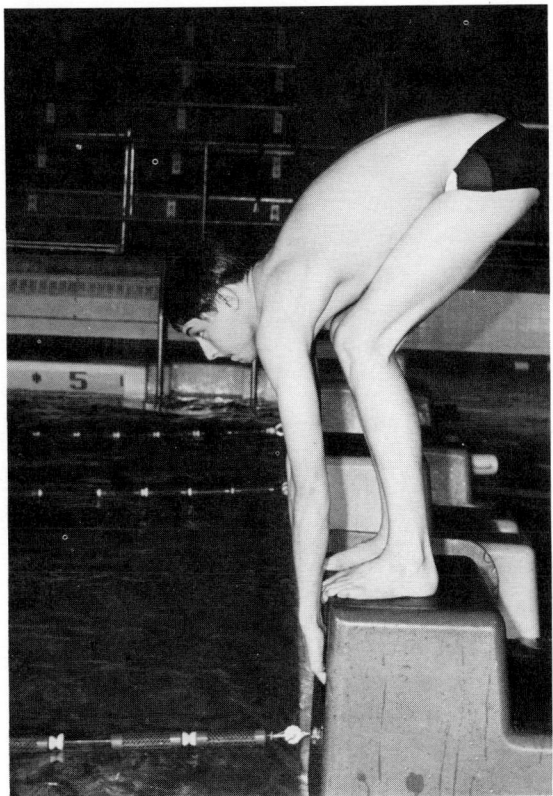

(a)

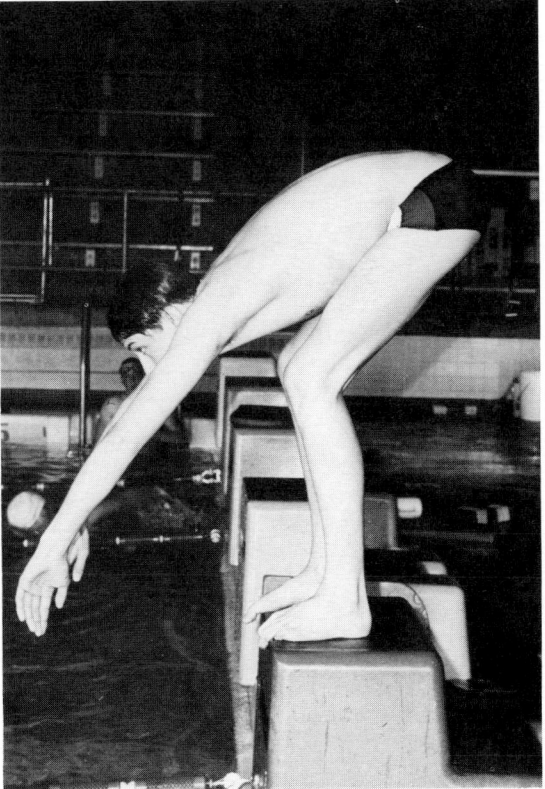

(b)

The elements of a forward start are comprised of three major parts: (1) starting position, (2) takeoff and flight in air, and (3) water entry. These elements involve a motionless stance before the takeoff; an effective takeoff and flight in the air with a downward angulation of approximately 15 to 20 degrees prior to entry; and a smooth water entry that exhibits a streamlined body stretch. Figure 10.11 illustrates full extension of arms, torso, and legs as the swimmer leaves the starting platform.

The quality of *flight* depends mainly upon the magnitude of force generated by the strength and power of the legs and the direction of that force off the platform. Swimmers using either the conventional or grab start tend to leave the platform with the head slightly higher than the legs; however, the ro-

tational forces acting upon the body allow the head to fall lower than the legs with the desired form attained at water entry. This procedure requires a vigorous extension of the hips, legs, and ankles sychronized with a circular-backward swing of arms, in the conventional type of arm swing. The swimmer should enter the water in an extended, streamlined position without hip flexion.

Irrespective of starting technique utilized, flexing of the hips or "piking" the body should be avoided because of its drag effect at the moment of water contact.

The grab technique in Figure 10.10a shows the hand grasp on the starting platform, as contrasted with the conventional position of arms and hands in front of the block. Recent studies support the grab start as a faster technique for leaving the platform than conven-

Figure 10.11 Flight in forward start

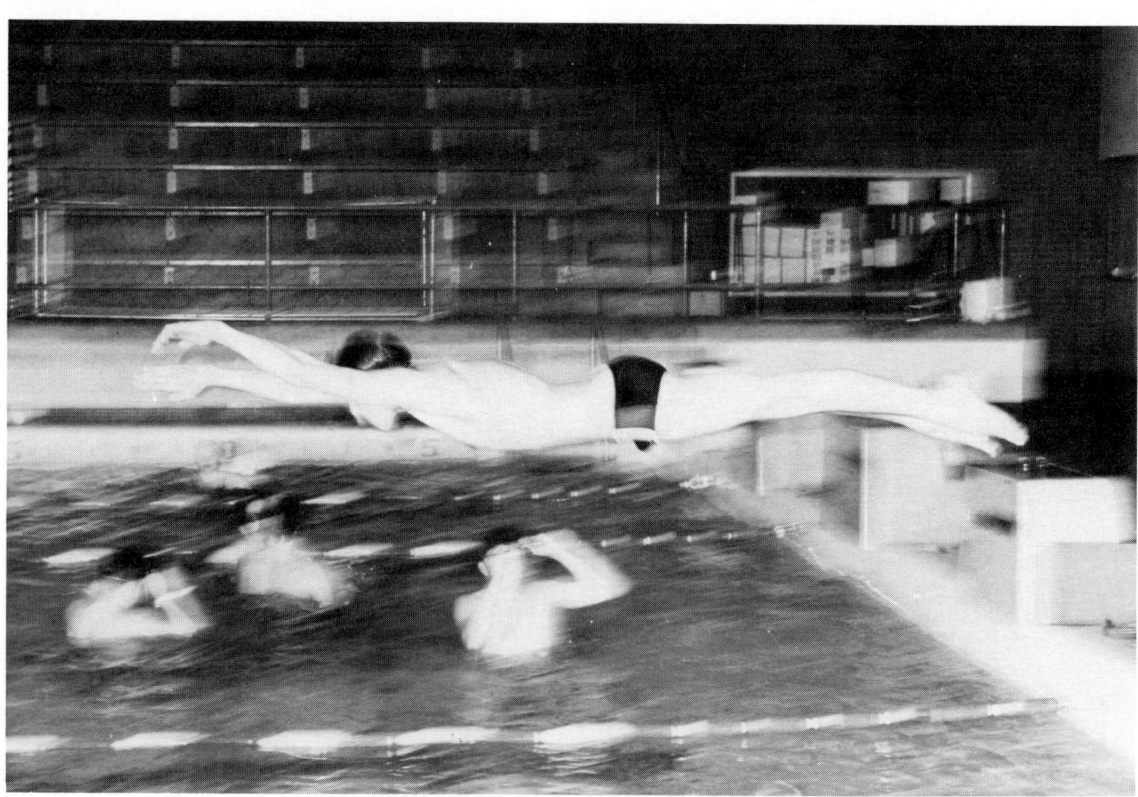

tional styles.[13],[14],[15] Most swimming coaches have accepted the premise that the grab start is superior to other techniques and this style is widely used in competition from high school to world class levels. The grab start allows the swimmer to better control balance and equilibrium while leaning forward with the center of gravity in front of the support base (feet). The forward lean in the grab start also permits the swimmer to drop the shoulders lower than in the conventional start. The overall effect allows the swimmer to take off with less resistance to resting inertia and at a lower flight trajectory. The greater support base allows the swimmer to move the center of gravity further forward without loss of balance. Forward lean and better balance control, in addition to the advantage of exerting greater force with the hands on the platform, favors the grab start over other contemporary techniques used in competitive forward starts.

Backstroke Start

The backstroke start is performed from an in-water position. Swimmers face the starting end of the pool with both hands grasping the starting platform or end-wall and both feet in contact with the wall at the starting end (Figure 10.12a). Any starting position may be assumed, but rules require that both hands and feet must be in contact with the pool end and the body must not be completely above the water. Swimmers must be motionless before the gun is discharged. Although significant changes have occurred with the forward start, little if any variations have been advanced for the mechanics of the backstroke start technique. The start is initiated by a forceful extension of the entire body pushing off backward with arms overhead in a streamlined gliding position. Swimmers vary in the magnitude of hip and arm flexion facing the starting platform. Certain competitors pull their chest close to the platform in a "hugging" position, whereas other back-

strokers may start from a partial standing posture with their head and shoulders over the block. Further research needs to be undertaken before any definitive generalization can be made about the superiority of the partial standing position over the full crouch stance. An interesting backstroke start was studied by Decker.[16] Figure 10.12b illustrates an experimental standing, screw-type start, as contrasted with the conventional backstroke method.

Swimmers and coaches are continually searching for ways and means of lowering times in racing events. Decker compared the conventional competitive backstroke start with a standing type backstroke method shown in Figure 10.12 to determine which of the two is faster. The experiment revealed that (1) the standing start is significantly faster than the conventional type, and (2) the experimental start also covers more distance on the takeoff when compared with the conventional in-water method. The implications of this study lends support to the view that backstroke swimming times would be cut noticeably if rules were altered to allow the standing screw-type start.

SWIMMING TURNS

Forward Turn

Historically, the forward turn developed in three stages: (1) open turn, (2) closed turn, and (3) flip or somersault turn. Each type is progressively faster in turning time. The open turn is described as a simple lateral turn to the left or right, with a breath taken as the preferred hand touches the end-wall. The closed turn is similar to the open type with the exception of breathing; the swimmer holds the head and face under the surface as the lead hand touches the wall and turns without an inhalation. The flip or somersault turn also eliminates the breathing component

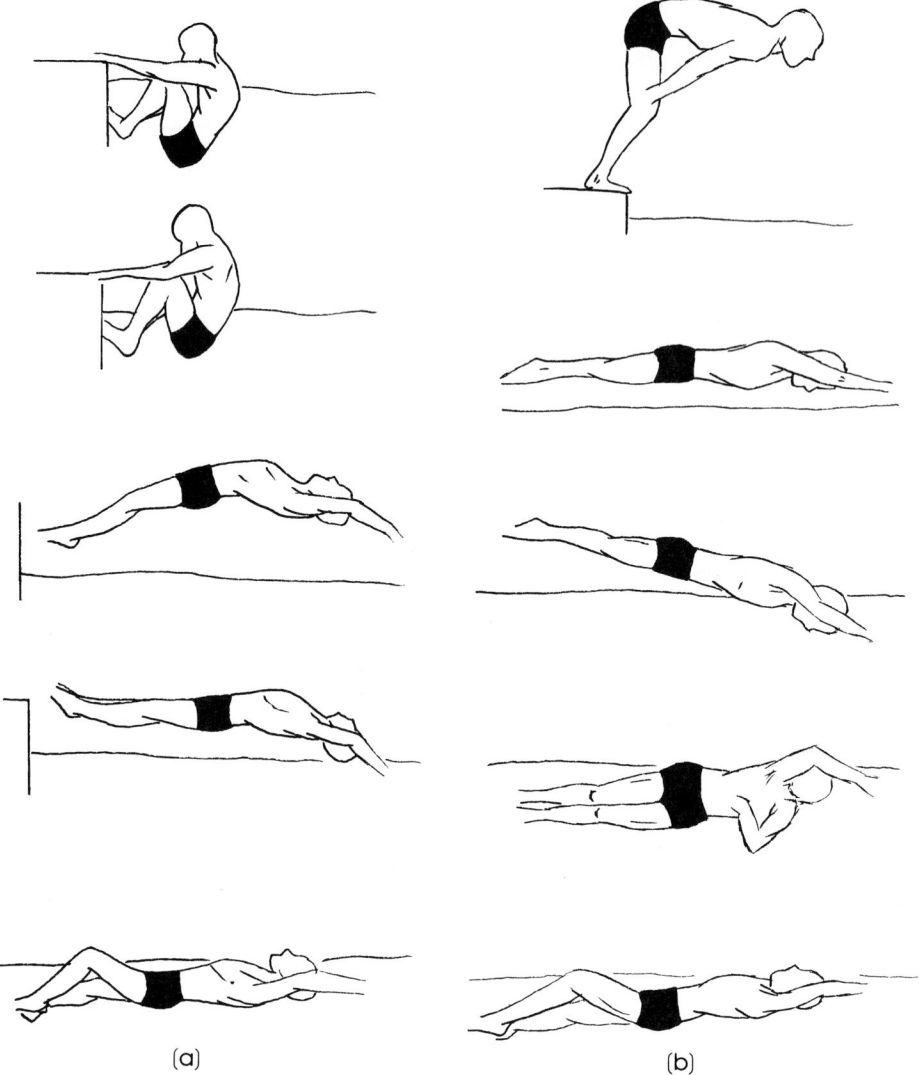

Figure 10.12 (a) Conventional backstroke start and (b) experimental backstroke start

and adds a half-twisting somersault motion without a hand or arm touch, as shown in Figure 10.13.

The front crawl stroke swimmer is relatively free to create and execute any method of turning because of a greater latitude in body contact with the end-wall before turning. Modern swimming competition has virtually eliminated the simple open and closed later-

al-type turns since these movements are significantly slower than the somersault maneuver. The flip or somersault turn is analyzed in the following section.

Certain mechanical principles apply to the correct execution of the flip turn. The following concepts are pertinent to an efficient turn: (1) compliance with Newton's first law, (2) speed of rotary velocity, and (3) reduction

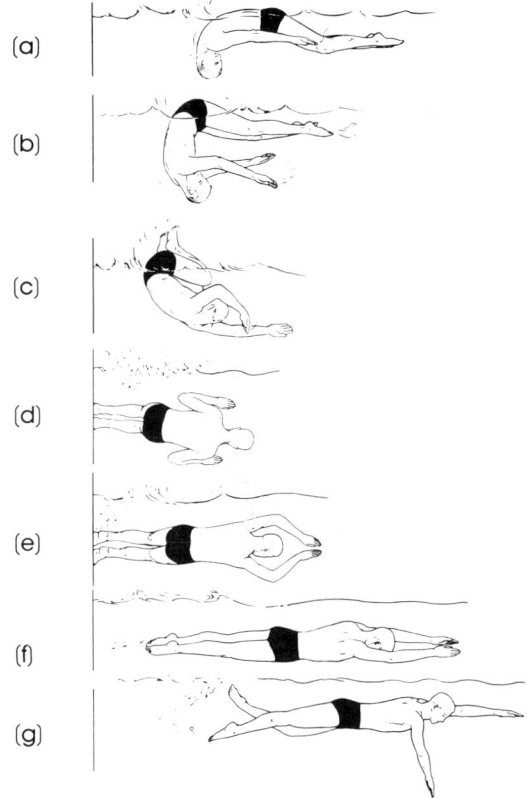

(a)

(b)

(c)

(d)

(e)

(f)

(g)

Figure 10.13 Forward somersault turn (from David Armbruster, Robert H. Allen, and Hobert S. Billingsley, **Swimming and Diving**, 6th ed., The C. V. Mosby Co., Saint Louis, Mo., 1973, with permission)

of body drag resistance. As the swimmer approaches the turn, horizontal speed continues to thrust the performer toward the wall because of Newton's law of inertia. This horizontal movement must be converted to an angular motion in the spinning action of the turn. A smooth ballistic transfer should be executed, simultaneously thrusting the head downward and hips upward without loss of speed (Figure 10.13a, b, c). The body should be close enough to the wall that the swimmer can assume a crouched position with knees flexed approximately 90 degrees (Figure 10.13d). The body should move in the direction of the turn in order to convert linear motion to rotary motion without deceleration,

thus preserving the effectiveness of Newton's law of inertia. The speed of the somersault is governed by the length of the radius through which the turn is executed. A long radius will require more time for the spin. A short radius hastens the speed of rotation. This concept can be translated by teaching knee flexion as the turn is initiated. Body drag is reduced by full extension of the body with arms on the push-off (Figure 10.13e, f). The thrust should be horizontal without any downward angular movement. Slight extension of the head and neck is desirable to allow for a gradual surfacing of the body, as the swimmer resumes a stroking action (Figure 10.13g).

The full flip may be described as a half-twisting somersault action as shown in Figure 10.13. Turning left or right depends upon the lead arm as the swimmer approaches the end-wall. If the swimmer is leading with the right arm forward, the twisting turn is made on the left side, and vice versa. Therefore, it is important for swimmers to learn to turn to both sides with equal proficiency since stroke alterations may cause the swimmer to enter the turn leading with either the left or right arm. Figure 10.13 exhibits a swimmer entering the turn with the right arm leading followed by a half-twisting somersault to the left as he completes the flip.

An interesting experiment analyzing two methods of performing the front crawl turn was conducted by Scharf and King.[17] These investigators compared the conventional flip turn using a two-arm glide push-off with a modified flip turn followed by a one-arm glide. Figure 10.14 illustrates the two types of turns studied. Results of the study revealed that the one-arm glide was significantly faster than the two-arm position shown by the steps 5 and 6 in Figure 10.14.

Although some evidence has demonstrated that the one-arm glide is a faster technique, this style has not been generally adopted by competitive swimmers. The skill pattern is quite different in the one-arm style, and per-

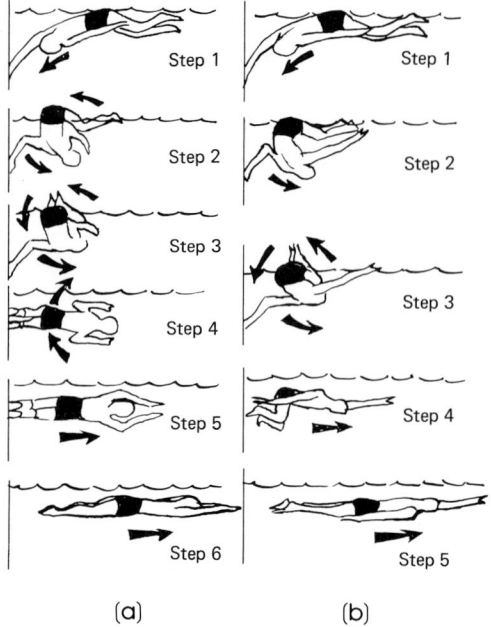

Figure 10.14 Forward turns: (a) two-arm glide method, (b) one-arm glide method (from William H. King and Raphael J. Scharf, "Time and Motion Analysis of Competitive Freestyle Swimming Turns," **Research Quarterly**, 35:37–44, March, 1964, with permission)

The two-arm glide, after the push-off shown in Figure 10.15, is generally utilized by competitive swimmers. The difference between the one-arm push-off and the conventional method of placing both arms overhead prior to the glide has been compared.[18] This experiment showed that the one-arm back glide technique is a faster procedure. Again, as in the front crawl turn, some evidence is presented supporting a one-arm glide over the two-arm mode, yet swimmers and coaches are hesitant to change from the traditional pattern to a different technique.

SPRINGBOARD DIVING

Fancy springboard diving is more directly related to acrobatic maneuvers found in tum-

Figure 10.15 Backstroke turn pattern (from David Armbruster, Robert H. Allen, and Hobert S. Billingsley, **Swimming and Diving**, C. V. Mosby Co., Saint Louis, Mo., 1973, with permission)

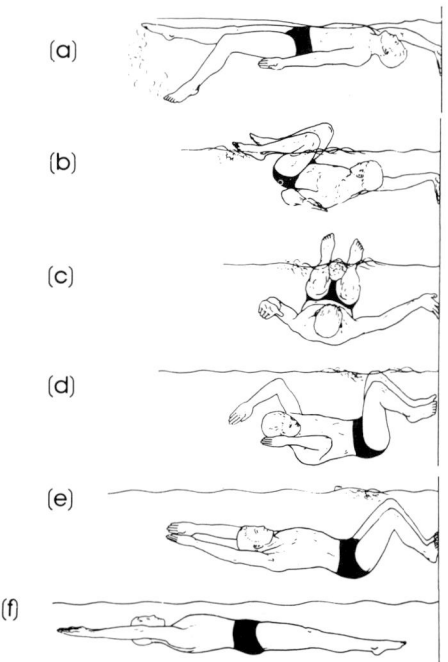

haps this variable is a reason that coaches are reluctant to change swimmers from the accepted older method to the newer technique.

Backstroke Turn

The competitive backstroke turn, commonly known as the "tumble" or "flip" turn, is actually a lateral movement left or right after the hand or arm touches the end-wall. The turn is made to the left if the lead arm into the turn is right and vice versa. Skilled backstrokers learn to turn left or right with equal proficiency since the approach may be made with either arm. Figure 10.15 illustrates the sequential pattern of the turn with the swimmer's right arm leading into the end-wall.

bling and trampoline activities than to swimming; however, since the sport must be performed in a natatorium, it naturally becomes an integral part of aquatic competition. Generally, springboard diving is executed from one- or three-meter boards. Most swimming pools are equipped with one-meter heights. Fewer facilities contain three-meter boards; therefore, the ensuing analysis pertains primarily to low board diving skills. Most divers are able to make a natural transition from low to high boards once basic mechanics of the forward running approach and standing backward takeoff are mastered. It is indeed far more difficult to transfer basic skills from the high to low board because of the different time permitted for execution of the dive. After low board techniques are properly acquired, similar procedures from the three-meter board apply, except at a slower rate of speed, since increased time is allowed for a smooth water entry.

Diving rules differ from tumbling and trampoline competition. Specified dives are listed in competitive rules, which means that contestants must perform only those dives listed in approved manuals. Each dive is assigned a particular degree of difficulty from a low of 1.2 for a forward dive to a high of 3.0 designated for a one-and-one-half somersault with a triple twist. Judges do not evaluate the difficulty of a dive. Performance alone is rated on a scale from zero to ten. Zero is considered a "failed" dive and ten is rated as "perfect." The score of each judge is multiplied by the degree of difficulty to arrive at a final rating figure. Therefore, judges in diving competition are concerned only with style and control, as contrasted with the judging of tumbling and trampoline routines, where the judge must consider difficulty of routines in arriving at a score. Competitors must be prepared to perform dives from five different groups: (1) forward, (2) backward, (3) reverse, (4) inward, and (5) twisting.

Generally, competition provides for certain required and optional dives in the program, depending on the level of competition. In addition to conforming with dive grouping, divers must execute selected dives in one of four positions: (1) tuck, (2) pike, (3) straight, or (4) free. Each position also carries an assigned degree of difficulty. Generally, dives performed in the straight position receive a higher degree of difficulty when combined with multiple somersaults and twists.

PHYSICAL CHARACTERISTICS OF A DIVER

Mesomorphic/Ectomorphic Tendency

Springboard diving is not strictly limited to an absolute physique type; however, obese persons and those individuals who have large heavy legs will find it difficult to achieve championship caliber in competitive diving. Tall slender persons appear to look more graceful in lay-out and twist dives; however, shorter individuals find forward and backward rotary moves around a horizontal axis an easier task because of a reduced radius of gyration. Divers usually reflect body characteristics similar to gymnasts and do not necessarily resemble the anthropometrical qualities of swimmers. A notation should be made about flexibility and diving performance. A controllable wide range of motion is desirable for divers, particularly at the ankle and foot. A clean "bulletlike" water entry is critical for superior performance; individuals possessing flexible lower legs and feet have a decided advantage in executing this final phase of all head-first dives.

DIVE PERFORMANCE COMPONENTS

Guidelines

A perfect dive is rated a score of ten. A perfect score is rarely awarded; however, any sound analytical approach should begin with an identification of basic elements. These component parts are *starting position, approach, hurdle* and *takeoff, execution,* and *water entry.* The total performance of a dive depends upon an uninterrupted sequential kinetic chain of movement from the starting position through the entry. An error in any component will affect some other element of the dive. For example, if a diver takes off from the board with excessive lean, a flattened parabolic flight curve will result, causing a decrease in height and excessive travel away from the board. If speed of rotation is too great in a forward one-and-one-half somersault, the diver will drop into the water beyond the desired vertical position, resulting in a "splashy" entry. An uneven projection "push" from both feet on the takeoff will result in flight execution and entry to one side, rather than directly in front of the board. Each component part must be judged immediately. The actual time required from take-off to entry of a dive from a three-meter springboard is 1.9 to 2.0 seconds.[19] Obviously, a one-meter dive takeoff/entry elapsed time is less since the dive travels one-third the distance.

DIVING MECHANICS

Although specific dives contain their own peculiar mechanical characteristics, the ensuing analysis applies to all the dives generally with an emphasis on basic principles governing each component of the *forward running approach* and the *backward standing takeoff.*

Forward Running Approach

The parts of a dive using the forward approach consists of *standing/starting posture, fast walk or run, hurdle step, takeoff, flight in air,* and *entry.*

Standing Starting Posture. The diver assumes an errect standing position, arms extended along the sides of the body with palms facing the thighs. Eyes should be focused at the end of the board. Eye focus on the end of the board aids in maintaining stability as the performer contemplates the elements of the dive to be executed "in toto." Principles of stability apply in this segment, which means that the line of gravity should be over the center of gravity, and the latter must be within its supporting base. Actually, most divers lean forward slightly, with most of the weight placed on the balls of the feet, thereby lessening the resistance of resting inertia, which must be overcome before the initial step is taken.

Fast Walk or Run. A minimum of three steps, in addition to the hurdle, are required by competitive diving rules. A diver initiating a three-step run with the left leg will naturally raise the right foot on the hurdle step, and vice versa. The run should project a natural movement similar to a fast walk. Forward momentum is generated by the run in forward dives. Momentum continues unless an abrupt change occurs in body position (Newton's first law). A slight lean of approximately 10 degrees accompanies the fast walking movement shown in Figure 10.16.

The center of gravity is slightly forward over the balls of the feet, with the arms leading the body forward, as the diver approaches the hurdle. The length of each step varies with the height of the diver and length of the board. The first step of most contestants is shorter, with each succeeding step slightly longer and faster than first.

Hurdle Step. The hurdle or fourth step in a three-step approach is critical to the takeoff action and flight that follows immediately. Figure 10.17 illustrates the correct arm and leg position as the diver jumps to the end on the board. The hurdle leg should be lifted as high as possible without loss of balance to attain maximum depression of the board. The

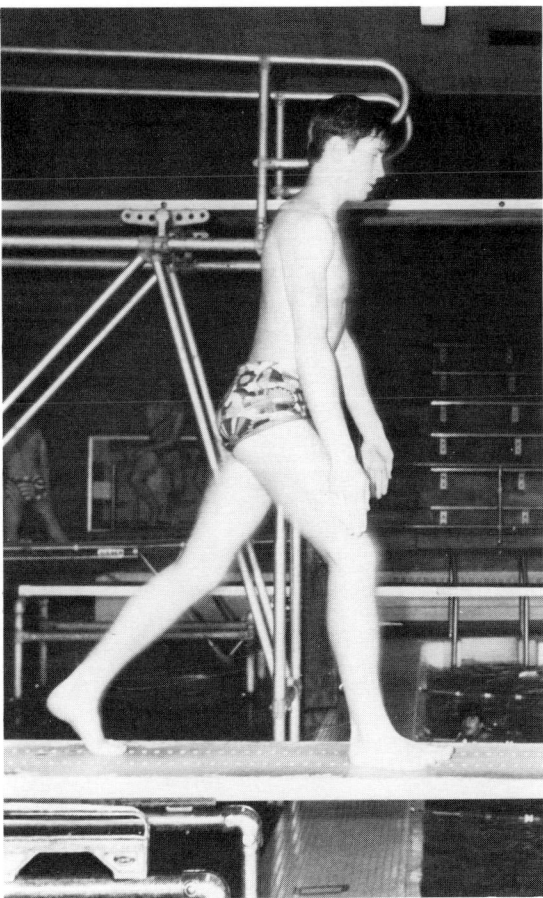

Figure 10.16 Forward lean in front running approach

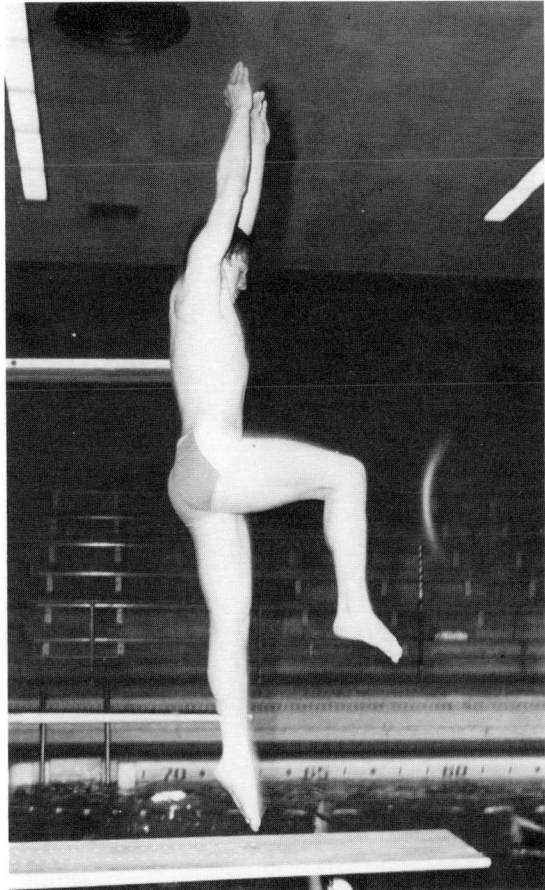

Figure 10.17 Hurdle in forward running dive

amount of board depression is one important factor that determines the height of the parabolic flight curve. The greater the depression of the board a diver can exert from the hurdle, the greater the force or upward thrust (Newton's third law). Force is equal to mass times acceleration. Since mass is constant for each diver, force can be augmented by increasing acceleration, which is facilitated by raising the height of the hurdle leg.

Takeoff. Synchronization of the arm and leg movements is an important mechanic of the takeoff. The upward sweep of the arms should precede the lift of the board during the hurdle in order to accelerate the rise of the body with the recoil of the springboard, as shown in Figures 10.18a and 10.18b.

The concept of "pushing" the board with the feet rather than "lifting" is an essential precept for maximizing the full effects of Newton's third law. The third law (action-reaction) principle is applied as the diving board pushes against the feet in equal and opposite direction to the downward and forward force of the body. The amount of lean on the takeoff depends on the dive description. Generally, dives that require little rotation accent slight body lean, exemplified by a forward header or "swan dive." In contrast,

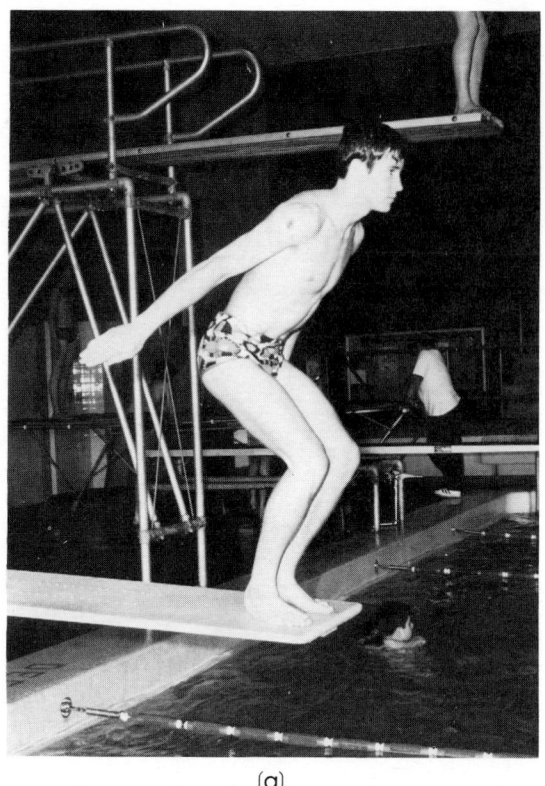
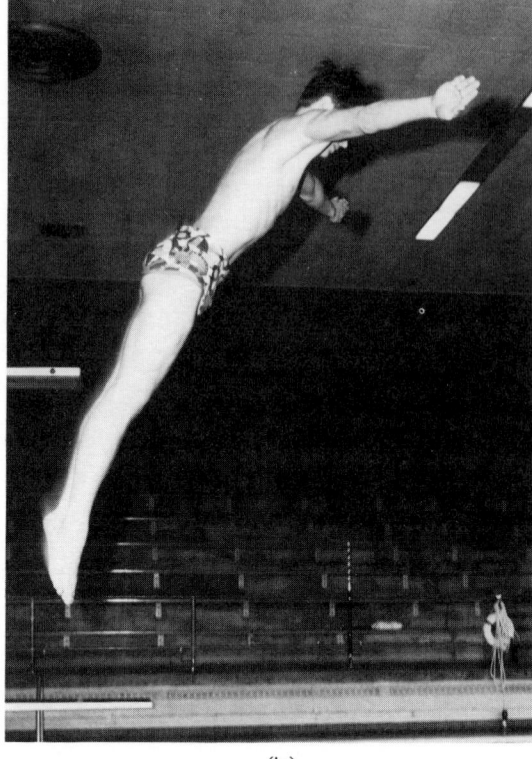

(a)   (b)

Figure 10.18 Arm and leg movements on takeoff

dives with spins such as the forward one-and-one-half somersault necessitate a forward lean of up to 30 degrees, contingent on the diver's style. Lean on the takeoff also has a direct bearing on height of the dive. The subsequent flight path of a dive is known as the *parabola*. A greater lean tends to flatten the parabola and subsequently to lower its height. The extent of lean not only affects dive height but also bears upon the diver's distance away from the board on the entry. Excessive lean results in added distance or travel away from the board. All dives should contain a minimum degree of body lean for safety purposes in addition to an emphasis upon the "lead effect" of the arms on the takeoff. Body lean must also be accompanied by a downward forward push of the feet in order to rotate sufficiently to effect a vertical

entry. Wilson[20] studied the topping technique of a diver falling forward in a rigid motion gaining linear and angular momentum during the flight path and demonstrated that the takeoff angle is approximately 50 degrees from a three-meter springboard. This angulation is necessary for a simple half rotation from the upright position to a vertical entry and points to the need for a downward force on the takeoff for dives utilizing slight leans such as the forward dive in the layout position.

Flight in Air. The flight of a dive is part of its execution. Characteristics of this phase are dependent upon the preceding movements of run, hurdle, and takeoff. Over 60 different dives may be performed in competition and each one diverges in movement form contingent upon *position*—tuck, pike, straight, or free—and *category*—forward, backward, reverse, inward, or twisting. Certain dives require rapid twisting and turning, such as the full twisting forward one-and-one-half somersault, whereas others reflect smooth graceful mechanics in execution, such as the forward dive in a layout position. Notwithstanding dive variations in quick or slow movements, execution should always project a sense of powerful and yet effortless movement to the critical eye of the judges and audience. Certain mechanical precepts apply to all dive executions irrespective of their differences in categories or positions. The following basic principles relate directly to the diver after leaving the board.

Parabolic Trajectory

The flight arc is determined by the force exerted upon the board and angle of lean on the takeoff. Once this flight path has been established, it cannot be changed in the air. Therefore each diver must determine his/her parabolic flight path objective before initiating the first step of the run. For example, if maximum height is desired, great force and minimum lean should be stressed. The resultant parabola will project a high arc with an entry close to the board. In contrast, multiple somersaults require greater body lean on the takeoff, which results in a lower parabolic curve and entry further away from the board. The diver who wishes both height and rotation on a chosen dive must sacrifice one for the other as optimum direction of both lean and force is sought for each particular dive.[21]

Somersault Dives

Somersault dives consist of spinning movements of the body rotating in a sagittal plane around a horizontal axis. The extent and speed of rotation is determined by (1) force exerted by the feet (push), (2) amount of lean

(trajectory), and (3) length of radius about the center of gravity. Divers can establish the radius of gyration by selecting a tuck, pike, or layout position. However, the force exerted (push) and lean (trajectory) concepts apply to all dives. A tuck dive has a shortened radius from its center of gravity and subsequently possesses greater rotary velocity. In contrast, dives in the layout position will not turn as fast because of the lengthened body posture, which slows down the speed of spinning. The speed of somersaulting or angular velocity depends upon the moment of inertia, which is the mass (diver's weight) times the square of the distance of the center of the mass to the axis of rotation. Figure 10.19 exhibits a diver rotating in a tuck position with a short radius of gyration and decreased moment of inertia.

Specific examples in other sports and motor movements are discussed in Chapter 5. The law of conservation of angular momentum applied to diving that increases or decreases the moment of inertia depending upon the length of the radius is illustrated by Figure 10.20 with an explanatory formula:[22]

Twisting Dives

Twisting dives consist of turning movements of the body in a horizontal plane around a vertical axis. Basically, twisting may originate from two starting points: (1) twists originating from the *board* and (2) twists originating in *air*. Dives such as the layout front dive with a half twist usually start their twisting movement on the takeoff, directly from the board. If the feet push left, the body will move right, which simply applies Newton's third law of action and reaction. Twisting or torque is produced by forces governing Newton's law of action–reaction from the board or free in air as described in Chapter 5. The principle of momentum transfer also arises when the diver twists from the board. As the arms, shoulders, and head rotate in the horizontal plane with the feet on the board, the initial

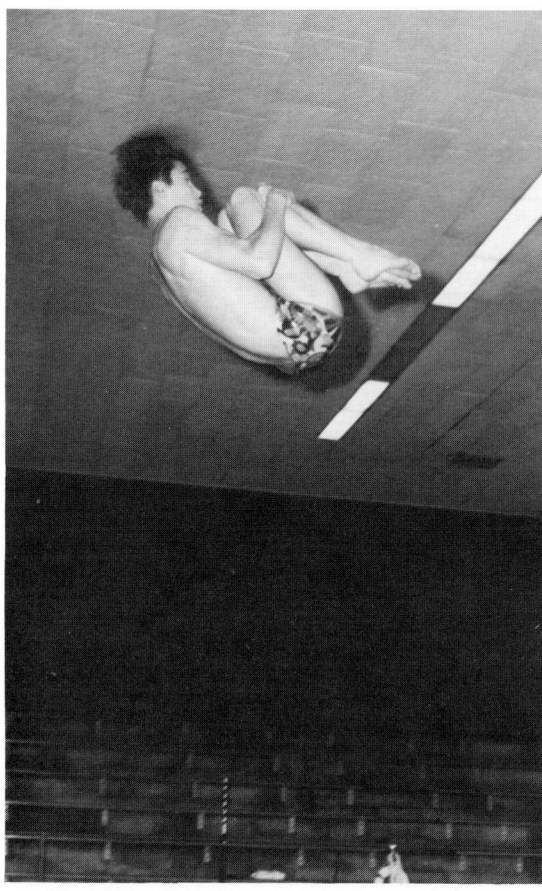

Figure 10.19 Decreasing moment of inertia and radius of gyration with a tuck somersault

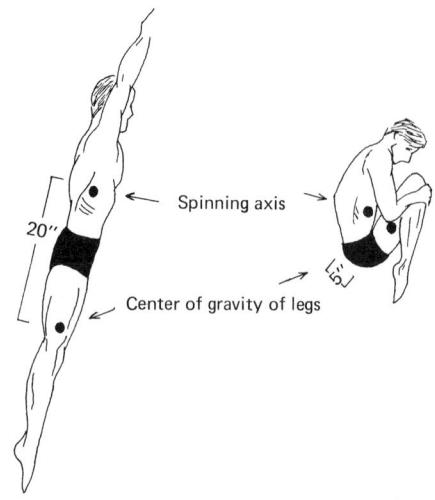

Figure 10.20 The effect of changing the radius of gyration. The formula for moment of inertia is $I = mr^2$.

I = moment of inertia
m = mass (weight)
r = radius (distance between the mass and axis of rotation)

Assume that a person's legs weigh 50 lb and the center of gravity of the legs is 20 in. from the spinning axis when the legs are straight. Since $m = 50$ lb and $r = 20$ in., then $mr^2 = 50 \times 20^2$ and

$I = 20,000$

If the legs are drawn into a tuck position and their center of gravity is then 5 in. from the spinning axis, then $m = 50$, $r = 5$, $mr^2 = 50 \times 5^2$, and

$I = 1,250$.

This means that when the legs are tucked, they will want to spin 16 times faster than when they are straight (from Charles Batterman, **Techniques of Springboard Diving**, MIT Press, Cambridge, Mass., 1968, with permission)

effect transfers and the entire body turns in the desired direction. Twisting from the board is less complicated than torque generated free in air. The board surface provides a source for absorption and establishment of direction; however, twisting left or right after the diver leaves the board entails intricate adjustments in body positions. McDonald[23] examined the twisting phenomenon free in air by observing the falling and turning movements of a former Olympic diver and described the body motions as a "cat drop." Figure 10.21 illustrates the sequential moves of a free fall starting from a hang position on the board and ending in completion of the turn.

The following description clearly shows the application of the effects of action-reaction when a body falls free in air, indicating that movement of one part of the body in one direction causes another segment to move in the opposite direction:

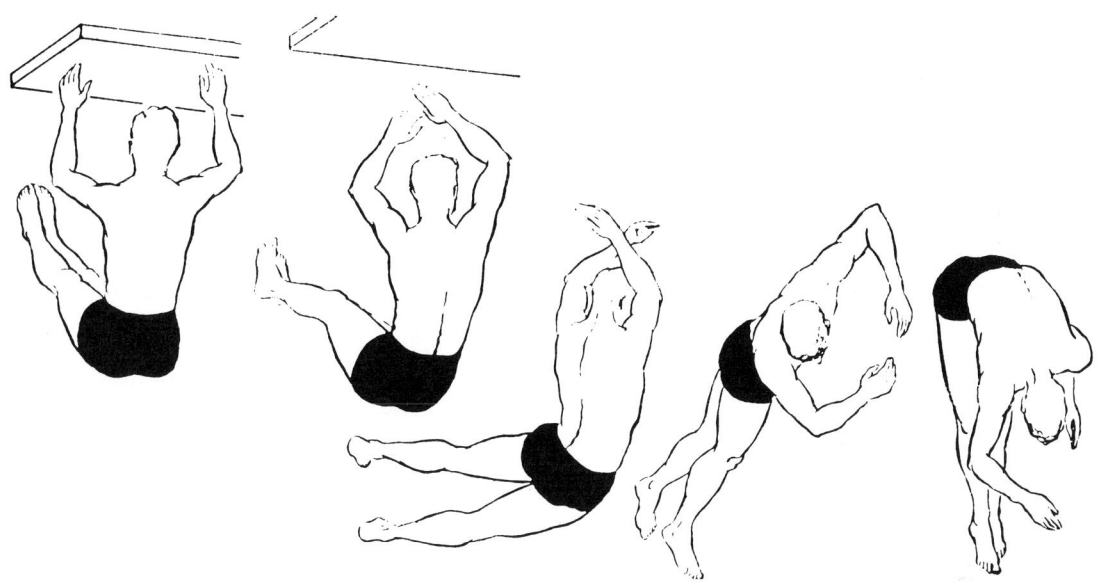

Figure 10.21 "Cat drop" twist maneuver—free in air (from Donald MacDonald, "How Does Man Twist in Air?" **New Scientist**, 10:501–503, June, 1961, with permission. This first appeared in **New Scientist**, London, The Weekly Review of Science and Technology)

Figure 10.21a shows the position just after release from the board. The body is flexed forward strongly at the lumbar spine and at the hips. Figure 10.21b reveals a stage early in the turn—the shoulders turning to the right and so are the legs. The body is straightening from its flexed position but it is being bent to the left. Figure 10.21c shows the turn half completed. The spine and legs are now strongly extended, and the bend to the left is most marked. Figure 10.21d shows the reverse process underway. The right side and front of the body are shortening so that the trunk is flexed and bending to the right. This brings the left shoulder over towards the right hip. Figure 10.21e shows the net result: the man has turned on his face and all that remains for him is to extend his arms to be in the final position analogous to that of a cat landing on its feet.[24]

The twisting is accompanied by the flexion in a forward-backward direction. If the left arm is swung forward and the right arm swung to the rear, a counter-rotation of the trunk to the left results. This rotating pattern is also shown by the swivel chair performance illustrated in Chapter 15. It should be noted, however, that man is limited in spinal column flexibility unlike the cat, which by natural endowment can far exceed human vertebral torque capabilities. Nevertheless, a diver's twisting motion in air is similar to a cat's motion sequence falling from an upside-down position, and turning over to land on the feet.

Entry into Water

The final and terminating phase of a dive is the entry. Since this part of a dive is the last component seen by the judges and audience, many performers and coaches place a great deal of emphasis upon the mechanics of executing a smooth, "bulletlike" entrance. All entries, head or feet first, should break the water surface near the vertical with a straight body alignment. A distinct pause showing a straight body posture is desirable immediately prior to entering the water. This pause is referred to as a "drop," which depicts substantial height and control in the execution of the dive. Figure 10.22 illustrates the extended position and "drop" prior to breaking the water surface.

A neat, clean-cut entry indicates control and poise, as the diver "lines the dive." In or-

Figure 10.22 Extending the body on the entry

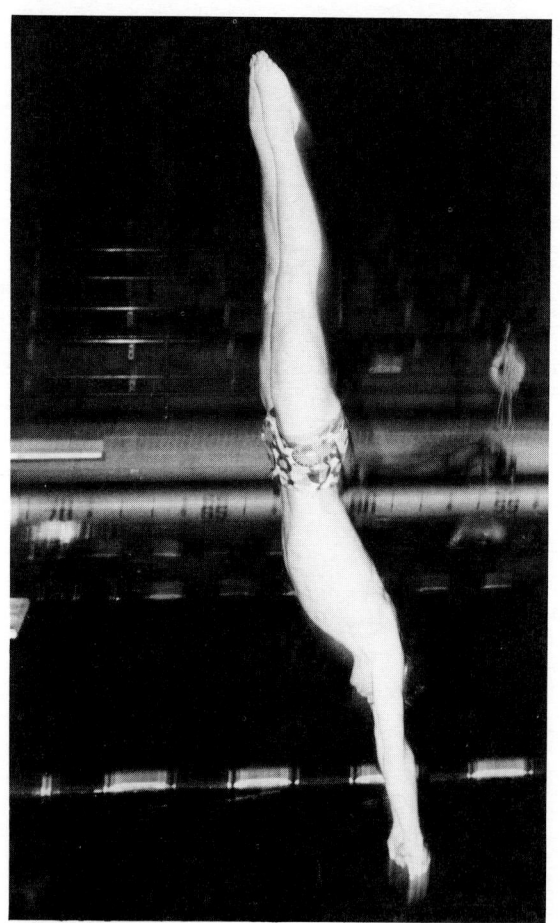

der to enter the water near the vertical mark, divers should begin their entry phase slightly before reaching the vertical position, since angular momentum is conserved after the diver leaves the board and continues throughout the dive. Rotary motion is present in all dives from the one-half turn used in the forward dive to the multiple spins of the forward two-and-one-half somersault. Two important aspects of mechanics affect the dive entry: (1) angular velocity and (2) Newton's third law. Angular velocity or speed of the spin can be changed since it depends upon the moment of inertia. Angular velocity can be adjusted by shortening or lengthening the radius of gyration, thus changing the body's moment of inertia, which is mass times the square of the distance of that mass to the axis of rotation. Therefore, angular velocity varies inversely with the length of the body. For example, a diver can speed up the spin of a forward one-and-one-half somersault in the pike position by simply assuming a "closed" pike rather than an "open" form; the radius of rotation is closer to the center of axis of the spinning body.

The application of control of angular velocity can be used to "save" dives. For example, if a dive is short (splash toward the board with too little spin) on a back dive, arching the back decreases the moment of inertia, thus speeding up the spin, and places the body closer to the vertical or 180 degree mark on entry. Newton's third law of action-reaction can be applied to effect a smooth entry. For example, if a diver's legs are over the head during the end of the flight in a swan dive, a movement of the arms and hands forward will cause a backward motion of the lower torso and legs. A forward thrust of the upper body and limbs causes the opposite or backward action of the lower body segments. Another example of action-reaction is exhibited by the diver performing a front dive in the pike position. Lowering the head between the arms will allow the hips and legs to move vertically above the shoulders, whereas holding or hyperextending the head forward causes a lowering of the hips and opposite action. The application of these mechanical principles can be a valuable aid to the diver in changing the entry position when a faulty run, hurdle, or execution has occurred, and thus "save" the entry.

Figure 10.23 (a) Starting position in backward takeoff. (b) Flight form of back dive in layout position

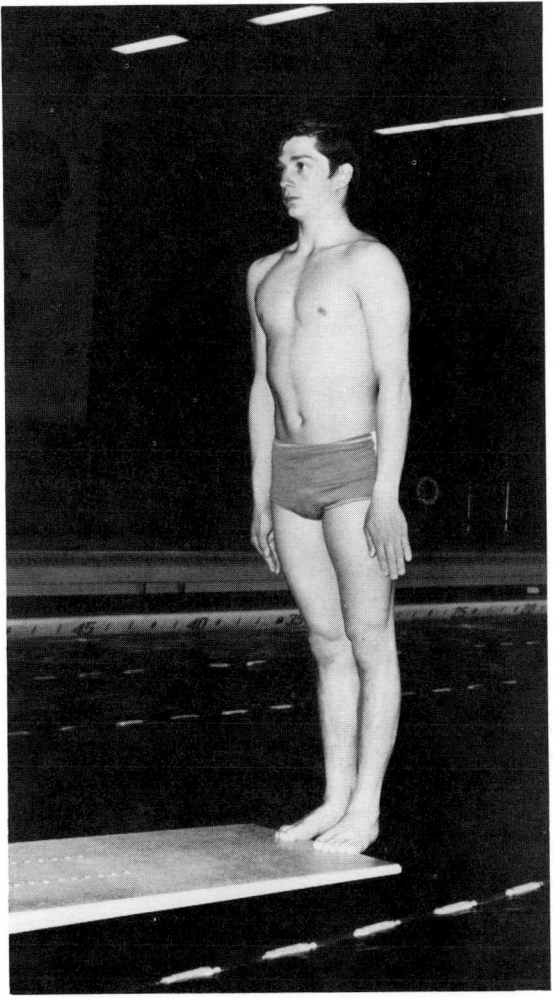

(a)

Standing Backward Takeoff Dives

Two types of dives are executed utilizing the standing backward takeoff, as illustrated by the starting position in Figure 10.23a and flight form in Figure 10.23b.

A balanced position, as shown in Figure 10.23a, is maintained for several seconds.

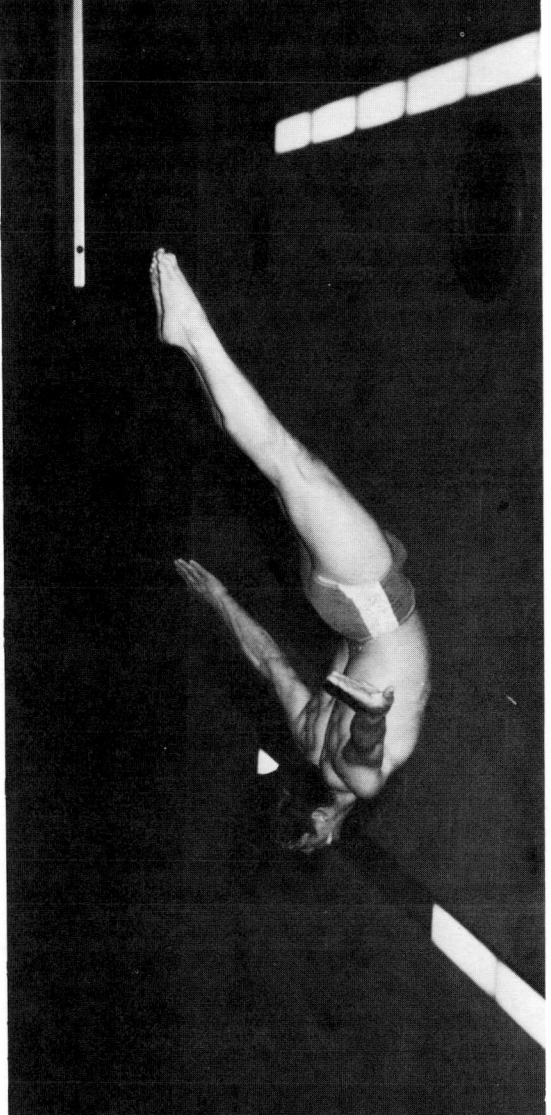

(b)

The time this position is held varies among divers.* The run and hurdle components in the backward approach are eliminated. The dive must depend upon body weight and neuromuscular coordination to complete an efficient takeoff, execution, and entry into the water. Attaining adequate height from a standing start is an important objective since the benefits of forward and upward momentum of the forward approach are not available. The major difference between backward dives, such as the backward dive layout, and inward dives, characterized by the back jackknife dive, is determined by the amount of lean on the takeoff. Less body lean is taken on inward or backward jackknife-type dives than dives that require backward rotation. Up to four rocking movements are usually taken by the diver in order to set the board in motion before it is fully depressed. A counterclockwise movement of the arms is coordinated with the depression and recoil of the board in such a way that the diver "rides" the board for maximum lift. The concept of "pushing" with the feet forward and downward simultaneously is also important to avoid hitting the board. Greater angular velocity is also required for full inward or backward somersault dives, and the diver must begin rotary action immediately on the takeoff to complete the necessary revolutions for a vertical entry. Newton's first law of continuous motion applies in the smooth ballistic motion of the arms and legs while depressing the board. The diver's lift phase depends on depression magnitude and also utilizes Newton's third law of action and reaction. Greater board depression causes more recoil and, thus, the diver receives a higher lift moving inward or backward depending upon the selected dive.

The execution and entry in backward standing dives are similar to the mechanics of

*Backward standing dives may also start with arms overhead; however, most divers utilize the posture of arms against the sides as shown in Figure 10.23a.

the running front approach. Vertical entries are made easier since the diver can use the board as a reference point for body alignment and stretch before breaking the water surface.

SUMMARY

Human locomotion in water is affected by anthropometrical characteristics of the human form including shape, size, body composition, flexibility, and skill factors. Archimedes' principle of weight and fluid displacement applies to bodies immersed in an aquatic medium.

Hydroplaning is desirable for certain sprint swimmers since lift forces are increased and drag forces are decreased.

The arm action generally contributes greater forward propulsive force than leg movements, except in breaststroke and butterfly stroke. The front crawl is recognized as the fastest stroke used by humans and entails a six-beat kick. All strokes utilize Newton's third law of motion where reaction forward is equal to the backward push or thrust of the body. The arm stroke in front crawl swimming is comprised of three major segments: (1) catch, (2) pull, and (3) recovery. Bent-arm pulling increases the mechanical advantage of the front crawl by allowing the upper arms to exert a greater force than in the straight-arm style.

Flexibility of the ankles in addition to large feet favors an effective flutter kick. Highly trained swimmers breathe on both sides of the body in the front crawl stroke.

Mechanically, the basic difference between the front crawl and the back crawl is in the breathing style. Similar to the front crawl, the bent-arm pull is favored by most swimmers. Mechanically, the bent-arm pull allows the arm to move overhead rapidly with greater propulsive force than the straight-arm style. The arm action in the back crawl consists of (1) recover, (2) entry and catch, and (3) pull and push elements.

The breaststroke is the most seaworthy of all strokes and entails the following sequence: (1) pull, (2) kick, and (3) glide. The major components of the breaststroke are (1) arm action, (2) leg action, and (3) breathing. Cinematographic analysis indicates that breaststroke arm pulling is a "sculling" action involving a sideward/backward motion of the hands. The breaststroke leg action is basically classified as of two types: (1) orthodox kick and (2) whip kick. The whip kick is considered faster than the orthodox technique. However, the orthodox kick, commonly called the frog kick, is easier to coordinate and is usually taught in beginner classes where speed is not the primary objective.

Two types of forward starts are employed in modern swimming: (1) grab start and (2) conventional start. Research supports the superiority of the grab start over conventional styles in takeoff speed. Full extension, rather than "piking," the body is desirable during the flight phase of grab and conventional methods.

Mechanically, the grab start allows the swimmer better control of balance and equilibrium while leaning lower and forward with the center of gravity in front of the base of support. The overall effect permits the swimmer to take off with less resistance to resting inertia and at a lower flight trajectory.

The back stroke start is performed from an in-water position facing the starting end of the pool. An experimental standing-type start, employing a "screw-type" turn on the takeoff, appears to be faster than the conventional in-water mode.

Three basic forward turns are utilized in competitive swimming: (1) open turn, (2) closed turn, and (3) somersault turn. The principal difference between the open and closed turn entails breathing mechanics. The somersault type is the fastest forward turn used by competitive swimmers. Efficient turns apply (1) preservation of Newton's first law, (2) speed governing rotary velocity, and (3) reduction of body drag resistance. Research supports the tuck-type body position as faster than the pike posture during the somersault maneuver. Research supports the one-arm glide push-off as faster than the two-arm technique in forward and back stroke turns.

Springboard diving is more directly related to acrobatic maneuvers found in tumbling and trampoline activities than to swimming.

A forward running dive is comprised of the following components: (1) starting position and walk, (2) hurdle, (3) takeoff, (4) execution, and (5) water entry. The total performance of a dive depends upon an uninterrupted sequential kinetic chain of movements from the starting position through the entry. An error in any basic component will affect the diver's water entry.

Principles of stability apply to the starting position in all dives. A slight forward lean lessens the resting inertia before the walk is initiated. Consistency of the run, hurdle, and takeoff is important for flight execution since these elements determine the height and parabolic dive path. A diver can exert greater force on the hurdle by acceleration of the forward run and by increasing the height of the hurdle leg. The concept of "pushing" the board rather than "lifting" the feet on takeoff is an essential precept for maximizing the effects of Newton's third law. Increasing forward body lean on the takeoff augments the speed of rotation while lowering dive height. The extent of body lean also affects entry distance from the board. All dives should contain minimum lean thresholds for a safe entry.

The parabolic flight curve, once established after leaving the board, cannot be changed. Tuck somersault dives spin faster and more easily than dives performed in the pike or layout position because of a shortened radius of gyration.

Twisting dives are turning movements of the body in a horizontal plane around a vertical axis. Twisting may be initiated directly from the board or started free in air after the takeoff. Newton's third law and the principle of momentum transfer affect twisting movements in the desired direction of the diver. Twisting free in air resembles the action of a cat falling from a height and illustrates the action–reaction concept of Newton's third law.

All dives, head or feet first, should enter the water near the vertical mark with straight body alignment. Dive entries may be "saved" by increasing or decreasing the moment of inertia and/or applying Newton's law of action–reaction.

Backward and inward dives are performed from a balanced standing posture facing the board fulcrum. Maximum height is gained when the diver "rides" the board on the lift phase. The lift of the board depends upon depression magnitude and utilizes Newton's third law of motion. Vertical entries are more pronounced in backward dives than in forward dives.

REFERENCES

1. Page, R. L., "The Role of Physical Buoyancy in Swimming," *Journal of Human Movement Studies*, 1:190-198, December, 1975.
2. Pendergast, D. R., diPrampero, P. E., Craig, A. B., Jr., Wilson, D. R., and Rennie, D. W., "Quantitative Analysis of the Front Crawl in Men and Women," *Journal of Applied Physiology*, 43:475-479, 1977.
3. Sheeran, Thomas J., "An Electrogoniometric Analysis of the Knee and Ankle in Competitive and Noncompetitive Swimmers," Unpublished Doctoral Dissertation, State University of New York at Buffalo, 1976.
4. Karpovich, Peter V., "Analysis of the Propelling Force in the Crawl Arm Stroke," *Research Quarterly*, VI:49-58, May, 1935.
5. Holmer, I., "Efficiency of Breaststroke and Freestyle Swimming," in L. Lewillie and J. P. Clarys (Eds.), *Swimming II*. Baltimore, Md.: University Park Press, 1975, pp. 130-142.
6. Magel, John R., "Propelling Force Measured During Tethered Swimming in the Four Competitive Swimming Styles," *Research Quarterly*, 41:68-74, March, 1970.
7. Atwater, Anne E., "Cinematographic Analysis of Human Movement," in J. H. Wilmore (Ed.), *Exercise and Sport Sciences Reviews*, Vol. I. New York: Academic Press, 1973, pp. 217-258.
8. Rackham, G. W., "An Analysis of Arm Propulsion in Swimming," in L. Lewillie and J. P. Clarys (Eds.), *Swimming II*. Baltimore, Md.: University Park, 1975, pp. 174-179.
9. Scheilauf, Bob, "A Hydrodynamic Analysis of Breaststroke Pulling Efficiency," *Swimming Technique*, 12:100-105, Winter, 1975.
10. Holmer, *op. cit.*, p. 133.
11. Yoshizawa, M., Tokuyama, H., Okamoto, T., and Kumamota, M., "Electromyographic Study of the Breaststroke," in Paavo V. Komi, (Ed.), *Biomechanics V-B*. Maryland: University Park Press, 1976, pp. 222-229.
12. Miyashita, Mitsumasa, "Method of Calculating Mechanical Power in Swimming the Breaststroke," *Research Quarterly*, 45:128-137, May, 1974.
13. Lowell, John C., "Analysis of the Grab Start and the Conventional Start," *Swimming Technique*, 12:66-69, 76, Fall, 1974.
14. Bowers, J. E., and Cavanagh, P. R., "A Biomechanical Comparison of the Grab and Conventional Sprint Starts in Competitive Swimming," in L. Lewillie and J. P. Clarys (Eds.) *Swimming II*. Baltimore, Md.: University Park Press, 1975, pp. 225-232.
15. Ayalon, B., Van Gheluwe, B., and Kanitz, M., "A Comparison of Four Styles of Racing Starts in Swimming," in L. Lewillie and J. P. Clarys (Eds.), *Swimming II*. Baltimore, Md.: University Park Press, 1975, pp. 233-240.
16. Decker, James, "A Time and Distance Analysis of Two Competitive Backstroke Swimming Starts," Unpublished Master's Project, State University of New York at Buffalo, 1969.
17. Scharf, Raphael, and King, William H., "Time and Motion Analysis of Competitive Freestyle Swimming Turns," *Research Quarterly*, 45:37-44, March, 1964.

18. King, William H., Jr., and Irwin, Leslie W., "A Time and Motion Study of Competitive Backstroke Swimming Turns," *Research Quarterly*, 28:257-268, October, 1957.

19. Piscopo, John, "Mechanical and Other Kinesiological Factors Affecting Dive Movements." Paper presented at the 60th National Convention of the American Association for Health, Physical Education and Recreation, Kansas City, Missouri, April, 1958.

20. Wilson, Barry D., "Toppling Techniques in Diving," *Research Quarterly*, 48:806-811, December, 1977.

21. Stroup, Francis, and Bushnell, David L., "Rotation, Translation and Trajectory in Diving," *Research Quarterly*, 40:812-817, December, 1969.

22. Batterman, Charles, *The Techniques of Springboard Diving*. Cambridge, Mass: The MIT Press, 1968, p. 22.

23. McDonald, Donald, "How Does a Man Twist in the Air?" *New Scientist*, 10:501-503, June, 1961.

24. *Ibid*.

SUPPLEMENTAL READINGS

Batterman, Charles, "Mechanics of the Crawl Arm Stroke," *Swimming World*, 7:4-5, 18-21, 1966.

Bober, T., and Czabanski, B., "Changes in Breaststroke Techniques Under Different Speed Conditions," in L. Lewillie and J. P. Clarys (Eds.), *Swimming II*. Baltimore, Md.: University Park, 1975, pp. 188-193.

Counsilman, James E., "Forces in Swimming Two Types of Crawl Stroke," *Research Quarterly*, 26:127-139, May, 1955.

Counsilman, James E., *The Science of Swimming*. Englewood Cliffs, N.J.: Prentice-Hall, 1968.

Durbin, Bruce B. (Ed.), *Swimming and Diving Rules*. Elgin, Ill.: National Federation of State High School Associations, 1980-1981.

Gabrielson, M. A., Spears, Betty, and Gabrielson, B. W., *Aquatics Handbook*. Englewood Cliffs, N.J.: Prentice-Hall, 1975, pp. 31-32, 66.

Hebbelinck, M., Carter, L., and DeGray, A., "Body Building and Somatotype of Olympic Swimmers, Divers and Water Polo Players," in L. Lewillie and J. P. Clarys (Eds.), *Swimming II*. Baltimore, Md.: University Park Press, 1975, pp. 285-305.

Jiskoot, J., and Clarys, J. P., "Body Resistance on and Under the Water Surface," in L. Lewillie and J. P. Clarys (Eds.), *Swimming II*. Baltimore, Md.: University Park Press, 1975, pp. 105-109.

Miller, Doris I. "Biomechanics of Swimming," in J. H. Wilmore and Jack F. Keogh (Eds.), *Exercise and Sport Sciences Reviews*, Vol. 3. New York: Academic Press, 1975, pp. 219-248.

Miyashita, M., "Arm Action in the Crawl Stroke," in L. Lewillie and J. P. Clarys (Eds.), *Swimming II*. Baltimore, Md.: University Park Press, 1975, pp. 167-173.

Ward, Thomas A., "A Cinematographical Comparison of Two Turns," *Swimming Technique*, 13:4-6, 9, Spring, 1976.

11 | ANALYSIS OF SELECTED SPORT SKILLS

CONCEPTS

1. Certain types of sport skills will demand greater emphasis upon internal mechanical elements, while other athletic activities will require greater attention to external mechanical aspects.

2. Each sport skill is unique, and an analysis will vary depending upon the specific nature of its movement pattern.

3. A kinesiological analysis of a motor performance entails two broad categories: (1) anatomical and (2) mechanical elements.

4. Qualitative analysis seeks gross information about a motor performance by observing film and videotape and is a popular method used by teachers and coaches.

5. Quantitative analysis entails the numerical calculation of data and is pursued by researchers where precision and exactness are required.

6. Whole dynamic movement of the body is a result of a sequential kinetic chain of linked joints.

7. Effective force in badminton is developed by creating a rhythmic pattern in the sequential kinetic chain from large joints to the smaller articulations of the body.

8. A racquet that possesses a high coefficient of restitution has greater speed of rebound on impact with the shuttlecock.

9. Muscles of the upper body—trunk, shoulder girdle, arms, and hands—are particularly important for grasping, pushing, pulling, and holding moves found in wrestling.

10. Quick movements can be facilitated by the wrestler keeping the center of gravity high and near the pivoting edge of his base in the direction of the movement.

11. When a wrestler desires more force with less effort in such moves as a body press combination, he should create a long force arm by extending the distance from the pivoting edge (fulcrum) to the point of force application.

12. Mechanically, cycling is a process of transferring rotary joint action, particularly of the trunk, legs, and feet, to the bike pedals creating a translatory motion of man and machine.

13. Riding low cycles at high speeds can be especially hazardous because quick changes in lateral deviations from the gravity center can occur with little time for the rider to correct the balance errors.

14. Running in baseball is similar to the sprint dash event; increasing the sprint stride and rate increases the speed of the runner.

15. Extending the arm on the forehand and backhand strokes in racquetball permits a longer lever from the shoulder to point of impact, with a resultant gain in speed of the racquet.

16. Direction and rebound of serves and placement of the ball depend largely upon the force, angle of incidence, and spin of the ball as it is struck by the racquet.

GENERAL CONSIDERATIONS

Literally hundreds of sport skills are offered in physical education programs. Selected sports found in a curriculum depend upon unique factors germane to a particular region or situation. Such elements as climate and facilities determine whether or not certain types of activities can be included in a program. Therefore, it is not unusual to find up to two-thirds of a physical education sports program contained within an inside setting in the North. Other conditions, such as facilities, faculty interest and expertise, schedules, and student interest also play an important part in deciding "what" and "when" sport skills should be included in regular class, intramural, and varsity categories.

Our discussion will focus on five sports; badminton, wrestling, cycling, baseball, and racquetball. Three sports are typically played indoors (badminton, wrestling, and racquetball); one sport is usually played outdoors (baseball); and one sport may be conducted indoors or outdoors (cycling).

A comprehensive analysis of these sports is not offered here, but, rather, our discussion presents a condensation of basic components that should be considered when examining the scientific characteristics of an activity. Certain types of sports will demand greater accent on internal mechanics; others require careful and minute evaluation of external mechanical factors. For example, putting in golf necessitates primary analysis of accuracy, timing, and neuromuscular coordination; on the other hand, performing handstand push-ups mandates an analysis of muscular strength as a central consideration. Each sport skill is unique. Its analysis will vary depending upon the specific nature of the movement. Certain sports require speed, others accentuate form.

The student should review the basic requirements of a skill, which include such variables as strength, speed, form, neuromuscular coordination, and accuracy, and assess the relative importance of these constituents for efficient performance of the activity under examination. Students should be selective in analyzing sport skills. Not all minute kinesiological analyses are applicable from a practical viewpoint. For example, in such activities as tumbling and swimming, the element of speed is essential for elite performance. This constituent is particularly related to flexibility. Therefore, the astute coach will focus on the most effective way to improve flexibility of body joints in order to enhance the speed proficiency of the performer.

PERFORMANCE CHARACTERISTICS

Elite athletic ability may be distinguished by a commonality of characteristics or features. As indicated earlier, each sport skill is unique, and the characteristics considered vary in their contribution to a successful performance depending upon the nature, description, and objectives of a given sport. Several common athletic characteristics are presented. Each of these variables is discussed in detail in other chapters of this text. The student should refer to the appropriate sections for an explanation of the performance components considered in the following paragraphs.

Strength Aspect

This component can be created internally and externally. Internal strength stems from the contractile strength of muscular fibers. Externally, strength or force is regulated by the type and manner in which implements and/or machines are utilized. How much strength is necessary for a given skill or task is a basic question. Some sports require more strength and power than others; nevertheless, all human movement must possess this basic ingredient before dynamic body action can result.

Endurance Aspect

How long can an individual sustain maximum effort? How important is this factor in swimming the 1500 meter event? Athletes who exhibit championship performance in such events must possess high levels of endurance, which require physiological efficiency in addition to the application of correct mechanical principles peculiar to the sport.

Body Type

It should be quite clear from the authors' explanations and discussions throughout this text that physique is an important factor in elite sport performance. Generally, it may be declared that mesomorphy, with some slight variations, is highly desirable for world-class performance of athletic skills.

Balance

Balance is an integral part of an efficient motor performance. As noted earlier, specific types of balance are categorized and identified according to the nature of the skill. Many examples of static, dynamic, upright, and inverted balance qualities are used in sport. A steady hand with body balance (static) is necessary when the individual is putting in golf. Dynamic balance is demonstrated by the football player catching a pass as he maneuvers his body without falling. Dynamic balance is involved in the act of walking, turning, and jumping. Therefore, this variable should be included in sport skill and analysis.

Agility and Neuromuscular Control

This performance characteristic is concerned with the ability of the individual to change body directions in a fluent and efficient manner. It is a combination of variables that includes balance, coordination, accuracy, speed, strength, and endurance functioning holistically. The amount of agility required varies from one activity or sport to another depending upon game play. For example, a downhill skier needs more agility and neuromuscular coordination than a cross-country ski specialist.

Speed and Accuracy

Speed and accuracy are basic ingredients of most motor skills. As explained in Chapter 4, speed and accuracy should be taught at the same time whenever these two elements are part of a required task. High jumping and hurdling events typify such a task. It should be noted that fatigue is a factor that restricts speed and accuracy.

Sensory Attention and Alertness

This characteristic is identified as a degree of keen awareness to sensations stemming from neural sensations of the nervous systems. Chapter 4 considers related aspects of this topic.

Rhythm Pattern

All sports contain a unique rhythm pattern that is associated with the fluency and style of its motion. Interpretive ice skating typifies one sport that demands a sense of rhythm as a foremost requirement for a winning performance.

Reaction Time

This stimulus–response phenomenon is a vital part of sports that require quick and accurate movements. The physiological mechanism is described in Chapter 4. It is recognized that certain sports demand more attention to this variable than other athletic skills. For example, sprint swimmers and track performers must develop a quick reaction response after the gun is fired on the start, whereas this variable is not as crucial to long-distance runners or swimmers.

Flexibility

The degree of flexibility necessary for performance efficiency also varies from one sport to another. This fitness parameter is of great importance in tumbling and high jumping. The implications of flexibility are further discussed in Chapter 14. The authors view this characteristic, not only as a therapeutic measure, but as an essential performance trait for effective mobility patterns of most athletic skills.

KINESIOLOGICAL CONSTRUCTS

Throughout this text we have explored and explained internal and external mechanics and numerous kinematic and kinetic aspects of activities. Now, the final task of the analyst is to apply these movement precepts for a better understanding of the *performer* and the *performance*. A kinesiological construct of a motor performance entails two broad categories: (1) *anatomical*, and (2) *mechanical*. A framework for analysis is indicated below:

Anatomical Aspects

A study of internal structure attempts to answer the following questions:

1. What muscles are responsible for the primary movement of the task or skill at hand? When determining functions, antagonists, neutralizers, and stabilizers should also be considered.

2. Which body joints and what type of lever classification are involved in the motor skill? The analyst will notice immediately that a single movement entails a number of joint motions in most sport skills. Identification of function of major articulations involved is sufficient for the practicing physical educator and allied health specialist.

3. How do body composition and physique affect the performance? This component entails an identification and classification of endomorphy, ectomorphy, or mesomorphy described in earlier chapters.

4. What kind of movement is involved in the skill? For example, is the action considered isotonic, isometric, or isokinetic? Further breakdown identifying concentric or eccentric muscular contractions should also be indicated.

5. What are the limiting factors of joint movements? Each major joint articulation should be identified according to synarthrodial, amphiarthrodial, and diarthrodial categories, since such structures impose anatomical restrictions on certain types of movements. For example, the shoulder joint is structurally designed to move in all planes, whereas the knee joint acts primarily in one plane. This anatomical consideration is especially relevant to safety and injury prevention.

Mechanical Aspects

The precision with which the analyst gathers kinesiological information will depend upon the purpose and utilization of the gained knowledge. Generally, practitioners are interested in *qualitative analysis* of the kind of data that stems from observations of film and videotape. The skill is subjectively analyzed from viewing the action on a screen. Such questions as, "When did the performer flex?" or, "At what point did the diver speed up the rotation of a somersault?" may be answered by observation of film and/or television. Researchers, on the other hand, rely on precision and exactness. This approach requires the numerical *quantification* of data and the application of mathematics and physics. Such instruments as the electrogoniometer, force platform, and electromyographic apparatus described in Chapter 15 are designed to give quantitative data about a motor skill. Instrumentation systems such as the motion analyzer provide numerical data about actions recorded from film. This type of analysis allows the investigator to take specific measurements of velocity, angulation, and motion displacement from a single motion picture frame.

Whether the analyzer selects qualitative or quantitative procedures, certain mechanical aspects should be considered when seeking answers of "why" a motion occurs in a particular manner. Several basic laws and principles should be applied to the performance. The analyzer should identify the following fundamental mechanical laws and principles:

1. Which of Newton's physical laws of motion apply to the movement? Frequently all three laws are involved in the total movement of a skill.

2. Which *kinematic* parameters affect the skill performance? These variables include descriptions such as time, displacement velocity, and acceleration without consideration of the forces acting on a body.

3. Which *kinetic* parameters affect the skill performance? Such descriptions and analysis of mass, force, and energy entail these elements in a kinesiological analysis. Kinetics deals with factors that initiate, alter, or stop movements and are considered by some kinesiologists as the highest level of biomechanical analyses of motion.

4. Is the movement angular or linear? It is possible that the performance may be a combination of both angular and linear classifications. For example, a forward roll contains angular and linear characteristics. These differentials should be indicated.

5. What kind of balance or equilibrium is involved in the motor skill? The instructor should determine whether the performance entails static, dynamic, upright, or inverted balance characteristics, which are described in Chapter 8.

SKILL OUTLINE

A general outline that can be used in analyzing a motor skill is presented by the authors for the practitioner. Although many different outlines are offered by other kinesiologists, the scheme indicated below can be employed by teachers and coaches seeking information about a particular motor performance.

General Outline of Motor Skills

1. Descriptive Analysis

Includes beginning or starting position, action during skill, and ending or terminal position. *Purpose* of the skill should also be indicated.

2. General Motor Classification

Includes identification of movement type; action on land or water; movement of *body* as a whole or striking an object with implement; body support with the body above or below the point of support such as support on parallel bars and swinging on rings; unsupported body action, such as found in tumbling and diving activities.

3. Muscular Analysis

Includes major muscle movers, stabilizers and antagonistic groups.

4. Internal Mechanical Factors

Includes such elements as lever types; flexibility; body composition; joint classifications and limitations.

5. External Mechanical Factors

Includes application of appropriate kinematics and kinetics, laws, and motion principles *outside* the body that affect the motor skill.

When using the above outline, the student should keep in mind that a principal objective is to *detect errors* in performance and then proceed to correct those errors by referring to the information gathered about the particular motor skill. It is also important to remember that human motion should be viewed as a continuum, that is, each position—*start, action,* and *terminal* points—is sequentially dependent upon the others from the initial point of movement to the follow-through action. For example, the entry of a dive or whether it is "short" or "long" can be caused by the degree of lean at the initial start before the run, hurdle, and takeoff from the board.

LINKAGE SYSTEM

An important concept in the mechanism of dynamic body motion entails the concept of *linkage of joints* from one articulation to another to provide a smooth flow of motion and balance in moving the whole body or striking an object with an implement. For example, the arm can be considered a series of segments or links beginning with the fingers and including the hand, wrist, elbow, and shoulder joints. Work on these segments is transmitted to the trunk and spine through a large musculoskeletal surface wherein there is an exchange of forces across a proximal fulcrum capable of generating massive energy.[1] Similarly, toes and ankle are links, together with the lower and upper leg that make possible the transmission of force into the hip from the feet in running and jumping movements. Each dynamic movement is a result of a sequential kinetic chain of linked joints. The analyzer should study and determine which joints and segments are germane to the motor skill performed and assist the performer to assume positions and movements that enhance

a *smooth rhythmic flow* of linkage from large body joints found in the trunk to the small articulations contained in the fingers and toes. It should be noted that kinetic chains of the upper extremities possess greater mobility (freedom of movement) than those of the lower extremities. For example, the hip joint linkage system moves through a lesser range of motion than the shoulder girdle kinetic linkage because of the restrictive characteristics of tendons and ligaments surrounding the pelvic area.

ANALYSIS OF SELECTED SPORT SKILLS

The ensuing discussion is limited to salient kinesiological aspects of each sport skill. The student should consult skill manuals in the specific sport described for detailed information concerning progression, teaching procedures, and strategies.

Badminton

The game of badminton, like tennis, is considered a member of the racquet sport family in which an implement is used for striking an object within a prescribed court area. The general outline presented earlier in this chapter, pointing out central movement principles and concepts applicable to the sport, is employed for the analysis.

Descriptive Analysis. Essentially, singles play is much faster than doubles play since a singles player must cover the entire court; in contrast, certain portions of the court are assigned to two persons in doubles. The following strokes are entailed in game play: service, forehand, backhand, clear, drive, drop, net, and smash.

General Motor Classification. Badminton is classified as a striking action with an implement from a solid surface. All three types of arm movements are involved: overarm, underarm, and diagonal or sidearm. The overarm pattern is typified by the *smash*, a short or long *service* stroke is executed with an underarm pattern, and a *flat drive* employs the sidearm pattern. Figures 11.1*a,* 11.1*b,* and 11.1*c* illustrate three different strokes that correspond to typical striking patterns.

The action of most strokes used in badminton is ballistic; that is, it is a follow-through movement. In the net shot, the wrist is held rigid. The bird rebounds off the racquet in the desired direction close to the net.

Muscular Analysis. Since badminton involves whole body movement, the muscles actually used comprise the entire system. However, certain areas are central to the sport, so specific muscle analysis is justified. Movements of the upper extremity, which provide the force for the strike, and actions of the lower extremity, which serve as force initiators in footwork, are presented.

Figure 11.1a   Overhead smash

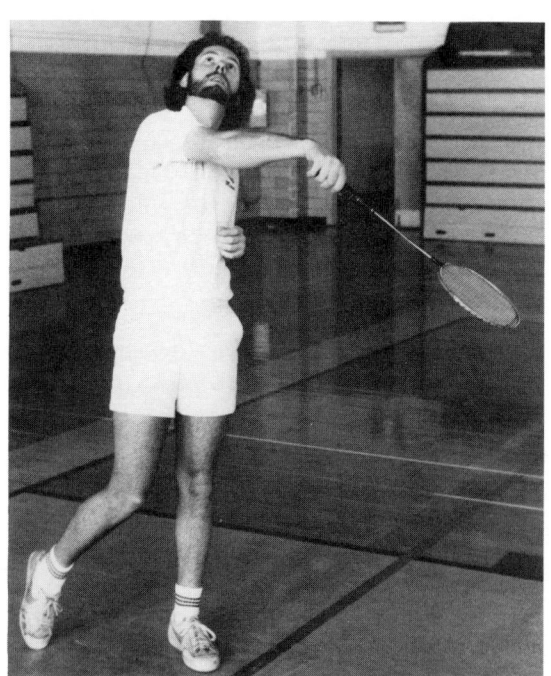

(a)

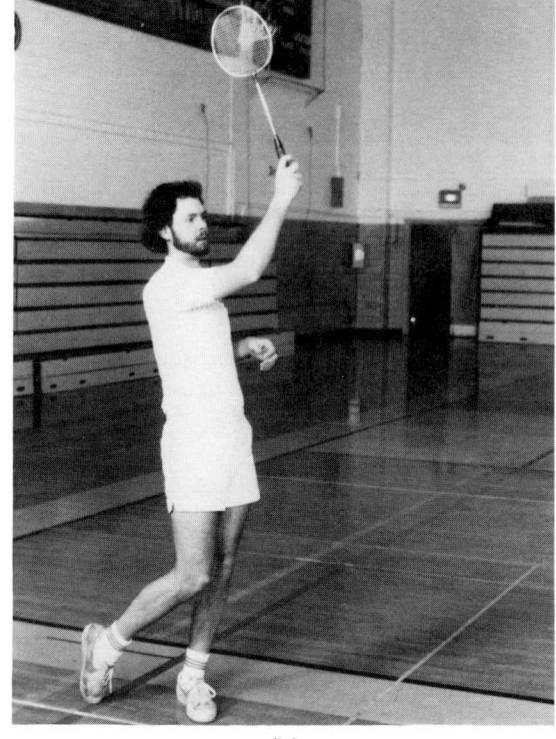

(b)

Figure 11.1b   Underhand service

Figure 11.1c   Sidearm flat drive

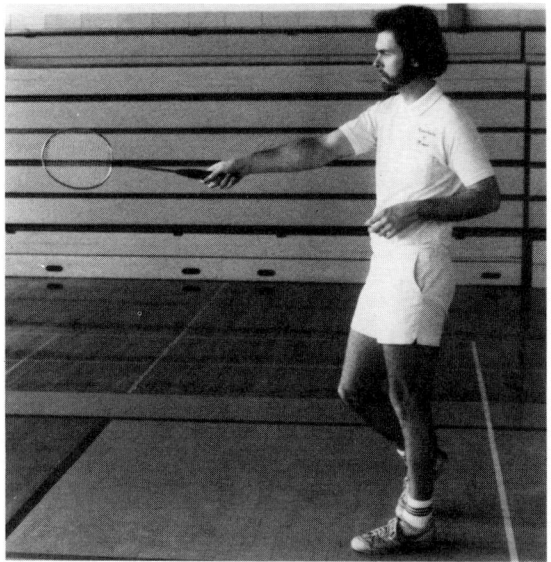

(c)

Muscles of the Upper Extremity

Considering the shoulder joint as a major articulation in the movement of the arm and the structural classification of this joint as diarthrodial-enarthrosis, muscles that move the humerus in all planes are responsible for the variations of strokes used in badminton. Each stroke should be analyzed separately because certain movements of this ball and socket joint require involvement of specific muscles as major and/or assistant movers. Major muscles may reverse their roles depending upon the action involved. For example, in badminton, the clavicular portion of the pectoralis major is a prime flexor (agonist) in the forehand flat drive; however, this segment of the pectorals becomes an extensor (antagonist) in a backhand drive stroke.

The principal shoulder girdle muscles of particular importance in badminton play are: *deltoids, supraspinatus, pectoralis major, coracobrachialis, subscapularis, lattissimus dorsi, teres major,* and *infraspinatus.*

The muscles of the *elbow* and *radioulnar joints* are also part of the link system moving the arm; therefore, these movers should be considered in the analysis. The following muscles are primarily responsible for flexion, extension, supination, and pronation of the elbow joint and lower arm: *biceps brachii, brachialis, brachioradialis, triceps brachii, supinator,* and *pronator quadratus.*

The muscles that flex, extend, abduct, and rotate the wrist are particularly critical in badminton. Wrist snap action and control depend upon the strength and flexibility of forearm flexors and extensors. The principal movers of the wrist are *flexor carpi radialis* and *ulnaris, extensor carpi radialis longus, brevis,* and *ulnaris.*

The thumb is an important appendage and, as described earlier, possesses a unique action called opposition. The placement of the thumb is vital in forehand and backhand strokes. In the forehand grip, the thumb wraps around the racquet handle, whereas in the backhand stroke, the thumb is placed in an extended position parallel to the handle. The major muscles of the thumb that control the grasp and tightness of the grip are as follows: *flexor pollicis longus* and *brevis, extensor pollicis longus* and *brevis, adductor pollicis longus* and *brevis, adductor pollicis* and *opponens pollicis.*

Muscles of the Lower Extremity

The myriad of movements in badminton require whole body action; therefore, muscles of the lower limbs are involved. The student may wish to examine minute muscles that are assistive in function to moving forward, backward, sideward, and turning. Specific actions of these muscles may be found in Chapter 2. However, our discussion is limited to the major movers of the hip, thigh, and lower leg. Each of the following muscles serves to flex and extend the knee; extend, abduct, and adduct the hip and leg; and flex and extend the ankle: *quadriceps, hamstrings, gluteals, adductors, gastrocnemius, soleus, tibilias anterior, flexor hallucis longus,* and *extensor hallucis longus.*

It can be seen from the muscular analysis of badminton that game play focuses largely upon the shoulder girdle, elbow, wrist, and hand for racquet and shuttlecock control, while lower limb actions are also necessary for moving the whole body from one point to another in the court area. From a muscular standpoint, badminton contributes minimally to abdominal strength other than toning the transversus abdominis, which is stimulated in forced expiration as the player reaches a rapid breathing state.

Internal Mechanical Analysis. Internally, four elements affect the quality of badminton game play: *levers, flexibility, body composition,* and *joint limitations.* Since movements of most body joints consist of levers of the third class, we can see at once that strength and power are not favored by internal lever construction. The exception to this structure characteristic is found in the execution of the backhand stroke shown in Figure 11.2. Extension of the elbow involves a first-class lever arrangement, through quick contraction of the triceps brachii.

Hitting the shuttlecock involves the concept of the open kinetic chain. Movement of the lever structures begins with the trunk and sequentially follows a rhythmic action flow from one internal lever to another, until the bird is propelled on contact with the racquet. The movement is *ballistic* if the stroke is a clear, smash, or drive, and *nonballistic* if the stroke is a net shot. Flexibility of the shoulder, elbow, and wrist joints is highly desirable since this factor adds to the range of motion in the arc or path of the arm moving as a whole. Elite badminton players are usually lean. Quick whole body movements can be performed by lighter individuals with greater efficiency and less effort since the force required to overcome resting inertia is proportional to the mass to be moved.

External Mechanical Analysis. An essential difference between tennis and badminton lies

Figure 11.2 Backhand stroke

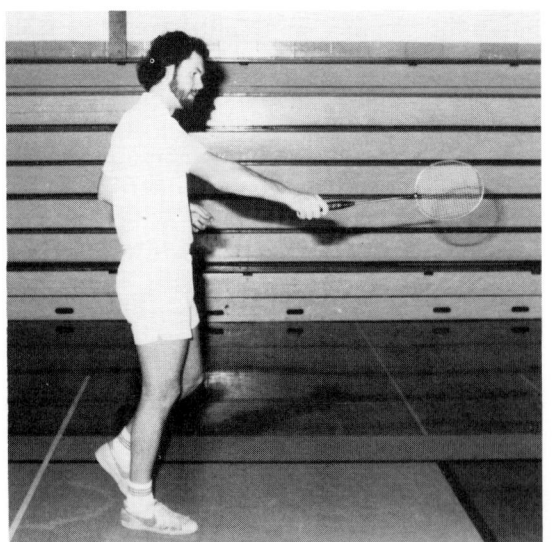

in the nature of the equipment used. Badminton racquets and shuttlecocks are much lighter than tennis racquets and balls. Therefore, less strength of the arm and hand is demanded in badminton. Primary importance is placed upon *speed, accuracy,* and *control of distance* of the bird. For example, a smash shot places emphasis upon force and downward speed of the struck bird. A net shot places critical importance on accuracy in placing the bird just over the net at a strategic point. A clear shot must have, not only accuracy in placement of the bird, but sufficient distance to the rear court as well. Air resistance affects the speed of the propelled bird. Generally, the higher the parabolic path of the shuttlecock, the slower and more vertical the drop of the bird in the opposite court. Flat drive shots are usually faster than high clear strokes.

Striking mechanics depend upon the type of stroke utilized. For example, in a single service stance using the forehand stroke, the left foot should be forward (right-hander) and point to the spot to which the bird is to be propelled. This is shown in Figure 11.3.

Ninety percent of the time, single service shots are played to the deep diagonal corner of the opponent's court.[2] When using the backhand stroke in the service, the right foot should be forward with the left foot to the rear and close to the center line as shown in Figure 11.2. Each stroke in badminton contains its own mechanical characteristics. The analyzer should assess the purpose of the stroke and then apply the appropriate principle. Several universal mechanical precepts are presented that generally apply to most racquet sports.

1. Increase force by developing a rhythmic pattern of a *sequential kinetic chain* from large to smaller joints of the body.

2. The force of impact is determined by the *speed* of the racquet at contact with the bird. Maximum momentum is gained

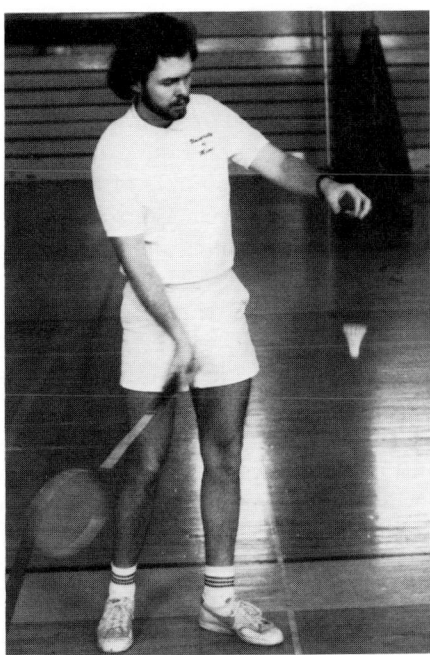

Figure 11.3 Singles service—forehand stroke

when the time and distance of acceleration are increased.

3. Extending the arm to full length increases the length of the lever arm, thereby allowing for greater potential in increasing the *linear velocity* of the racquet head.

4. Body weight should be moving *forward* at the striking moment to gain speed.

5. A heavier racquet, handled with control, possesses greater *potential striking force*, since the greater the mass, the greater the probability of developing more kinetic energy.

6. Use of a quality strung racquet that possesses a strong *coefficient of elasticity* will improve the speed of rebound.

7. A firm grip will enhance control of *placement* of the shuttlecock.

Wrestling

The sport of wrestling is categorized as a combative activity and is universally found in competitive athletics around the world. Our discussion will center around the kinesiological principles rather than the rules and regulations that govern the sport. The student should refer to the National Collegiate Athletic Association and the Amateur Athletic Union guides for specific legalities and illegalities concerning the conduct of competition.

Descriptive Analysis. The purpose of freestyle wrestling is to win a match by securing a fall by pinning both shoulders of the opponent for two seconds or scoring more points than the other contestant. When a fall does not occur in any period, the referee shall award the match to the contestant who has earned the greatest number of points. Wrestling skills include such moves as stances (upright and kneeling), holds and counters, take-downs, rides, escapes, breakdowns, and pins.

General Motor Classification. Wrestling may be classified as motor skill whereby the whole and/or segmental parts of the body are meeting varying sustained degrees of resistance on a solid land surface. The ability to act and react quickly in offensive and defensive moves is a vital skill component for effective wrestling. Two important attributes for a winning performance are the development and maintenance of muscular endurance and the application of correct internal and external mechanical principles.

Muscular Analysis. A well-planned progressive muscular strength and endurance program should be an integral part of developing proficiency in wrestling. Although we feel that the application of scientific principles of motion should be paramount, the implementation of those principles depends upon the energy created by the force of muscle power and endurance. The term *grappler* probably emanated from the typical motion pattern of the wrestler, whereby the contestants are continually grasping each other in various moves and countermoves. Muscles that surround the upper extremities, i.e., upper trunk, shoulder girdle, arms, and hands, are vital for grasping, pushing, pulling, and holding moves. A notation should be made about the neck muscles. Nearly all novice wrestlers lack strength in the neck.[3] Therefore, it is quite common to observe contestants practicing "bridge" exercises whereby the participant moves his head forward and backward and from left to right from the position in Figure 11.4.

Hand strength is also an important factor in wrestling. Contestants are constantly maneuvering from one position to another. Although specific techniques are prescribed to break away from a held hand, strength of the hand flexors and extensors is necessary in order to gain control of the wrestler's own hands.

Leg strength also contributes to efficient wrestling. Correct use of the legs can be applied as an effective weapon in the offensive wrestler's repertoire. For example, a wrestler can develop a powerful take-down by hooking one leg around the ankle of his opponent and driving forward. Of course, proper leverage and correct application of force in the movement must be performed in addition to a quick and vigorous thrust in the hooking action of the leg.

It can be seen from the above discussion that muscular strength of the upper body, shoulder girdle, arms, hands, and legs is important in the wrestler's conditioning program. Such activities as pull-ups, dips on the parallel bars, rope climb, bridge exercises, forearm curls (forward and reverse), running (cardiorespiratory endurance), and quadricep and hamstring exercises against resistance are recommended for the development of strength in wrestling muscles.

Figure 11.4 The bridge (courtesy of Niagara County Community College, Sanborn, N.Y.)

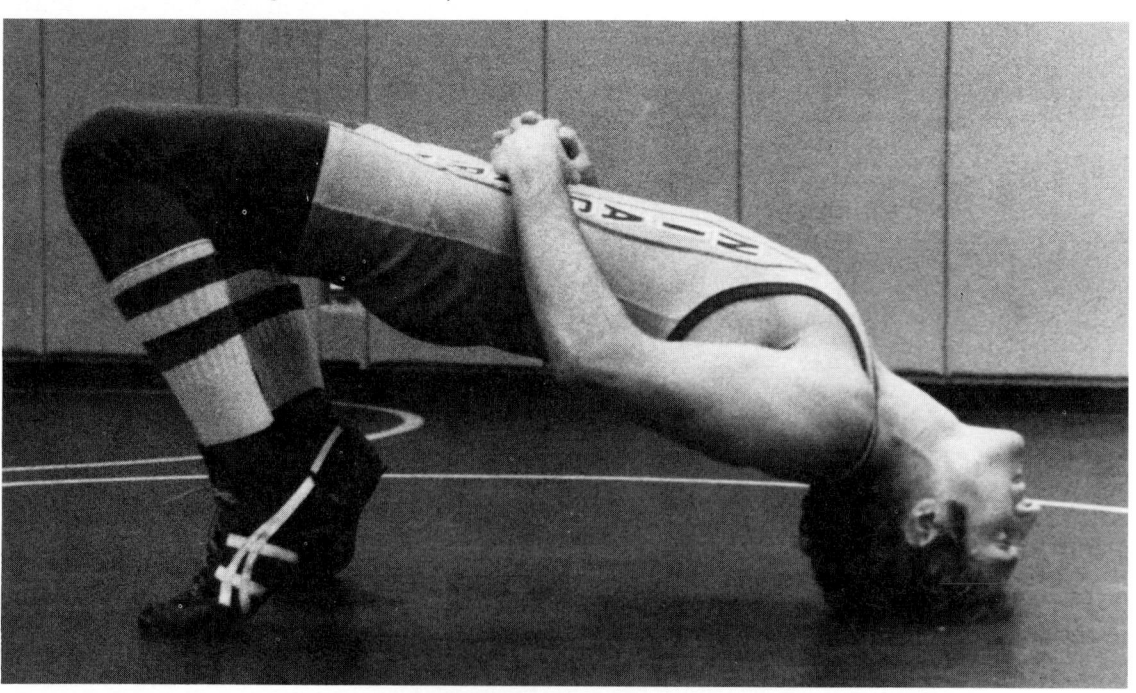

Internal Mechanical Analysis. Internally, body composition, flexibility, and lever types affect wrestling performance. From a stability standpoint, a heavier individual possesses greater stability than a lighter wrestler simply because of his greater mass. Wrestlers are found in all shapes and sizes. Although lighter competitors are anatomically less stable, this structural delimitation can be overcome by using correct external mechanical maneuvers. For example, the lighter wrestler can widen the distance between his feet in the open stance position to avoid being thrown off balance. In this example, stability is enhanced by increasing the width of the support base. The physique of a competitive wrestler favors mesomorphy. Hirata[4] found that Olympic contestants were not as stout as weight lifters. Not all superior wrestlers are powerful, burly individuals. Since wrestling contains many holds and moves, a variety of physique types can be successful in the sport. For example, the short, stocky person can concentrate on mastering holds that require great strength of arms and shoulders. Tall individuals have the advantage of using their legs for hooking maneuvers, setting up takedowns, and pins. Individuals who are extreme endormophs are handicapped in wrestling because their strength is not proportional to body weight.

Flexibility of the shoulders, trunk, and legs can be an important asset in augmenting speed and preventing muscular strains and joint sprains. Leighton[5] investigated seven groups of highly skilled athletes in swimming, baseball, basketball, track, weight lifting, gymnastics, and wrestling. It was interesting to note that wrestlers showed a pattern of lowest flexibility among the seven athletic groups measured, being high in only eight out of 30 joint movements. These were *neck* flexion, extension, and lateral flexion; *shoulder* adduction, abduction, and rotation; and *elbow* flexion and extension movements. The above study does suggest that neck, shoulder, and arm flexibility is an important factor among skilled wrestlers. The student should remember that flexibility is specific to a particular joint and that a common degree of flexibility in all joints does not exist.[6]

External Mechanical Analysis. Unlike the runner or swimmer, who is repeating a sequence of motion patterns against a relatively constant force, the wrestler is working against a changing situation entailing a variety of positions and forces.

The application of *motion, balance, leverage, speed,* and *position* are important external mechanical elements for successful wrestling.

Motion

The offensive wrestler is one who continually drives forward. A backward motion places the wrestler in a defensive position and gives the opponent an advantage. Elite wrestlers are in a constant state of motion, attempting to maneuver to position advantage. Movements forward, left, or right are offensive. Since the wrestler is striving for continuous movement, force application in the proper direction with sufficient speed is a prime consideration for offensive combat. The student will recall, from Chapter 6, four principles for the production and application of force: *magnitude, direction, point of application,* and *time* over which the force is applied. Each of these factors can be applied to wrestling. For example, in order for the wrestler to increase his magnitude of force, he should increase his speed, since force equals mass times acceleration. This principle is particularly important for lighter wrestlers.

The initial take-down move is of vital importance in the outcome of a wrestling match. Maertz[7] investigated the effect of the initial take-down on the outcome of wrestling matches and found that 76 percent of 2465 matches were won by wrestlers who secured the initial take-down. *Speed* along with balance and leverage was considered necessary for a successful take-down.

Numerous examples are found in wrestling where force can be maximized by applying it at correct angles in the desired direction over a time period. The student is referred to Chapter 6 for descriptions of related force principles.

Balance and Stability in Wrestling

Most experts agree that balance and stability are essential mechanical elements for controlled moves in wrestling. Several points drawn from Chapter 8 can be applied to wrestling.

1. Stability is proportional to its base area.

Whenever the wrestler is standing with his feet together, he can be easily thrown off balance and overturned. However, if the wrestler stands with feet about 24 to 36 inches apart and one foot ahead of the other, his base of support is enlarged, and therefore his opponent will find him more difficult to move (Figure 11.5). The same principle can be applied in the wrestler's down position with the hands placed shoulder width apart and with both knees and feet in contact with the mat. In addition to increasing the support base with hands apart, the center of gravity is lowered by keeping the hips below shoulder height. This position provides a firm and stable base.

2. Lowering the center of gravity above its base increases stability (nonpivoting base).

In wrestling, because of changing moves and positions, the height of the body's center of gravity over its base is continually changing. Therefore, whether the wrestler is standing or crouching, he should attempt to keep his gravity height as low as possible. Figure 11.6 illustrates a stable de-

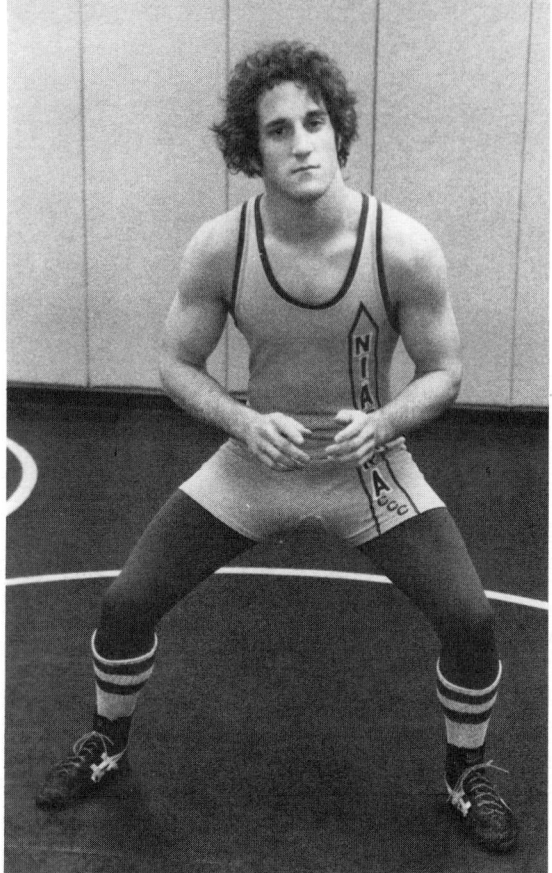

Figure 11.5 Wrestler's position standing with legs apart enhancing stability (courtesy of Niagara County Community College, Sanborn, N.Y.)

fensive position with buttocks held close to the base of support.

3. Stability in a given direction depends upon the horizontal distance of the center of gravity from its pivoting edge or base.

An example of the above principle is applied when a wrestler starts a take-down move using a leg tackle and decides to change his tactics at midpoint. The wrestler can stop his forward thrust without losing control, if his center of gravity is focused on the rear foot rather than the forward leg. In this situation, the gravity center, when transferred from the forward

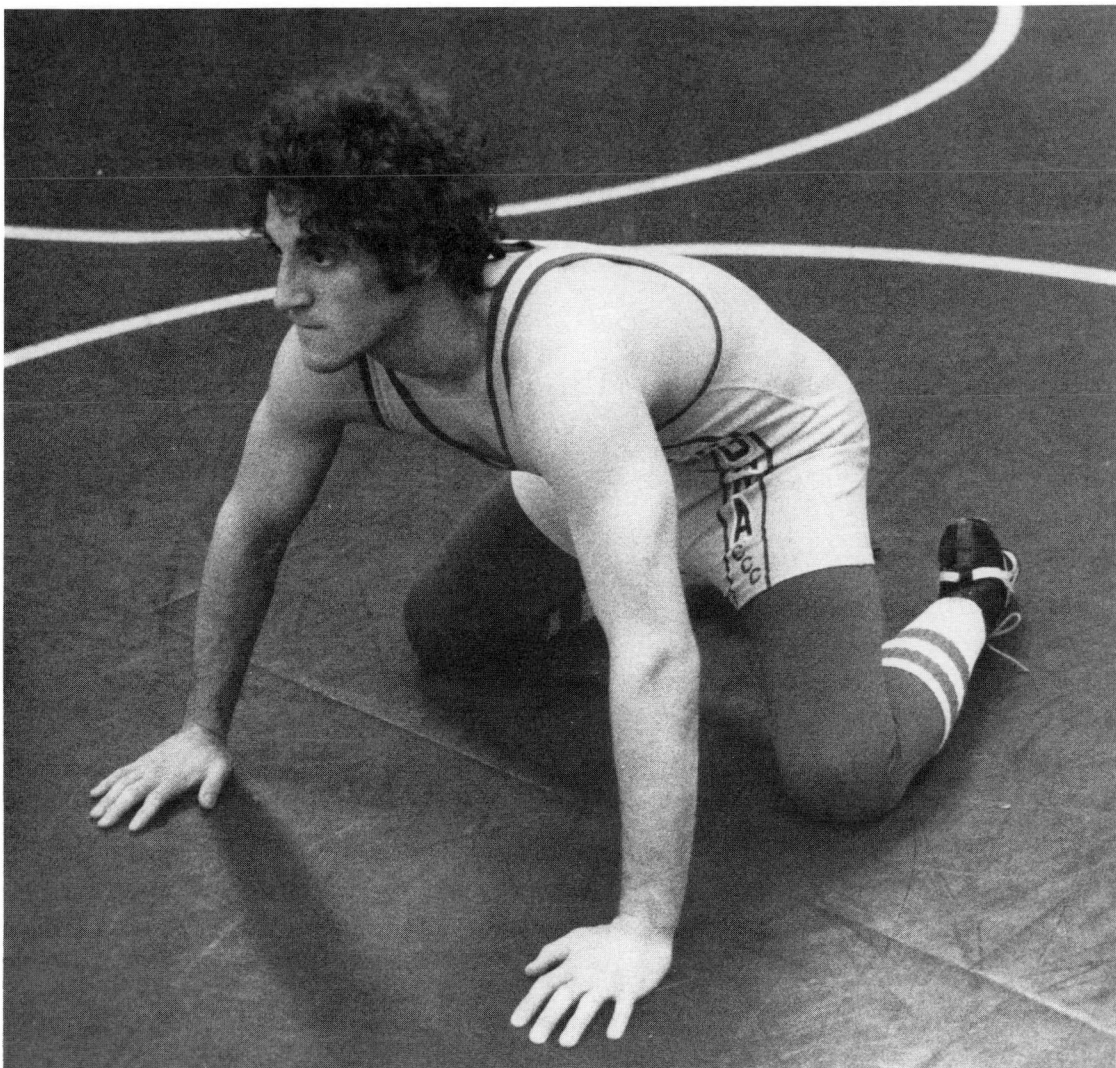

Figure 11.6 Wrestler's defensive position with buttocks held close to the base of support (courtesy of Niagara County Community College, Sanborn, N.Y.)

foot to the rear foot, is farther away from its pivoting edge in the direction of movement and the wrestler is less likely to lose his balance and fall forward.

4. Stability is increased when the line of gravity falls near or directly over the base center.

The wrestler in an open leg stance, with one leg placed slightly forward, is maximizing his stability by allowing his body weight to fall within the center of his stance; thus, it would be more difficult for his opponent to push or pull him off balance.

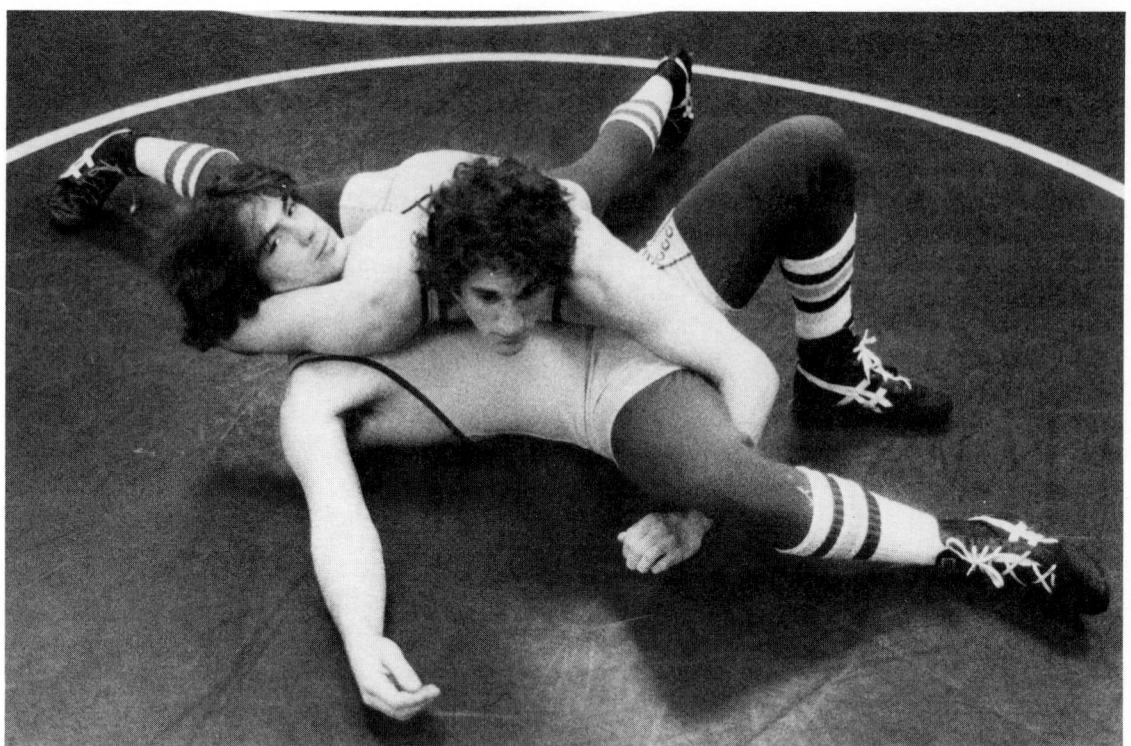

Figure 11.7 Applying the second-class lever in a pinning movement (courtesy of Niagara County Community College, Sanborn, N.Y.)

It can be seen, from a balance stability aspect, that certain principles can be applied to wrestling such as:

a. A wrestler's body is on *balance* or *stabilized* when his gravity center falls within its base.

b. Quick movements can be facilitated by the wrestler keeping the center of gravity high and near the pivoting edge of the base in the *direction of the movement*.

c. The wrestler should keep his center of gravity *low* and support base as *large* as possible when seeking immobility in a particular position.

d. If a wrestler desires to *stop quickly* when moving in a forward motion, he should *increase* his support base and *lower* his gravity center.

Leverage in Wrestling

Applying correct leverage outside the body can be one of the greatest assets of a wrestler, especially in the absence of strength. In wrestling, the application of the second-class lever is demonstrated when the wrestler is attempting to pin his opponent in a body press pin combination. In this instance, the *fulcrum* is the opponent's shoulder on the mat, and *force* is applied to the opposite shoulder by the offensive wrestler in an attempt to pin. The *defensive* wrestler is applying *resistance* to his opponent's body, forcing upward or "fighting" the pin as shown in Figure 11.7.

When the wrestler desires more force with less effort, he should create a long force arm. This is well demonstrated by Figure 11.7, which illustrates the offensive wrestler exerting his greatest force upon the defensive's wrestler's shoulder, thus extending the distance from the fulcrum to the application of force. The offensive wrestler has strengthened his *moment* or *torque arm* and has gained a *mechanical advantage* over his opponent. On the other hand, it may be desirable to overturn an opponent quickly. In this case, a short force should be created. For example, when executing a half nelson, the wrestler places his left arm under his opponent's left arm with the forearm behind the opponent's neck. Rather than applying the force on the neck, it is diverted to the shoulder, thereby hastening the turning action since a shorter force arm moves faster than a longer one.

Cycling

Bicycling is emerging as a popular activity in schools and colleges from elementary to university level. The sport has universal appeal from youth to senior citizens. A sampling of successful programs have been reported in the *Journal of Health, Physical Education and Recreation.*[9] This attests to the growing popularity of the sport. Curriculum offerings range from informal leisure-type programs for older persons in retirement settings to formally structured courses at universities.[10-12] The popularity of bicycling has created the need for a better understanding of bicycle mechanics including both machine and human aspects. Since millions of persons of all ages have taken to the road, accidents have increased to major proportions. A monitoring system of 119 nationwide hospital emergency rooms for injuries associated with consumer products, including sports and recreational equipment, revealed that bicycling and bicycle equipment are a leading cause of accidents.[13] Therefore, with the gain in popularity of bicycling and its accompanying safety risks, we believe that the inclusion of cycling is justified in a physical education program. The ensuing discussion is focused upon basic applied analysis of techniques for the improvement of efficent cycling.

Descriptive Analysis. Two general types of bicycling forms are identified: *recreational* and *racing.* Racing is further divided into *road racing* and *track racing.* Mechanically, the cyclist is transmitting rotary joint action, particularly of the trunk, hips, legs, and feet, to the bike pedals creating a translatory motion of man and machine.

Road races are held on an open road or a closed racing circuit. The most familiar type of road racing event is the *massed start* race (Figure 11.8) where a group of riders start together, pedal for a predetermined distance, and the first rider to finish is declared the winner. Massed start racing pits riders against each other in head-to-head competition.

Perhaps the most famous massed start road race is the "Tour de France," a multiple-stage road race that stretches for 2600 miles from Lille to Paris over grueling territory including the Pyrenees mountains.[14] Another type of road racing is called *cyclo-cross* racing. The bicycle riders start together as in a massed start road race; however, their course is routed through woods, streams, and remote paths. The bicyclers use special bikes with high bottom brackets and knobbed tires for greater traction and chain wheel guards to combat mud friction. Cyclists pass through bogs of mud and sand that force the racers to dismount and carry their bicycles on their backs. Actually, cyclo-cross is a combination of cross-country running and cycling.

Track races are held on a velodrome track and may involve individuals or teams in a variety of events. Sprint racing (Figure 11.9) is a phase of track racing and may range from a distance of 500 to 1000 meters. Bike handling and maneuvering, in addition to speed and stamina, are important qualities of the sprint racer.

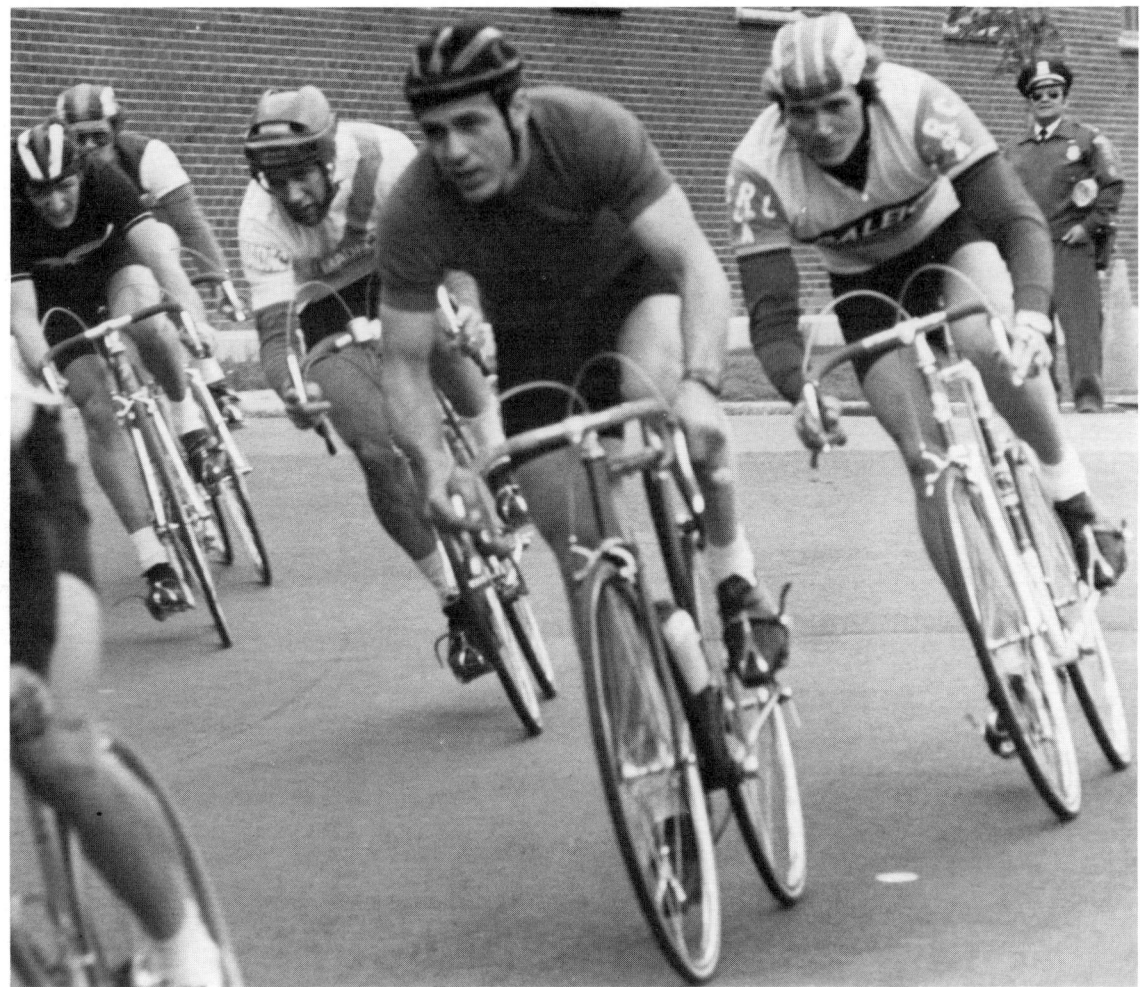

Figure 11.8 Massed start road race: (a) criterium-style circuit (courtesy of House of Wheels, Williamsville, N.Y.)

General Motor Classification. Cycling may be classified as a motor skill in which the individual is working with a machine from a ground or floor surface creating a translatory motion. Cycling is a sport requiring a positive ratio of performance between man and machine for efficient movement. It is a combination of rotary and translatory movements. Rotation is achieved by the joints of the performer and the wheels of the bicycles to produce rectilinear (straight-line) or curvilinear (curved-path) motion.

Muscular Analysis. Essentially, muscles of the lower trunk, legs, and feet are involved in bicycle recreational riding and racing. Some action of the pectoralis major, rectus abdominis, and erector spinal muscles are involved in the balancing aspect of riding.[15] The following muscles play a significant role in the pedaling action:

1. Rectus femoris
Flexion of the thigh on the hip and extension of lower leg at the knee

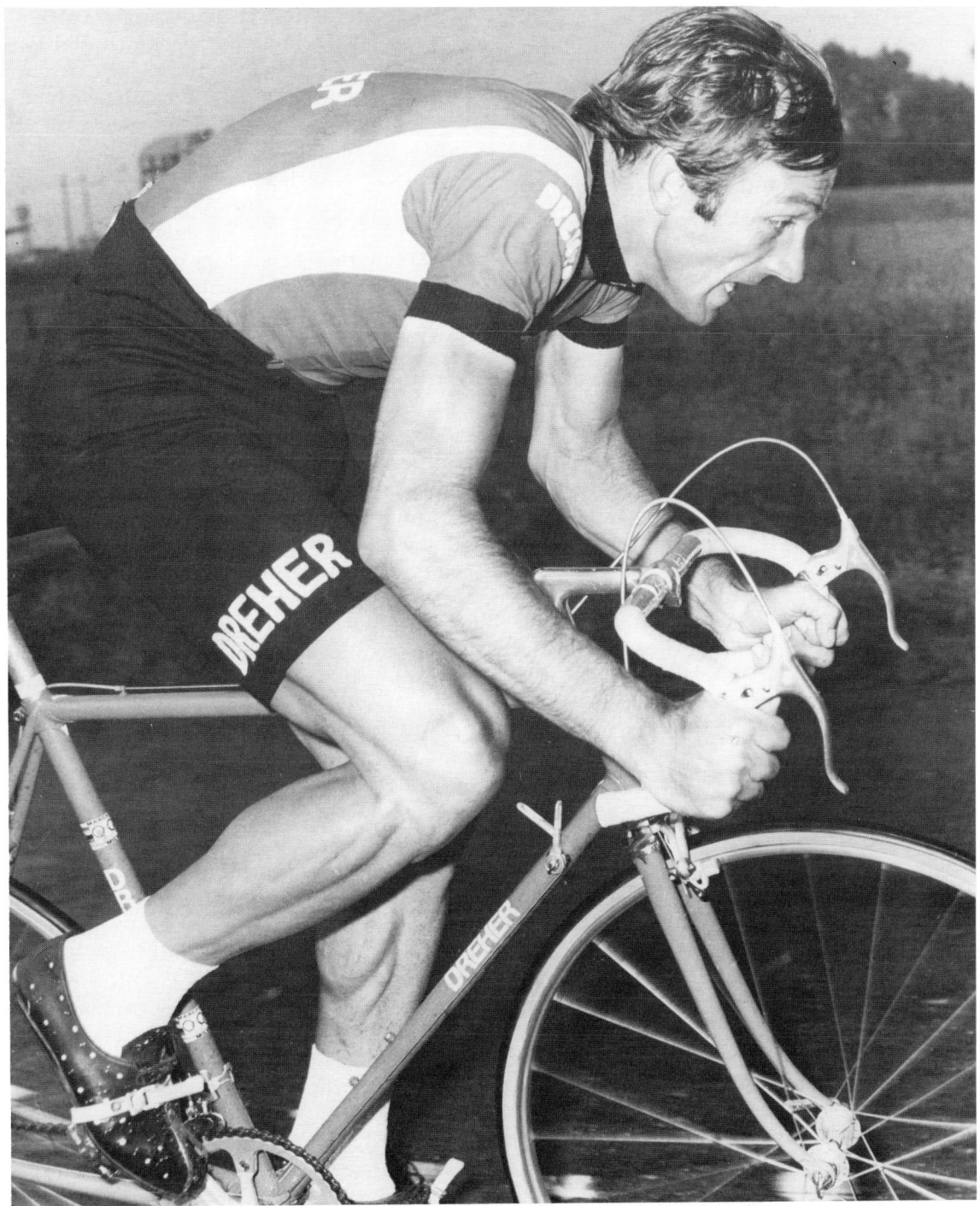

Figure 11.9 Sprint racing (courtesy of House of Wheels, Williamsville, N.Y.)

ANALYSIS OF SELECTED SPORT SKILLS **413**

2. Sartorius
Flexion and lateral rotation of hip and knee

3. Gluteus maximus
Extension of the hip

4. Tensor fasciae latae
Flexion of thigh at the hip and extension of the knee, and some synergistic action

5. Biceps femoris, semitendinosus and semimembranosus
Extension of the hip, and flexion of the knee

6. Tibialis anterior
Dorsiflexion of the foot as well as inversion

7. Gastrocnemius and soleus
Plantar flexion of the foot

Rasch and Burke[16] point out that one hip extensor (gluteus maximus) is not called into action until the hip is flexed 45 degrees unless there is a strong resistance when the angle is less. This explains, in part, why cyclists stoop forward for the advantage of a crouching start in sprint racing. Other flexors and extensors of the lower body also assist in the movements of the hip, leg, and feet; however, our discussion is limited to the analysis of the major movers.

Internal Mechanical Analysis. The build of racing cyclists follows a pattern of shorter height than the average physique with stout characteristics for sprint races and lean qualities for longer distances such as the 4000 meter road race.[17] Speed and muscular endurance are desirable elements for the competitive cyclist. However, these components apply to a different degree, depending upon the event.

For example, leg, hip, and back strength are required to provide the explosive force needed for climbing hills and high-geared speed. Muscular endurance, which involves cardiorespiratory condition, is essential for long cross-country races.[18] Although the lower extremities provide the major source of pedaling force, muscles of the upper extremities, which include the pectorals, biceps, triceps, and flexors of the fingers, are used in up-hill stretches.[19] Thus, internally, competitive cycling requires ample muscular strength and endurance. Cycling is akin to endurance-type activities such as running, speed skating, cross-country skiing, rowing, and swimming. However, the duration of most cycling races far exceeds these related sports. Training and conditioning should include aerobic and anaerobic regimens, as well as progressive resistive-type programs.

External Mechanical Analysis. Bicycling involves balance and equilibrium in motion. Riding a bicycle requires maintenance of upright dynamic balance while coordinating man and machine. The cyclist must sustain balance while riding with a relatively high center of gravity (weight of the body on the seat) and narrow base of support (wheels of the bike). It would seem that a mini-bike is easier to control and balance than a regular sized bicycle because greater stability is contained by the mini-bike's lower center of gravity. However, the student will recall from Chapter 8 that it is easier to maintain and correct balance errors on a larger bicycle because the speed of movement of the center of gravity decelerates as its distance above the base lengthens. Applying this principle to cycling, the mini-bike with its lower center of gravity will tip over faster than the regular bicycle and, therefore, is more difficult to control in the event of balance loss. Riding low motor skooters at high speeds can be especially hazardous because lateral deviation of the gravity center develops quickly and the rider has little time to react and correct balance errors.

Forward momentum of the cycle and maintenance of the line of gravity within tolerable limits of the support base are essential ingredients for efficient riding. Balance is maintained partly by the use of the front wheel; that is, if the rider starts to fall to the right, the front wheel is turned slightly to the right with the weight shifted to the left. If the fall starts toward the left, the movement is reversed.

Body posture is another important consideration in competitive cycling. Experienced racers agree that the best pedaling position occurs when the center of the knee is over and just behind the pedal-center when the crank is parallel to the ground. This position is achieved by adjusting the seat angle and height and is dependent upon the height of the rider. Shorter cyclists will ride with lower saddle heights. Saddle height significantly influences the range of plantar flexion of the ankle. Therefore, if a rider seeks to improve ankle flexibility, the height of the seat should be raised to a point where pedaling efficiency is not lost. The student is referred to reference 20 for an excellent review of bicycle frame construction, further details about somatotype, and various riding positions.

Baseball

The mechanical elements of *pitching, batting,* and *hitting* are explained in Chapter 7. Base running and running between bases are discussed in the subsequent section.

Base Running. Base running techniques are similar to sprint training methods. However, different forces act on the runner when running to first base and running between bases. The mechanics of running to first base are not as complicated as running from one base to another, since the latter entails control of centrifugal forces. Also, running between bases involves control in starting and stopping. Several basic factors are considered in the following paragraphs.

Running to First Base. At the outset, it should be noted that people do not run precisely the same way. James and Brubaker[21] point out

that because of variations in anatomic structure, anthropometric proportions, muscular strength, posture, training, and even mental attitude, running patterns can differ among individuals. From a physique identification, baseball players may be classified as mesomorphic with a slight tendency toward endomorphy. High levels of joint flexibility are characteristic of baseball players. Baseball players and swimmers possess similar patterns of flexibility.[22]

Several salient mechanical elements are indicated below with particular reference to *running to first base*:

1. Running to first base is similar to a sprint dash event.

2. Increasing the sprint stride distance and rate increases the speed of the runner.

3. Slight trunk lean in front of the center of gravity enhances speed and reduces air resistance.

4. A forceful push of the rear leg is essential for gaining speed.

5. High knee lift and long running stride enhance efficient running.

6. Increased speed is gained when more force is exerted in the horizontal rather than the vertical direction.

7. Firm contact should be made on the ball of the foot when landing.

8. Efficient starts emphasize primary force exerted in the horizontal direction and depend principally upon the strength of hip, knee, and foot extensor muscles.

9. Step length has a greater effect on running speed than step frequency.

10. Foot placement on landing should be directed beneath the center of gravity, thereby decreasing the amount of deceleration.

11. When running to first base, the runner should not jump on his last stride since this movement will slow down his horizontal speed.

Running between Bases. Basic sprint running mechanics also apply to running between bases. Two aspects of running between bases and/or running for home plate are noteworthy for analysis: (1) base runner's starting position and (2) control of centrifugal forces.

The runner should be in position ready to move toward the next base or return instantly. The starting position is illustrated in Figure 11.10.

Several important descriptive and mechanical elements are indicated as follows:

1. Feet are shoulder width apart with weight evenly balanced over both feet for quick movement either way—next base or return to present base.

2. Body in semicrouch position with eyes focused on the ball; position helps to reduce air resistance on the thrust.

3. Arms hanging loosely to allow for quick thrust in either direction.

4. Angulation of lead foot about 45 degrees to allow for better balance and pivoting action on movement.

5. Hands relaxed with thumb and index finger gently touching—helps reduce tension of forearm and hands.

Control of centrifugal force must be considered since the base runner turns from one base to another. Principles of lean apply here. The base runner must develop skill in keeping the radius of the circular running path small without decelerating speed. As discussed in Chapter 6, the problem of controlling centrifugal force is greater when the radius of turn becomes smaller. This force tends to pull the athlete off course. An example of a runner attempting a sharp turn and applying the formula $F = wv^2/gr$ is presented in Chapter 6. The runner should stay as close to base line as possible when turning. This action will require some slowing of speed as the runner rounds the base.

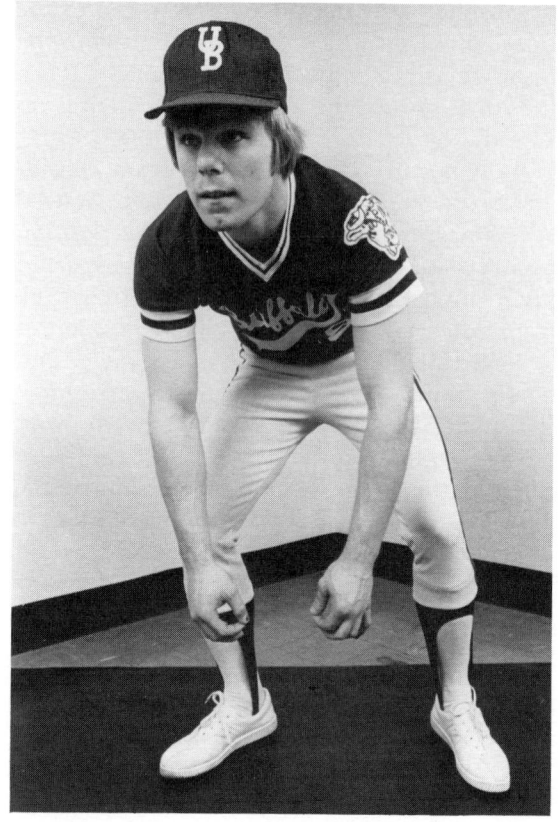

Figure 11.10 Base runner's starting position (courtesy of *Athletic Journal*, Evanston, Ill.)

Racquetball

The game of racquetball is the newest of racquet sports. The popularity of the sport is probably due primarily to the relative ease in learning, as compared to tennis, handball, badminton and similar striking activities. In addition, it can be played with vigor and finesse at all ages, from novice to championship levels.

General Description. Racquetball is a *striking* activity. The game may be played by two, three, or four players. A *singles* game is played by two persons. Our discussion will consider the descriptive analysis, muscular analysis, and mechanical elements of singles play. The game is won by the first player scoring 21 points. The server may serve from any place within the service zone and must remain in the zone until the ball passes the service or short line. The player bounces the ball on the serve, strikes it so that it hits the front wall first, so that on the rebound it hits the floor behind the service line, with or without touching a side wall. A *fault* occurs on the serve when the ball strikes both side walls or the ceiling after hitting the front wall. In singles play, two faults result in a *side out*, which retires the side. The purpose of the game is to win on each rally by serving or returning the ball in such a manner that an opponent cannot return the ball before it bounces twice on the floor. A point is scored when the server wins a rally.

Muscular Analysis. Like badminton, racquetball entails whole body movement. The muscle descriptions in the badminton section also apply to racquetball. However, the student should remember that the implement and ball used in racquetball are much heavier and demand a greater magnitude of propelling force upon ball impact with the racquet. The linkage system from lower limbs, trunk, shoulder girdle, arms, and hand supplies the linear force in propelling the ball to the wall. The anterior muscles of the shoulder girdle and arms, including the *anterior deltoids, pectorals, coracobrachials, forearm flexors,* and *wrist flexors* are prime movers in the forward swing movements. The posterior muscles of the shoulder girdle and arms including the *serratus anterior, posterior deltoid, supraspinatus, forearm extensors,* and *wrist extensors* are major movers in the backward swing action. The student should refer to Chapter 2 for specific muscular descriptions and actions of the shoulder girdle, arm, wrist, and hand.

Internal Mechanical Analysis. Internal lever classification of the upper extremity in racquetball is identical to that in badminton; that is, in a forward swing motion, flexion of the upper arm, forearm, and wrist forms a lever of the third class. However, when extending the elbow in a backhand movement, a lever of the first class of the elbow is ordered by triceps extension. Although forward swing and backward swing motions of the shoulder girdle and lower arm are third- and first-class levers, respectively, both types favor speed and range of motion at the expense of force because muscular insertions are close to the fulcrum in each case, and, consequently, the involved levers possess a long resistance and short force arm arrangement. The racquet extends the lever arm further and allows greater potential for the development of speed in the swinging motion; however, more strength is needed for control of the added weight of the implement; consequently, the player should never select a racquet that exceeds his strength capabilities. A principal difference between racquetball and badminton entails the weight of the racquet and the flight of the bird and ball. Since the implement and ball used in racquetball are heavier than the racquet and shuttlecock utilized in badminton, strength of the upper extremity, particularly in the wrist, is of greater importance in racquetball.

Flexibility of the upper extremity and trunk is a valuable internal articulation quality, since a flexible player can increase his speed by allowing the racquet to follow a greater range of motion in offensive and defensive shots. Although a definitive somatotype is not indicated, the leaner athletic-type body build favors the motor abilities of quickness, speed, and stamina necessary for skilled play in racquetball. Activities such as tennis and badminton, which are in the racquetball sport category, favor the ecto-mesomorphic or lean athletic-type body build.[23] It seems that the lighter individual with a strong mesomorphic component has a physique advantage when the individual is seeking championship caliber competition.

External Mechanical Analysis. The principles of *stability, force production,* and laws governing *ball rebound* are found in racquetball. These principles are considered in Chapters 6 and 7. Concepts and laws that most directly deal with the sport are discussed in the following section.

Two basic strokes are used in racquetball: *forehand* and *backhand*. These strokes require different grips. The forehand is grasped so that a "V" made by the thumb and forefingers is positioned on top of the handle, as shown in Figure 11.11.

Figure 11.11   Grip in forehand stroke

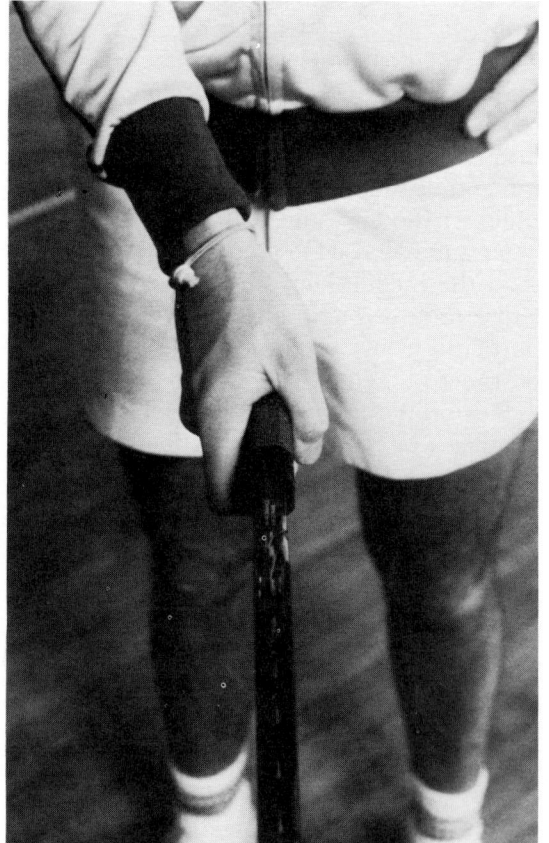

The hand should be placed with a slight separation between the forefinger and middle finger. This positioning allows greater hand control of the racquet. The handle of the racquet should not be placed too deeply in the palm of the hand since such a grasp would restrict the mobility of the wrist in ballistic follow-through actions. The grip position for the backhand stroke is similar to the forehand grasp except that the "V" formed by the forefinger and thumb is positioned on the left side of the racquet, as shown in Figure 11.12.

Stability Aspects

Factors affecting dynamic upright balance are involved in the myriad of movements in all directions as the racquetball player maneuvers from one position to another on the court. Depending upon the specific shot, the player should maintain stability by lowering his stance, with a comfortable distance between the legs to widen the support base. The weight of the body should be on the balls of

Figure 11.12   Grip in backhand stroke

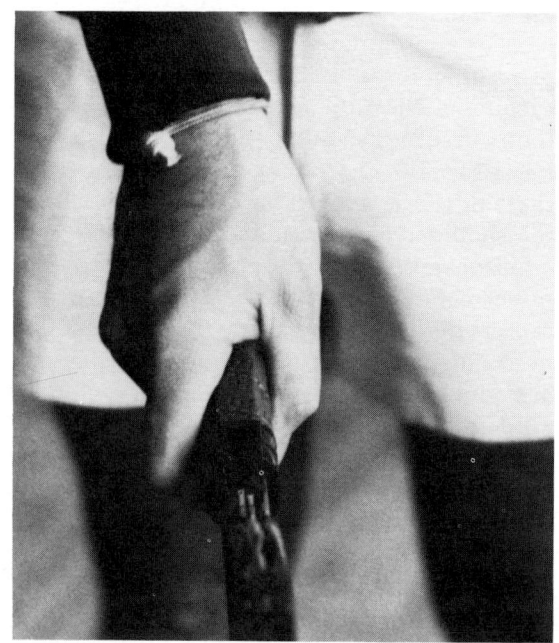

the feet. This will allow the player to move quickly in any direction without losing balance. When moving, the player should take short steps and attempt to keep his weight well balanced in an open stance. Sensory mechanisms of vision, proprioception, and kinesthesia also affect upright dynamic balance skills found in racquetball. The student is referred to Chapter 8 for a detailed discussion of these elements.

Force Aspects

Whether the player is executing a forehand or backhand shot, if the objective is to gain speed, the swing should be made from the shoulder (fulcrum) with an extended arm. This technique allows the longest lever possible and a resultant gain in velocity. The sequential kinetic chain action from the trunk to the hand helps to create the force necessary for long court shots. The greater the speed, the greater the force that can be imparted to the ball. A *firm* (moderate) *grip* should be applied in forehand and backhand shots to assure minimum recoil of the racquet and sufficient transmission of force from the body to the implement and ultimately to the ball. Hatze[24] investigated the magnitude of forces and reactions of the hand during and after ball impact in tennis. Studying a highly skilled player, he found that a tight grip increases both the impulse imparted to the ball and the power of the stroke. A contrary action was found for a loose grip. However, concurrent with greater power, the amount of vibration increased with the tight grip. A tight grip may be desirable for top players, but beginners should not hold the racquet too tightly because of increased vibration and resultant loss in accuracy. Although this investigation pertained to tennis, similar conclusions may well apply to racquetball. It appears that a *moderately tight grip* is best for novice players; this provides a balance between imparting force and receiving vibrations to the hand from the ball upon impact.

Other external mechanical elements influence the application of force in racquetball. Several salient points are as follows:

1. Move forward in the direction of the ball and focus the strike so that the muscles of the shoulders can exert their greatest force upon impact.

2. Use a heavier racquet (individual strength permitting) since heavier mass of the implement has greater striking force potential.

3. Use a ball and racquet that possess a high coefficient of restitution (elasticity) for gaining maximum speed.

4. The speed of the striking implement should greatly exceed the speed of the oncoming ball.

5. The speed of the racquet is affected by the amount of force applied and length of time the ball is held on the strings.

Ball Rebound and Placement

Directing the ball to certain court areas depends upon its angle of incidence and angle of rebound. Accuracy in placing the ball entails the application of rebound and general spin principles. These principles have been presented in Chapter 6, and the player should remember that the angle of rebound depends upon the angle of incidence in the flight of the ball. The spin of the ball also affects its direction; and finally, the grip firmness at impact influences the angle of the racquet and the projected force, which subsequently regulate the direction and distance of the struck ball.

SUMMARY

Each sport is unique and its analysis will vary depending upon the specific nature of the movement. The basic requirements of a sport skill should be determined and include such variables as strength, speed, form, neuromuscular coordination, and accuracy.

Athletic ability is characterized by a number of attributes. These features are muscular strength, endurance, balance, somatotype, agility and neuromuscular control, speed and accuracy, sensory attention and alertness, rhythm pattern, reaction time, and flexibility.

A kinesiological analysis of a motor performance entails two broad categories: (1) anatomical and (2) mechanical. The anatomical aspect includes an analysis of internal structure and muscles involved, joints and lever classification. The mechanical aspect may be analyzed from a qualitative or quantitative perspective. Such information, derived from observations of film and videotape, may be analyzed qualitatively. Collection of data and its numerical quantification, which yield precise and exact information about parameter constituents, constitute quantitative analysis. The application of the following mechanical aspects is usually considered in sport analysis: Newton's laws of motion, kinematics, kinetics, motion classification, and balance.

A general outline includes descriptive analysis, motor analysis, major muscular analysis, internal mechanical factors, and external mechanical factors.

The concept of body joint linkage and its role in athletic performance were considered with an example of how the sequential kinetic chain of linked joints functions from large joint structures of the trunk to small articulations of the fingers. It was pointed out that kinetic chains of the upper extremities possess greater mobility than kinetic chains of the lower extremities.

The latter part of this chapter dealt with kinesiological analysis of badminton, wrestling, cycling, baseball, and racquetball.

Such factors as rhythmic kinetic chain, striking force, impact, coefficient of elasticity, effect of mass and speed, and leverage were explained. Racquet grip firmness and its effect on power and vibration were discussed. Common errors in grip technique in badminton were also noted.

Selected offensive and defensive moves were analyzed in wrestling. It was emphasized that the ability to act and react quickly in various movements is a vital skill component for effective wrestling.

The external application of motion, balance, leverage, speed, and position was discussed and related to offensive and defensive wrestling. It was pointed out that the application of correct leverage outside the body can be one of the greatest assets of a wrestler, especially in the absence of strength.

Two general types of cycling were considered: (1) recreational and (2) racing. Mechanical aspects of road racing and track racing were discussed. Mechanically, the cyclist transmits rotary joint action, primarily of the trunk, hips, legs, and feet, to the bicycle pedals creating a translatory motion of man and machine. The effect of trunk riding position and saddle height upon the action of the hip muscles and ankle joint motion were described. Balance control was discussed in relation to riding low- and high-type bicycles. It was pointed out that riding low motor scooters at high speeds can be especially hazardous because of the development of lateral deviation in the gravity center from the rider's base of support.

Two components of baseball were considered: (1) base running and (2) running between bases. It was pointed out that internal and external mechanics of running to first base are similar to a sprint dash event. Although basic sprint running mechanics also apply to running between bases, two other factors were added for analysis: (1) starting position and (2) control of centrifugal forces.

Finally, racquetball was examined. Muscular analysis and internal and external mechanical aspects were considered. The basic forehand and backhand strokes were analyzed. Other selected mechanical elements of stability, force, spin, and ball rebound and placement were delineated.

REFERENCES

1. Nicholas, James A., Grossman, Robert B., and Hershman, Elliott B. "The Importance of a Simplified Classification of Motion in Sports in Relation to Performance," *Orthopedic Clinics of North America*, 8:510, July, 1977.

2. Hoffman, Ron L., "An Instructional Unit in Advanced Badminton," Unpublished Master's Project, State University of New York at Buffalo, 1975, p. 11.

3. Stone, Henry A., *Wrestling*. New York: Prentice-Hall, 1945, p. 32.

4. Hirata, Kin-Itsu, "Physique and Age of Tokyo Olympic Champions," *Journal of Sports Medicine and Physical Fitness*, 6:207-222, December, 1966.

5. Leighton, Jack R., "On the Significance of Flexibility," *Journal of Health, Physical Education and Recreation*, 31:27-28, 80, November, 1960.

6. Clarke, Harrison H. (Ed.), "Joint and Body Range of Movement," *Research Digest*. Washington, D.C.: President's Council on Physical Fitness and Sports, Series 5, No. 4, October, 1975.

7. Maertz, Richard C., "The Initial Takedown and Wrestling Outcomes," *Athletic Journal*, 52:54-56, September, 1971.

8. Blaettler, Richard B., "Stability—An Important Factor in Wrestling," *Athletic Journal*, 48:54-56, October, 1967.

9. Bailey, Dot, et al., "Bikes, Feature on Cycling Program," *Journal of Health, Physical Education and Recreation*, 45:93-98, September, 1974.

10. Stone, William J., "A Cycling Program for Senior Citizens," *Journal of Health, Physical Education and Recreation*, 45:97-98, September, 1974.

11. Baker, Jack, and Arnold, Linda, "Physical Fitness in a College Course," *Journal of Health, Physical Education and Recreation*, 45:95-96, September, 1974.

12. Gensemer, Robert E., "About Bikes," *Journal of Health, Physical Education and Recreation*, 45:10-13, May, 1974.

13. Esch, Albert F., "The National Electronic Injury Surveillance System (NEISS)," in Timothy Craig (Ed.), *The Medical Aspects of Sports: 15*. Chicago: American Medical Association, 1974, pp. 13-18.

14. Saunders, David, "Blood and Thunder in the Tour de France," *International Cycle Sport*, 48:8, May, 1972.

15. Desipres, M., "An Electromyographic Study of Competitive Road Cycling Conditions Simulated on a Treadmill," in Richard C. Nelson and Chauncey A. Moorehouse (Eds.), *Biomechanics IV*. Baltimore: University Park Press, 1974, pp. 348-355.

16. Rasch, Philip J., and Burke, Roger K., *Kinesiology and Applied Anatomy*, 6th ed. Philadelphia: Lea and Febiger, 1978, p. 274.

17. Hirata, *op. cit.*, p. 14.

18. Coetis, J. E., "Above Average Exercise Capacity in Competitive Cyclists," *Journal of Physiology*, 80:97, June, 1972.

19. Rodoni, Adriano, *Cycling and Its Scientific Applications*. Rome: F.I.A.C., 1972, p. 39.

20. Sullivan, Mark, M., "A Survey of Mechanics, Human Performance and Cycling Technique," Unpublished Master's Project, State University of New York at Buffalo, 1974, p. 43.

21. James, Stanley L., and Brubaker, Clifford E., "Biomechanical and Neuromuscular Aspects of Running," in Jack H. Wilmore (Ed.), *Exercise and Sport Reviews*, Vol. 1. New York: Academic Press, 1973, p. 202.

22. Clarke, *op. cit.*, p. 10.

23. Willgoose, Carl E., "Body Types and Physical Fitness," *Journal of Health, Physical Education and Recreation*, 27:26-77, 79, September, 1956.

24. Hatze, Herbert, "Forces and Duration of Impact, and Grip Tightness During the Tennis Stroke," *Medicine and Science in Sports*, 8:898-95, Summer, 1976.

12 POSTURAL PRINCIPLES

CONCEPTS

1. Adaptations enabling man to maintain the erect position were begun over 70 million years ago when his remote ancestors became arboreal.

2. The abdominal muscles are the most important muscles involved in maintenance of posture from the point of view of prevention of lordosis, visceral and circulatory ptosis, and low back pain.

3. Because of the position of the thoracic cage anterior to the body's line of gravity, it is important to maintain the tone of muscles that lift the thoracic cage.

4. One postural standard should not be applied to all people because of individual variations in body type, weight distribution, structural anomalies, disease, congenital defects, and injury.

5. Static posture refers to held positions such as standing or sitting, while dynamic posture refers to the many segmental alignments of the body during the thousands of movements of the human body.

6. Differences in walking patterns arise out of structural differences such as the length, thickness, and shape of bones, range of motion in joints, and distribution of body weight.

7. During the sprint, the feet strike the ground under the center of gravity and the horizontal component of force is as great as possible. Furthermore, the body is inclined forward 20

to 25 degrees, the arms are flexed, and the knee is flexed during the swinging phase.

8. When lifting, the object raised should be kept as close as possible to the body's line of gravity throughout the lift.

9. Shearing forces upon lumbar vertebrae are less when lifting with the trunk nearly vertical than when lifting with the trunk inclined forward.

10. Heavy lifting with the body rotated may produce injury to the vertebral column or the spinal rotatores.

11. Long continued participation in certain sports or occupations can cause postural deviations.

12. Certain sports activities may be utilized to correct specific postural deviations.

13. Scoliosis begins as a C curve and develops into an S curve.

14. When muscles are not used in maintenance of vertical alignment of body segments, excessive stress is placed upon involved ligaments, which may become stretched.

15. The stimuli for maintenance of postural tonus arise from the labyrinthine righting reflexes, optical reflexes, reflexes acting on the head, proprioceptive reflexes, plantar reflexes, and stretch reflexes.

16. Postural deviations are classified as either structural or functional.

17. It is possible for students to pass the plumb line test and yet exhibit poor posture.

GENERAL CONSIDERATIONS

Man's remote ancestors, 70 million years ago, made the first step toward establishing him as the dominant animal of the world when they began to escape their enemies by climbing into trees and swinging by their "hands" from limb to limb. During the millions of years that generation after generation spent suspended by their arms, the hind legs were gradually extended in line with the body, the mobility of the shoulder girdle was increased, the length, strength, and movements of the forelimbs were increased and, of greatest importance, a hand adapted for grasping began developing. Other anatomic adaptations slowly came about that made it easier to stand erect. The anterior-posterior diameter of the thoracic cavity decreased, moving the center of gravity backward. The frequent hanging position with the forelimbs hyperflexed and in line with the trunk caused the scapula to move backward so that in the standing position the arms could hang at the side of the trunk (see Figure 12.1). These changes presented some advantages for man's ancestors when they returned to the ground. They could stand erect and maintain balance for longer periods because of the greater extensibility of the hip joints and the backward displacement of the center of gravity. This enabled man's ancestors to look over the tall grass and bushes to see their enemies and to spot game for their own food. The erect position also freed their hands to utilize implements.

Over the millennia, the standing position produced additional structural changes in man's predecessors. The foot had to bear the entire body weight. The weight was no longer borne exclusively on the toes. The foot became broader and longer. The pelvis rotated so that the limbs and vertebral column formed a straight line rather than a right angle. This caused the extensor muscles, and particularly the gluteals, to become much larger and stronger. The pelvic bones became shorter, thicker, and broader. The quadriceps became larger and stronger to prevent the knee from flexing upon impact with the ground when walking, running, or jumping. The lumbar curve of the vertebral column developed to facilitate the erect position. No species other than mankind has a lumbar curve. That ontogeny recapitulates phylogeny is demonstrated in the development of the S curve from the C-shaped curve of the spine of the infant. Before it learns to walk, an infant's spine forms a C-shaped curve. This postural characteristic makes it difficult for the infant to position the legs and trunk in a straight line relationship, which is manifested when the infant tries to walk. The knees are flexed and the trunk is inclined forward due to inability to extend the hip joints. After the lumbar curve is developed, the erect position is easier to assume.

In quadrupeds the abdominal muscles are called upon to hold the vertebral column in alignment. In the erect position, this becomes the work of the extensors on the back; consequently, the abdominals deteriorate. In quadrupeds the abdominals are assigned the task of maintaining the C curve of the spine. This results in the maintenance of abdominal tone and strength. In quadrupeds the abdominal viscera, which hang from the horizontal dorsal walls by their mesenteries, are held in place by the abdominal wall. In the erect position, the viscera are suspended from vertical dorsal walls and can no longer rest against the horizontal abdominal wall. The weight of the organs causes a downward thrust toward the pelvis, stretching the mesenteries and causing the upper organs to impinge upon the lower ones. The abdominal muscles must be under tension to hold the organs in place. Unfortunately, they tend to weaken, particularly during middle age and senescence, with a resultant protrusion of the lower abdomen. This condition is known as *visceral ptosis*.[1] It may be characterized by

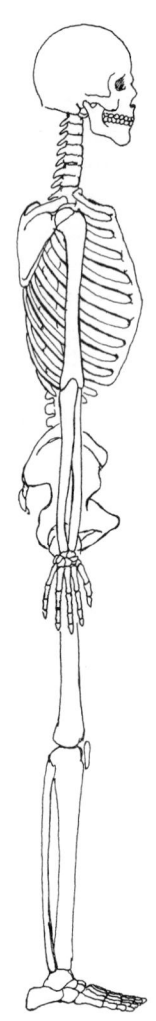

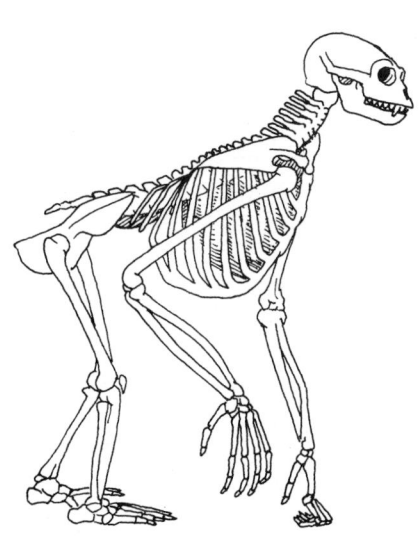

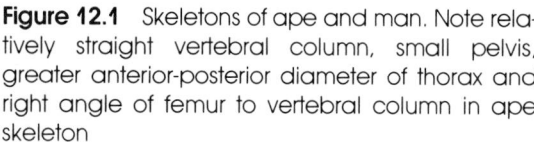

Figure 12.1 Skeletons of ape and man. Note relatively straight vertebral column, small pelvis, greater anterior-posterior diameter of thorax and right angle of femur to vertebral column in ape skeleton

nervous irritation due to the stretching of blood vessels and nerves. Blood vessels in the digestive organs become dilated, resulting in pooling of venous blood.

A common health complaint of adult men is *low back pain*. This is one of several penalties man has paid for assuming the erect position since he is the only mammal showing evidence of problems in the lumbar area. Low back pain is usually associated with chronic increased inclination or forward tilt, which increases the lumbar curve. It will be recalled (see Chapter 2) that the abdominal muscles, which insert on the pubis, cause the pelvis to rotate on its frontal-horizontal axis in the direction of decreased inclination or backward tilt. Weak abdominals will permit the powerful erector spinae, rectus femoris, tensor fasciae latae, and iliotibial bands to pull the pelvis into a position of increased inclination and to pull the lumbar spine into a hyperextended position. As a result of the tilted articulation between the sacrum and the fifth lumbar vertebrae, the weight is placed principally on the dorsal aspect of the lumbar vertebrae and its tendency to slip forward is increased. This lumbosacral strain is often, erroneously, referred to as a sacroiliac strain.

In quadrupeds the thoracic cage hangs directly downward from the vertebral column, making breathing relatively easy. In the erect position, the weight of the thoracic cage must be continuously held in position and be lifted with each inspiration. During the middle years and senescence of most people, when muscles begin to lose tone, the ribs sink and vertebrae become compressed due to the continual pull of gravity. As indicated in Chapter 14, many people show a decrease in height of one or more inches over their life span. This process can be decelerated, to some extent, through maintenance of muscle tone into advanced age.

The erect position has also made it more difficult for the venous blood to return to the heart. Venous blood in the human must have sufficient pressure behind it to push it upward against the pull of gravity. Cooper[2] reports that after standing without moving (other than sway) with the feet together for more than 15 minutes, the individual may faint due to an insufficient supply of blood to the brain. Even in the most rigid position of attention, the body sways, and the longer the position is held, the greater the sway. The "milking action" of alternately contracting and relaxing muscles alludes to the pressure exerted upon blood vessels when muscles contract, squeezing the blood vessel against adjacent tissue, forcing the blood from the area squeezed. Valves in the veins permit the blood to flow only toward the heart and prohibit its flow away from the heart. Because of this structure, the blood can flow only toward

the heart when the veins are squeezed. Body sway is caused by muscular contractions. These muscular contractions help in returning blood to the heart and in preventing cerebral anemia. However, as Cooper's research shows, sway is inadequate in prevention of fainting after 15 minutes. Continuous stationary standing should be avoided, if possible. However, when it cannot be avoided, fainting can be prevented by repeated alternate contraction and relaxation of the muscles of the legs.

When man assumed the erect position, the center of gravity was elevated, making it necessary that continuous muscular action be utilized in maintaining balance. The muscles used in maintaining posture are called the *postural muscles.*

Everyone is aware of posture. Many professionals study posture—anthropologists, orthopedic surgeons, artists, actors, dancers, fashion models, sculptors, psychologists, and physical educators. Each views posture differently. Further, the human body assumes many different postures. The obese, frail, muscular, tall, short, and orthopedically handicapped all must assume different postures for most efficient functioning. Obese people usually lean backward to shift the center of gravity backward so that it is over the feet. Women in late pregnancy often do the same. Extremely obese people tend to waddle as they walk, and to minimize this lateral motion they take short steps. Frail people assume the "fatigue slouch" in which the center of gravity is over the feet but the several body segments zigzag so that the stress is on the ligaments rather than the muscles. The energy cost of this position is about 30 percent less than that of the position of attention. Many athletes assume postures of extreme relaxation because they have learned how to conserve energy. Tall girls and women (before ERA) have tended to slouch to make themselves appear shorter. Short men tend to stand in good posture to make themselves appear taller. Orthopedic handicaps, such as a short leg, require that compensatory curves be formed in the vertebral column in order to place the center of gravity over the points of support. Steindler[3] points out that ectomorphic body types with long, narrow backs possess spines that are able to withstand little stress. In these types, the lumbar spine sits high upon the sacrum, which appears to be longer than normal. The lumbar curve is flattened and the muscular development of the lumbar area is inadequate to withstand stresses of any magnitude.

Elsewhere Steindler[4] observes that mesomorphic types are most prone to develop round upper backs while ectomorphs tend to develop flat backs (see pgs. 450 & 454). He also states that endomorphs are most prone to round hollow backs with no compensatory kink at the lumbosacral junction, but with the entire lumbar area in lumbar lordosis.

It is well known that posture varies according to psychological state. Actors, artists, and sculptors make use of this phenomenon. Dejection, sadness, humility, a slovenly attitude, elation, joy, or pride can all be portrayed through various postures. Undoubtedly, a reciprocal relationship exists between posture and emotions. An erect, alert, aesthetically pleasing posture can make a favorable first impression upon others by representing self-confidence and self-assurance. A fatigue slump may be interpreted as laziness and incompetence.

For many years physical and health educators have been almost compulsively obsessed with posture. Many tests and measures of posture have been devised and widely used. Published postural standards were universally adopted and much time has been spent in attempting to bring all students up to these standards. Much of this has been done with almost no research evidence of the phyiologic or functional advantages of good posture. We can suspect that this occurred because of the convincing rationale presented by those who were interested in promoting good posture and because everyone has a posture. The dearth of conclusive research will probably continue because of the problems cited earlier—variety of body types, physical anomalies, the need for lifetime studies, and the fact that all people assume thousands of postures during the course of a day.

However, there is value in making efforts to meet postural standards if it is recognized that a measure of posture is only a starting point, and that the posture adapted to the individual is the best posture. Measures of standing posture can be regarded only as points of departure because a great many postures are assumed by everyone during the course of each day. Moreover, some variability in postural standards must be accepted because of the variety of physiques.

STATIC AND DYNAMIC POSTURE

Static Posture

Static posture refers to held positions, such as sitting and standing. A long-accepted criterion of perfect alignment, which is now being questioned, has been the plumb-line test. From the side view, when a plumb line is dropped even with the ear lobe, it should pass through the center of the shoulder, the middle of the hip, and slightly behind the patella and fall in front of the outer malleolus. For many people, this is an efficient posture that maintains the individual bones and the body segments in balanced and attractive alignment with a minimal expenditure of energy. However, for some, this posture would require excessive muscular tension. For example, those with an unusually large thorax or women with large breasts carry a larger amount of weight forward of the acromion process of the shoulder. Consequently, the center of gravity of this mass is further forward than it is on the average. If these people are to meet the criteria of the plumb-line test, it would be necessary to maintain a continual powerful contraction of the sacrospinalis, rhomboids, and part III of the trapezius. A balanced position for this segment of the population is one in which the upper back is rounded. In others, the clavicle may be longer or shorter than average. A long clavicle will force the scapula and shoulders backward, while a short one will pull the scapula and shoulders forward to create a round-shouldered position.

When the differences between the anterior and posterior vertical dimensions of vertebrae are greater than average, and the vertebrae are lying squarely on one another, efforts to diminish the spinal curves will cause the anterior borders of some vertebrae and the posterior borders of others to separate. Obviously, this structural condition can be determined only through an x-ray. Postural tests merely inform the examiner that the subject does not meet the criteria of the postural test. These tests do not indicate the reason for failure to meet the criteria. In some cases, efforts

to improve posture may do more harm than good.

Fait[5] has pointed out that differences in the location of the acetabula influence the direction and amount of tilt of the pelvis. Pelvic tilt contributes to the amount of the lumbar curve. If the acetabula are farther forward than usual, decreased inclination or backward tilt of the pelvis will result producing a flatter back. If, on the other hand, the acetabula are further back than is typical, increased inclination or forward tilt of the pelvis resulting in an increased lumbar curve will result. (Figure 12.2)

Dynamic posture refers to the thousands of different segmental alignments of the body assumed during daily movements in routine activities and while at work and play. It has been assumed that if standing posture is efficient and aesthetically pleasing, dynamic postures will also be efficient and aesthetically pleasing. The authors believe that if static posture is at an optimal level, the probability that dynamic postures will be good is enhanced. However, since a multitude of other factors are involved, there can be no guaran-

Figure 12.2 Pelvic positions: (a) normal, (b) forward (downward) tilt, (c) Backward (upward) pelvic tilt

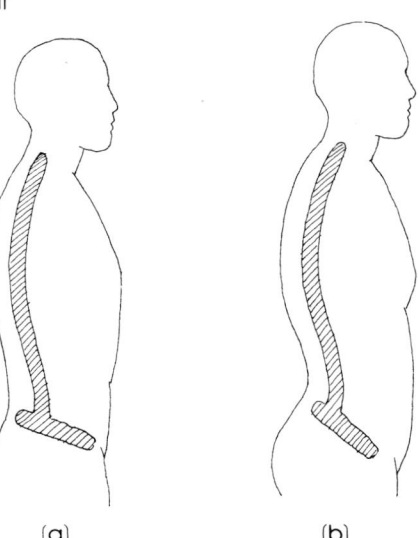
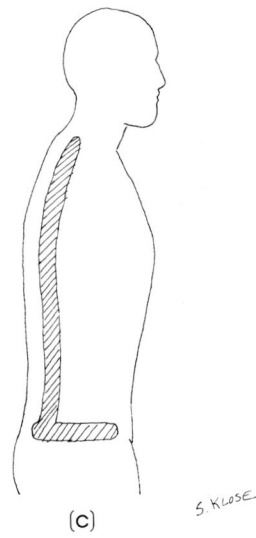

(a)   (b)   (c)

S. KLOSE.

tee that good static posture will assure desirable dynamic posture.

Sitting Posture

Sitting could be classed as a second type of static posture although, like standing, and as everyone has observed, no one sits motionless very long. When sitting at a desk, drawing board, or bench for work purposes, the head and eyes must be brought over the work; consequently, the trunk must be inclined forward from the hips with the head, neck, and trunk in a relatively straight line. The buttocks should be placed far back in the chair and the weight should be distributed over the entire underside of the thighs (Figure 12.3). When sitting in a chair to rest, the body should be supported by as much of the chair

Figure 12.3 Desirable sitting posture

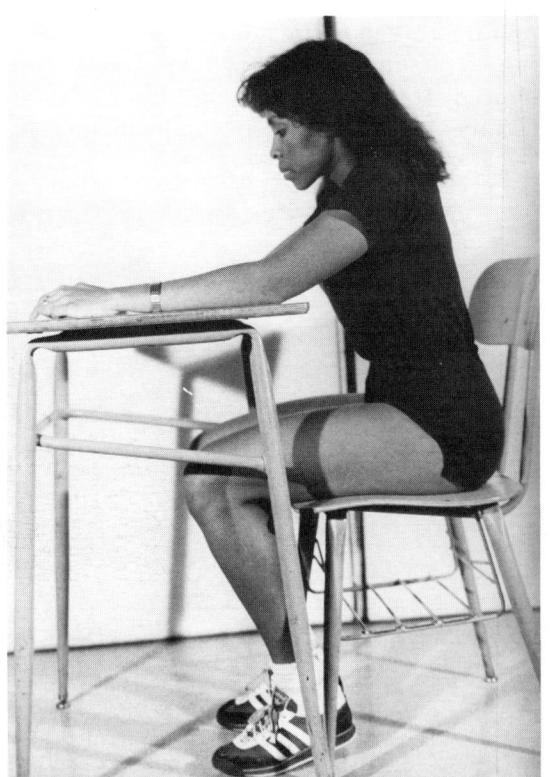

as possible. The buttocks should be against the rear of the chair, as should the entire back. The weight should not be shifted to one side; the shoulders and back should not slump, and the leg should not be curled up on the seat.

Dynamic Postures

There are, of course, thousands of dynamic postures. Discussion of all the varieties would require volumes. We will discuss three of these—walking, running, and lifting.

Individual differences in patterns of walking are observable during childhood. These differences arise out of structural differences such as the length, thickness, and shape of bones, range of movement in joints, and distribution of body weight. It is likely that the body, in its innate wisdom, selects the patterns of movement most efficient for the particular structure.

Walking

When one thinks about his or her walking patterns, tension is developed and rhythm and coordination are upset. This is because walking is a reflex action. Reflexes control movements of both the limbs and trunk in resisting the downward pull of gravity. Good reflexes, normal flexiblity of the joints, and stability of the body are essential to efficient walking patterns.

Walking is initiated by a relaxation of the plantar flexors to permit the center of gravity to move forward so that the body is unbalanced (Figure 12.4a). One foot will move forward to receive the body weight. As this foot makes contact, the center of gravity of the forward falling body moves forward over the new point of support due to the push from the rear foot (Figure 12.4b, c). The off-balance position of the body and the push off the rear foot provide the horizontal component of force necessary to overcome the standing

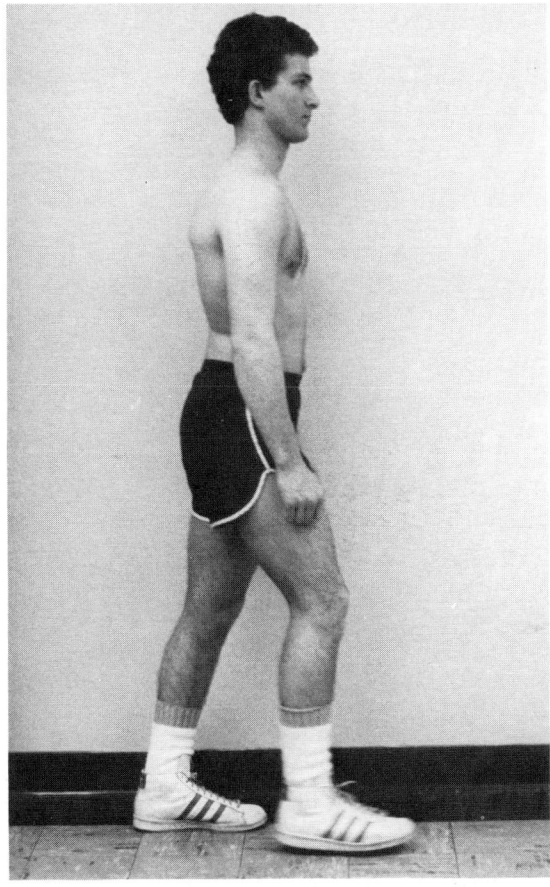

Figure 12.4 Walking (a)

Figure 12.4a Center of gravity forward of supporting left foot

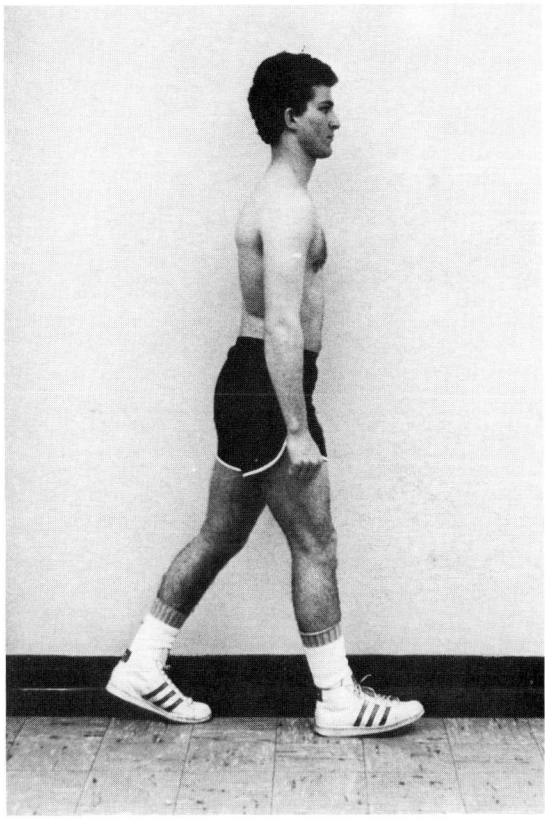

(b)

Figure 12.4b Center of gravity moving forward over new point of support—right foot

inertia of the body (Figure 12.4d). During walking, each leg acts like a pendulum swinging first with the hips as the axis during the swinging phase and then with the foot as the axis and the pendulum in an upside-down position during the supporting phase.

The alternate movements of hip flexion at one end of the lever (the entire leg) and dorsal flexion of the ankle joint (in which the lower leg moves closer to the foot) at the opposite end is converted into linear motion of the body. Because there is a decrease in the speed and, consequently, in the momentum of each leg as the heel strikes the ground,

inertia must be overcome at each step and a new push-off is required.

Each leg passes through two phases: the *swinging phase* and the *supporting phase* (Figure 12.4e). The supporting phase extends from the time the foot touches the floor to begin restraining the forward momentum, through the time the center of gravity moves over the foot, and until the foot begins to leave the floor after it pushes off in the backward thrust of the foot and leg. In the swinging or recovery phase, momentum and gravity are principally responsible for causing the leg to swing forward (Figure 12.4f). Muscular contraction initiates the movement, making this a ballistic-type movement. Since both feet are in contact with the floor at the same

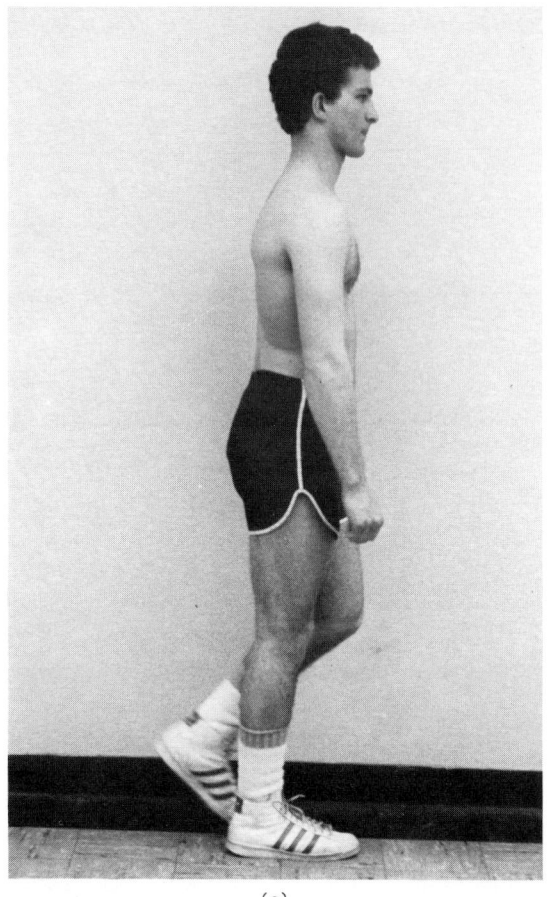

(c)

Figure 12.4c *Right foot receiving body weight; center of gravity has moved forward over this foot*

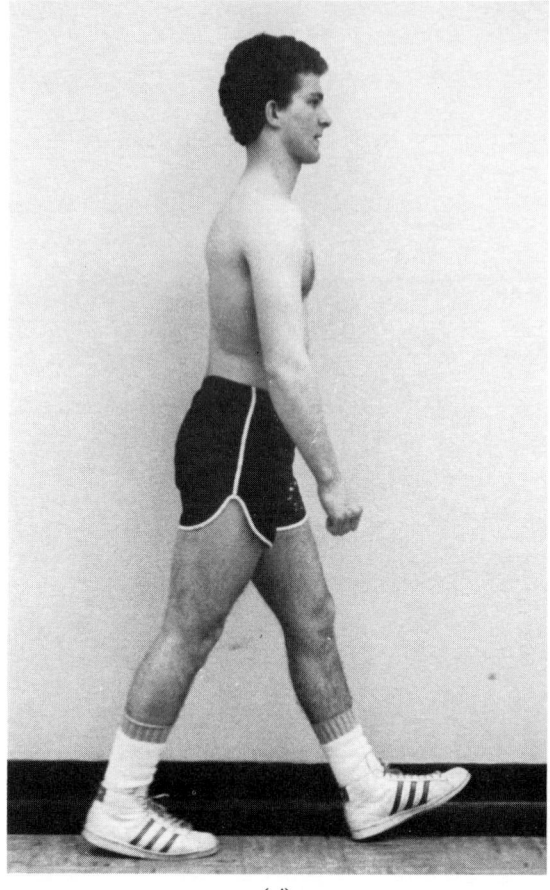

(d)

Figure 12.4d *Right foot providing forward component of force along with forward inclination of body; right arm swings forward as left leg swings forward*

moment, there is a period of double support (Figure 12.4g). This period of double support occurs when one foot is striking the floor at the beginning of the restraining movement and the other is completing its propulsive phase. When running there is no period of double support. Additionally, in running, there is a period of nonsupport when neither foot is in contact with the supporting surface. The faster one is moving, the greater the forward inclination of the body.

Too great a vertical component of force during the propulsive phase will cause the body to bounce up and down while walking. This is wasteful of energy. Bounce is further

minimized by flexion of the knee as the center of gravity passes over the supporting leg.

As one side of the pelvis and the leg on the same side move forward during the swinging phase, the shoulder and arm on that side of the body move backward while the shoulder and arm on the opposite side swing forward. Arm swing in the anterior-posterior or sagittal plane minimizes shoulder rotation. Arm swing across the body in the oblique plane serves to further minimize trunk rotation caused by pelvic rotation and support of the

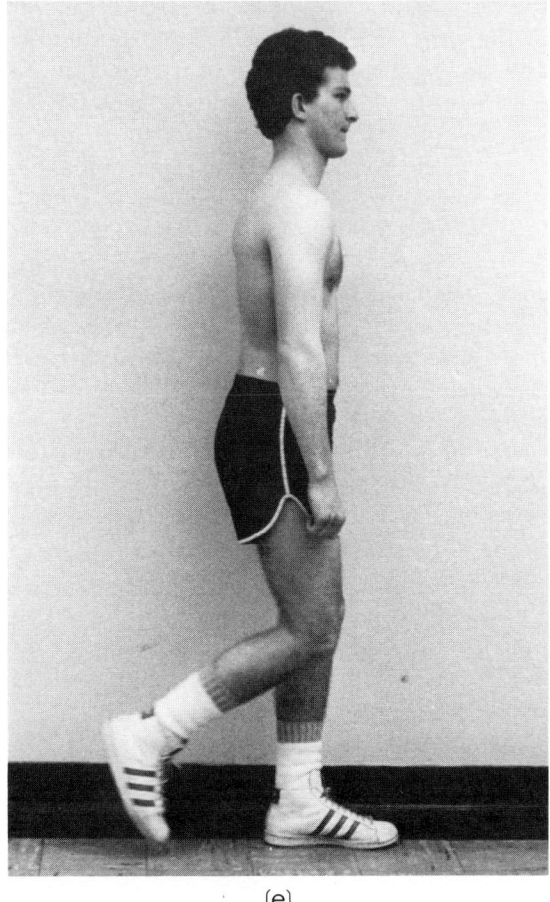

(e)

Figure 12.4e Left leg in supporting phase, right leg in swinging phase

body first on one leg and then the other. The broader the shoulders relative to height, the more the arms tend to swing across the body. As the speed of walking is increased, the arm swing becomes more vigorous and the elbows are flexed more fully to shorten the radius of rotation of the arms and facilitate more rapid movement of the arms.

Stability during walking is enhanced by increasing the lateral distance between the feet; however, if this distance is too great, the body sways and a weaving gait is produced. The most efficient procedure is placement of the feet so that their inner borders fall along a straight line.

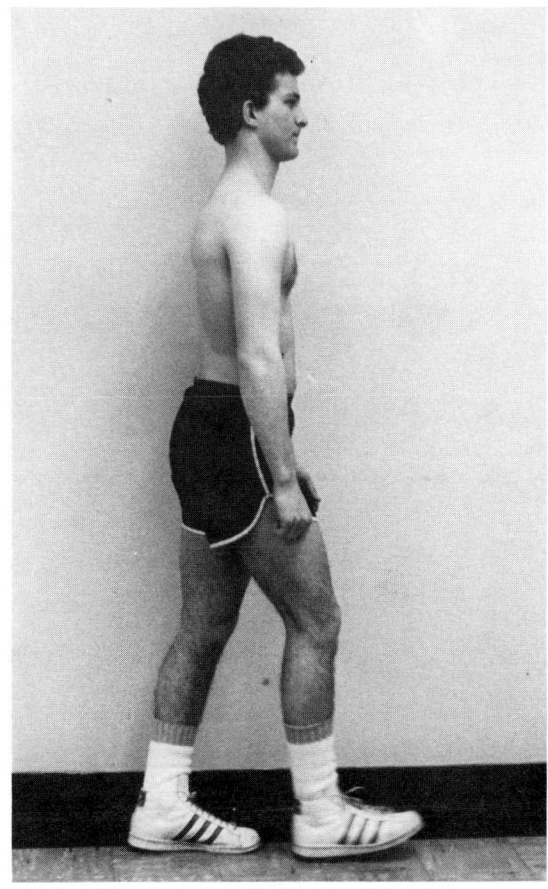

(f)

Figure 12.4f Pendular action of legs with axis of right leg now at hips while axis of left leg is at foot

Following are some common walking errors:

1. Swinging the legs excessively in a lateral direction.

2. Excessive toeing in or out. Rasch and Burke[6] indicate that the normal range is from 10 degrees toeing-in to 20 degrees toeing-out with the majority of individuals toeing-out 7.5 degrees on the average.

3. Excessive shifting of weight to the supporting foot.

4. Excessive forward inclination of the trunk from the hips.

5. Forward head.

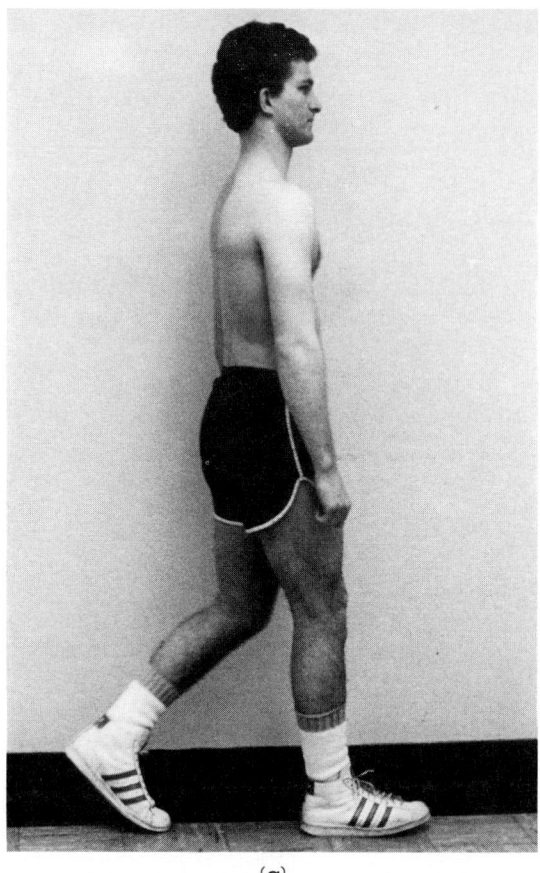

(g)

Figure 12.4g Period of double support

6. Holding the arms and shoulders excessively rigid to minimize the arm swing.

7. Swinging the arms excessively in a lateral direction.

8. Excessive vertical component of force during push-off.

Running. The major differences between walking and running have been pointed out. In running there is no period of double support and there is a period when neither foot is in contact with the supporting surface. Other differences are that in the run, the foot strikes the ground almost directly under the center of gravity instead of in front of the body and the horizontal component of force is greater in the run. Also, the pelvis is carried lower, and during the push-off of the foot and extension of the knee, the angle between the leg and the ground is smaller to facilitate an increase in the horizontal component of force.

As speed increases, the amount of inertia to be overcome decreases. Inertia is greatest during the start and acceleration. To increase the horizontal component of force during the start in sprints (Figure 12.5), spiked shoes and starting blocks are used. In the crouched position of the start, the thrust is more nearly in a horizontal direction. Also, when the hips are flexed to this degree, the powerful gluteus maximus is called into play on extension. This muscle does not extend the hip when the hip is in full extension as when running.

Figure 12.5   Crouch Start
Figure 12.5a   Starting position

(a)

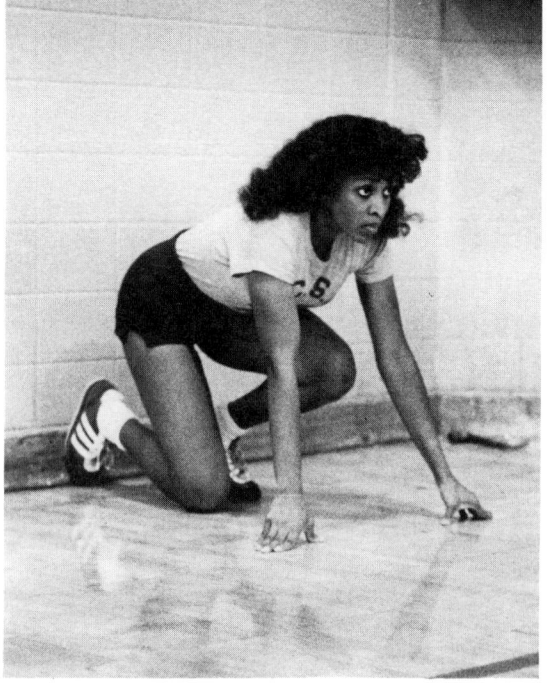

The first steps in a sprint should be relatively short and as forceful as possible. As the body accelerates, the hips extend until at full speed the body is inclined between 20 and 25 degrees to the ground. The arms flex to shorten the radius of rotation and, consequently, the time required to pump them back and forth is reduced. For the same reason, the knee is flexed during the swinging phase as the leg is moving forward. The restraining phase of the walk is eliminated since the foot contacts the ground directly under the center of gravity of the body. Force is applied immediately and continues until the foot leaves the ground. Increase in the length of stride, up to an optimal point, and speed of leg movement account for increases in speed. As has been pointed out (Chapter 5),

acceleration is directly proportional to the force producing it. Therefore, the greater the muscular power available, the greater the potential acceleration.

The leg should be extended during the propulsive phase in order to utilize as long a lever as possible. The reader will recall that the longer the lever, the greater the linear speed at the end of the lever when the angular velocity is the same. All movements should be as nearly directly forward and backward as possible since lateral movements of the arms, legs, and trunk detract from forward propulsion.[7]

Lifting. Postures, or body alignments, are of great importance in lifting most effectively and without injury. The weight should be kept as close to the line of gravity as possible

Figure 12.5b Short step with right leg. Arms pumping vigorously. Note angle of body and consequent large horizontal component of force.

(b)

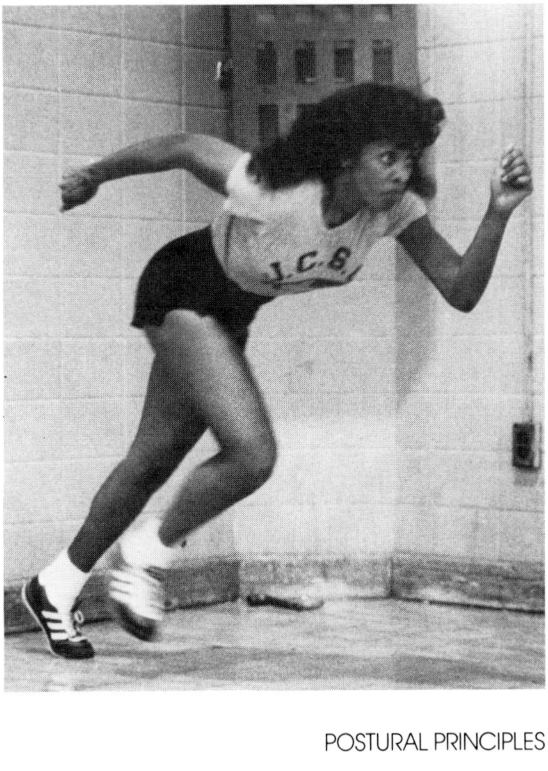

Figure 12.5c Elbows flexed to shorten radius of rotation to speed arm action

(c)

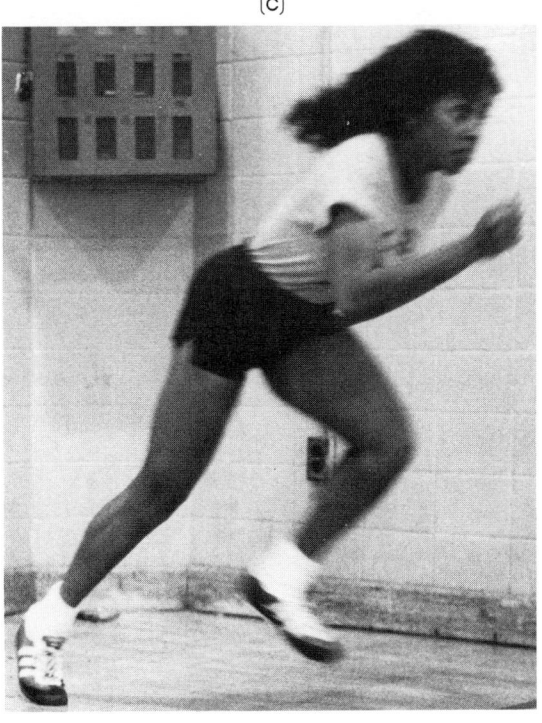

in order to shorten the lever arm. The student will recall that R × RMA = F × FMA. Because most levers in the human body are third-class levers with very short force moment arms and since the length of these bony structures cannot be changed, tremendous force must be generated by muscles to overcome even relatively small resistances. The shorter the resistance moment arm, the less force required to overcome the resistance. The closer the resistance or weight to be lifted is to the body's center of gravity, the shorter will be the RMA. Furthermore, when lifting with a shorter resistance arm, the shearing forces upon vertebrae and surrounding soft tissue are less, decreasing the probability of injury. The closer the lifter is to the weight to be lifted, the more nearly vertical is the spine. Shearing forces are less when the spine is vertical than when it is flexed.

One should avoid lifting with any part of the body rotated or lifting in such a manner that it will be necessary to turn the body while supporting the weight. These procedures necessitate spinal rotation, which will greatly increase shearing forces. They will also place great stress on the small spinal rotators.

The feet should be kept flat on the floor and spread about 12 inches apart to increase stability. Stability permits the lifter to focus his attention on the object to be lifted. Loss of balance makes it necessary to use smaller muscles not adapted to lifting of heavy weights.

The Clean and Jerk Lift

The strongest muscles should be utilized in this lift. These are usually the extensors of the knees. Champion weight lifters, when cleaning and jerking 400 or more pounds to arm's length overhead, demonstrate this principle very well, as Figures 12.6 and 12.7 show. It will be noted that at the start of the lift, the lifter's feet are under the bar to place his center of gravity as close to the weight as possible (Figures 12.6a and 12.7a). The knees are for-

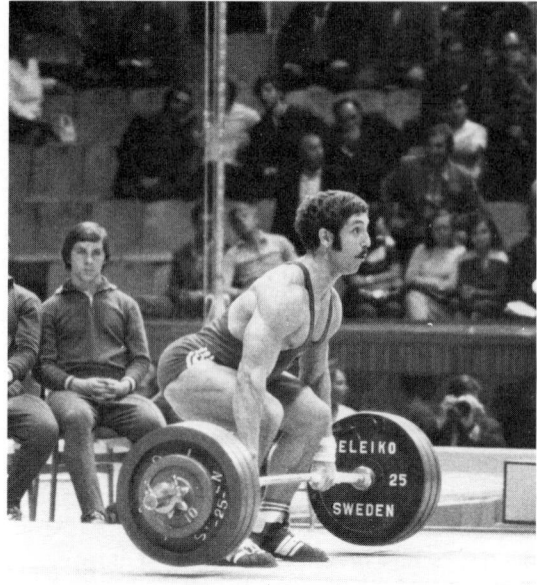

(a)

Figure 12.6   Clean and Jerk—Squat Style
Figure 12.6a   Feet in line and under bar, shoulders above bar, knee joints at right angle

Figure 12.6b   Pull is directly upward, knees have extended

(b)

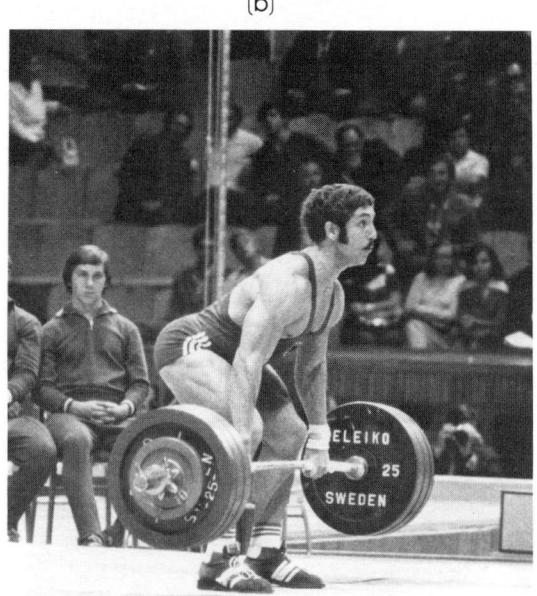

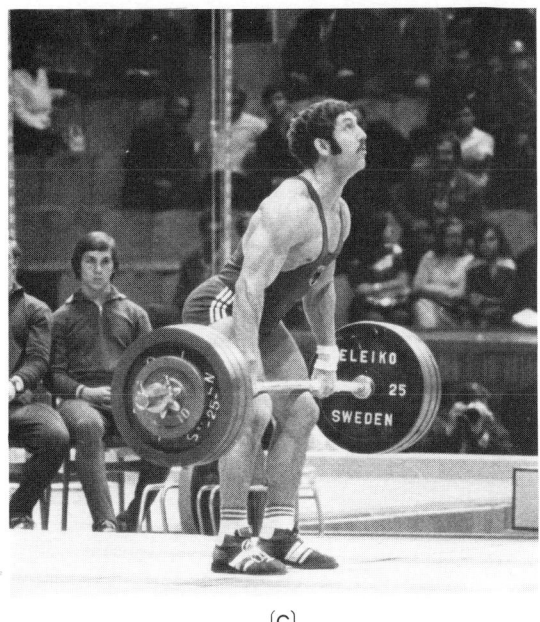

(c)

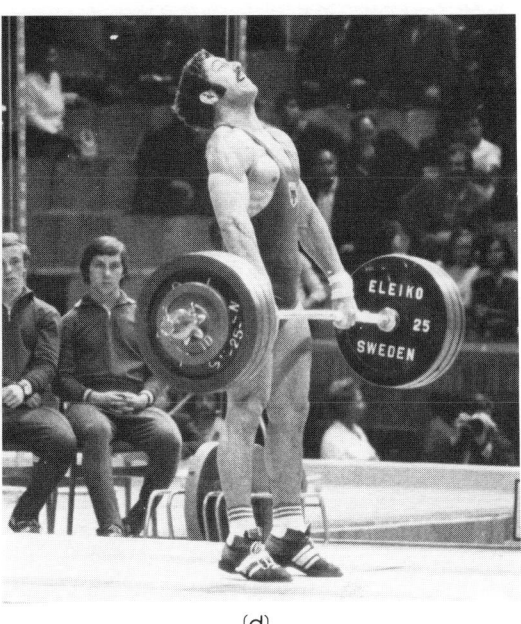

(d)

Figure 12.6c Bar momentarily resting on thigh, note head position

Figure 12.6d Hips and knees have extended, shoulders elevating, feet plantar flexing

Figure 12.6e Dropping under the barbell, wrists rotating under bar, center of gravity of bar over the feet

Figure 12.6f Elbows forward, humerii horizontal, trunk vertical

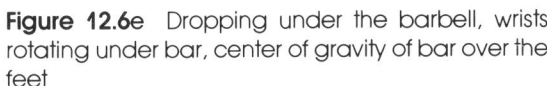

(e)

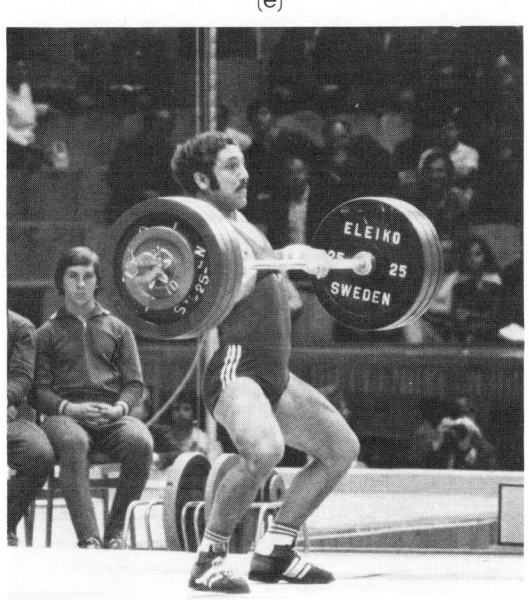

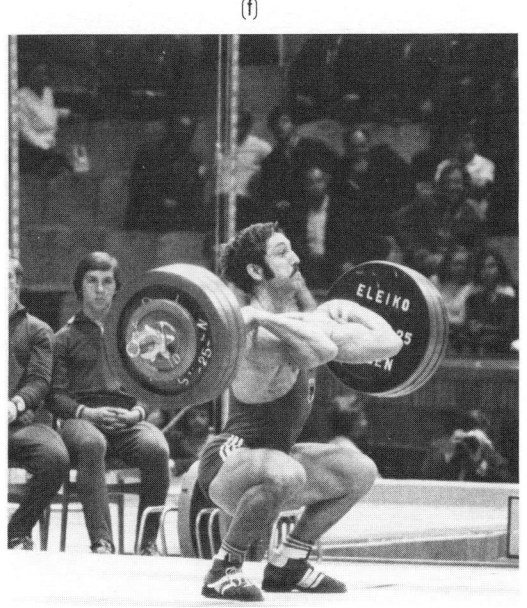

(f)

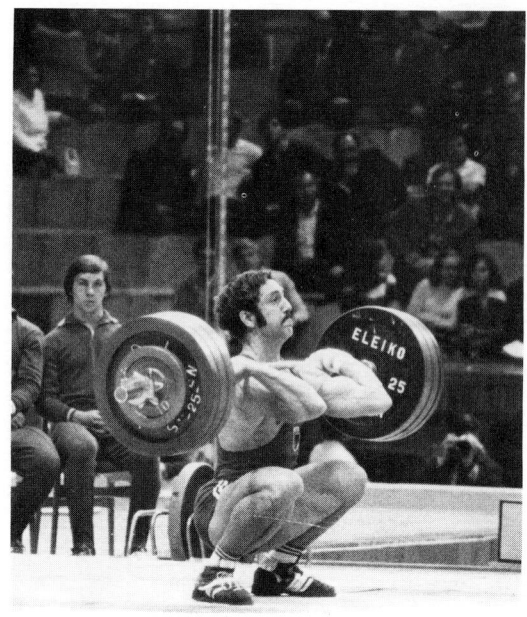

(g)

Figure 12.6g Full squat, bar across shoulders

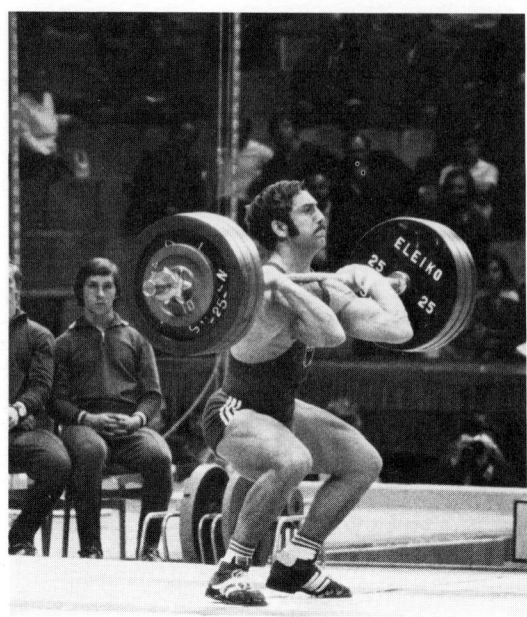

(h)

Figure 12.6h Knees and hips extending

Figure 12.6i Erect position

Figure 12.6j Knees have flexed slightly and are now beginning to extend, note bend in bar

(i)

(j)

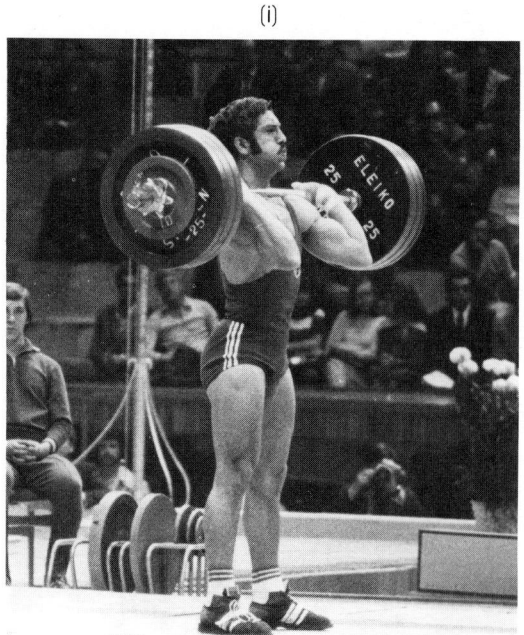

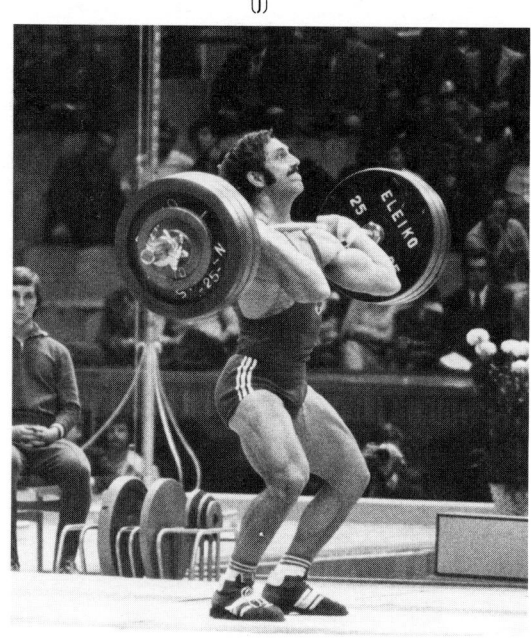

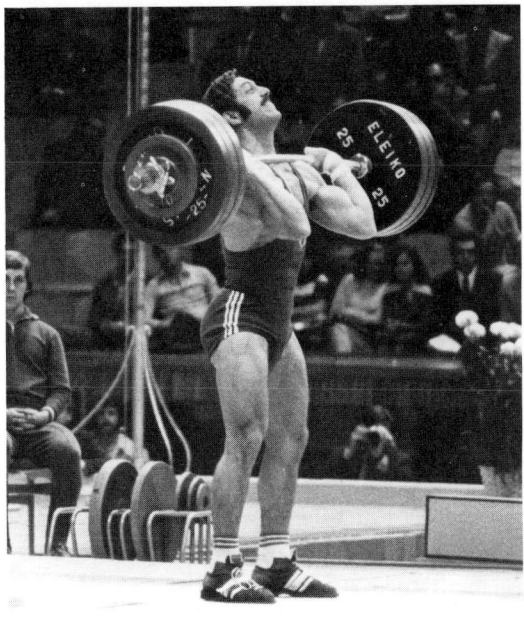

(k)

Figure 12.6k   Bar still has upward momentum

Figure 12.6m   Split completed. Note that center of gravity of bar is in a vertical line passing through the arms, shoulders, spine and pelvis

(m)

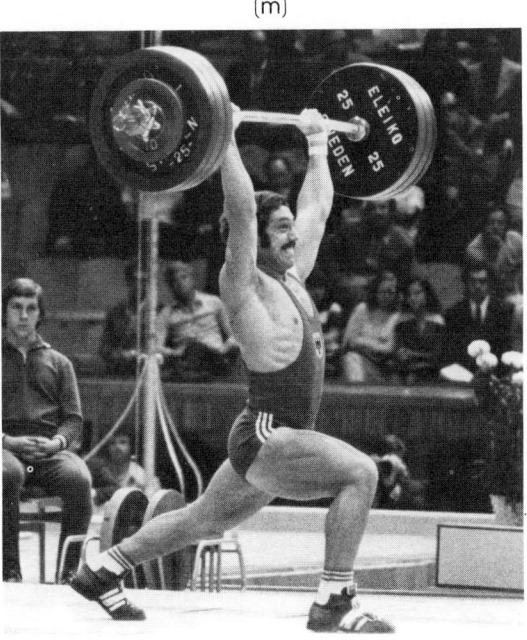

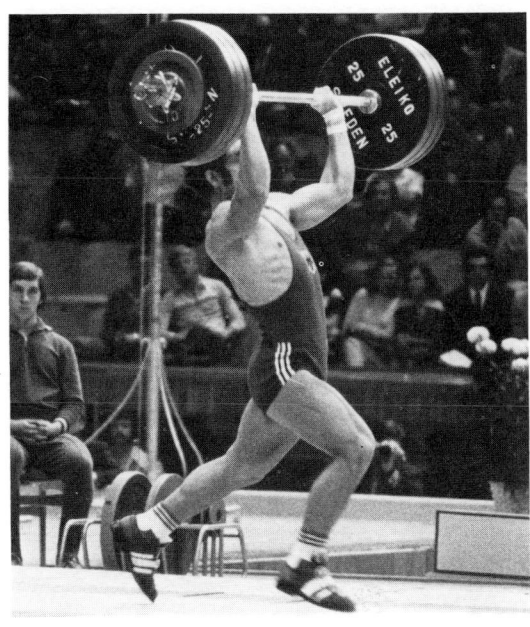

(l)

Figure 12.6l   Dropping under the upward moving bar, arms extending, note feet are off platform

Figure 12.6n   Lift completed

(n)

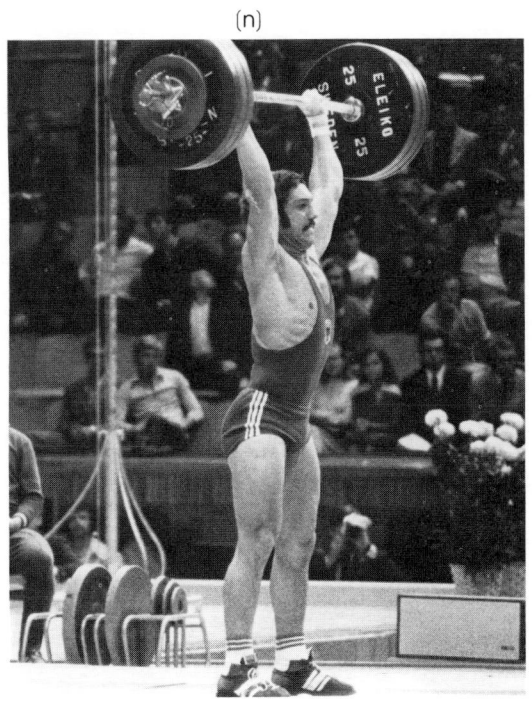

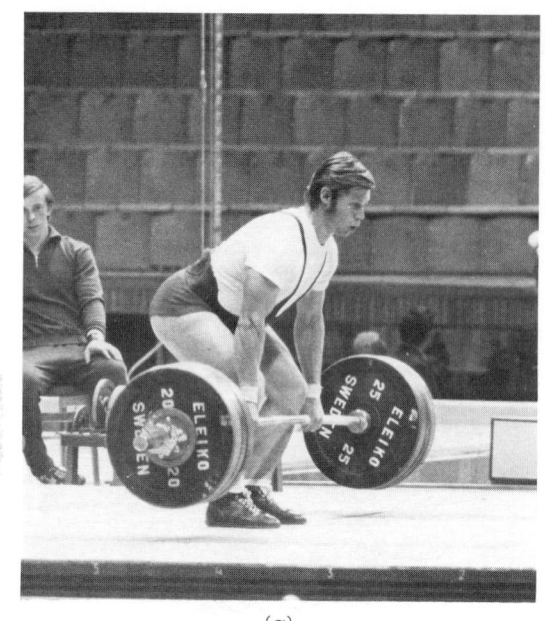

(a)

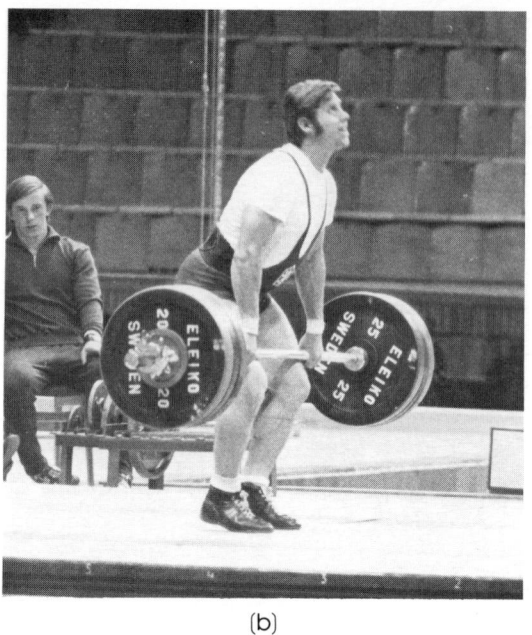

(b)

Figure 12.7 Clean and Jerk—Split Style
Figure 12.7a to 12.7c Procedure is identical to squat style

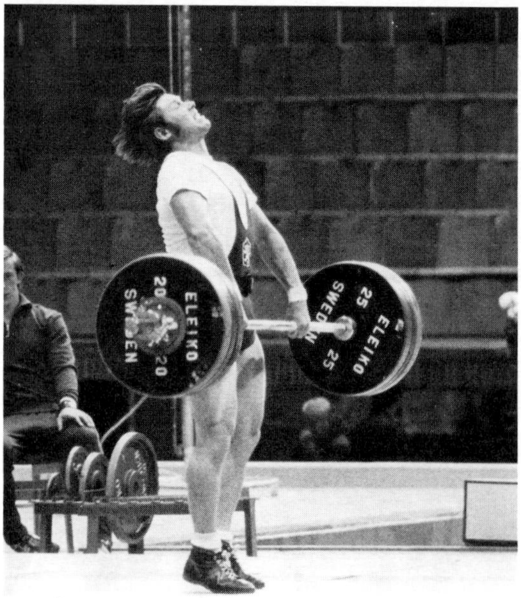

Figure 12.7d Dropping under the bar into the split

(c)

(d)

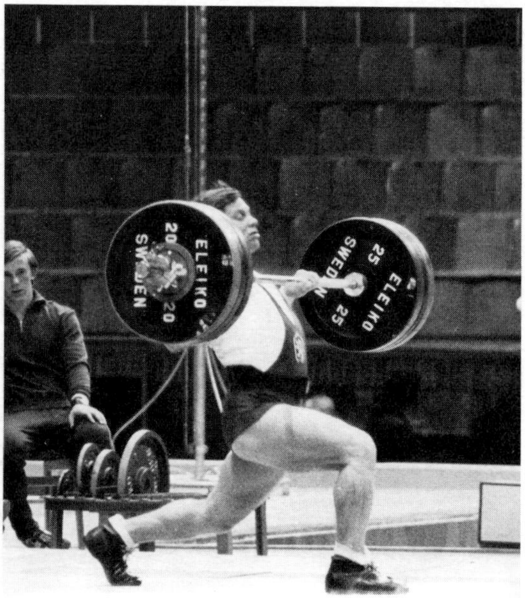

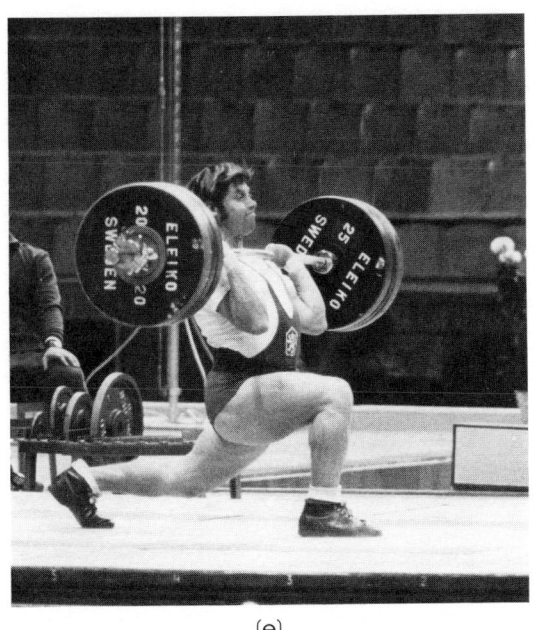

(e)

Figure 12.7e Full split. Note degree of hyperextension of left hip and flexion of right hip. A great range of movement in the hip joints is required in this style

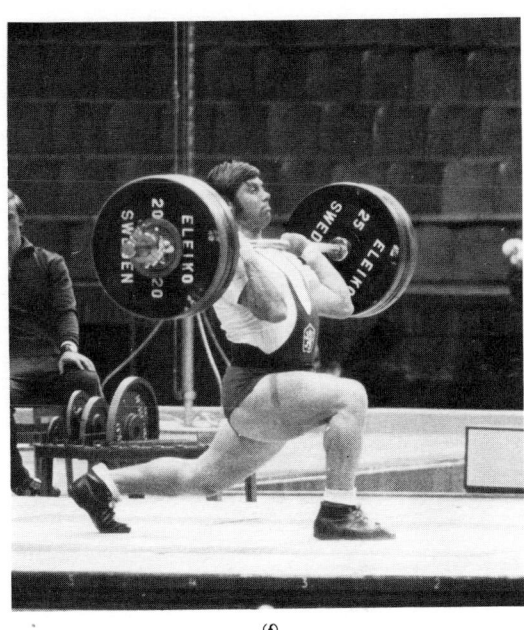

(f)

Figure 12.7f to 12.7h Moving into the erect position

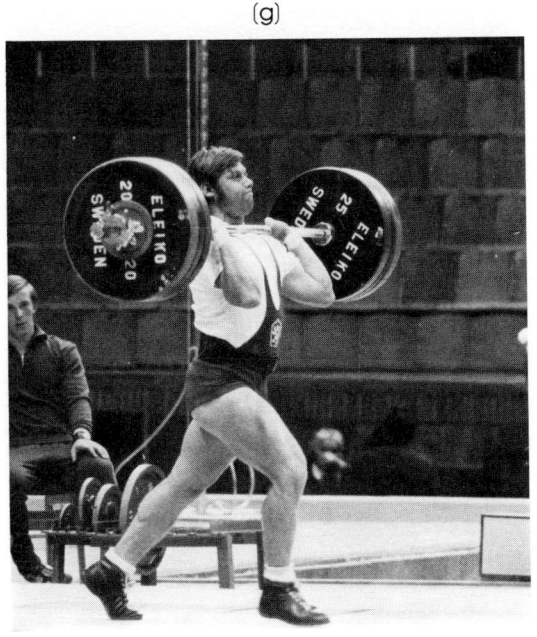

(g)

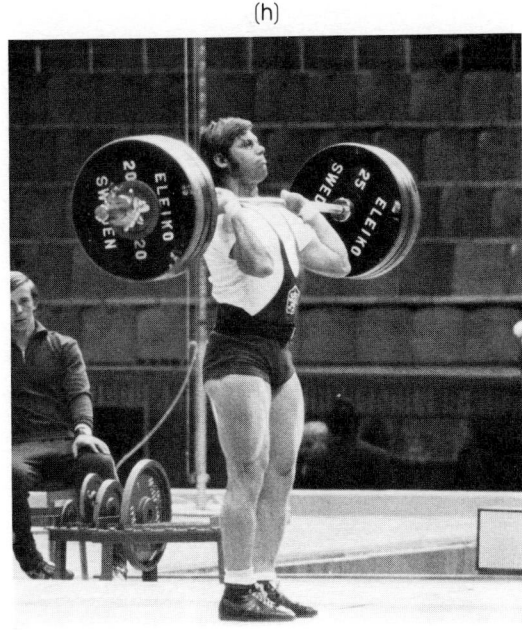

(h)

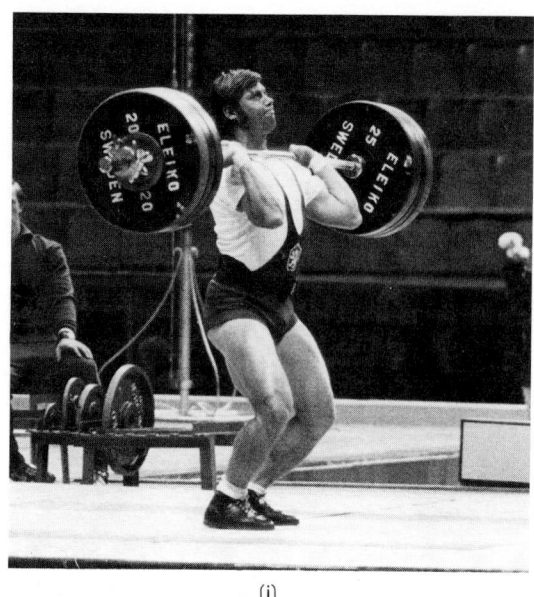

(i)

Figure 12.7i Knees and hips flexing in preparation for "kick"

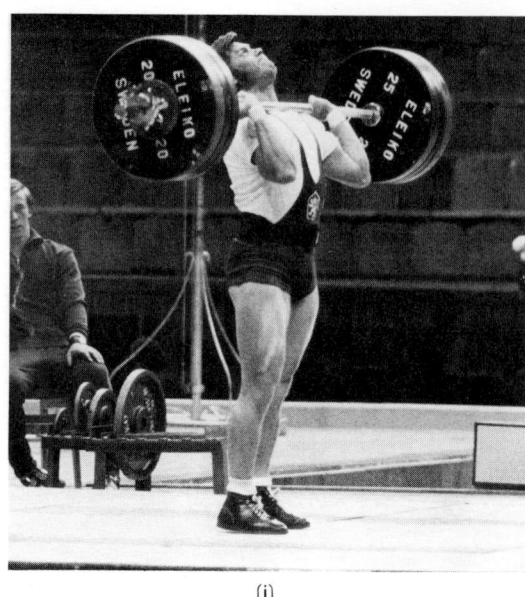

(j)

Figure 12.7j Knees and hips extended, feet plantar flexing

Figure 12.7k to 12.7l Splitting under the bar

(k)

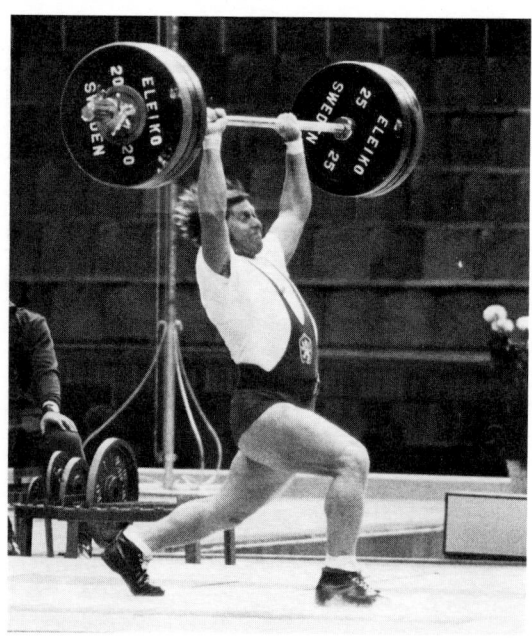

(l)

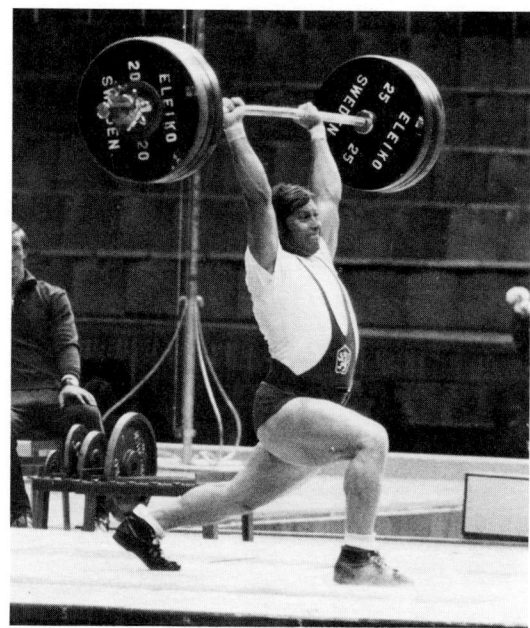

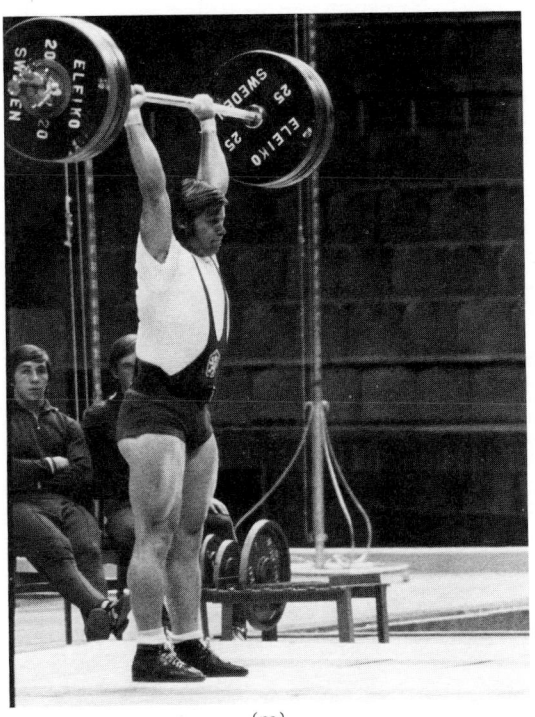

(m)

Figure 12.7m Lift completed

ward of the bar. The arms are perpendicular in order that the pull will be directly upward. The arms remain extended, serving as cables, while the powerful knee extensors overcome the inertia of the barbell and start it on its way upward (Figures 12.6*b* and 12.7*b*). The body's center of gravity is raised as the knees and hips are extended (Figures 12.6*c, d* and 12.7*c*), and then the knees and hips are quickly flexed to drop the body under the upward-rising barbell as the hands are rotated under the barbell while the elbows and shoulders are flexed (Figures 12.6*e* and 12.7*d*). After the barbell's inertia has been overcome via knee and hip extension and is already moving upward, the shoulders are elevated and the elbows are flexed to continue the upward movement initiated by the knee extensors.

After the barbell is resting across the chest while in a squat position (Figures 12.6*g* and

12.7*e, f*), the knees are extended (Figures 12.6*h–k* and 12.7*g, h*). Next, the knees are flexed slightly, followed by an explosive extension of the knees to start the barbell upward (Figures 12.6*l* and 12.7*i, j*). After the barbell has been started upward, the center of gravity of the body is dropped by means of a split of the legs or a squat (Figures 12.6*m* and 12.7*k, l*). As the body drops under the bar, the arms are extended under the bar. The legs are then extended in the squat style, or the feet are brought together in the split style (Figures 12.6*n* and 12.7*m*). Decreased inclination of the pelvis and the forward head should be noted. These positions insure that the line of gravity of the weight passes vertically down the vertebral column and through the bones of the arms and legs to minimize shear forces. It also minimizes the muscular force that must be utilized in supporting the weight. Throughout the lift, the major force is provided by the most powerful muscles—the knee extensors.

The principles followed by the weight lifter should be observed by workers who are called upon to lift or move weights (see Figure 12.8). When an object must be lifted from a shelf overhead, one foot should be placed somewhat behind the other in the event the horizontal momentum of the object, as it is pulled off the shelf, forces the lifter backward (see Figure 12.9). Under these circumstances, it is difficult to maintain stability because the center of gravity of the lifter has been raised due to the weight, and the horizontal component of force of the object moves him off balance. During this process, the pelvis should be in a position of decreased inclination.

MUSCULAR ASPECTS OF POSTURE

Muscular strength and flexibility beyond the average are not necessary for the maintenance of good posture. However, weak muscles tire more quickly and allow gravity to

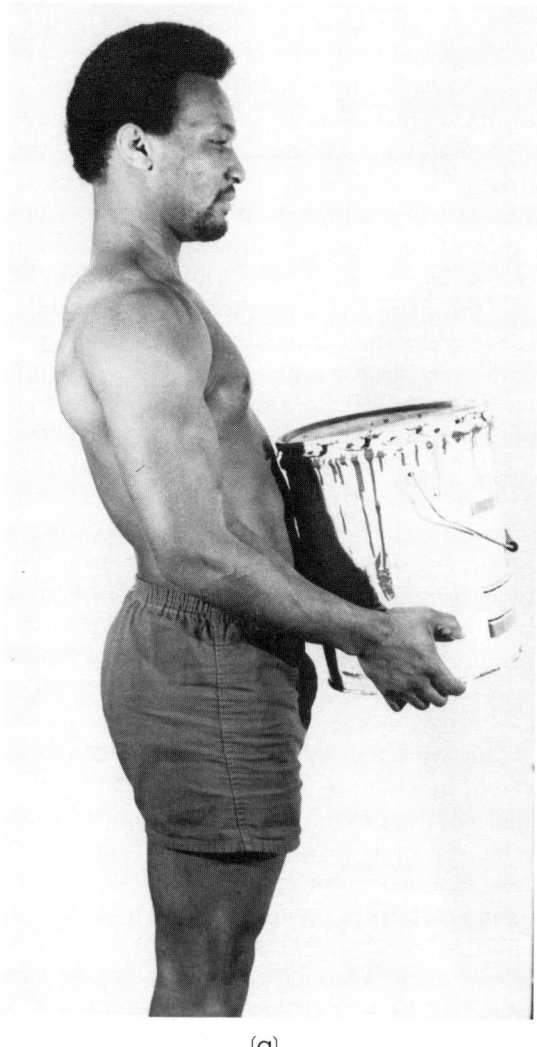

(a)

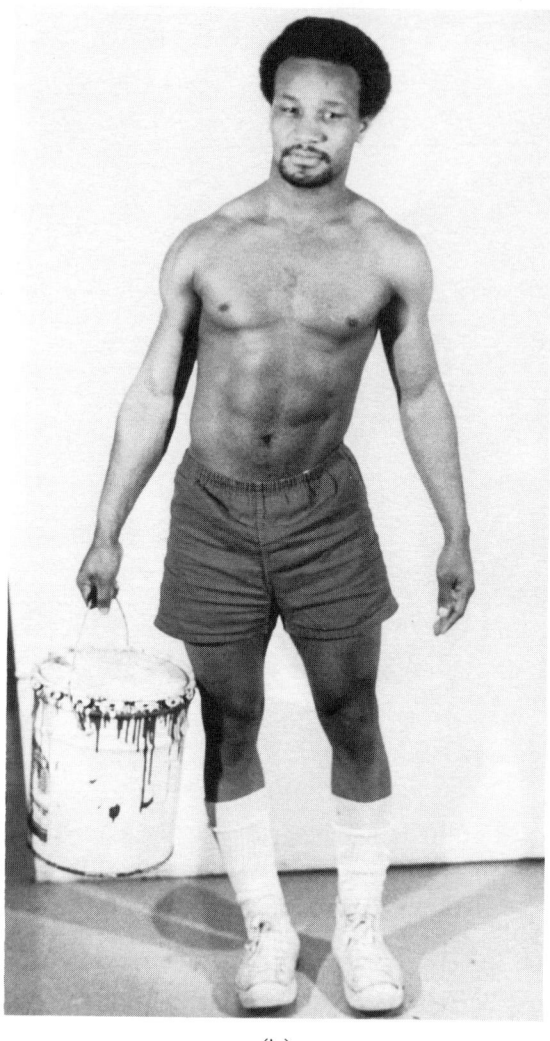

(b)

Figure 12.8a Trunk angled backward to counter-balance weight of paint bucket

Figure 12.8b Trunk inclined sideward to move center of gravity over feet

pull the body segments downward into a zig-zag relationship with one another. The result is that continuous stress is placed on the ligaments and shearing forces are exerted on the vertebrae. Consequently, a modicum of strength is required, particularly of those muscles involved in maintenance of posture.

Among the most important of these muscles are those of the abdominal wall. These include the abdominis rectus, internal and external obliques, and transversali. The rectus abdominis is the only longitudinal anterior muscle controlling the amount of the lumbar curve. This long flat muscle extends from the lower part of the chest to the pubis. One of its major duties is to decrease pelvic tilt and thereby to flex the lumbar spine. In addition to its rotational pull on the pelvis, it

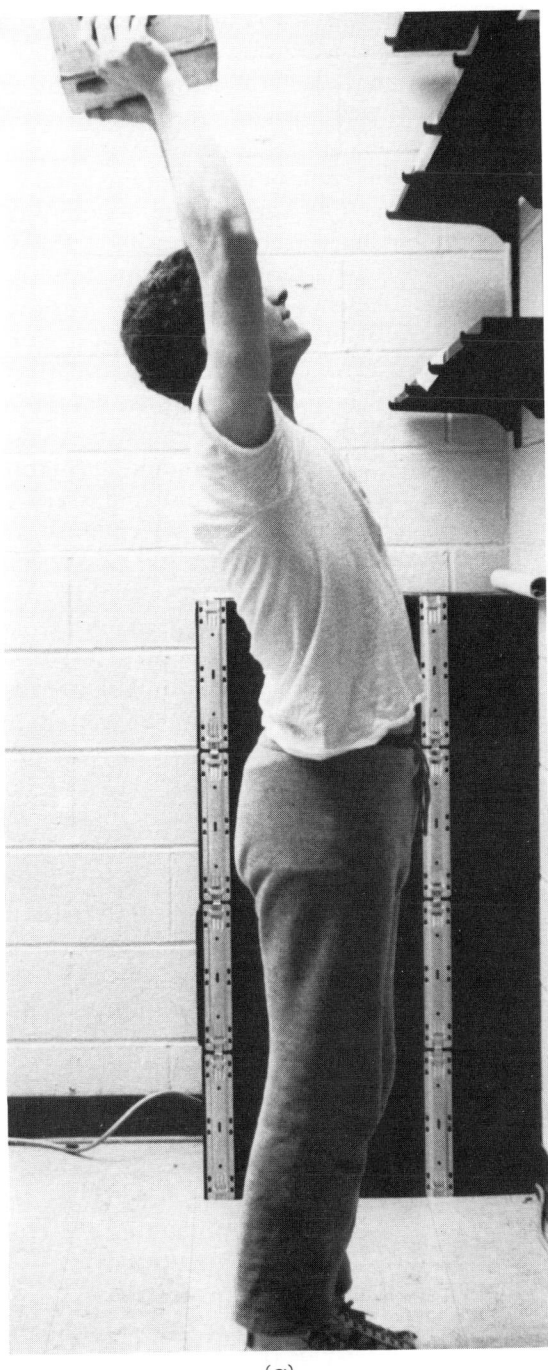

(a)

Figure 12.9a Incorrect method of lifting a weight from a shelf. Elevated center of gravity and backward tangent of force may cause loss of balance.

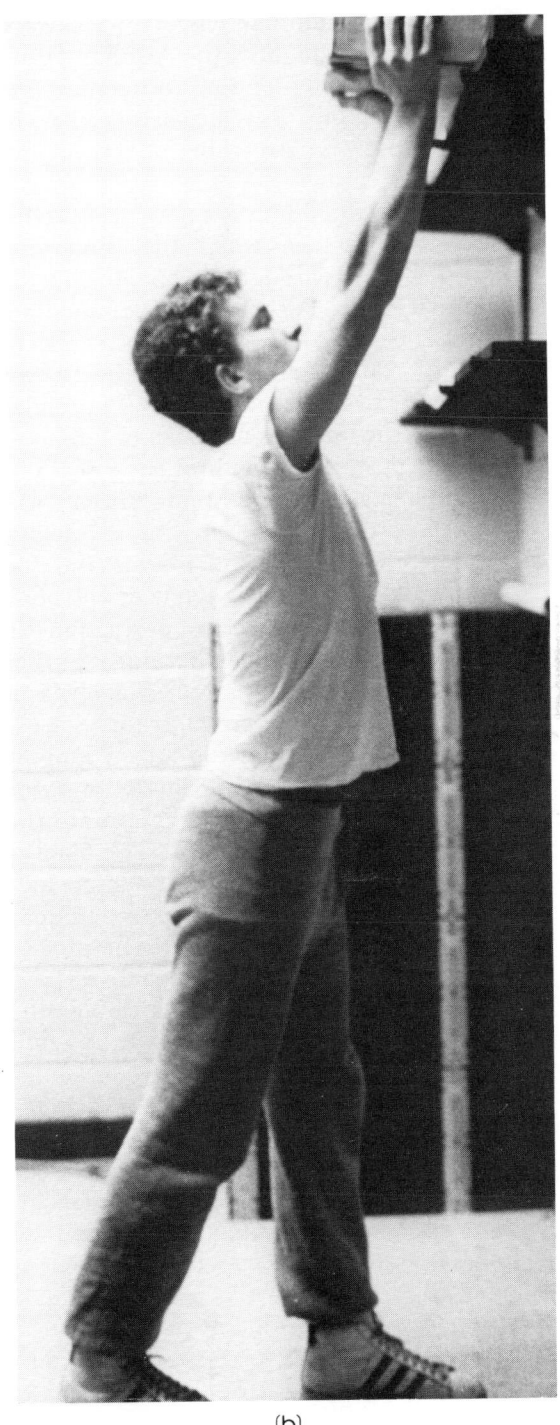

(b)

Figure 12.9b Correct method

pushes the abdominal viscera backward against the sacrum and the lumbar vertebrae, thus, not only tending to decrease the lumbar curve, but also supporting the viscera. This prevents stretching of the visceral mesenteries.

Weak abdominal muscles may also predispose one to hernia in which the abdominal viscera protrude through an opening in the abdominal wall. Although the immediate cause may be a blow to the abdomen, violent coughing, straining at stool, or a fall, the real cause is weakness of the abdominal musculature. Once the opening has been enlarged as a result of pushing through of the viscera, a hernia is likely to recur. Minor surgery will correct this problem.

While standing, the abdominals and the sacrospinalis contract alternately as the body sways back and forth. Other opposing muscle groups engage in the same alternate contraction and relaxation. The muscles involved in the legs include the gastrocnemius, soleus, tibialis anterior, extensor digitorum longus, and peroneus longus. The tibialis anterior and extensor digitorum longus maintain the position of the tibia on the talus. The plantar muscles of the feet, such as the abductors hallucis, minimi digiti, and adductor hallucis, contract reflexively. In addition to helping to maintain balance, these muscles help to keep the bones of the feet in position, although the plantar ligaments assume the major portion of this responsibility.

In the shoulder area, the trapezius, rhomboid, and levator adduct the scapulae while the serratus and pectoralis major and minor abduct the scapulae. When the scapular adductors are weak or become stretched due to long held positions as occurs in some occupations, a condition known as *round shoulders* can develop. This position shifts some of the body weight forward, necessitating a compensatory curve in another part of the body.

Reading, writing, sewing, mechanical drawing, and typing are some of the activities during which the scapulae are abducted for long periods. It would be well for those heavily engaged in these activities to participate in recreational activities that stretch the serratus and pectoralis muscles and shorten and strengthen the rhomboids, trapezius, and levator muscles. The backstroke in swimming, archery, fencing, and horsemanship are some examples of activities that accomplish this objective. These people may also, periodically during the day, perform several stretching and isometric exercises. Several of these exercises are described later in this chapter.

Many cases of round shoulders are associated with "winged scapulae" (Figure 12.10). In this condition, the scapulae are in a position of upward tilt in which they are turned on their frontal-horizontal axis so that the posterior surface is turned slightly upward and the inferior angle protrudes from the back.

An imbalance in the deeper muscles of the vertebral column that rotate the vertebrae can result in lateral curvature of the column. This is called *scoliosis* (Figure 12.11). Lateral curvature is always associated with rotation of the vertebrae. The condition usually begins with a single C curve, which may extend the entire length of the spine or only a portion of it. With a lateral curvature, the head is tilted sideways; consequently, the righting reflexes will cause the upper part of the spine to bend in the opposite direction in order to place the head in a vertical position. In time, this produces an S curve in the spine. The preceding simplified explanation of scoliosis is adequate for physical educators. Physical educators should always work under the direction of an orthopedic surgeon when conducting exercise programs for students with scoliosis.

The muscles involved in scoliosis are the semispinalis, multifidus, and rotatores. When the member of the muscle pair on the right side of the vertebrae is stronger than its opposite member on the left side of the vertebrae, the vertebrae will usually be rotated, causing a concavity on the left side. In most cases, the concavity is on the side of the weaker muscles. However, in a few cases, the muscles on the side of the convexity are weaker.

12.10 Winged scapulae.

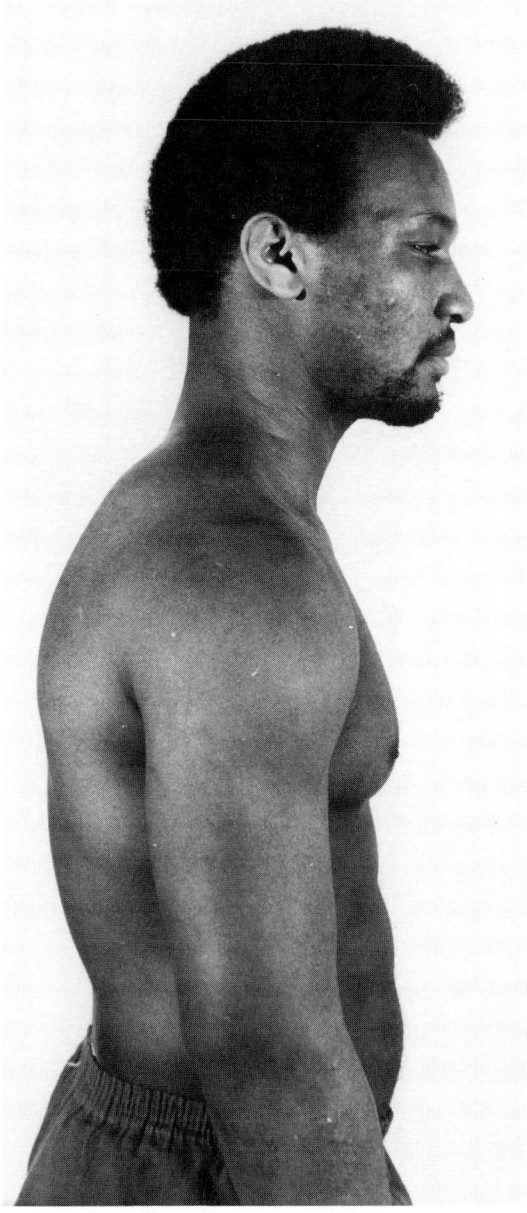

MECHANICAL ASPECTS OF POSTURE

The body is composed of a number of segments that, in the erect position, are all balanced one upon the other. With respect to posture, the important segments are head, trunk, thighs, legs, and feet. Muscles are the first line of defense in maintenance of posture. When the vertical alignment between adjacent segments is lost and the angle between these segments decreases below 180 de-

Figure 12.11a Scoliosis. Note protruding right scapulae, lateral curvature to the right in the thoracic area and slightly elevated right hip

(a)

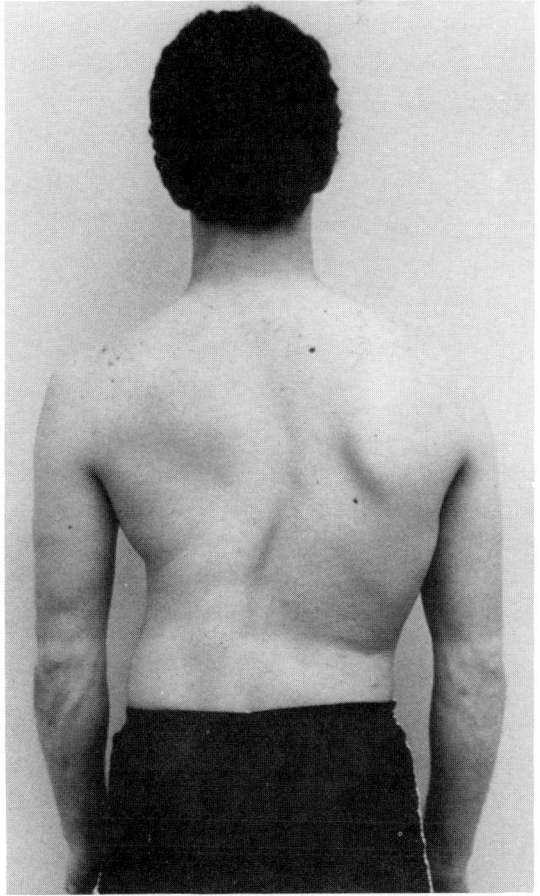

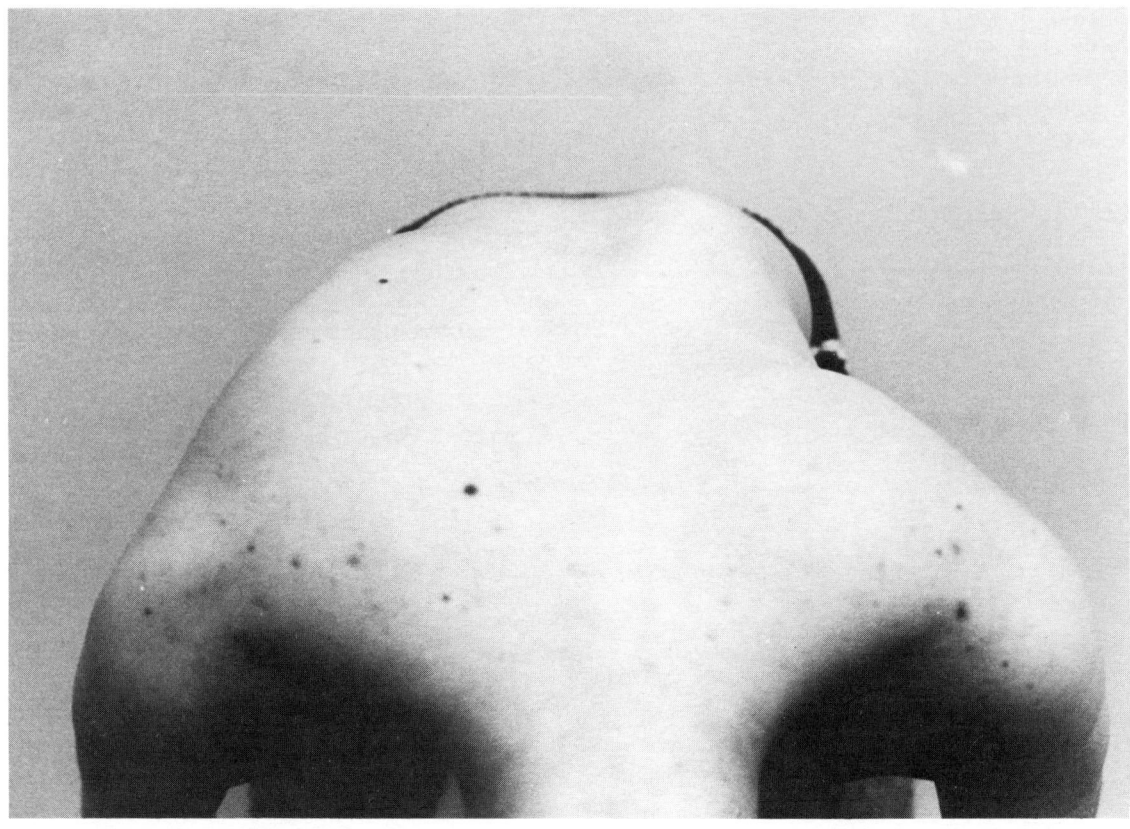

(b)

Figure 12.11b Scoliosis. Subject has bent forward. Note difference between right and left side

grees, stress is placed on the ligaments. When the muscles are called upon to bring the segments into vertical alignment, the work required becomes greater as the angle between the segments decreases. This is illustrated by a comparison of the amount of force required to hold a broom by one end vertically with that required to hold it horizontally. As the broom moves from the vertical toward the horizontal position, an increasing amount of force is required. This is because the length of the resistance arm of the involved levers increases from the vertical to the horizontal position. Consequently, a position of vertical alignment of the several body segments is more economical of energy expenditure than one in which the segments are in a zigzag relationship. However, if the postural muscles are excessively flaccid as in the fatigue slouch, expenditure of energy will be minimal but damage will be done to ligaments and the intervertebral disks.

Base of Support and Posture

The wider the base of support, the greater the stability in the direction of movement. Balance can be more readily maintained when the feet are spread apart in the plane of movement or anticipated impact than it can when they are held together. Equilibrium can be maintained when the line of gravity falls within the base of support. It will be recalled from a previous discussion that the nearer the line of gravity to the center of the base of support, the greater the stability. This condition will exist when the body segments are vertically aligned. When carrying objects in front of the body, it is necessary to angle the trunk backward to maintain the line of gravity between the points of support (Figure 12.8a). When carrying objects on one side of the body, it is necessary to angle the body sideward and to abduct the arm opposite to the side of the weight (Figure 12.8b). This will place the line of gravity between the points of support.

When a force, such as wind, is acting on the body, one must lean into this force a proportionate amount. When one is anticipating impact of a force that will upset balance, the line of gravity should be moved to the edge of the base of support in the direction of the impending force. The feet should also be aligned more nearly in the direction of the impending force. In some instances, as in racing starts, it is advisable to move the line of gravity to the most forward position of the base of support. This will make possible the quickest start and one with the least expenditure of energy (e.g., see Figure 12.12).

In the erect position, the extensor muscles carry the major share of the load. The junction of the fibula and tibia with the talus is behind the center of the foot and also behind a perpendicular line from the body center. As a result, the tibia and fibula are inclined forward about two to three degrees from a perpendicular line passing through the center of the body. In order to maintain the center of gravity, or body center, over the center of support, there must be constant contraction of the muscles that plantar flex the feet—the gastrocnemius, peroneus brevis and longus, soleus, and tibialis posterior. Muscles of the hip joints, back, shoulders, and neck must also be in a state of continuous contraction. The sustained contraction of the muscles that maintain posture is called *postural tonus*.

Figure 12.12 Football lineman's position. Center of gravity is near forward edge of base of support to facilitate quick start

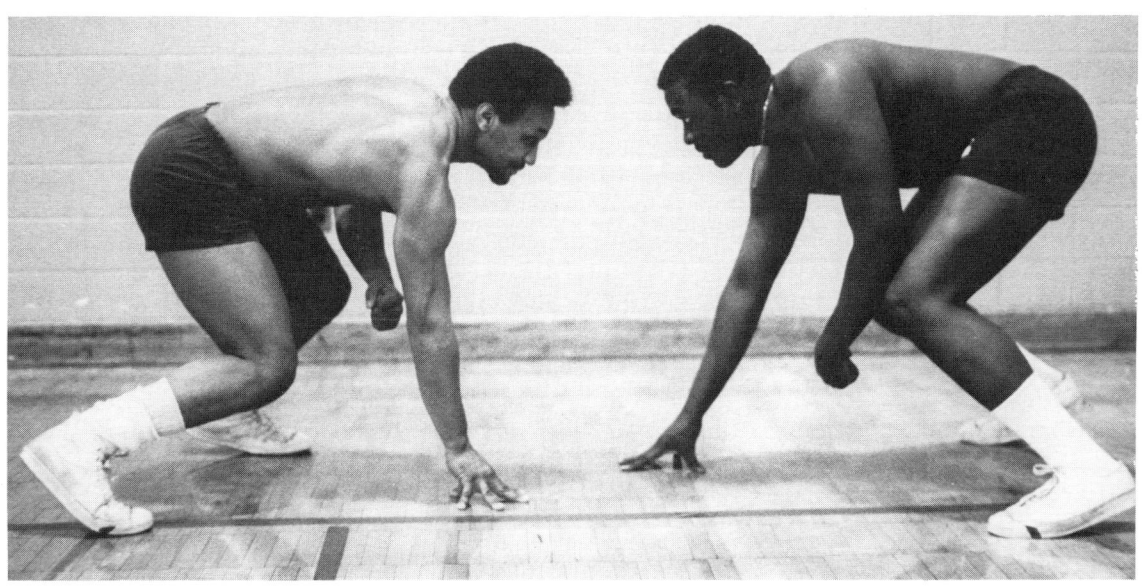

It is necessary that these muscles be continually excited if they are to maintain tonus. The stimuli can arise from every sensory organ of the body; however, the major stimuli arise from several sources: (1) labyrinthine righting reflexes, (2) visual or optical reflexes, (3) reflexes acting on the head, (4) proprioceptor or kinesthetic sense, (5) plantar reflexes, and (6) stretch reflexes. For a more detailed discussion of the neural aspects of postural tonus, the reader is referred to Chapter 4.

Head Positions and Posture

Changes in postural positions can be induced by movements of the head. Changes in the position of the head produce stimuli acting upon the receptor organs of the labyrinth in the inner ear. These stimuli produce changes in the tonus of muscles of the trunk and limbs. When the head is tilted backward, the abdominal muscles relax, the extensors of the trunk contract, the shoulder girdle is adducted, and the flexors of the knee joints contract. Flexion of the neck produces the opposite results. Lateral flexion and rotation of the head produce an increase in limb extensor tone on the side to which the head is flexed or rotated and a decrease in extensor tone to limbs on the opposite side. When an athlete steps sideward, he first turns and flexes his head to the side of the step. This increases extensor tone on the side of the step to prepare the leg on that side to receive the body weight. Head positions clue an opponent to forthcoming movements of an athlete. Athletes in some sports such as boxing, soccer, and ice hockey should learn to overcome these reflex actions.

Within the fluid in the semicircular canals of the ears are found tiny particles of calcium called *otoliths*. When the head is tilted, the otoliths touch the walls of the canals and brush against the many hairlike sensory nerves that line the canal. This creates impulses that inform the brain of body position.

The body also tries to retain its field of vision. When the head is tilted backward, the eyeballs move downward. When the head is tilted forward, the eyeballs move upward. When the head is turned sideward to the left, the eyeballs move to the right. This helps gymnasts, divers, skaters, and dancers to maintain their orientation and minimizes sensations of dizziness.

Visual impressions inform the person of his body's relationship to the objects around him. A back somersault is easier than a front somersault because, in the back somersault, the gymnast can see the mat during the last three-quarters of the movement to know when to open up. In the front somersault, the thighs are in the line of vision to the mat and, consequently, the gymnast must depend upon clues from sources other than the visual to inform him of his position. Sports such as gymnastics and diving develop the *labyrinthine and proprioceptive reflexes*, while sports such as basketball, baseball, and soccer develop *eye–muscle coordination*. In order to achieve most complete development of all the reflexes, children should participate in a variety of sports. The rationale could be offered that this will enable the child to become more proficient in the sport of his or her choice. In the sports that develop primarily the labyrinthine and proprioceptive reflexes, there are instances when visual clues are utilized, and, conversely, in sports that develop primarily reflexes beginning with visual stimuli, there are occasions when the athlete must place high reliance upon the labyrinthine and proprioceptive reflexes. For example, a view of the goal or of teammates may be obstructed due to other players, yet skilled players are able to make accurate passes or shots as a result of proprioceptive reflexes, memory of the location of the goal, and judgments of a teammate's speed and direction.

Plantar reflexes inform the individual of

the relative pressures on the various areas of the plantar surface of the feet. When the pressure on the heels increases, the dorsi flexors of the ankle and the flexors of the vertebral column contract, and when the pressure on the toes increases, the opposing postural muscles contract.

The *stretch reflex* is well-developed in the postural muscles. When the body segments begin to be pulled out of vertical alignment due to the pull of gravity, the muscles involved in maintenance of posture begin to be stretched. They immediately contract to maintain posture. The *extensor thrust reflex* is responsible for the contraction of the extensors of the knees and hips when pressure is placed on the soles of the feet.

POSTURAL DEVIATIONS

Classifications

Postural deviations are classified as either *structural* or *functional*. In a structural deviation, the shape of bones has been modified and, consequently, the condition cannot be rectified without surgery or having the part placed in a cast or brace for a period of time. Obviously, corrective exercises alone cannot correct this condition. Most postural deviations, except those resulting from congenital defects, injury, or disease, begin as functional disorders. In functional disorders, only soft tissues, such as the muscles and ligaments, are involved. However, if the condition is not corrected, bony changes gradually occur; that is, the condition becomes structural. Functional postural deviations can be corrected through exercise and educational procedures.

Causes

Injury to bone, ligament, or muscle will weaken support at the point of injury. In the effort to relieve the injured part from the stress of weight bearing, postural adaptations will be made. For example, if the ankle or knee has been sprained, body weight will be shifted to the unaffected leg and the spine will assume a lateral curvature. During the time the injury is healing, postural habits may be formed that persist after the injury has healed. Coaches and physical educators should assume the responsibility for insuring that this does not occur by informing their injured students of this phenomenon.

Diseases. Diseases such as rickets, tuberculosis of the bones, or poliomyelitis may cause muscles or bones to lose their strength or range of motion. The antagonists of paralyzed muscles gradually shorten and pull the bones out of desirable alignment. Hereditary disorders such as spina bifida, congenital hip dislocation, osteochondrosis, wryneck, spondylolisthesis, cerebral palsy, and muscular dystrophy cause severe postural problems. Exercise programs for people suffering from these problems are beyond the scope of this text. Surgical procedures such as decreasing or increasing the length of muscles or tendons, removing or grafting bone, and transplanting of tendons may be used, in combination with braces and exercises to alleviate these conditions.

Other causes of poor posture are faulty habits, muscular weakness, or psychological problems. Posture, like many other routine activities of life such as ways of speaking, eating, walking, or sleeping positions, is a habit formed early in life. Family members, idols, and teachers provide models that may be emulated. Visual and hearing defects may cause postural deviations because the child, in straining to see or hear, twists or inclines the head or the entire body. Certain occupations, such as those where a weight is carried on one side of the body or where the head and trunk are bent over a desk, may lead to postural problems.

Muscular Weakness. Muscular weakness results in a fatigue slouch because this position requires the expenditure of less energy. Participation in vigorous leisure activities will prevent this problem from arising. The development and promotion of excellent school physical education and community recreation programs and work such as that done by the President's Physical Fitness Council and the many sports federations promoting and facilitating youth participation in a variety of sports will go a long way toward decreasing the incidence of muscular weakness.

Psychological Causes. When a person feels dejected or depressed, that person usually informs others of his emotional state through posture. The shoulders slouch, the head hangs, and the body gives to the pull of gravity. When a person feels confident, elated, or joyous, the posture is erect, the head is held high, the shoulders are pulled back, and the general impression is one of vitality. There can be no denying that there is a reciprocal relationship between emotional state and posture. Physical educators should point out this relationship and the influence of this aspect of "body language" upon the impression made upon others—particularly those of the opposite sex when they are between 12 and 22 years old.

Postural patterns may be symptoms of personality problems or emotional disturbances. Shyness and lack of confidence may be manifested by a drooping posture or the cocky posture of a short man may be overcompensation for feelings of inferiority.

Lordosis

An exaggerated lumbar curve caused by a forward tilt of the pelvis is called *lumbar lordosis* (Figure 12.13*a*). Lumbar lordosis is often associated with kyphosis (see Figure 12.15*b*), which is an exaggerated thoracic curve. One condition gives rise to the other because of the necessity for keeping the body

weight centered over the point of support. There is also hyperextension of the knees. An increase in the lumbar curve brings the spinous processes closer together and decreases the size of the openings between the vertebrae (foramina) through which the spinal nerves pass. This may cause pain due to the pressure placed upon the nerves. This pain may be "referred" to another area, usually the leg.

Flat Back

In flat back (Figure 12.13*c*) there is more than normal backward tilt of the pelvis and a

Figure 12.13 Postural deviations: (a) lordosis, (b) ptosis, (c) flatback

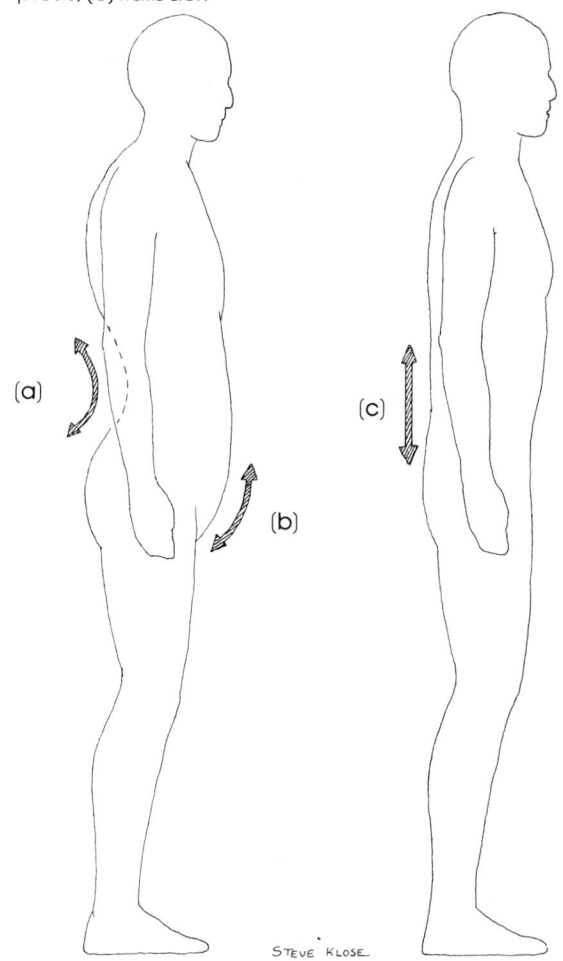

STEVE KLOSE

consequent decrease in the lumbar curve. Some believe that a flat back decreases the effectiveness of the shock-absorbing mechanism of the spine. In this condition, the hamstrings are shortened while the hip flexors and the iliofemoral ligaments are lengthened.

Forward Head

In this condition the neck is flexed and the head is held forward and downward (Figure 12.14*b*). "*Poke neck*" or *cervical lordosis* (Figure 12.14*c*) is a similar condition except that the head is held up. Many nearsighted people suffer from "poke neck." Postural exercises are of little help in correcting the latter condition. Forward head is usually associated with an increased thoracic curve. Occasionally, twisting or lateral flexion of the neck is present in this condition.

Round Shoulders

In this condition the scapulae are held in an abducted position and there is an increased thoracic curve (Figure 12.15*a*). Postural exercise programs are usually successful in correcting the condition. Round shoulders may be caused by structural differences such as relatively short clavicles or a large thoracic cage. These cases cannot be corrected nor should efforts be made to correct them. The condition is often associated with a forward head.

Protruding Shoulder Blades

In this condition the scapulae are in a position of upward tilt in which the posterior surfaces face slightly upward and the inferior angle protrudes from the back. The condition may be associated with round shoulders and round upper back. Inadequate strength in the muscles of the upper back is often a cause.

Round Upper Back

Round upper back, also called *thoracic* or *dorsal kyphosis* (Figure 12.15*b*), is a condition of increased curve in the upper back. Insufficient strength of the spinal extensors permits the spine to give to the pull of gravity resulting in an increased thoracic curve. In this position, the sternum is depressed and the rib

Figure 12.14 *Postural deviations of the cervical spine: (a) normal head position, (b) forward head, (c) cervical lordosis*

(a) (b) (c)

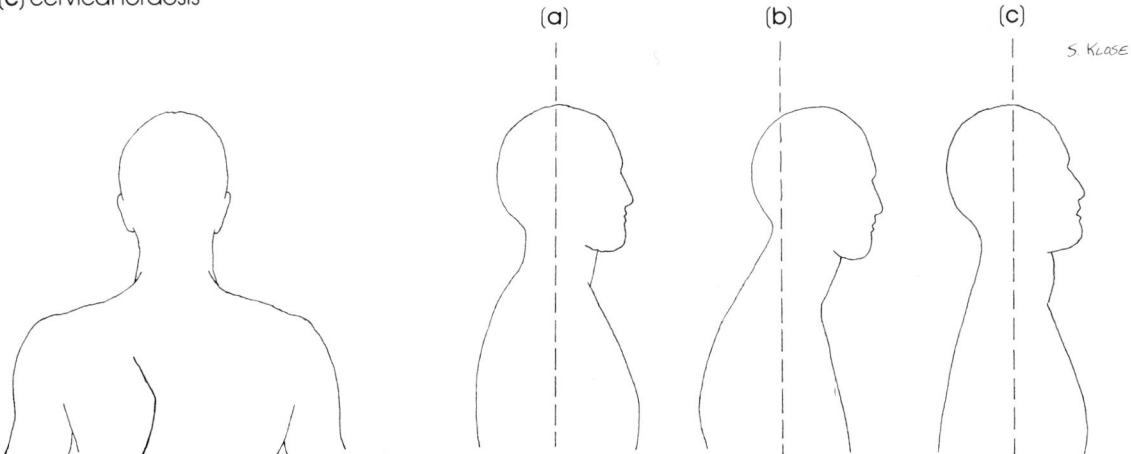

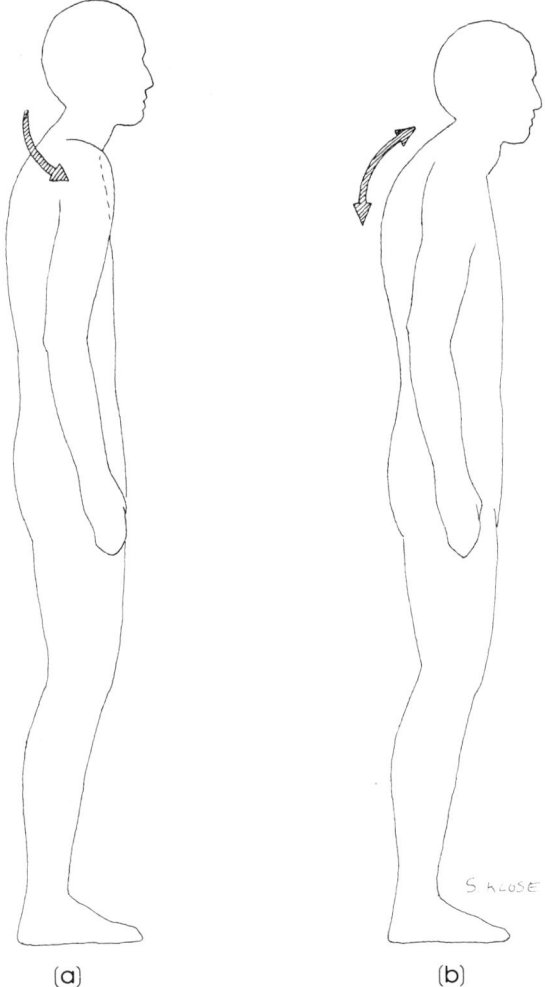

(a)   (b)

Figure 12.15 (a) Forward or round shoulders, (b) kyphosis

cage is lowered, resulting in a decrease in the thoracic volume. Exercises that strengthen the spinal extensors and stretch the flexors of the spine wil contribute greatly to correction of this condition.

Scoliosis

A lateral curvature of the spine in which there is longitudinal rotation of the vertebrae is the condition known as scoliosis. At its in-

ception, scoliosis is usually functional, as indicated by disappearance of the lateral curvature when the subject hangs by the hands. Ultimately, if poor posture continues, the condition becomes *structural*. At this point correction is extremely difficult and complex, and, for this reason, all cases of scoliosis should be referred to a physician. In cases of structural scoliosis, corrective exercises may produce a compensatory curve rather than correction of the primary curve. Scoliosis is sometimes the result of unequal visual or auditory acuity. In these cases, the student will habitually rotate the trunk and seek to place the stronger eye or ear in a more favorable position. For this reason, all students with scoliosis should be screened for unilateral vision and hearing defects. Seats and desks not adjusted to the proper height may force students to sit with a lateral curvature of the spine. Seating equipment should be checked to insure that adjustments are appropriate for the leg and trunk length of the individual student.

Scoliosis may be caused by defects in bone structure, damage to vertebrae, ligaments, or muscles due to diseases, a short leg, a flat or pronated foot, paralysis of the spinal muscles on one side, or a muscular development that is stronger on one side of the spine than it is on the other.

As has been pointed out earlier, the lateral curvature may be either a C curve or an S curve. If the convexity of the C curve is to the left, it is called a left C curve. In this case, the person's right shoulder will be lower than the other while the right hip will be higher than the left hip. In a right C curve, the convexity is to the right and the left shoulder will be lower and the left hip higher. Left C curves are usually present at birth while right C curves usually are those that develop after birth.

The upper curve in an S curve is referred to as the *primary curve* because the curve in the upper spine is usually present first. In most S curves, the primary curve is to the left and the right shoulder and hip are lower than their counterparts on the opposite side of the body.

Treatment of scoliosis may require use of corsets, adjustable frames, casts, and muscle re-education. Muscle re-education should be under the supervision of a physician. It should be pointed out that many postural deviations, whether anterior-posterior or lateral deviations, are caused by hereditary influences, and these problems involve the utilization of medical devices or instruments such as the Milwaukee and Boston braces.

Foot Defects

Each foot is made up of 11 intrinsic muscles, the tendons of 12 muscles whose bellies lie outside the leg, over 100 ligaments, tough protective fascia, and yards of blood vessels and nerves. The structure of the feet enables them to withstand the cumulative impact of hundreds of tons each day and to continue this throughout a lifetime. The feet deserve more consideration than they normally receive.

Flat feet are not necessarily painful or functionally inefficient. The feet of some people exhibit a loss of the arch only during weight bearing. This condition is not regarded as pathological unless there is loss of function or pain. Some people have a pad of fat on the plantar surface of the feet, which obliterates the arch even though the bones are in an arched position. *Pes planus*, or *true flat foot*, may be hereditary or congenital. It may not be pathological if no discomfort or functional inefficiency is present.

Functional flat feet, however, are the result of weak and stretched muscles, ligaments, and fascia. Discomfort and diminished functional capacity usually are present. Corrective exercises will ameliorate this condition.

Pronated feet are characterized by a toeing-out position of the feet, a prominent internal malleolus, a flat longitudinal arch, a curved tendon of Achilles, and, possibly, flat feet. This condition can usually be corrected through exercises and retraining in habits of standing and walking. *Pes cavis* is a defect in which the longitudinal arch is rigid and greatly exaggerated. *Pes equinous* is a condition in which the heel is raised due to permanent plantar flexion of the feet, which forces the individual to walk on the toes. These are two variations of *talipes* or *clubfoot*. Other talipes conditions are *calcaneus* (heel lower than the toes), *valgus* (toes and sole of foot turned out), *equinovarus* (a combination of talipes varus and talipes equinus), *calcaneovarus* (a combination of talipes calcaneus and talipes varus), *varus* (toes and sole of foot turned in), *equinovalgus* (a combination of talipes valgus and talipes equinus), and *calcaneovalgus* (a combination of talipes calcaneus and talipes valgus). When treatment is begun early, braces are effective in treating talipes if the deformity is mild. In many cases, however, surgery is necessary.

POSTURAL EXERCISES

Before an exercise program for improvement is begun, it is of great importance that the students be sufficiently motivated toward improvement of posture. It will be necessary for students to perform the exercises outside of class time and that the exercises be continued beyond the end of the semester. The time available during a one-semester class in physical education is inadequate to effect changes in posture. Additionally, other objectives such as improved organic fitness, improvement in sports or recreational skills, and improvement in social skills must be met.

The first step is to orient the student to the criteria of good posture and to help him or her experience the kinesthetic feel of desirable postural mechanics. The exercise program should begin only after determination that the deviation is functional rather than structural and after all pathological causes have been ruled out. At the beginning the exercise program should be mild but should continuously and progressively increase in intensity and duration with each exercise session.

Exercises for Lordosis

1. **Wall Sit (Figure 12.16).** A bench is placed against the wall. The student sits on the bench and pushes the trunk backward so that the lumbar area presses against the wall.

2. **Floor Sit (Figure 12.17).** The student sits on the floor with back against the wall and legs extended and presses the lumbar area against the wall.

3. **Flat Back (Figure 12.18).** While lying supine on the floor, the knees are flexed moving the feet upward toward the buttocks. While so doing, the back is pressed against the floor. The legs are next extended while the back is kept against the floor. Do 4 or 5 repetitions.

4. **Lying Tucks (Figure 12.19).** While in a supine position, draw the knees to the chest. Later, wrap the arms around the legs and pull the legs toward the chest. Do 10 to 25 repetitions.

5. **Hamstring Stretcher (Figure 12.20).** Sit on the floor with legs extended and straddled. The ankles are grasped and the trunk is pulled downward. Repeat 10 to 20 times.

Exercises for Flat Back

1. **Elvis' Pelvis.** Alternately, increase and decrease pelvic tilt. Increase pelvic tilt vigorously and quickly but decrease pelvic tilt gradually and passively.

2. **Back Bend (Figure 12.21).** Lie on the back with feet under the buttocks and the

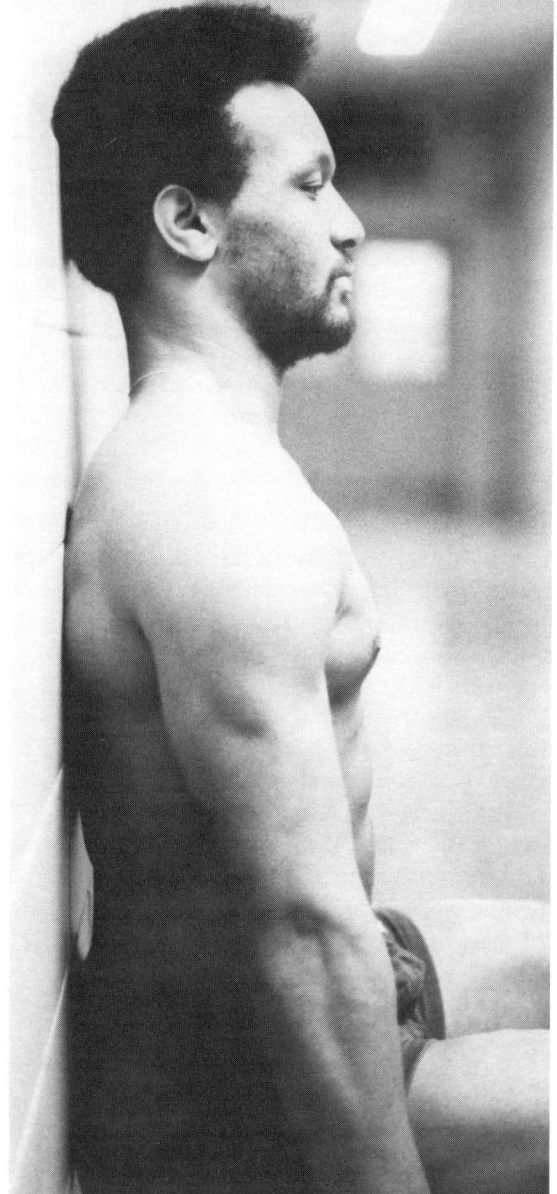

Figure 12.16 Wall sit

palms of the hands on the floor above the head with fingers pointing toward the feet. Extend arms and legs to push up into a back bend. A spotter can stand alongside with hands under the subject's lumbar area in the event the arms collapse. This exercise

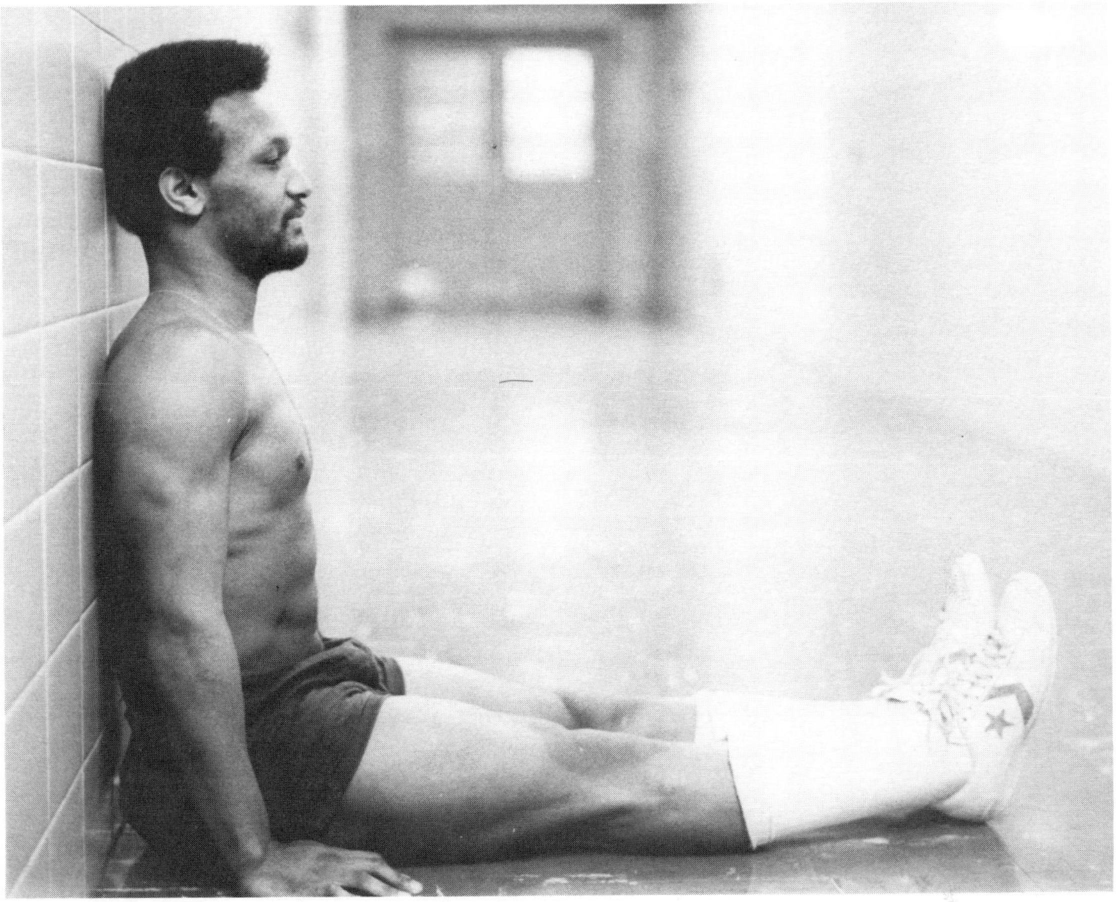

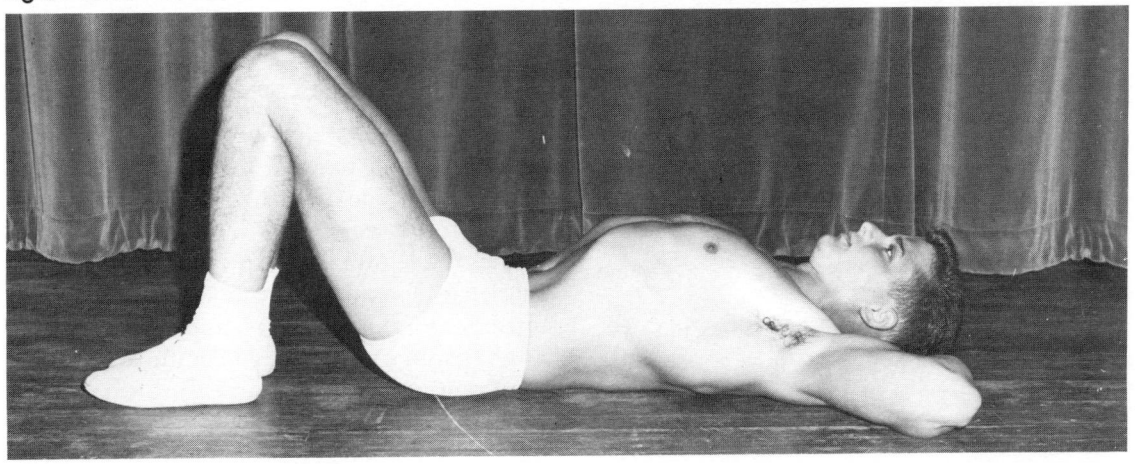

Figure 12.17 Floor sit

Figure 12.18 Flat back exercise

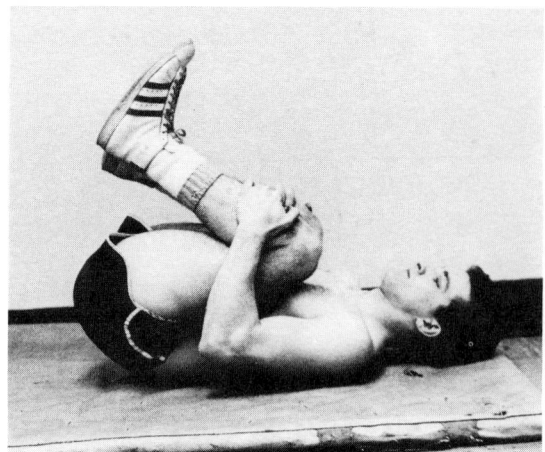

Figure 12.19 Lying tucks

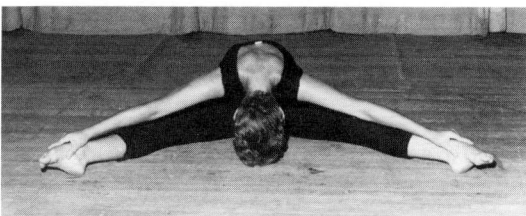

Figure 12.20 Hamstring stretcher

Figure 12.21 Back bend

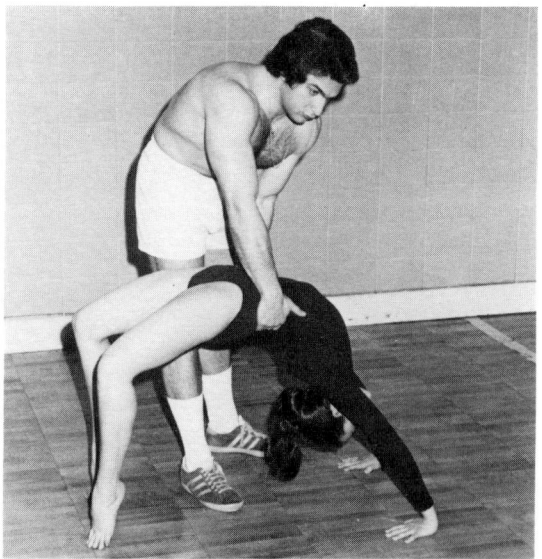

stretches not only the lumbar muscles but also those of the cervical, thoraxic, hip, and shoulder areas.

3. **Belly Out (Figure 12.22).** Stand with the back against the stall bars. Grasp a bar at about head level, or slightly higher, with the palms facing forward. Push the belly forward as far as flexibility will allow, extending the arms and legs at the same time. This exercise stretches the muscles and ligaments of the shoulder, hip, and thoracic areas as well as those of the lumbar area. Like the preceding exercise, it may also be used as a corrective exercise in cases of round upper back and round shoulders.

4. **Scale Push (Figure 12.23).** The student stands facing the wall with the feet approximately two feet from the wall. The hands are placed against the wall at chest height. A partner standing behind the student grasps one leg at the knee with one hand and at the ankle with the other and pushes upward and forward in line with the long axis of the bones of this leg. The push should gradually increase in force until the subject indicates tolerance limits have been reached. The position should be held 6 seconds. Both legs should be exercised. This exercise stretches the tendons of the muscles of the lumbar area and the hip extensors.

5. **Scale Bend (Figure 12.24).** The student stands approximately three feet from the wall with the trunk parallel to the floor and the hands placed against the wall. The partner grasps the knee and ankle of one leg and pushes the leg forward-upward for 6 seconds. Both legs should be stretched. Stretches the hip extensors, hamstrings, and muscles of the lumbar spine. The partner should apply pressure gently, gradually increasing the stretch until the student indicates tolerance limits have been reached.

APPLIED ASPECTS OF KINESIOLOGY

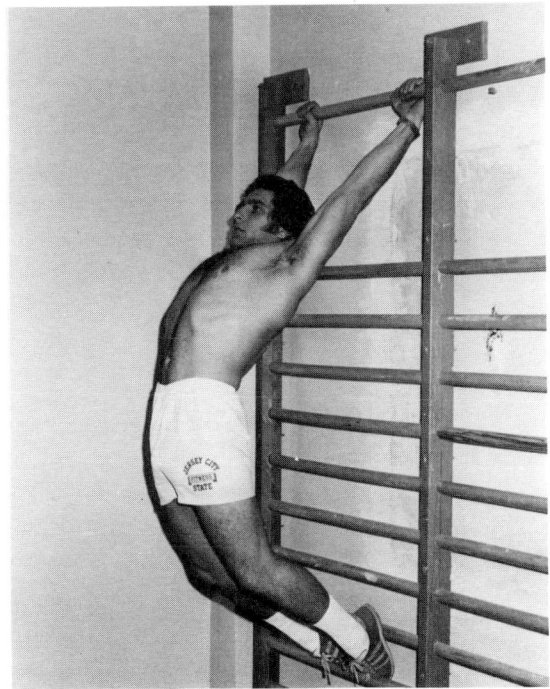

Figure 12.22 Belly-out exercise

Figure 12.23 Scale push

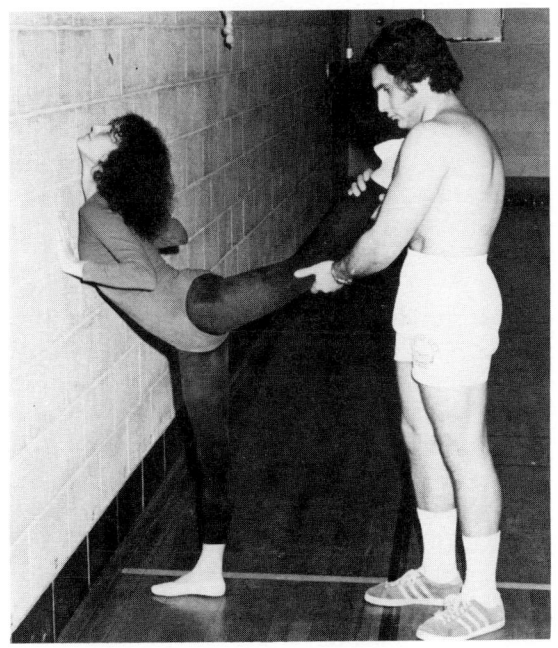

6. Chest Raiser (Figure 12.25). The student begins in a prone position with hands clasped behind the neck. A partner straddles the student's knees with her knees facing in the same direction and places her hands on the student's pelvis. The student pulls his chest and head upward as far as he is able and then returns to the starting position. Do 10 to 20 repetitions. Strengthens the cervical, thoracic, and lumbar extensors.

Exercises for Forward Head

1. Book Balance. The student walks about while balancing a book on top of the head. The chin should be tucked in.

Figure 12.24 Scale bend

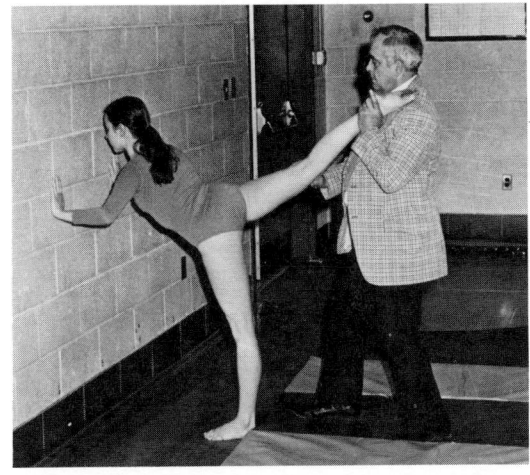

Figure 12.25 Chest raiser

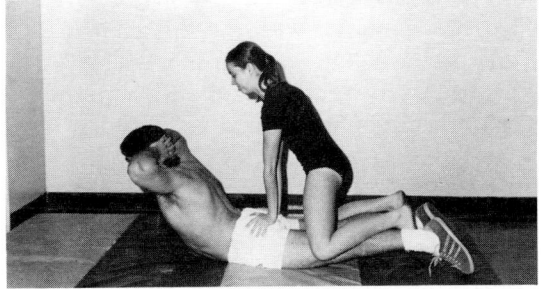

2. **Neck Press.** The hands are clasped behind the neck and the arms pulled forward while the head is pressed backward. Hold for 6 seconds.

3. **Wrestler's Bridge.** The student begins in a supine position. Feet are drawn up under the buttocks and then by pressing the head backward against the mat and pushing the hips upward, the body is lifted off the mat until it is supported only by the head and feet. Do 5 to 7 repetitions. See figure 11.4 in Chapter 11.

4. **Neck Wrestle.** The student lies prone. The partner kneels alongside, their heads facing, with both hands on the back of the partner's head. The student attempts to lift his head against the resistance provided by his partner. Hold for 6 seconds.

5. **Neck Iso Exercise (Figure 12.26).** The student holds a wide belt or towel against the back of the head as illustrated. He endeavors to push his head backward against the resistance provided by his arms through the belt. Hold for 6 seconds.

Exercises for Round Shoulders

1. **Elbow Pull.** The student places the fingertips behind the neck with the upper arms horizontal. The elbows are pulled backward as forcefully as possible and the position is held for 6 seconds.

2. **Backward Elbow Punch (Figure 12.27).** The student stands with the fists clenched in front of the chest and the elbows elevated. The elbows are pulled backward explosively in a horizontal plane. Do 10 to 20 repetitions. Stretches the pectorals while strengthening the trapezius, deltoids, and lower serratus.

3. **Chest Pull (Figure 12.28).** The student wraps each end of a twisted towel around

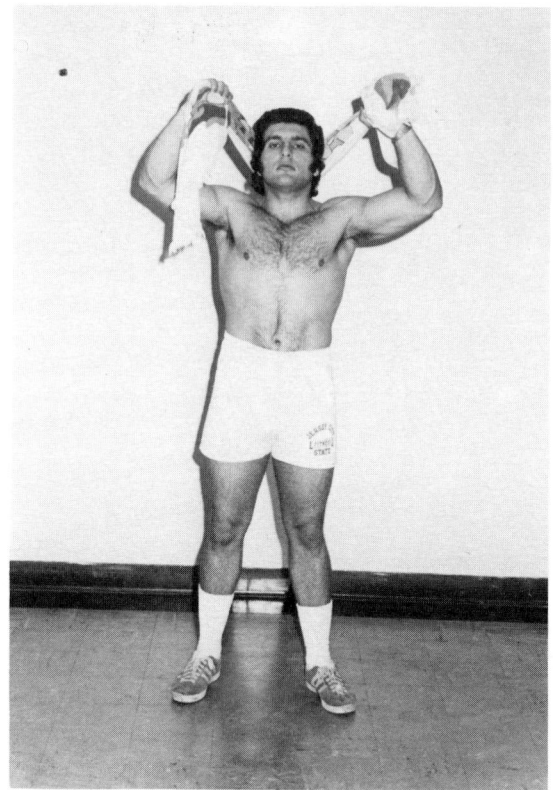

Figure 12.26 Neck iso exercise

each hand in such a manner that the hands will be two to eight inches apart when the hands are held in front of the chest. Holding his elbows up, the student endeavors to pull the towel apart for six seconds. Develops the posterior deltoids, lower serratus, and rhomboids.

4. **Assisted Horizontal Extensor-Abductor (Figure 12.29).** The student sits on the floor with legs extended and straddled and arms extended sideward at shoulder level with the palms facing forward. A partner kneels on one knee behind the student facing him, places one knee against his back, grasps his arms at the elbows, and exerts a steady backward pull in the horizontal plane. The subject should avoid resisting the pull but should inform the partner when his tolerence has

been reached. Hold for six seconds. Stretches the pectoralis and anterior deltoids.

5. Assisted Shoulder Hyperflexor (Figure 12.30). The student sits on the floor with the legs extended and straddled and arms extended overhead. A partner kneels on one knee behind him with the other knee against his back. He/she grasps his elbows and applies a steady backward pull to the arms. The subject should not resist the pull but should let the partner know when tolerance has been reached. Hold for six seconds.

6. Hang. Hang by the hands from a horizontal bar, horizontal ladder, or rings with the arms extended for as long as possible.

Exercises for Protruding Shoulder Blades

1. Elbow Downer (Figure 12.31). The student places clenched fists at the shoulder while holding the upper arms above the horizontal (Figure 12.31a). The elbows are pulled vigorously downward while holding the head up and fists back (Figure 12.31b).

Figure 12.27 Backward elbow punch

(a)

(b)

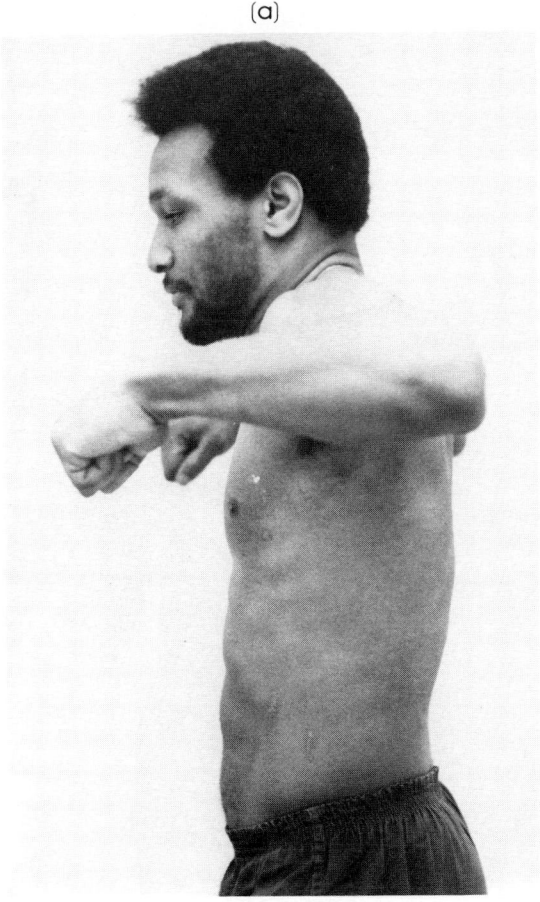
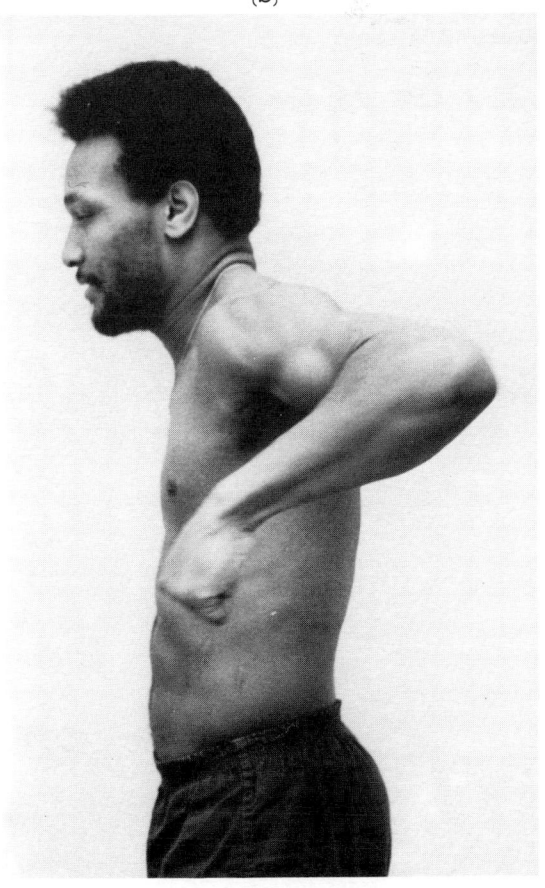

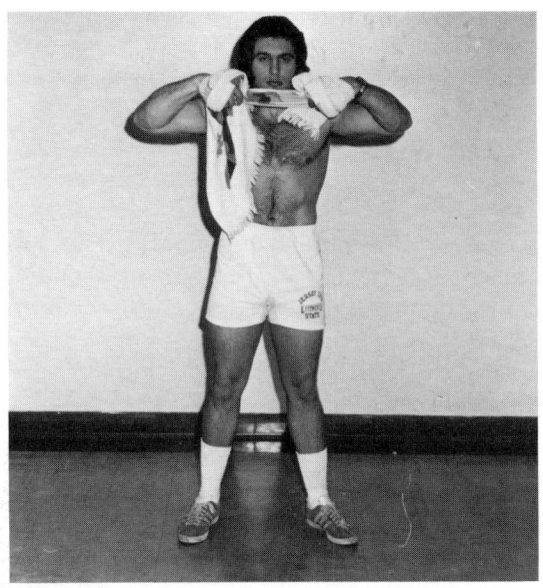

Figure 12.28 Chest pull

Figure 12.29 Assisted horizontal extensor-ab-ductor

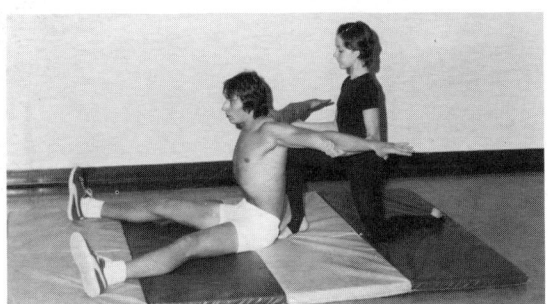

Figure 12.30 Assisted shoulder hyperflexor

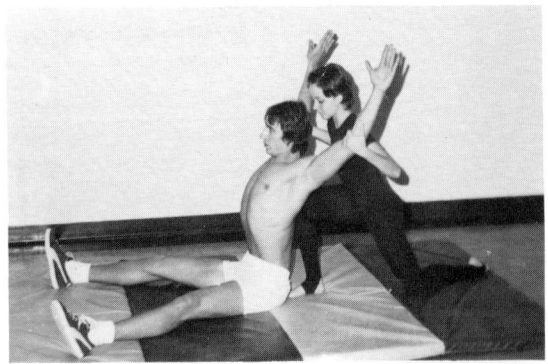

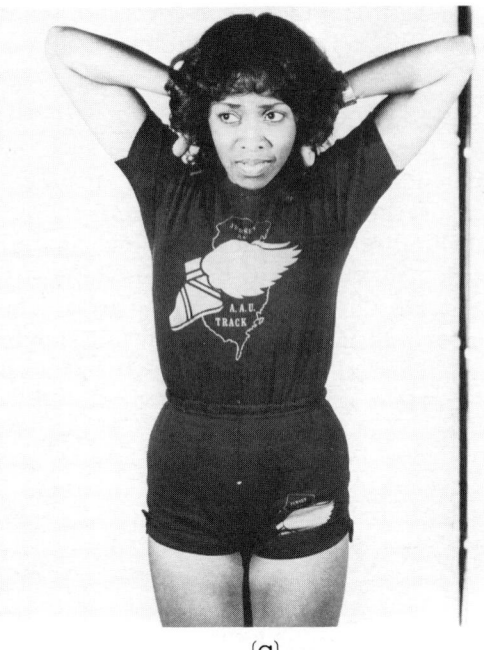

(a)

Figure 12.31 Elbow downer

(b)

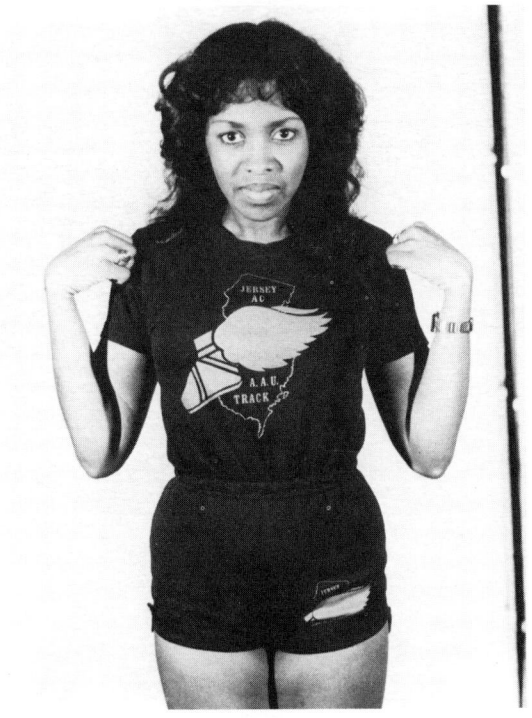

2. **Backward Throw.** The student stands with feet apart and arms at sides with the fists clenched. Arms are moved forward, upward, and backward behind the head while rising on the toes as the arms are directed overhead.

3. **Corner Stretch (Figure 12.32).** The student stands a foot or more from the corner of a room, places the palms against each wall with the arms horizontal at shoulder height, and leans forward with back straight until the chest is in the corner.

4. **Dumbbell Stretch.** The student lies supine on a narrow bench with feet on the floor. A dumbbell is held in each hand and the arms are extended sideward at shoulder level. The student avoids resisting the pull of the dumbbells and allows the weight to stretch the muscles of the chest.

5. **Bent-over Rowing (Figure 12.33).** The student stands with feet apart, legs extended, and trunk parallel to the floor. A barbell is held in the hands with arms extended and is then pulled to the chest and lowered to the starting position. A weight with which only 6 to 10 repetitions can be done should be used. As strength increases enabling the student to execute more repetitions, the resistance should be increased 5 to 10 pounds.

6. **Assisted Shoulder Hyperextensor (Figure 12.34).** The student sits on the floor with legs extended and straddled and the arms extended downward and backward behind the trunk. A partner stands behind and facing him, grasps his arms just above the elbows, and pulls slowly upward. The student should not resist the pull but should inform his partner when the limits of his tolerance have been reached. The partner should pull easily at first, gradually and slowly increasing the force.

Exercises for Round Upper Back

1. **Hands-up (Figure 12.35).** The student begins in a supine position with knees flexed, feet on the floor, and arms extended at the sides of the body with palms up (Figure 12.35a). The arms are moved along the floor to a position above the head (without increasing the lumbar curve (Figure 12.35b) and then returned to the starting position.

2. **Human Bow.** This exercise is begun in a prone position with arms extended beyond the head. The student then raises the head, trunk, and arms by arching the upper back. The abdomen should maintain contact with the mat. This can be facilitated by utilization of a partner who kneels straddling the subject's knees and who holds the lower back down by means of hand pressure against the pelvis.

3. **Chesty (Figure 12.36).** The student interlocks fingers behind the lower back and extends the arms, endeavoring to bring the elbows closer together. Hold for six seconds. Throughout the exercise, the head should be held up and the lower back should be held in position.

4. **Upper Back Stretcher (Figure 12.37).** The student sits on the floor with legs extended and straddled and hands clasped behind the head. A partner kneels on one knee behind and facing him, places the other knee between the shoulder blades of the student, grasps his elbows, and, while pushing the knee forward, pulls the elbows backward. This exercise stretches the thoracic spine, the pectorals, and the anterior deltoids. Hold for six seconds. The pull should be strong and steady, gradually increasing in force.

5. **Wing Lifts.** The student lies prone on a narrow bench while holding a dumbbell in each hand. The dumbbells are lifted side-

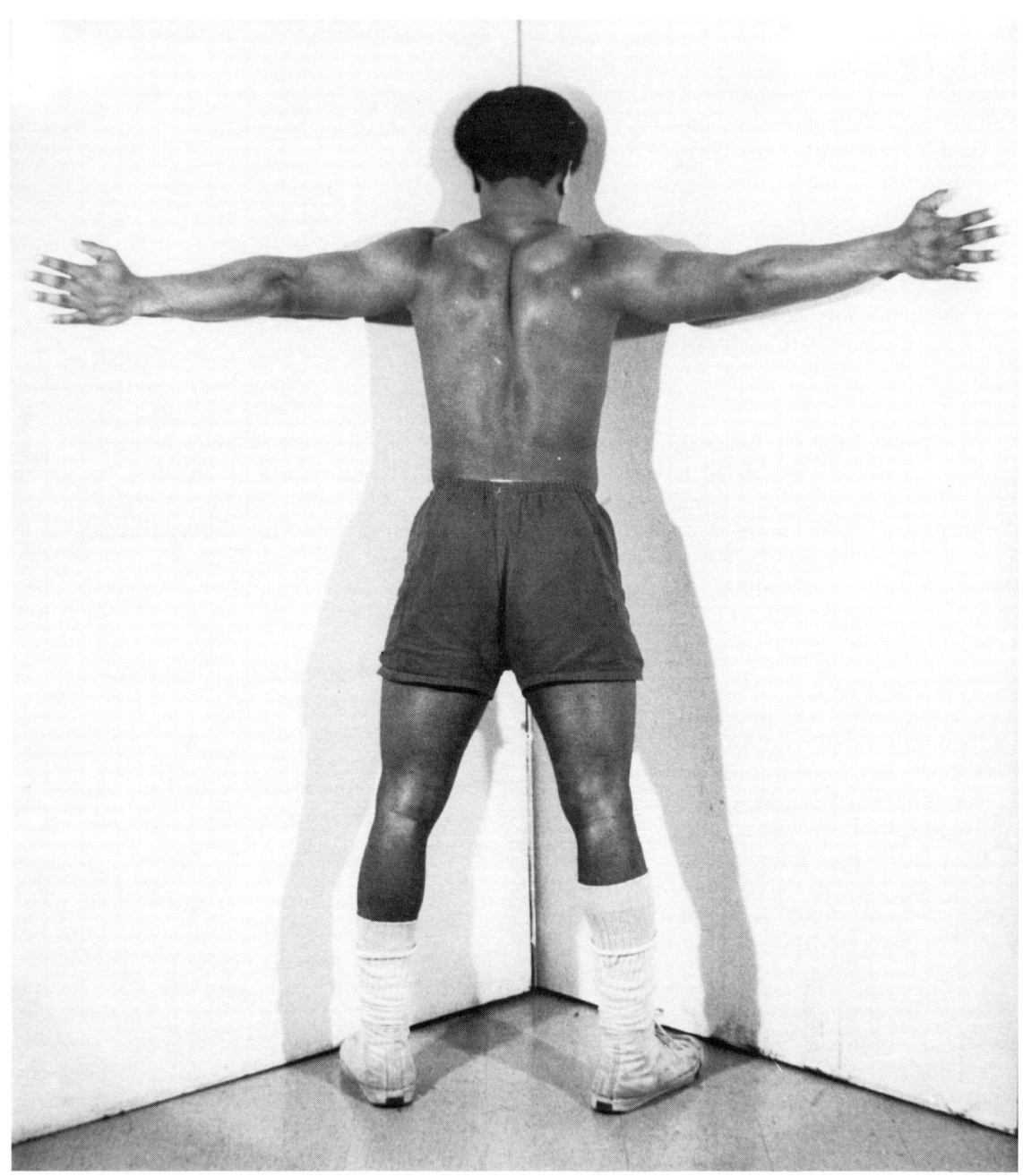

Figure 12.32 Corner stretch

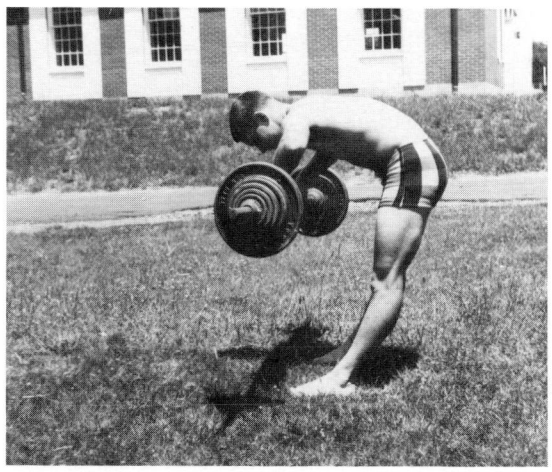

Figure 12.33 Bent-over rowing

ward as high as possible with the arms extended and then dropped downward with minimum resistance. Mats may be placed on the floor to prevent damage to the floor. Six to ten repetitions should be done with 60% to 70% of the maximum amount that can be lifted in one effort.

Exercises for Scoliosis

The reader is reminded, once again, that exercises for scoliosis should be given only under the direction of a physician.

Exercises for a C Curve with Convexity to the Left. When the convexity is toward the right, the instructions should be reversed.

1. **Hang.** Hang by the hands from a chinning bar, stall bar, or rings.

2. **Left Hand Push.** Standing with the right hand on the hip, push the extended left arm downward alongside the body as hard as possible. The body should be erect throughout the exercise. Hold for six seconds.

3. **Rib Push (Figure 12.38).** Standing with the right arm extended upward over the head, place the left hand against the ribs at the side of the body, push against the ribs and bend the trunk to the left. Push for six seconds.

4. **Lateral Thoracic Stretch (Figure 12.39).** Stand with the right side toward the stall bars, place the left hand against the left hip, grasp the stall bar over the head with the right hand, and allow the body to fall toward the right while continuing to hold the stall bar. Hold stretch for six seconds.

5. **Uneven Hang (Figure 12.40).** Face the stall bars and with the left hand grasp the highest bar that can be reached. Grasp a lower bar with the right hand, pull the feet off the floor and hang for six seconds.

6. **Reversed Fencer's Lunge (Figure 12.41).** From a stand, lunge forward with the left foot while maintaining the right foot in position. The left knee should be fully flexed while the right leg is extended rearward in line with the trunk. Raise the right arm to place it in line with the trunk while stretching the left arm backward.

Figure 12.34 Assisted shoulder hyperextensor

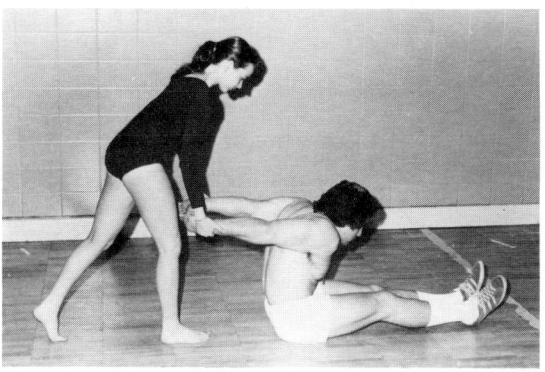

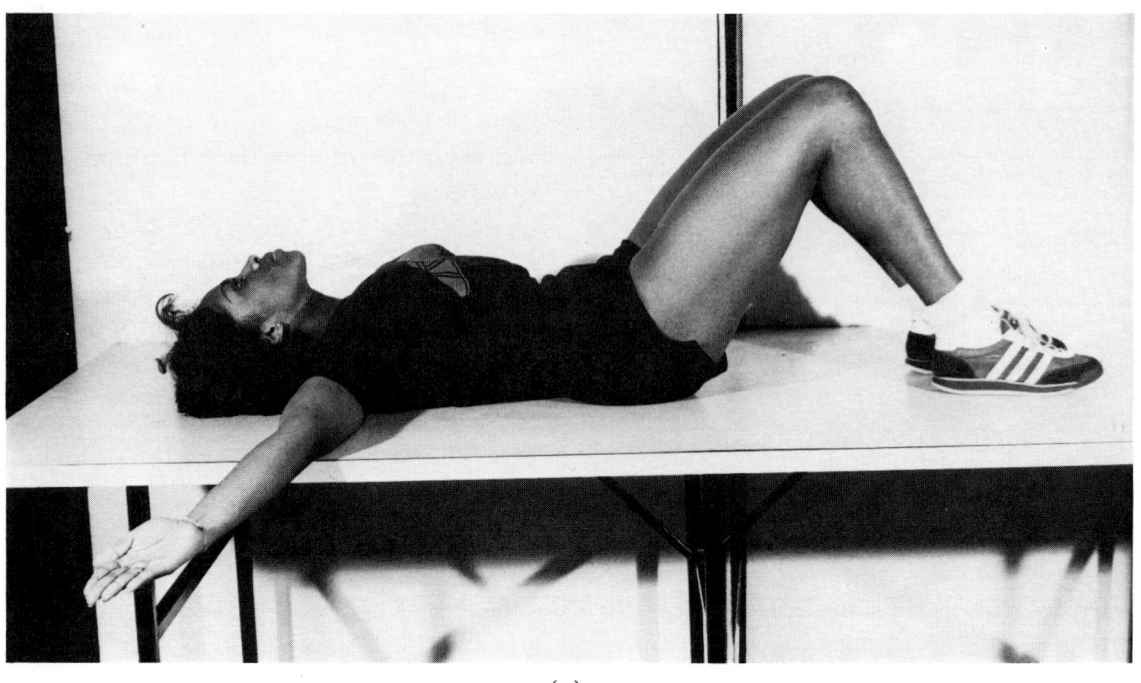

(a)

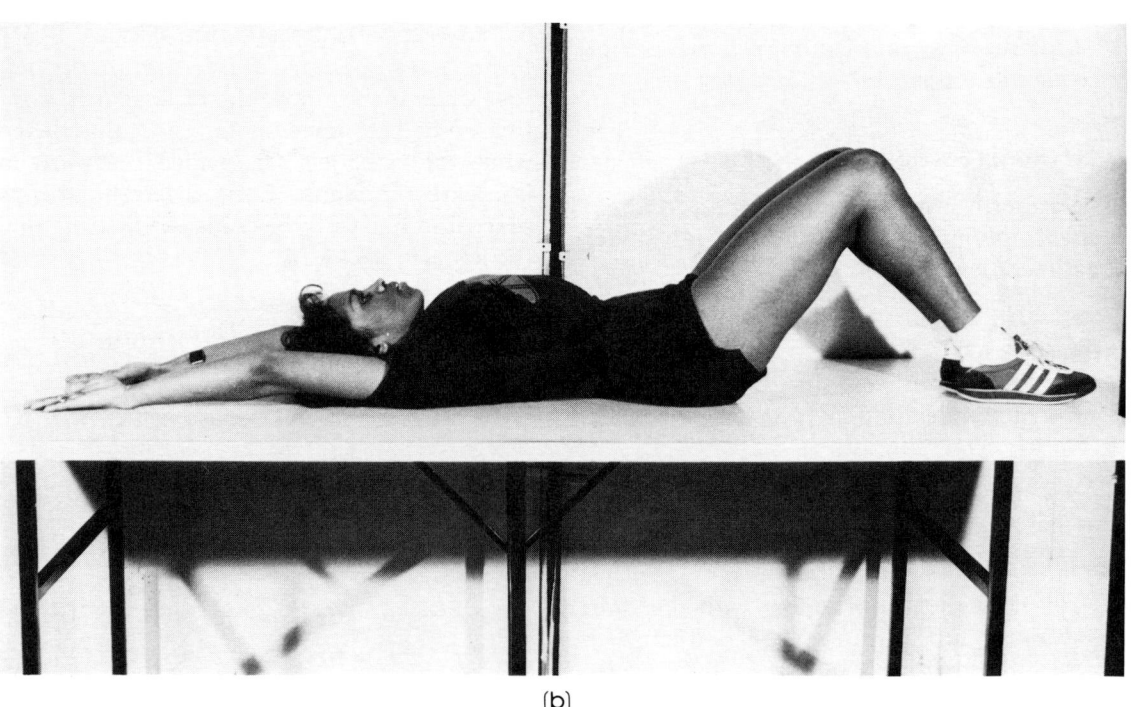

(b)

Figure 12.35 Hands-up exercise

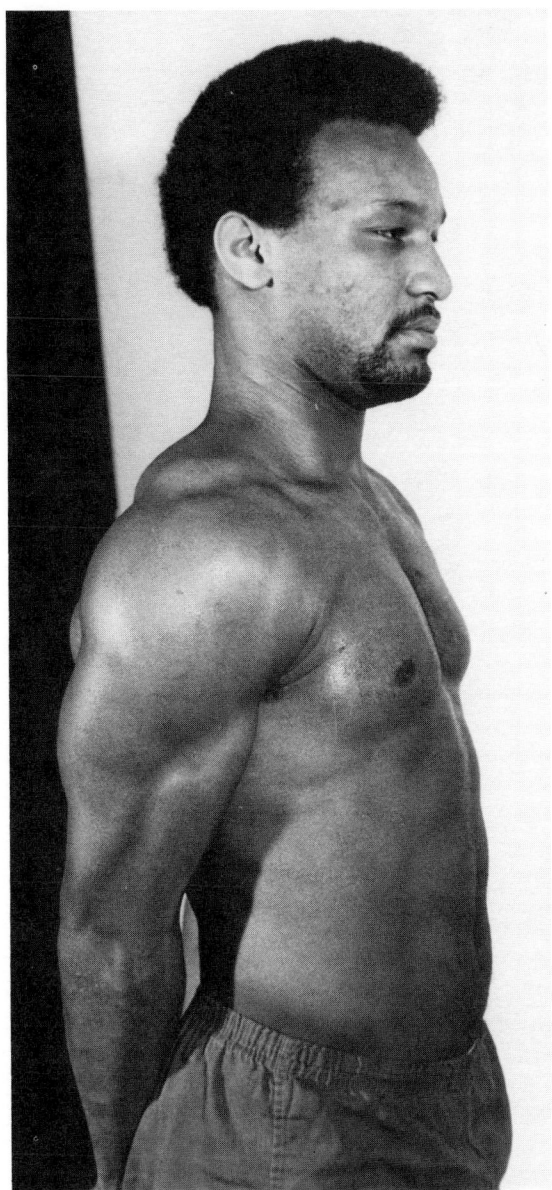

Figure 12.36 Chesty exercise

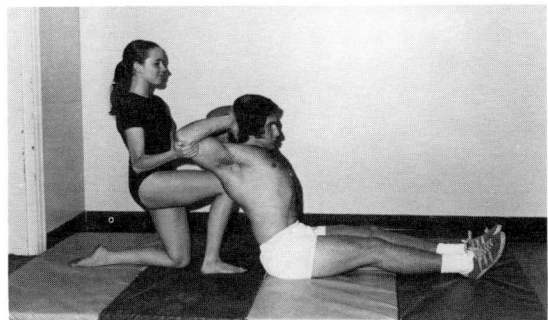

Figure 12.37 Upper back stretcher

Figure 12.38 Rib push

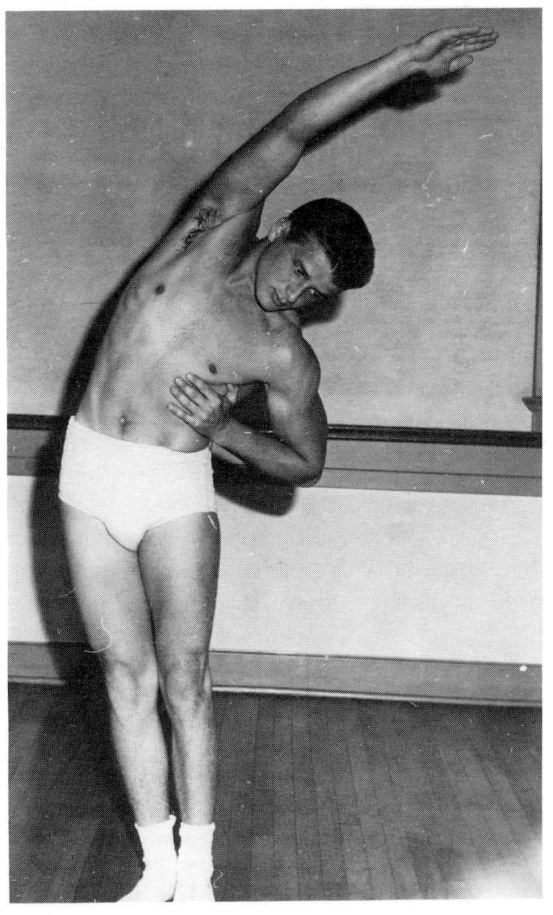

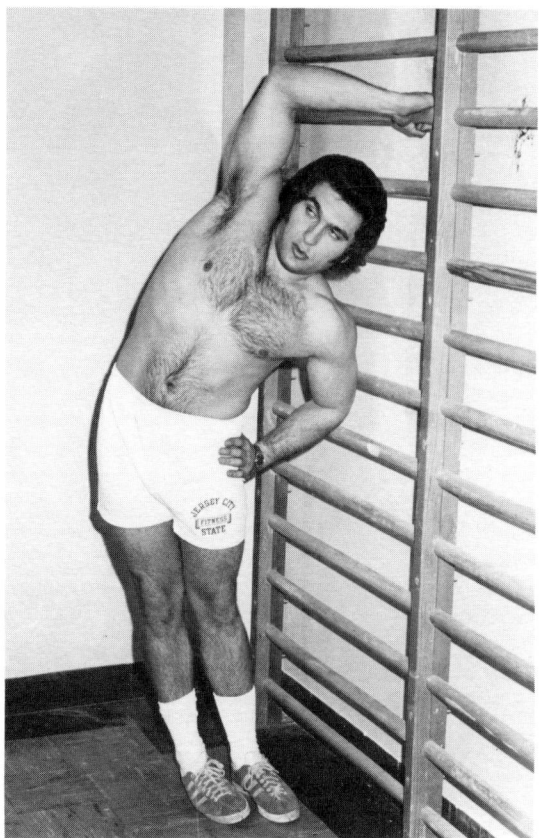

Figure 12.39 Lateral thoracic stretch

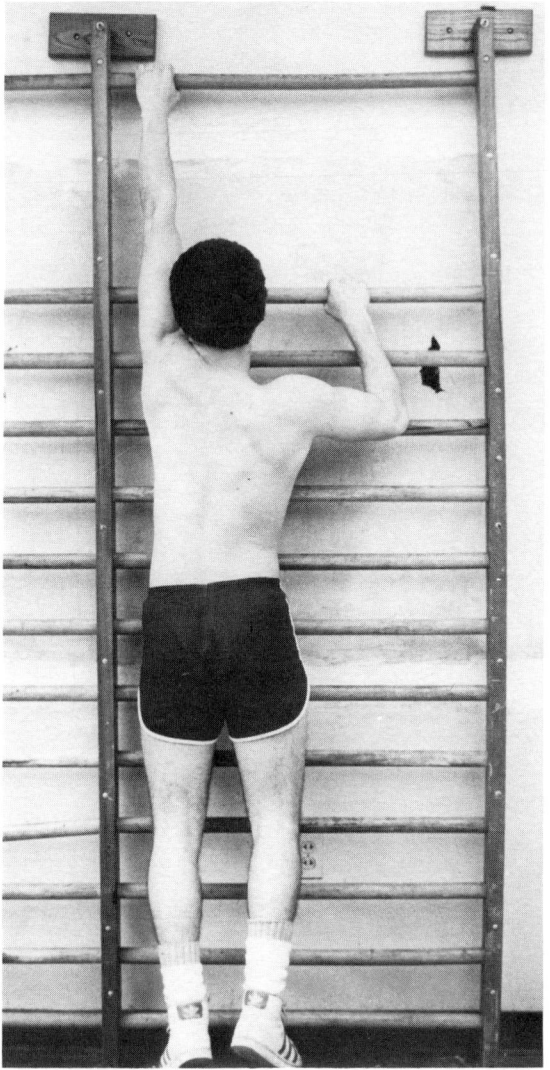

Figure 12.40 Uneven hang

Exercises for an S Curve (with left dorsal and right lumbar curve. Reverse the exercises for opposite curves).

1. **Lying Tuck.** While in a supine position, pull knees to the chest, wrap arms around the knees, and hold for one minute.

2. **Torsion Stretch (Figure 12.42).** While in a supine position, stretch the right arm upward beyond the head and at the same time stretch the left leg across the body.

3. **Creeping.** Walk on hands and knees on a mat moving continuously to the left. As the left arm moves forward, move the right knee forward and vice versa. Take increasingly long steps.

4. **Prone Arch (Figure 12.43).** While lying prone on the floor with the hands clasped behind the back, extend the arms forcefully while arching the body upward as far as possible. A partner can hold down the ankles or thighs.

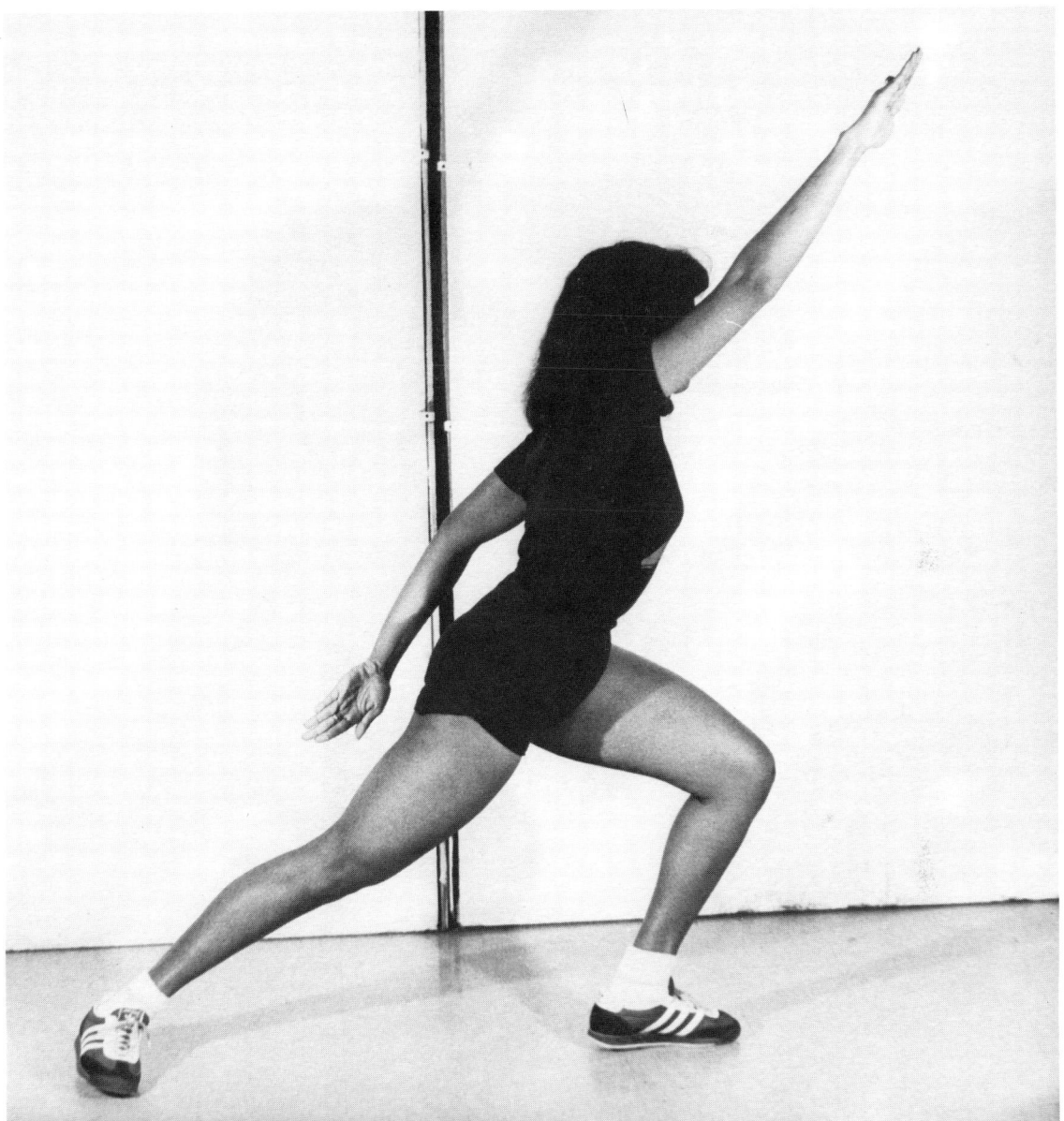

Figure 12.41 Reversed fencer's lunge

5. Front Support. Adjust the horizontal bar or one parallel bar to hip height. Grasp the bar with a front grip and push downward on the bar until the feet are off the floor.

6. Crooked Hang (Figure 12.44). Face the stall bars and grasp a bar at reaching height with the left hand. Grasp a bar two rungs lower with the right hand. Slowly slide the

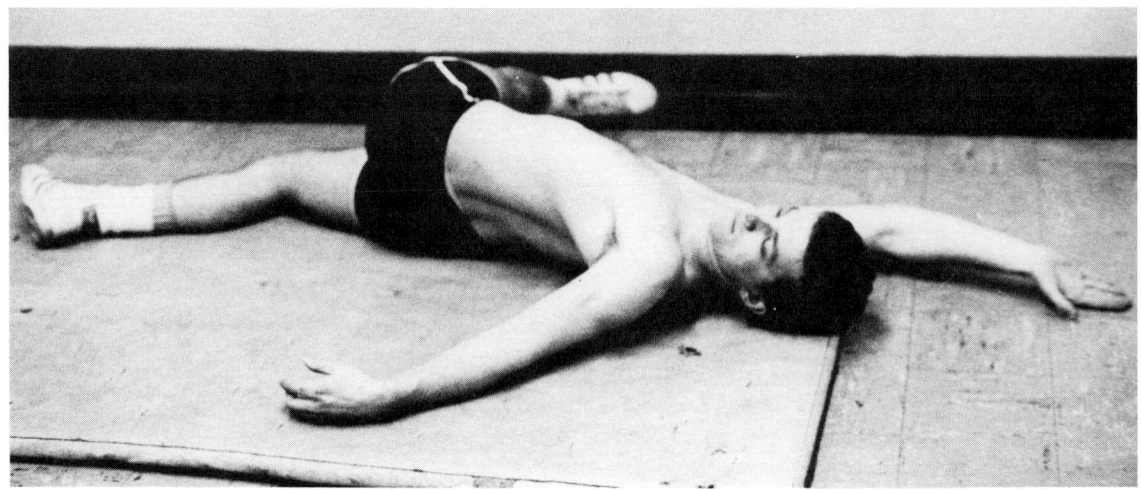

Figure 12.42   Torsion stretch

Figure 12.43   Prone arch

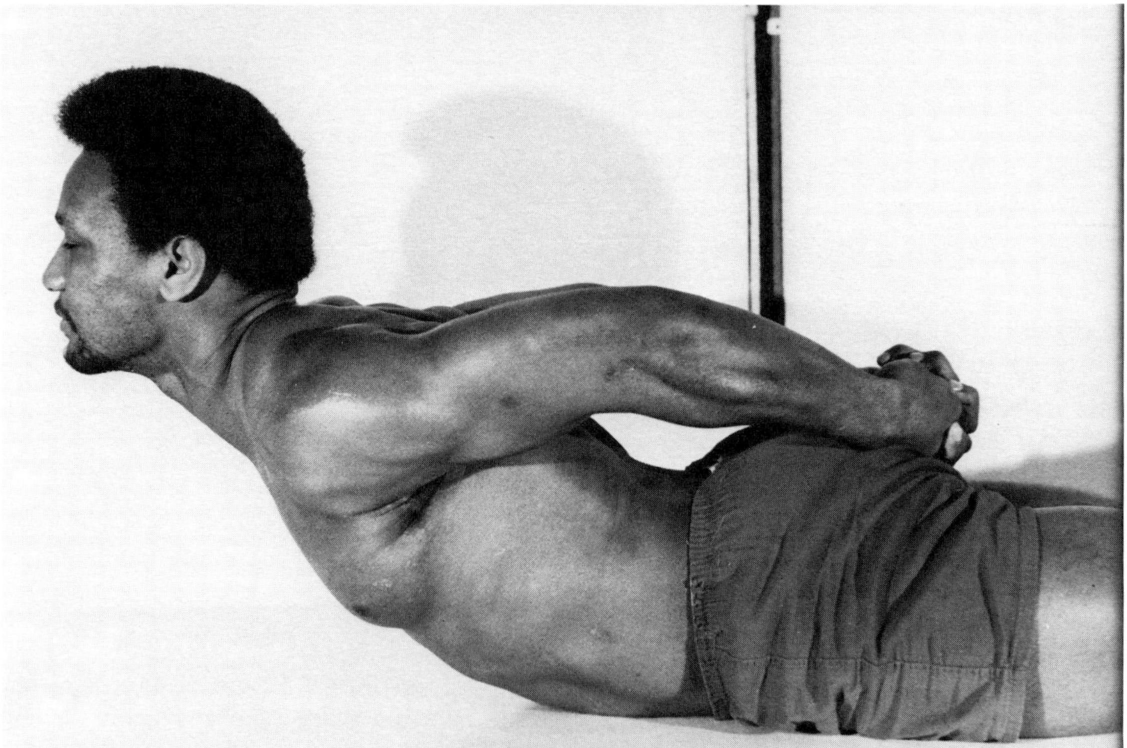

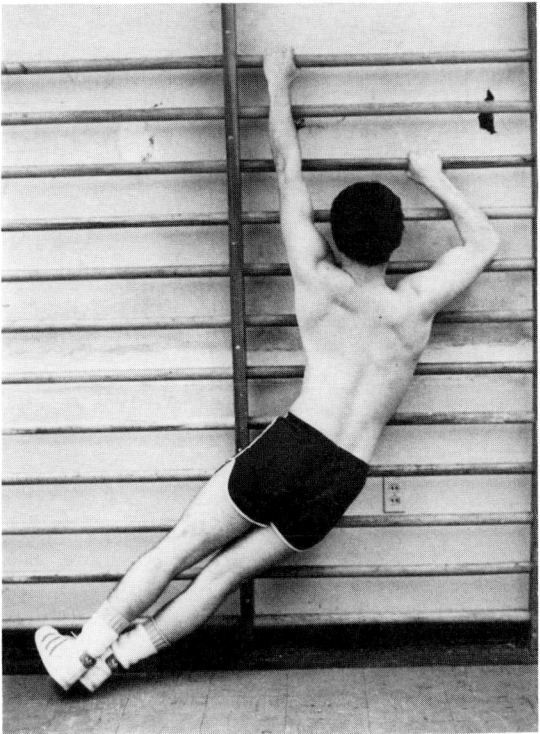

Figure 12.44 Crooked hang

feet toward the left until the body is hanging in a curved position.

Note: Some of the preceding exercises are from: Hollis F. Fait, *Special Physical Education*, W. B. Saunders Company, Philadelphia, 1978, Fourth Edition, pp. 376–381.

SUMMARY

When man's early ancestors became arboreal, structural changes occurred over the millennia that enabled him to become the dominant animal, but these changes also caused several health problems from which modern man suffers. Among the structural changes were (1) an increased range of mo-

tion in the direction of extension of the hip joints, (2) an increase in the mobility of the shoulder girdle, (3) an increase in the mobility of the hand and wrist adapting the hand for grasping, (4) a decrease in the anterioposterior diameter of the thorax, (5) a backward displacement of the scapulae, (6) a broadening and lengthening of the foot, (7) a shortening, thickening, and broadening of the pelvic bones, (8) development of the lumbar curve, (9) an elevation of the center of gravity, and (10) an increase in strength and size of the gluteal, quadricep, and extensor muscles of the vertebral column and a decrease in the strength and tone of the abdominal muscles.

The erect position freed man's forelimbs, enabling their use in performing a variety of tasks, while the increased mobility of his wrist, hand, and fingers enabled the fashioning and use of tools. Many anthropologists attribute the development of man's brain to the maneuverability of the hand, which enabled the use of tools.

The erect position, however, has caused man to suffer some aches and pains not suffered by other animals. The most common of these is low back pain usually due to increased inclination of the pelvis. Visceral ptosis and greater difficulty in returning blood to the brain are other problems created by the erect position.

Structure and body-type differences, obesity, pregnancy, injuries, birth defects, and illness produce necessary changes in alignment of body segments and of posture. In some cases orthopedic devices can aid in solution of these problems. Psychological states, self-concept, the state of mental health, and emotions also influence postures.

Long-used tests of static posture, such as the plumb-line test, do not take into consideration anatomic differences such as an unusually large thorax or breasts, short clavicles, the relationships between the anterior and posterior vertical dimensions of vertebrae, and the location of the acetabula on the horizontal dimension. Most posture tests evaluate only erect static posture. Erect static posture is assumed for only a tiny fraction of the total time of each day. Thousands of postures are assumed during the course of each day by every person. Three dynamic, or moving, postures were discussed: walking, running, and lifting.

Walking is a reflex action in which each leg acts like a pendulum with the axis of the pendulum at the hip joint during the forward swinging phase and with the axis at the foot (and the pendulum upside down) during the support phase as the body moves forward over the foot. Walking, unlike running, involves a period of double support when both feet are simultaneously in contact with the ground. Eight common walking errors were presented.

It was pointed out that running differs from walking in that in the run there is no period of double support, there is a period of no support, the foot strikes the ground directly under the center of gravity rather than forward of it, the horizontal component of force is greater, and the pelvis is carried lower. Details of the sprint start and run were presented and kinesiologic analyses were made.

When lifting weights, the weight should be kept as close to the line of gravity as possible to decrease the length of the resistance moment arm and the shearing forces upon the lumbar vertebrae. A mechanical analysis of the clean and jerk used in competitive weight lifting was made.

The role of a number of muscles in the maintenance of the alignment of body segments to which they are attached was discussed. The muscles that must be stretched and those that must be strengthened in the prevention and correction of such conditions as visceral ptosis, hernia, round shoulders, winged scapulae, lordosis, and scoliosis were

presented. Work and sports activities that may contribute to development of postural deviations or that may be used to ameliorate these conditions were also discussed.

The rationale for maintenance of vertical alignment of body segments, adjustment of the center of gravity so that it is centered on the base of support, and displacement of the center of gravity to the edge of the base of support under certain circumstances (racing start, an impending impact, or wind) was presented. The stimuli for maintenance of postural tonus arise from the labyrinthine righting reflexes, visual or optical reflexes, proprioceptive reflexes, plantar reflexes, stretch reflexes, and reflexes acting on the head. The manners in which these reflexes influence body positions as well as procedures for their development were discussed.

The differences between structural and functional postural deviations were explained. The causes of postural deviations may be injury, diseases, or hereditary disorders. In most of these cases, surgical procedures and the prescription of braces in addition to exercise is necessary. Other causes of poor posture are faulty habits, muscular weakness, psychological problems, visual and hearing defects, and occupations that require assumption of certain positions for long periods of time. Each of these cases was discussed.

Postural conditions such as lordosis, flat back, forward head, round shoulders, protruding shoulder blades, round upper back, and scoliosis, and foot defects such as pes planus, functional flat feet, pronated feet, pes equinus, pes cavis, and talipes were defined and their causes explained. The interrelationships between several of these conditions was discussed.

A number of exercises for each of the postural conditions were presented. Several general suggestions were made for the initiation and conduct of this exercise program.

REFERENCES

1. Steindler, Arthur, *Kinesiology of the Human Body under Normal and Pathological Conditions.* Springfield, Ill. Charles C Thomas, 1955, pp. 234–235.
2. Cooper, John M., and Glassow, Ruth B., *Kinesiology*, 4th ed. St. Louis: C. V. Mosby, 1976, p. 192.
3. Steindler, *op. cit.*, p. 170.
4. *Ibid.*, pp. 232–233.
5. Fait, Hollis F., *Special Physical Education*, 4th ed. Philadelphia: W. B. Saunders, 1978, p. 363.
6. Rasch, Philip J., and Burke, Roger K., *Kinesiology and Applied Anatomy*, 6th ed. Philadelphia: Lea and Febiger, 1978, p. 395.
7. Saito, M., Kobayashi, K., Miyashita, M., and Hoshikawa, T., "Temporal Patterns in Running," *Biomechanics IV* (R. Nelson and C. A. Morehouse, editors). Baltimore: University Park Press, 1974, pp. 106–111.

13

KINESIOLOGICAL CONCEPTS OF INJURY PREVENTION

CONCEPTS

1. The formula for kinetic energy (½ mass × velocity squared) indicates that with respect to the human body, velocity is the important consideration in prevention of injury since the body mass cannot be changed.

2. The principle of conservation of energy requires that the work done to absorb the kinetic energy of a moving body be equal to the kinetic energy. Since work done is force times the distance over which it is applied, the work done or force times distance = $\frac{1}{2} mv^2$.

3. A falling body accelerates at the rate of 32.2 ft/sec/sec; therefore, the greater the height from which an object falls, the greater will be its kinetic energy upon landing or being caught.

4. The greater the time over which kinetic energy can be absorbed, the less the probability of injury.

5. Injury may be prevented by decreasing the length of a lever arm through which a potential injury-producing force acts.

6. Soft tissues of the human body, such as muscle or fat, possess greater elasticity than bone and, for this reason, injury may be prevented by turning or twisting to receive an impact upon the buttocks, thighs, or shoulder rather than an area where bone is near the surface.

7. Muscular strength must be adequate, with respect to the distance through which force is applied, to absorb the kinetic energy possessed by an object (ball, football, etc.) or the human body (during a dismount, jump, etc.).

8. Strong muscles contribute to prevention of injury to joints and bones by providing more padding as well as furnishing a greater stabilizing component of force to joints.

9. The thoracic cage, because of its mobility, flexibility, and curved surface, can absorb a surprising amount of force without injury.

10. Injury can be prevented by distributing an impact over a greater surface area since there will then be less force per square inch.

11. "Spearing" and use of helmets with face and nose guards greatly increase the probability of cervical fracture, severing of the spinal cord, and paralysis.

12. Basketball players, due to their high center of gravity and, consequently, greater propensity for falls, suffer principally from injury to the wrists, elbows, and head.

13. Since the advent of the rigid plastic boot used in skiing, the incidence of sprains and fractures of the ankle have decreased while fractures of the tibia and fibula have increased.

14. Molded face masks used by ice hockey goal tenders provide little protection, while wire masks provide the greatest protection of all types of masks.

15. Little League pitchers are prone to suffer traumas of the shoulder and elbow joints and the surrounding muscles due to forceful pronation and supination of the forearm and inward and outward rotation of the humerus.

16. The spotter should stand as close to the performer as possible in order to keep his forearm or entire arm more nearly vertical so that greater lift force can be provided due to a shortened resistance arm.

17. Injury resulting from landing on water can be minimized by entering the water vertically, with the body streamlined and stabilized.

GENERAL CONSIDERATIONS

Physical education and athletic programs use vigorous physical activities as their educational media. Force is utilized to propel the body through space, to propel an implement, or against an opponent to force him off balance or to push him out of the way. Dynamic balance must be maintained as the body moves through unusual positions. These factors increase the probability of injury. They make it more likely that a person will suffer an injury while engaged in sports than while engaged in sedentary activities. It is likely that it is this risk factor (and the inherent challenge of avoiding injury while accomplishing the physical skill) that is attractive to many sports participants.

That the incidence of injury has not been considerably higher than it has is a testament to the effectiveness of physical education teachers, sports coaches, and manufacturers of sporting goods. However, although injuries will never be completely eliminated, their frequency could be substantially lowered through improved design of athletic equipment, more rigorous standards of physical conditioning, and improved instructional and coaching procedures. The science and the study of kinesiology can contribute to all three of these areas. Kinesiology is concerned with force, impact, absorption of force, ki-

netic energy, rebound, equilibrium, range of movement of body joints, and torsion and stress limitations of bones and muscles. All of these are important considerations in the prevention of injury.

An understanding of the kinesiologic principles involved in these considerations will enable those involved in teaching various forms of human movement to decrease the incidence of injury among their students. They will be able to deduce the most effective techniques for absorbing force and impact, the part of the body with which to accept an impact, procedures for maintenance of dynamic balance, and techniques for decreasing the probability of injury when falling into water. They will be better able to appraise the force-absorption qualities of protective equipment and, consequently, to make more informed decisions when purchasing sports equipment.

ABSORPTION OF KINETIC ENERGY

The application of force is necessary to give an object impetus or to cause it to move. After the object is in motion it possesses kinetic energy due to its motion. The greater the object's velocity, the greater its kinetic energy. Further, the greater the object's mass, the greater its kinetic energy. This relationship is shown by the formula for kinetic energy:

$$KE = \tfrac{1}{2}\, mv^2$$

When the object stops moving, it no longer has any kinetic energy.

To absorb the kinetic energy of a moving object requires that the amount of work done be equal to the kinetic energy of the object. Work done equals the product of the weight (or force) times the distance it is moved. Where F = force and d = distance through which the force is applied, the formula

$$Fd = \tfrac{1}{2}\, mv^2$$

illustrates that to absorb the kinetic energy of an object, the force must be greater as the distance through which it is applied is decreased. Conversely, the greater the distance through which force is applied, the less force necessary to absorb the object's kinetic energy.

When a gymnast dismounts from the apparatus and his body is dropping toward the mat, the kinetic energy within his body at the moment the mat is contacted will equal ½ mv^2. The gymnast's mass is constant but his velocity will be dependent upon the height from which he drops. His acceleration during the drop will be 32.2 ft/sec/sec. He will absorb this kinetic energy through eccentric contractions of his hips, knees, and plantar flexor muscles. In the event there was a horizontal component of force, he must, if he is to maintain equilibrium, land with his feet forward of his forward-moving center of gravity. He can maximize the distance through which the kinetic energy is absorbed by landing with his knees and hips almost, but not quite, fully extended. His muscles must possess sufficient strength to generate force adequate to absorb the kinetic energy through the distance available through eccentric muscular contraction (see Figure 13.1). For additional information regarding kinetic energy see Chapter 6.

The baseball or football player when catching the ball reaches outward toward the ball to increase the distance over which the kinetic energy of the ball may be absorbed. Upon receiving the ball, the arm is flexed and, if the ball's velocity is very great, the body is rotated and a step backward is taken to further increase the distance.

The probability of injury to the shoulder joint is increased when catching a line drive with the arm extended overhead because of the long resistance lever. The moment of force, in this case, is the product of the force of the impact and the perpendicular distance from the shoulder joint to the ball's line of flight at the moment it is caught. To prevent injury, the player can shorten the lever arm immediately after catching the ball by flexing his elbow slightly. He can also reach forward before catching the ball and, after it contacts his glove, allow his arm to be carried backward.

INJURY AND REBOUND PRECEPTS

When two objects collide, they rebound from one another. The direction, speed, and distance of the rebound is determined by both objects' elasticity, mass, and velocity, friction between the objects, rotations, and the angle at which they meet, as explained in Chapter 6.

The elasticity of an object is its ability to return to its original size and shape after the impact, force, or stress is removed. The change in shape or distortion is called *strain* and is determined by the amount of force or stress acting on the object. Some materials have greater resistance to distortion than others and regain their original shape after being deformed. Steel can withstand considerable stress. Sheetrock cannot. A rubber ball has considerable elasticity and will quickly regain its original shape after an impact. A ball of putty will not. The soft tissues in the human body possess considerably more elasticity than do bones. For this reason, it is preferable to receive an impact on the soft tissues than on an area where the bone is near the surface. A kick to the shin bone is likely to inflict greater injury than a kick of equal force to the posterior side of the lower leg, which is well protected by soft tissue—the gastrocnemius and posterior tibialis muscles. When a fall or receipt of a blow is eminent, injury can often be prevented or minimized by turning the body or moving so that the impact is received by an area with ample soft tissue such as the buttocks, arms, or thighs.

Although there is relatively little soft tissue on the chest, blows of considerable force can

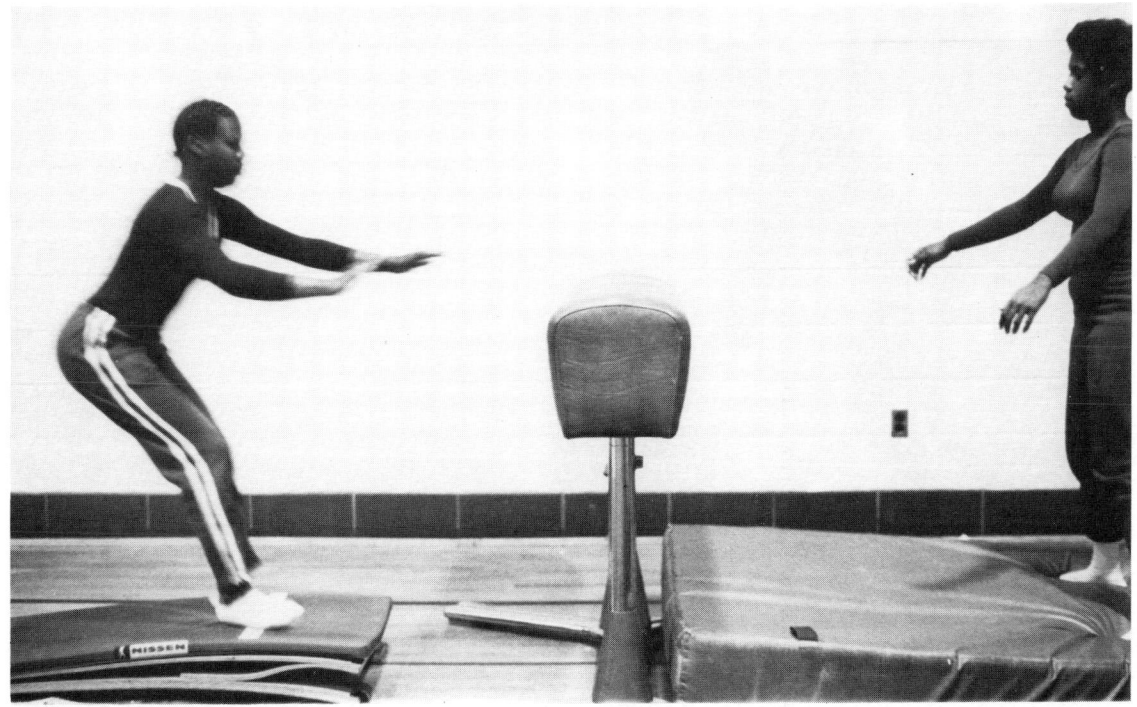

Figure 13.1   Straddle Vault over Side Horse
Figure 13.1a Note angle of legs (blocking action) to convert horizontal momentum into a vertical direction

be received in this area without injury due to the construction of the thoracic cage. The bowed shape of the ribs, their cartilaginous attachments, and the mobility of the sternum due to one end being free give the thoracic cage considerable elasticity.

The learning of gymnastic skills has been made considerably safer by the use of "crash pads"—mats 6 to 12 inches thick. These mats have much elasticity and, consequently, absorb the impact of the human body quite well. Catcher's mitts utilize the same principle. The thick padding increases the distance over which the ball's kinetic energy is absorbed and also distributes the impact over a greater surface area.

Injury can often be prevented by distributing the force of an impact over a greater surface area. If 500 pounds of force is focused on an area of one square inch, the force of impact equals 500 pounds per square inch. If this 500 pounds of force is distributed over an area 10 inches by 10 inches or 100 square inches, the impact force will be only 5 pounds per square inch. Professional wrestlers and karate experts utilize this principle when they land on the entire surface of the upper back and slap their arms backward into the mat. Trampolinists utilize the principle when performing the front drop or seat drop, as do tumblers when they drop backward with legs extended to move into a backward roll with legs extended. The principle is widely applied in the design of protective equipment used in football and other sports. Thigh, hip, and shoulder pads and helmets all serve to distrib-

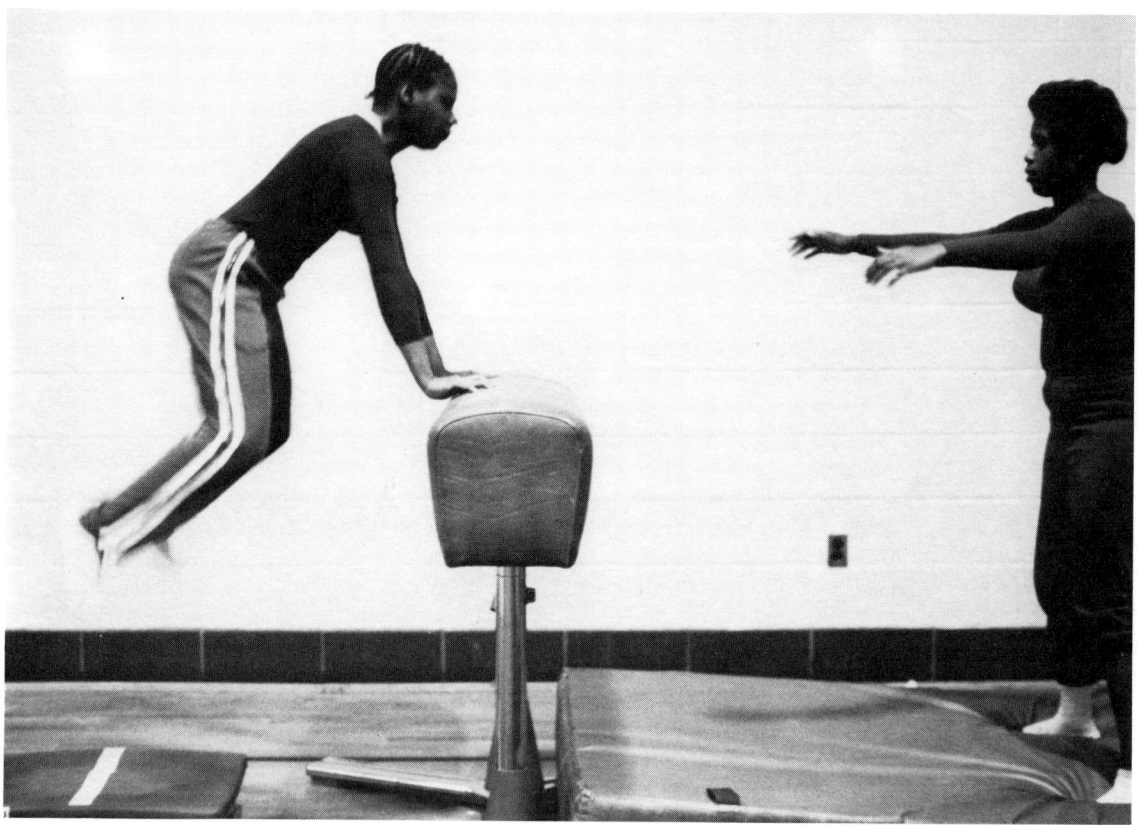

Figure 13.1b Arms angled backward at moment of contact with horse to further direct forward momentum in an upward direction

ute the force of impact over a greater surface area.

If time, position, and other factors permit, injury may be prevented by receiving the impact of a fall over a large surface area. It may be possible to turn to receive the impact over the entire lateral aspect of the leg or to fall backward to receive the impact on the entire posterior surface of the legs. Competitive volleyball players demonstrate application of both the principle of receiving the impact over a greater surface area and of receiving the impact over a greater period of time when they dive to make spectacular saves. They dive headfirst to strike the ball with their fists

and then receive the impact on the anterior side of their forearms, chest, and then the abdomen, the segments striking the floor in quick succession. Both the time and the size of the area receiving the impact are increased through this technique.

PREVENTION OF INJURY IN SELECTED ACTIVITIES

According to a report of the U.S. Consumer Product Safety Commission,[1] there were 41,709 team sport injuries requiring hospital treatment in 1974. Half of these injuries were to people in the 15 to 24 year age group.

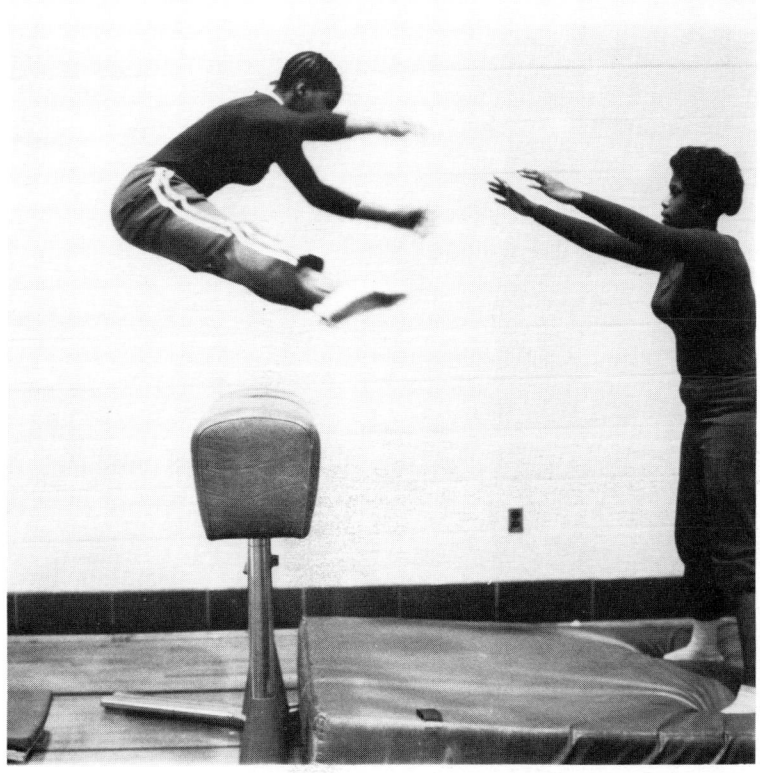

Figure 13.1c Hip flexion and knee extension have brought feet over the horse

Eighty-six percent of these injuries were to males. It can be anticipated that the percentage of females whose injuries require hospital treatment will increase as their number as participants in sports increases.

Football

Klafs and Arnheim[2] estimate that a high school football player participating in a full season of practice and games has a 20 percent chance of being injured during the season and an 8 percent chance of suffering a serious injury. By multiplying the number of annual participants in football by the current injury ratios, they estimate a total of 200,000 to 600,000 injuries to football players. Accord-

ing to the New Jersey State Safety Council,[3] an estimated 300,000 children and adults are treated in hospital emergency rooms, and about 20 people die annually as a result of football-related injuries. Forty percent of these injuries occur among 15- to 19-year-old males. The incidence of injuries in football is higher than in any other sport.

The Committee on Injuries and Fatalities of the American Football Coaches Association indicated in its 1975 report that during 1974 there were a total of 19 fatalities in football, that more fatal injuries occur to defensive players than to offensive players, that 10 injuries to the head, neck, and spinal cord were fatal, and that 55 percent of the direct fatalities were to players 16 to 18 years old.

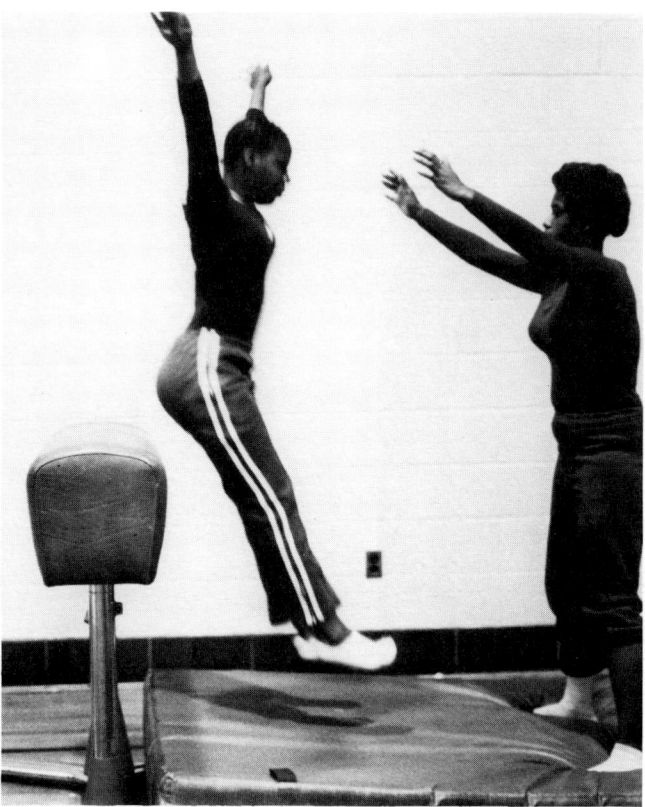

Figure 13.1d Landing about to be made with the center of gravity behind the feet, forward momentum will carry center of gravity over feet as knees and hips flex to absorb impact

They also reported that 33 percent of the fatalities occurred during tackling, 15 percent during ball carrying, and 10 percent during blocking. The location of injuries that culminate in death occur most frequently to the head and face (66 percent), while the spine is the location of 18 percent and the abdominal-internal area is the location of 11 percent.

Twenty-five percent of football injuries are the result of a player receiving a hard blow from the helmet, shoulder pad, or shoes of another player. The incidence of injuries due to this cause could be lowered if shoulder pads and helmets had a soft external padding to cushion blows. Sprains and strains account for 30 percent of the injuries, severe bruises and scrapes for another 30 percent, broken bones for 22 percent, and serious cuts for 10 percent.

The importance of mastery of the fundamentals and of development of strength is pointed out by the high percentage of injuries among young players. Proper execution of tackling and blocking, in particular, must be given high priority. "Spearing" with the head during blocking and tackling is one of the most dangerous practices in football because of the great potential for head, neck, and spinal injuries. Spearing places tremendous compression and shearing forces upon the vertebrae. These forces may fracture the vertebrae, sometimes resulting in severing of the spinal cord by the sharp edges of the fractured vertebrae. Lateral forces upon the head and neck during orthodox blocking and tackling also place stress upon the neck. Strengthening of the muscles of the neck will decrease the probability of suffering a cervical injury. Football players should contract the neck muscles isometrically while executing blocks or tackles.

Helmets should not be used as offensive weapons. Face and nose guards attached to helmets, because they increase leverage, cause the force delivered to the chin to be 30 percent to 100 percent greater than the original force. When force is applied to the nose or face guard in a lateral direction to produce rotation of the spine, the area receiving this force is the side of the neck, which has the least muscular and ligamentous support. When this force is applied with the neck in either flexion or extension, the rotational shear forces may produce a cervical dislocation or a fracture-dislocation of the cervical vertebrae.

Forceful and rapid flexion of the neck, as often occurs during spearing, produces a wedging force on adjacent vertebrae. The force of the impact is focused on the anterior edge of the vertebrae, increasing the probability that the vertebral body will be crushed and the laminae and pedicles will be fractured. Bone fragments may be forced into the spinal canal with the potential for producing paraplegia or death.

Spearing can also force the neck backward beyond its limits in hyperextension, usually fracturing the spinous processes of the sixth or seventh vertebrae.

Basketball

The rate of injuries in basketball is second only to football. Basketball players are usual-ly tall. This places their center of gravity high above the floor, decreasing their stability. When leaping under the basket during close and rough play, body contact below the hips is likely to capsize the player. Injuries to the wrists, elbows, head, ankles, and fingers are most frequent among basketball players. Injuries to the Achilles tendon occur as a result of quick stops, starts, or change of direction. Acromioclavicular separation or fracture of the radius results when a player brings his arms forcefully downward across the extended arms of a player who is shooting the ball. Lacerations and abrasions from falling with forward momentum are fairly common.

Fatigue causes decrements in agility and coordination, thus increasing the probability of a fall or collision and consequent injury. For this reason, basketball players should undergo a through conditioning program to develop both endurance and strength. Strength work should focus on development of the legs, back, shoulders, and arms. It is recommended that players wear light hip pads and knee guards. Those with weak ankles should have them wrapped or taped, while those with weak knees should be provided with a properly fitted brace.

Skiing

There are currently over 4,000,000 skiers in the United States. Ellison[4] estimates that as many as 200,000 injuries occur each season. He points out that as skiing continues to gain popularity, the number of beginning skiers will increase and, consequently, the incidence of injuries will increase. Requa and co-workers[5] found the overall injury rate to be 9.3 per 1000 skier-days. (A ski-man day is the total number of skiers on the slopes on a given day). The mean number of days lost (from work or school) for all injuries was 12.5. Sprains are the most common injury (56 percent) while fractures account for 12 percent of all injuries. Lacerations are the type of injury most frequently reported to the ski patrols. Bruises are infrequently reported either to physicians or the ski patrol but do occur rather frequently. The lower extremity suffered 78 percent of the bruises while bruises to the knee accounted for 24 percent.

Accidents on the ski slopes are of two basic types—falls and collisions. Falls occur in fairly predictable ways and consequently produce fairly predictable injuries. Most skiing injuries are sprains and fractures of the lower limbs.

The skier's body possesses considerable kinetic energy from high velocity, which must be converted into strain energy to produce a sprain or fracture (see Figure 13.2). This usually occurs when there is sudden deceleration due to digging the tip of the ski into the snow. Often this occurs when the skier encounters a mogul, a three- to five-foot mound of packed snow. Deceleration of the forward end of the inside edge of the ski forces the leg into external rotation as the front end of the ski turns outward. The body weight is on the opposite foot and momentum carries the skier downhill. The externally rotated leg is forced into abduction and the leverage of the fixed ski combined with the skier's momentum imposes tremendous forces upon the knee joint, tibia, and fibula when they are levered over the rigid boot top.

In a situation such as illustrated above, if the skier can bring his left shoulder forward and right shoulder rearward to cause the body to rotate toward the right, the forces on the right knee and leg will be diminished and an injury may be avoided. Without this rotating motion, the situation described usually results in fracture of the lateral malleolus, spiral fracture of the tibia and fibula, and sprains of the knee and ankle.

Sometimes the front tip of the ski catches in the snow in such a manner that the skier is thrown forward (see Figure 13.3) with the result that the lower leg is levered over the rigid top of the boot, resulting in tearing of the Achilles tendon or the peroneal retinacula, dislocation of the peroneal tendons, and fracture of the tibia and fibula.

When the skier falls forward, the arms are extended to "brake" the fall. The impact may produce a fractured forearm or dislocation of the shoulder joint. This is more likely if the snow is hard packed. However, it should be pointed out that the incidence of other types of injuries is *decreased* on hard packed snow. The reason for this is because most skiing injuries are caused by twisting or torsion rather than impact. Situations creating torsion forces are most likely to occur on wet and heavy snow, less likely to occur on powder snow, and least likely on icy slopes. Torsion forces occur when a part of the ski becomes fixed in the snow.

Beginning skiers, who tend to cross the skis, are most likely to suffer injuries caused by internal rotation of the legs. In these injuries the outside edge of the ski becomes fixed in the snow, causing the ski and the leg attached to it to rotate inward. Internal rotation may result in ankle sprains, fracture of the medial malleolus, or fracture of the tibia.

Ellison[6] states that nine out of ten skiing injuries involve the lower limb, primarily at three sites: the ankle, lower leg, and knee. Modern rigid high plastic boots have significantly decreased the incidence of ankle injuries. However, because the newer boots protect the lower portions of the leg, the force during a fall is projected to a higher level on the tibia and fibula, where a greater force is required to fracture the bones. When fracture of the tibia and fibula at the higher and stronger level does occur, it is usually a comminuted fracture with severe soft tissue damage. Consequently, fractures of the tibia and fibula are the most severe fractures in skiing.

When the inside edge of the ski is caught, the force of external rotation-abduction rotates the talus between the medial and lateral malleoli. Sometimes the rotating talus drives the lateral malleolus backward with sufficient

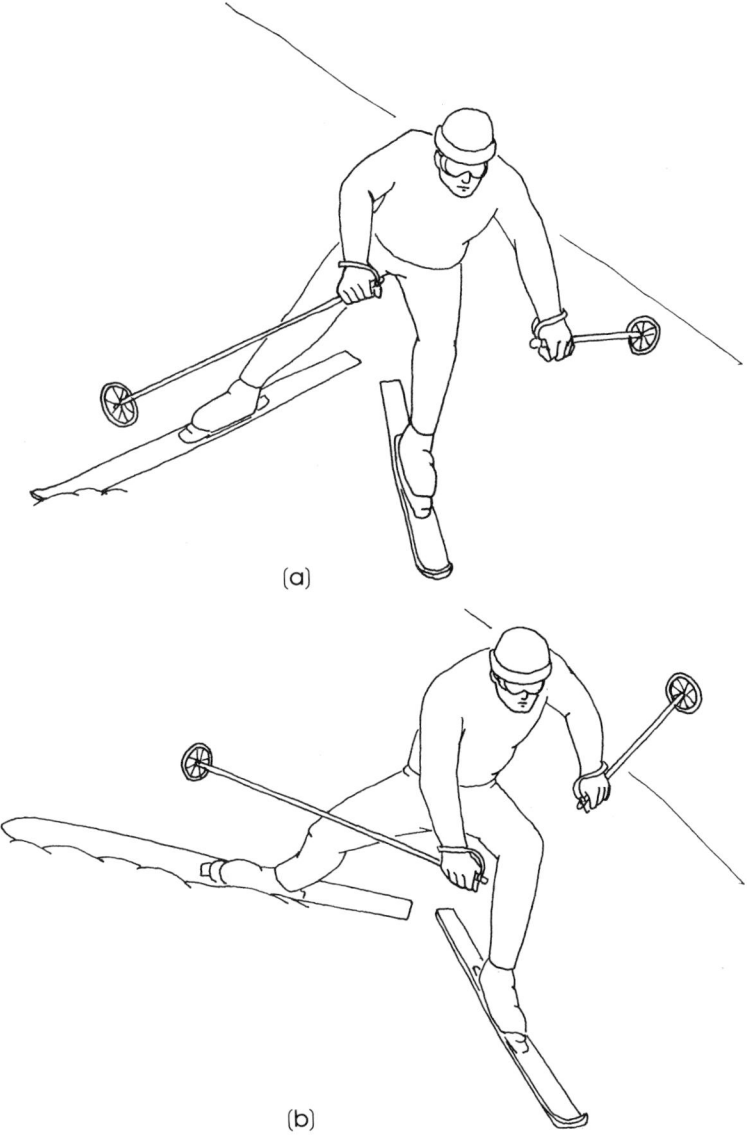

(a)

(b)

Figure 13.2 (a) Tip of right ski is decelerated, weight shifts to left ski, which continues downhill as right leg externally rotates and abducts; (b) leverage of ski plus forward momentum increase forces upon the knee and lower leg

force not only to tear the anterior deltoid and anterior tibiofibular ligaments but also to cause a spiral oblique fracture of the tibia and fibula. Increasing use of the high plastic boot has substantially decreased the incidence of this type of injury since it is virtually impossible for the talus to rotate in this type of boot.

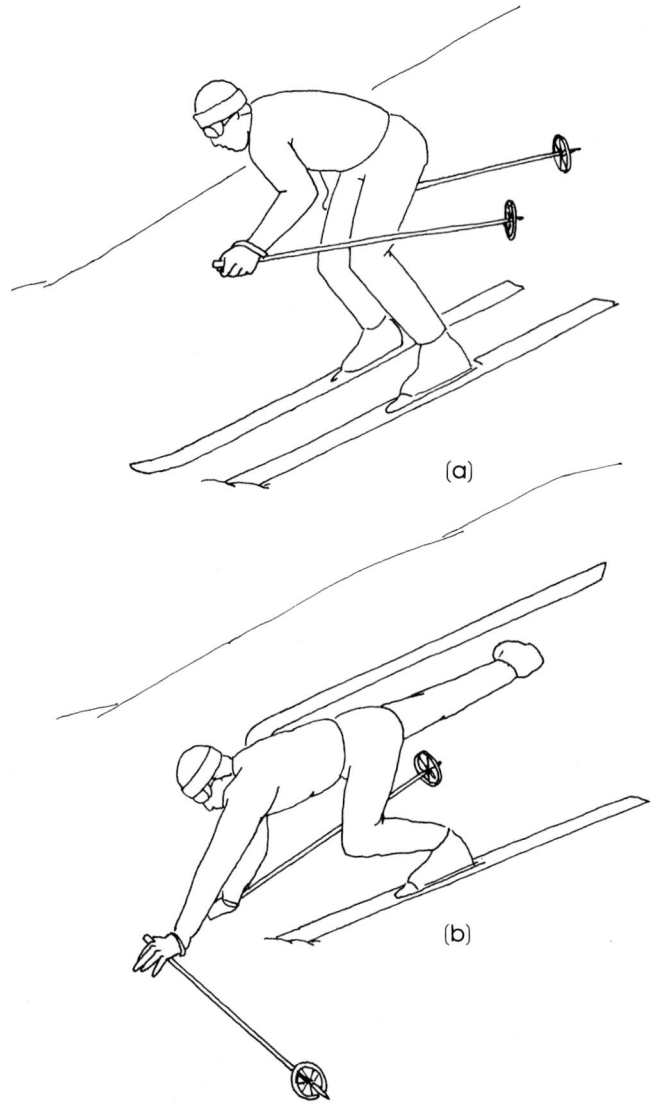

Figure 13.3 (a) Tip of the ski digging into the snow during rapid downhill descent; (b) skier thrown forward abruptly with lower leg suddenly and forcefully levered against the rigid boot top

The femur is seldom fractured in skiing. When it is, the fracture usually occurs in the area of the trochanter, on hard packed snow, and as a result of a collision. Fractures of the femoral neck are most common among older skiers.

Forward falls on hard packed snow where the skier extends the arms to catch the impact on the hands sometimes cause fracture of the tuberosity of the humerus or, if the skier is holding the ski pole when his hand impacts against the snow, fracture of the first metacarpal bone of the thumb. This type of fall can also produce dislocation of the shoulder.

Abrasions on the face most commonly occur after a forward fall when snow is granular, corn, or frozen. Contusions occur as a result of falls on ice or hard packed snow when a body area where the bone is near the surface impacts against the skiing surface. Backward falls on the sacrococcygeal area in a sitting position are one of the more common causes of contusions.

Ice Hockey

Ice hockey has a relatively large accident rate. Athletic directors, coaches, and equipment managers can contribute to a decrease in the incidence of athletic injuries through the judicious selection of equipment, and particularly protective equipment. This is as true in the case of selection of equipment for ice hockey as it is for any other sport. It is especially important to select face masks for ice hockey goaltenders that have maximum impact-attenuating properties.

The possibility is great that the goaltender will be struck in the face by the sharp-edged, hard rubber puck, which achieves speeds as high as 110 mph. There is presently a great variety of face masks of a wide array of shapes, sizes, and materials. This variety is due principally to the lack of design recommendations since neither the federal government or manufacturers have established procedures to evaluate the effectiveness of goaltenders' masks.

Norman and his colleagues[7] investigated the relative impact-attenuating qualities of several commercially available face masks. They found that none of the face-molded masks provide adequate protection against all blows. Their study showed that more than 75 percent of the total load transmitted through a mask from a direct blow to a contact point arrives on the contact point; that is, the mask does not disperse the load very ef-

fectively. It was found that the wire mask achieved the objective of both force dispersion and reduction and at the same time prohibited loads from reaching the vulnerable right forehead and cheek. It was also shown that the shape of the mask, particularly the reinforcing effects of raised ridges, plays a more important role in distributing impact loads than does the type of material from which the mask is made.

Baseball

Baseball has a low accident rate. The number of participants in Little League, Pony League, sandlot games, high school, and college conferences totals well over a million. In view of this large number of participants, it is surprising that a larger number of injuries are not reported. Klafs and Arnheim[8] state that 96 percent of injuries in baseball occur to the arm and hand, leg and foot, head and neck. Most of the injuries to the arms and legs are caused by poor sliding techniques and uneven playing surfaces. Injuries to the head and neck usually are the result of a blow with the bat or the ball or collision between two players.

Pitching subjects the shoulder and elbow joints to stresses of great intensity and, consequently, accounts for a considerable number of chronic injuries to these joints. Great torque forces are imposed upon the elbow and shoulder due to the inward or outward rotation of the forearm and humerus used to give the ball greater speed and to cause it to curve. If this action is improperly executed over a long period of time, the rotator cuff muscles, long head of the biceps brachii, pronator teres, anconeus, and deltoid muscles may become damaged.

During the preparatory phase of the pitch, when the arm is brought backward or cocked, there is powerful external rotation of the humerus and as a result tendinitis may develop in the biceps, triceps, and shoulder rotators.

During the delivery, the pectoralis major and latissimus dorsi muscles come under powerful contraction and, as a result, tendinitis of these muscles sometimes develops. Osteochondrosis of the proximal humeral epiphysis and fracture of the proximal end of the shaft of the humerus are so common among Little League baseball players that these conditions have come to be called "Little League shoulder." "Little League elbow" is a condition produced by compression forces acting on the radiohumeral joint to produce changes in the joint that may result in an aseptic (bacteria-free) destruction of tissue of the radial head or osteochondritis dissecans of the capitulum of the humerus where it articulates with the radius. It has been pointed out earlier that the bones grow at the epiphyseal ends and that the bones are not yet completely ossified during adolescence. Consequently, the bones of adolescents are susceptible to injury. Pitchers of all ages are prone to suffer from bony spurs on both the radius and ulna. The follow-through phase of the pitch contributes to few traumas except when a "breaking" pitch is used frequently. In this pitch there is forceful pronation of the forearm as the pitch is completed, with the potential of causing trauma to the pronator teres.

Soccer

On a worldwide basis, soccer has long had the largest number of participants of any sport. In recent years it has experienced a phenomenal growth in the United States. Although body contact is not permitted and no protective equipment is utilized, the injuries incurred are much like those of football. Because of the sudden stops and starts, rapid accelerations, and quick change of direction required, injuries to the knees and ankles and shin splints are quite common. There is also a high incidence of facial lacerations and eye injuries resulting from heading the ball and player collisions.

Gymnastics

The incidence of injury in gymnastics is highly related to the knowledge, experience, and degree of conscientiousness of the instructor or coach of this sport. The rapid growth of gymnastics resulting from the televising of world and Olympic gymnastic championships with the resultant shortage of qualified instructors, the movement toward holding teachers accountable, and the discovery by attorneys of the potential for large contingency fees resulting from law suits for injuries occurring in physical education classes, all converged to create great concern among physical educators and equipment manufacturers about safety in gymnastics in particular and physical education activities in general. Leaders in gymnastics were among the first in any sport to make organized efforts to decrease the incidence of injuries.

These efforts were initiated with the formation of the United States Gymnastic Safety Association (USGSA) in 1975. "Guidelines to Safety in Gymnastics," a workbook, was compiled by members of this new organization led by Cap Caudill and John Fiore. The success of this publication resulted in the decision to develop a certification program in safety in gymnastics and to publish the *Gymnastics Safety Manual*.[9] This manual, edited by Eugene Wettstone, consists of twelve chapters written by recognized authorities in gymnastics on such topics as facilities and supervision, selection and use of equipment, spotting methods and safety equipment, clothing and personal equipment, utilization of visual aids, warm-up, progressions, and medical and legal responsibility. Leaders in other sports should follow this trailblazing effort in order to decrease the incidence of injuries in all sports, particularly in high-risk activities. High-risk activities can make life more interesting, exciting, and challenging, and can provide learnings about one's self and others that can be provided by no other medium.

The instructor should develop in students the habit of checking on the security and safety of the equipment before using it. This should be done after every adjustment for width or height of the piece of equipment. Some class time should be spent in teaching students to absorb the impact of the body. Beginning students should jump from progressively higher heights starting at one foot and progressing to three or four feet. They should be taught to absorb the impact by means of eccentric contraction of muscles that plantar flex the feet and that extend the knees and hips. The extensor muscles of these joints should resist the impact through eccentric contraction. The shoulder, forward, and backward rolls in tumbling and their variations should be taught before initiating instruction on the gymnastic equipment in order that participants develop kinesthetic awareness during rotational movements of the body. Further, students will be able to utilize these rolls to increase the time over which impact is absorbed in the event of a fall from gymnastic equipment with horizontal as well as vertical momentum.

Baley[10] makes the following suggestions regarding breakfalls:

1. When catching the weight on the hands during a backward fall, the fingers should be pointed forward in order that the elbows can flex on impact. This will increase the time and distance for absorption of impact.

2. The face should be turned in the direction of the fall if possible.

3. The chin should be tucked in or the face turned sideward just prior to impact in a forward fall.

4. The body should be tucked immediately after landing to go into a forward, backward, or sideward roll if at all possible.

This distributes the impact over a greater period of time.

5. Well-padded body parts such as the buttocks or thighs should contact the surface if possible.

Baley[11] also indicates that students should be taught that they have the following responsibilities with regard to their own safety:

1. Develop an amount of strength, power, flexibility, and endurance necessary to the successful achievement of the move or combinations of moves they are attempting to learn. (A student needs adequate arm and shoulder girdle strength to be able to swing in a straight-arm support on the parallel bars.)

2. Observe all safety rules.

3. Learn skills in their progressive order of difficulty. (See Chapter 4 for rationale.)

4. Master fundamentals.

5. Warm up properly.

6. Be willing to spot and coach others.

7. Be willing to ask others to spot.

8. Avoid "horse play."

9. Use the necessary amount of carbonate of magnesium to increase friction and thereby decrease probability of slipping.

10. Possess the courage to follow a skill through to its completion once it has been initiated.

11. Possess knowledge of and sufficient skill to apply the principles of breakfalling in the event of an error. There are two principal methods by which to lessen probability of an injury as a result of a fall. These are:

    a. distributing the impact over a greater area.

    b. distributing the impact over a greater period of time.

It is inadvisable to present here all the necessary points on spotting procedures. Readers should refer to the many excellent textbooks on gymnastics for detailed procedures. However, we will present a few of the more important points:

1. Protect the head first.

2. Be prepared to provide additional rotational force and at the same time to check overrotation.

3. Additional force is provided during a forward somersault by pushing on the back above the center of gravity and during a backward somersault by pushing below the center of gravity. Overrotation is checked in both somersaults by applying force above the center of gravity in a direction opposite the rotation.

4. Lift is provided, in the case of a low somersault, by applying force at the center of gravity.

5. Whether spotting by hand or with a hand belt, the spotter must stand close to the performer so that his lifting force is more nearly vertical.

6. Tension caused by fear can increase the probability of commiting an error and thereby contribute to a fall. Effective spotting allays fear and, consequently, contributes to improved performance since it permits the performer to concentrate on the mechanics of execution of skill. However, the ultimate goal is to perform the move unassisted; therefore, the gymnast must progress as rapidly as possible toward independent execution while at the same time being kept safe. Independent execution can be delayed by keeping the gymnast in the safety belt excessively long. This dilemma can be circumvented by progressively decreasing the amount of assistance given the gymnast as he masters the move. For example, in learning a front salto or somersault in tumbling, the gymnast should use three spotters—two manning the safety belt and one standing at the anticipated point of landing to check for overspin. As the gymnast masters this skill, the spotter for overspin should be removed and then one manning the belt. Next, the move can be done with two hand spotters, then with one hand spotter, then with a hand spotter in readiness but providing no lift, and finally with a hand spotter a step away.

7. The spotter must focus his or her attention fully upon the performer.

8. The performer must inform the spotter when he or she is about to initiate the move.

9. The spotter must understand the mechanics of the move.

10. In moves such as flyaways from the horizontal bar or vaults over the side or long horse, the spotter must be prepared to move in a horizontal direction in order to be positioned alongside the performer when assistance is required.

11. When using the hand belt, the spotter should grasp the rope with one hand near the swivel and wrap the rope around the opposite hand about one to three feet from the swivel. This distance will vary according to the height attained by the performer during the move. The rope should not be wrapped around the hand that is grasping the rope near the swivel since it is often necessary to slide this hand along the rope.

12. The ropes on safety belts should be held neither so taut as to restrict the performer's movements nor so slack as to get in his way. During running approaches in tumbling, the ropes should be held loosely during the run but tightened as the move is executed.

13. If a twisting belt is not available for use in learning moves with twists or rotation around the vertical axis, the ropes may be crossed in front of or behind the body so that they will unwind as the move is executed. It is obviously of great importance that the spotter and performer be certain that the ropes are crossed in the correct manner.

14. Always continue spotting through the move until its completion (including the landing).

15. Spot from below the parallel bars so that the arm will not be trapped between the performer and the bar, possibly resulting in a fracture.

The most successful gymnastics coaches insist on the mastery of skills at each level of difficulty before urging gymnasts to the next highest level of difficulty. Those called upon to teach or coach this activity should study the numerous textbooks on the subject, attend clinics, and become certified by the United States Gymnastics Safety Association.[12]

Students in gymnastics classes and those who are members of gymnastics teams should be presented relevant information from kinesiology and anatomy. They should understand the structural limitations of the cervical and shoulder areas and of the wrists and ankles and the movement limitations of the knees and elbows. They should also understand rotational forces, momentum, and absorption of impact; the influence of rotational forces and momentum upon best body positions for maintenance of balance; trajectory; and Newton's laws of motion.

Mats provide the last line of defense against injury in gymnastics. For this reason, they should be carefully selected when purchasing, in ample amount, and be properly utilized. The mat specifications of the several gymnastic conferences and associations vary due, principally, to the various skill levels that they serve. The higher the level of skill, the less the thickness of mat permitted. Mats vary in thickness from 1 to 12 inches.

Mats should provide good traction, be resistant to water, and provide color contrasts so that gymnasts can orient themselves as they approach the mat from somersaults and twists. Mats should be kept clean and in a state of good repair.

The National Safety Council has indicated that the incidence of accidents in rebound tumbling is one of the lowest of all school physical education activities.[13] However, a few of the accidents have been extremely serious ones resulting in quadriplegia due to injuries to the spinal cord in the cervical area. These injuries often occur during high bouncing and when the trampolinist attempts somersaults before having mastered the skills prerequisite to learning this skill. Piscopo[14] pointed out the hazards in teaching somersaults in physical education classes as long ago as 1966. He stated that this skill should be reserved for the skilled and competitive performer. Spinal cord injuries may also occur because of under- or overrotation while attempting somersaults. The cervical area is the most mobile of all areas of the vertebral column.[15] The vertebrae in the cervical area are the smallest of all the vertebrae and, consequently, most vulnerable to fracture. When they are fractured, the sharp jagged edges of bone may sever the spinal cord or do serious neurologic damage. Injury may occur as a result of hyperextension when the forehead strikes the bed or floor while rotating forward around the horizontal axis in a front somersault, or it may occur as a result of hyperflexion as would occur if the trampolinist overspun a backward somersault, landing on the back of the head. A compression fracture could occur if he/she dropped vertically downward onto the top of the head.

Injuries in rebound tumbling could be almost totally eliminated if proper procedures were followed. The two principle factors in prevention of injury are proper spotting and mastery of fundamentals. A minimum of four spotters, one on each side of the trampoline, should be used at all times. Spotters should not attempt to catch the performer but should push him back onto the bed as one would a beach ball. They should focus their attention on the performer at all times and should not carry on a conversation while spotting.

Skills should be learned in their progressive order of difficulty. Each skill should be mastered before moving on to the next, more difficult skill. At least 19 skills and their variations should be mastered before attempting somersaults. These skills are described in several textbooks.

BALANCE/EQUILIBRIUM PRECEPTS AND INJURY PREVENTION

As has been stated in Chapter 8, balance and equilibrium are important elements when considering safety and injury prevention. The physical educator or coach must determine why the student fell or lost balance.

Stability is increased by lowering the center of gravity. The expert canoeist who changes from a position of sitting on the seat to kneeling or sitting on the floor of the canoe when rough water is encountered is behaving according to this precept. Through this act the center of gravity of the canoe is lowered, making it less likely that the canoe will capsize and that the canoeist will experience a cold, wet plunge. A skier can decrease the probability of an injury-producing fall when balance is momentarily lost by flexing the knees and hips to assume a squatting position, thereby lowering the center of gravity to regain balance. A gymnast finding himself with an excessive horizontal component of force or momentum after a dismount can often retain his balance by dropping into a squat position in addition to hopping forward. A wrestler increases his stability by lowering his center of gravity by bending his hips and knees.

Stability and, therefore, safety in sports is increased when the base of support is widened in the direction of an impending force. When the gymnast dismounts with excessive for-

ward momentum, he/she can prevent an embarrassing headlong fall and perhaps an injury by stepping forward with one foot to absorb the linear force. The defensive lineman is less likely to be knocked down by the onrushing offensive player if he will widen his base of support in the direction of his opponent's charge. The shortstop is less likely to be bowled over upon catching a line drive if he widens his base of support in the direction of home plate. Also, his hand will sting less since he will be provided a greater distance through which to decelerate the ball and to absorb its impact.

Maintenance of balance of a vertically segmented body is most easily accomplished when the center of gravity of each weight-bearing segment lies in the line of gravity or in which deviations in one direction are exactly balanced by deviations in the opposite direction. The human vertebral column is an example of a vertically segmented body. Less stress is placed upon ligaments of the vertebral column when the vertebrae are in a straight-line relationship. In the doubles and triples balancing events of sports acrobatics there are many stunts such as a three-high stand on shoulders or high hand-to-hand balance where maintenance of the balanced position requires that the center of gravity of each segment lie in the line of gravity. Beginners in this activity must expend considerably greater muscular force to maintain the balanced position because they are not aware of an imbalance as soon as the experienced and skilled balancers. In some static balance or hold moves in gymnastics, such as the V seat or scale, the center of gravity of various body segments fall outside a line perpendicular to the center of the base of support. If the center of the base of support is viewed as the fulcrum of a first-class lever, then it will be understood why the weight of the segment on one side times the distance of this segment's center of gravity to the line perpendicular to the center of the base of support must equal the weight of the segment on the other side of this line times the distance from the segment's center of gravity to the line. The law of levers is operative to facilitate accomplishment of balance skills where the weight on one side of the fulcrum is considerably greater than that on the other side.

Dynamic balance is also maintained by counteracting the weight of one body segment on one side of the line of gravity with the weight of another segment on the opposite side. As the punter's kicking leg swings forward of the line of gravity, his trunk is inclined rearward to counterbalance the weight (and momentum) of the kicking leg. If one's foot slips out from under the body on an icy pavement, the arms or other body segments will move in a direction opposite to that of the foot to maintain balance.

The relationship of the line of gravity of the body to the base of suport should be such as to facilitate the desired action. In most instances, such as in racing starts or the football lineman's position, the line of gravity should be forward of the center of the base of support. In others, such as in vaults over the long or side horse or the basketball player's reversal of direction, the line of gravity should be behind the center of the base of support. In the case of vaults, the momentum generated during the run will carry the line of gravity forward after the landing; therefore, the vaulter should land with his center of gravity behind his feet in order to control his balance after landing. In the case of a quick reversal of direction, as demonstrated many times by basketball players, the player must lean backward as he or she brakes to a stop in order to facilitate quick reversal of direction and to avoid a headlong fall as forward momentum carries the center of gravity beyond the base of support. For more detailed discussions, see Chapters 6 and 8.

Friction between the supporting surface and the feet will enhance stability. This principle becomes readily observable when one attempts to run on ice, where friction is minimal. Falls in football and soccer are more frequent when the grass is wet than when it is dry. Wearing of cleats helps to minimize the probability of slipping and falling. Wet areas on basketball floors decrease friction and can result in falls producing severe injury. Dust and dirt on gymnastic or wrestling mats can decrease friction between the athlete's feet and the surface of the mat. This can cause the athlete's feet to slip out from under the body when an attempt is made to accelerate or to stop quickly as in starting a run, stopping after a vault or dismount, or attempting a take-down.

The quality of the sense of balance is related to the state of mental and emotional health. For this reason, when ill, athletes should refrain from participating in dangerous activities that require a high level of balancing ability.

In gymnastics, points are deducted for an uncontrolled landing after a vault or dismount. In a well-executed dismount, the gymnast lands with the feet together, the trunk erect, the knees separated, and the arms extended forward-sideward. Although some of these requirements are in violation of the balance precepts we have expounded, they enhance safety in the sport because they place a premium upon a well-executed flight, precision, and control. If gymnasts were not penalized for uncontrolled landings, they would be encouraged to attempt dismounts and vaults of a level of difficulty beyond their present level of ability.

FORCE REDUCTION WHEN FALLING INTO WATER

Water cannot be compressed. It can, however, be separated. Therefore, the greater the surface area of the body contacting the surface of the water at one moment, the greater the discomfort. Water is most easily parted by the human body when entry is made with as small an area as possible (fingertips or toes) and with the body streamlined and almost perpendicular to the surface of the water. A diver should enter the water a few degrees short of the perpendicular, since body rotation will continue into the water. This is true whether the body is rotating forward or backward. Although body extension prior to entry into the water decreases the speed of rotation, rotation continues, although more slowly, even after the hands or feet have entered the water. The entry of the hands and arms into the water slows rotation further and the center of gravity of the body is moved forward in a front or inward dive and backward in a back or reverse dive. This movement of the body's center of gravity is due to the hands or feet becoming a point of pivot upon entry since they somewhat fix that end of the rotating lever (the body).

As the hands enter the water, the shoulder joint should be stabilized to prevent strain to the shoulder joint and so that the arms will not be forced out of alignment with the body. At the same time, the body should be stretched to maximum length with no arch and no hip, knee, or shoulder flexion. This will streamline the body so that it enters with a minimum of resistance. The head, trunk, and legs should fall into the "hole" made by the hands and arms. The abdominal and extensor muscles of the back contract isometrically to stabilize the hip joint in a position of extension as the entry is made.

The extended position should be maintained until the bottom of the pool has been reached or until momentum has been substantially decreased. If any part of the body is either flexed or hyperextended while it is moving at a high rate of speed through the water, excessive strains may be imposed upon the joints involved. Neck, back, or shoulder strains may be caused by lifting the head or arms or arching the back too soon in an effort to return to the surface quickly. Shoulder

strains can also occur as a result of holding the arms too wide on dives with a head-first entry.

A depth of 10 feet for the one-meter board and of 12 feet for the three-meter board is required to insure that the diver will not strike the bottom with excessive force. On feet-first dives, the momentum should be absorbed at the bottom of the pool in the same manner as jumping from a height on land; that is, the landing should be made on the balls of the feet, and the feet should be dorsiflexed while the knees and hips are also eccentrically flexed. In dives with head-first entries, the elbows should be flexed as the hands contact the bottom, and then the feet should be brought to the bottom by flexing the hips and knees as in a snapdown from a handstand.

The position of the body as it enters the water is determined principally by the quality of the takeoff from the board and secondarily by correct body mechanics during execution of the dive and during entry. A takeoff with a low and flat trajectory will almost inevitably result in a flat or shallow entry. Opening up either too soon or too late will also cause the diver to slap the body against the water. As anyone who has experienced a "belly-whopper" knows, this is both painful and embarrassing. However, when "belly whoppers" occur from a one-meter board these slaps and stings rarely produce injuries more serious than redness and minor discomfort. A flat entry from a three-meter board, however, may result in broken blood vessels, internal damage, black eyes, and a bloody nose. A slap against the side of the head, which is more likely to occur in twisting dives, can cause serious damage to the inner ear. For this reason, all twisting dives should be mastered from the one-meter board before being tried from the three-meter board.

The uninitiated believe that dives are easier from the three-meter board because more time is provided. The additional time provided is very small because the body accelerates at the rate of 32.2 ft/sec/sec. Additionally, the impact force is considerably greater from the three-meter board.

Divers seldom strike the board, but when they do a serious injury often results. The diver should maintain sight of the end of the board throughout the approach and hurdle. The approach and hurdle should be smooth and under control. An excessively long pre-hurdle step creates balance problems and puts the diver too near the end of the board. To compensate, the diver leans backward or flexes the hips during the hurdle thereby upsetting both alignment and balance. Hip flexion during the hurdle and a backward lean produce a lift either directly upward or backward, bringing the diver onto or too close to the board. During the approach, all body segments should be vertically aligned. Heavy pounding on the heels and a flat-footed landing from the hurdle must be avoided. The first results in poor balance and control and the second may cause the diver to skid off the end of the board. The approach and hurdle must be practiced and mastered since it is a part of every running forward and reverse dive. Failure to master this basic technique will result in failed dives and can result in injury. The reader is referred to Chapter 10 for a more detailed discussion of diving techniques.

Other causes of injury include lack of familiarity with the depth and obstructions at the bottom of the pool, efforts to progress too rapidly, fatigue, collisions with swimmers under the board, and great courage combined with little intelligence.

SUMMARY

The potential for injury in sports activities is greater than it is in routine daily activities because in sports, considerable muscular force is utilized, impact must be absorbed, and balance must be maintained. The element of

risk is undoubtedly one of the characteristics of sports that make them attractive.

That the incidence of injury has not been greater is a testimonial to the work of physical educators, coaches, and manufacturers of sporting goods and equipment. However, the incidence of injury could be considerably decreased through greater study and effort. The study and application of principles of kinesiology can contribute greatly to a decrease in the number of injuries.

The nature of kinetic energy is symbolized by the formula $KE = \frac{1}{2} mv^2$. The amount of work that must be done to absorb kinetic energy is dependent upon the force and the distance through which this force is applied, as illustrated by the formula $Fd = \frac{1}{2} mv^2$. The two formulas also show that the amount of work done and the absorption of an amount of kinetic energy are equal. The formulas indicate the importance of increasing the distance over which kinetic energy is absorbed.

The probability of an injury during execution of some athletic skills can be decreased by shortening the length of the lever arm through which an impact acts upon a joint.

Elasticity is an object's ability to return to its original size and shape after an impact, force, or stress acting upon it is removed. Soft tissues of the body such as muscle or fat possess greater elasticity than does bone. For this reason, when a blow or fall is imminent, it is preferable to adjust the body so that the impact is received on soft tissue such as the buttocks, shoulder, or thigh rather than an area where bone is near the surface. In addition to providing a greater amount to the stabilizing component of force of the muscle's pull upon a joint, strong muscles, since they are larger, can provide greater protection against fractures because they provide greater absorptive power just as does a thicker mat or glove.

The thoracic cage, because of its mobility and the bowed shape of the ribs, can absorb a surprising amount of force without injury.

Prevention of injury in selected activities was discussed. Football shows the highest incidence of injuries.

The incidence of injuries could be decreased by mastery of fundamental skills and elimination of "spearing."

Basketball players suffer injuries to the wrists, elbows, head, and fingers principally as a result of falls since they are more prone to falls due to their relatively high center of gravity. Injuries to the Achilles tendon and sprains of the ankles are also fairly common among basketball players.

In skiing, falls and collisions result in sprains and fractures of the lower extremities. Most injuries occur on wet, heavy snow when the tip of the ski digs into the snow. The incidence of sprains or fractures of the ankle has declined since the introduction of the rigid plastic shoes, but the incidence of more serious comminuted fractures of the lower legs has increased because the force is projected to a higher level—the tibia and fibula. The mechanism of a variety of accidents in skiing was described.

Injuries in ice hockey are the result of personal physical contact or being struck with the hockey stick or puck and occur principally to the head or skin. Sportsmanlike play and utilization of the best protective equipment are the most important requirements for decreasing the incidence of injuries in ice hockey. Most currently used goaltender's face masks provide inadequate protection. The wire face mask provides the best protection.

Baseball has a low accident rate. Most of the injuries are to the arms and legs and result from poor sliding techniques and uneven playing surfaces. Pitchers are prone to chronic traumata of the elbow and shoulder joints due principally to vigorous pronation and supination of the forearm and rotation of the humerus. "Little League elbow," bone spurs, and trauma of various muscles was discussed.

Injuries in soccer are principally to the knees and ankles due to sudden stops and starts and change of direction. Facial lacerations and injuries to the eye resulting from heading and collisions rank next in frequency.

Injuries in gymnastics and trampolining could be substantially reduced through insistence upon mastery of skills at each level of difficulty before the participant moves to the next level of difficulty and through utilization of proper spotting procedures. This requires that the coach or instructor of gymnastics possess the necessary knowledge. The newly formed USGSA is helping to disseminate this knowledge. Furthermore, students in gymnastic classes and members of gymnastic teams should be taught relevant kinesiologic principles as they apply to gymnastics.

Balance/equilibrium precepts for prevention of injury were next presented. Illustrations of application of these precepts were provided.

Injury prevention when landing in water requires procedures that differ in some respects from those recommended when landing on the ground or floor. The most important precept is that the body must be streamlined and vertical when entering the water. This is because water is not compressible. The body should be a few degrees short of a vertical position as it begins to enter the water in somersaulting dives because it continues to rotate after the feet or hands have entered the water even though the speed of rotation is considerably slower in the extended than in the tucked or piked position.

REFERENCES

1. *A.C.S.M. Newsletter* 9.4, "Team Sports Heads Consumer Products Injury List," 1974.
2. Klafs, Carl E., and Arnheim, Daniel D., *Modern Principles of Athletic Training*, fourth edition, St. Louis: C. V. Mosby, 1977, p. 5.

3. Hughes, James F., Editor, *Safety Briefs*. New Jersey State Safety Council, Vol. 36, No. 2, November, 1974, p. 3.

4. Ellison, Arthur E., "Skiing Injuries," *Clinical Symposia*, Vol. 29, November 1, 1977, CIBA.

5. Requa, Ralph K., Toney, Jack M., and Garrick, James G., "Parameters of Injury Reporting in Skiing," *Medicine and Science in Sports*, Vol. 9, No. 3, 1977, pp. 185–190.

6. Ellison, *op. cit.,* p. 7.

7. Norman, R. W., Thompson, Y. Sze, and Hayes, D., "Relative Impact-Attenuating Properties of Masks of Ice Hockey Goaltenders," *Biomechanics IV*. Nelson, Richard C., and Moorehouse, Chauncey A., (eds.) Baltimore: University Park Press, 1974.

8. Klafs and Arnheim, op. cit., p. 9.

9. Wettstone, Eugene, Editor, *Gymnastics Safety Manual.* The Pennsylvania State University Press, University Park & London, 1977.

10. Baley, James A., *Handbook of Gymnastics in the Schools*. Boston: Allyn & Bacon, 1974, p. 35.

11. *Ibid.*

12. United States Gymnastics Safety Association, 424 C Street, N.E., Capital Hill, Washington, D. C. 20002.

13. National Safety Council, *Rebound Tumbling*, a report prepared by the Public Safety Committee, National Safety Council, Chicago, Illinois, March 1961, p. 2.

14. Piscopo, John, "Clues to Safety on the Trampoline," *Journal of Health, Physical Education and Recreation*, 37: 51–61, April, 1966.

15. Piscopo, John, and Hennessy, Jeff, "Trampoline Safety," *Journal of Health, Physical Education and Recreation,* 47: 33–36, April, 1976.

14 MOBILITY PATTERNS, FITNESS, AND AGING

CONCEPTS

1. Joint mobility is a component of dynamic physical fitness equally important to elite athletes and handicapped individuals seeking improvement in basic motor skills.

2. The degree of flexibility on various joints is not necessarily related.

3. Flexibility norms are rough guides in assessing flexibility and should not be interpreted as absolute standards.

4. When designing physical fitness programs for athletes, the specific physical fitness qualities required for success in the athlete's sport should be considered.

5. Strength and power, flexibility, balance, and endurance are dissimilar qualities and require different modalities for most efficient development.

6. Analysis of muscle involvement in specific exercises is essential if exercises are to be properly prescribed for development of specific muscle groups.

7. Aging is irreversible. It is an inescapable retrogressive process of structural, functional, and chemical changes in the human organism.

8. The rate of change due to aging can be slowed to a significant degree by maintaining sensible standards of physical fitness.

9. Fat loss due to aging tends to be centripetal; that is, fat is lost early and to a greater degree from the extremities and maintained longer on the trunk.

10. Strength development and maintenance for persons over 50 serves two basic purposes: (1) to maintain muscle tone for good posture and (2) to provide energy source of force for efficient movement.

11. Using the "direct line of pull" principle assists individuals with strength decrements to move more efficiently and with less effort.

12. The pectorals, abdominals, pelvic and hip extensors are particularly vulnerable to weakness among older people.

13. The intrinsic stability of the spine diminishes with age because of disk changes; however, the extrinsic support is alterable by strengthening abdominal, thoracic, and spinal skeletal muscles.

14. New motor skills can be learned by older persons provided they are encouraged to perform in a slower manner and at their own pace without pressure.

GENERAL CONSIDERATIONS

Mobility is an indispensable condition of motor skills and athletic sport. An essential ingredient of mobility is joint and muscular flexibility. The following discussion explores

494

kinesiological mechanisms of human structural and functional flexibility factors as they pertain to the maintenance and improvement of fundamental movements surrounding the everyday living environment of the individual as well as investigating salient points that accompany fitness and the process of aging.

Flexibility is viewed by the authors as one component of dynamic fitness. Other kinesiologists deem this quality to be a therapeutic or corrective measure and become concerned when gross deviations from the average range of motion occur that obviously impede the mobility patterns of the individual. Simply stated, flexibility is defined as the range of a joint articulation or set of joints. The assessment of flexibility includes measurements of flexion, extension, abduction, rotation, and circumduction. It has been shown that joints have specific degrees of flexibility not related to each other. Flexibility shown by one joint does not reflect the range of movement that can be obtained in other joints.[1] Joint structure, ligaments, and tendons are but a few physical determinants that aid or hinder range of movement. The biceps brachii, located at the upper anterior portion of the humerus, is a major flexor of the forearm. The antagonistic triceps group is located posteriorly and considered a prime forearm extensor. The elbow joint can flex only when the triceps relaxes and the biceps concentrically contracts. If some condition causes the triceps to tense to the slightest degree, it will be more difficult to shorten the biceps. Skeletal muscles must be in a relaxed state to achieve maximum motion motility. In addition to somatotype and structural and training modalities, the authors believe that a basic relationship exists between tension, anxiety, and one's flexibility pattern. Whelan[2] investigated the relationship between anxiety and flexibility of adolescent males and found a consistent degree of positive correlations between tension and flexibility performances in certain upper and lower body segments (shoulder and hip joints). Other data from his study show that as anxiety levels increase, joint flexibility decreases. Few studies, if any, have pursued the association between tension and flexibility. Rathbone[3] is one of the few educators who draws attention to the anxiety/flexibility relationship by stating:

Almost without exception, tense individuals have restrictions in joint flexibility. In the early states, this flexibility may be due solely to the inability of muscles to relax sufficiently to make possible full range of movement. In later states, the joint structures may become so tightened that flexibility cannot be regained.

Some research has been conducted exploring the relationship between anxiety and motor tasks, which is akin to joint mobility. Muscular spasticity and rigidity increase during a period of stress.[4] One investigator found that subjects with low levels of anxiety required less time to perform certain motor skills than high-anxiety persons, and also that the former group was able to perform better than their high-anxiety counterparts.[5] The study also showed that the differences became more pronounced as the complexity of the skill increased. These findings support the premise that psychic factors have an important influence in muscle tone regulation, which affects the range of joint motion. Tense individuals may well possess "stiff joints." Although limited research indicates a linkage between the physical and emotional aspects as these components affect flexibility, more research is needed before definitive generalizations can be made.

Structural and Functional Aspects of Mobility

The articulating biomechanical structures of man are made up of bone, tendon, ligament, fascia, and cartilage. *Bone* provides the rigid physical support for joint articulation. *Tendons* serve as attachments to muscle, bone, or another tendon, ligament, or fascia and have the function of conveying the pull from one bone to another segment. *Ligaments* contain bundles of fibers richly supplied with *collagen* (protein substance), which gives joints tensile strength and limits the extent of separation and thereby assists in preventing injury. Ligaments are strong, pliable, and inextensible (incapable of being stretched) yet tough fibers that hold joints together. *Fascia* is composed of superficial and deep fibrous connective tissues of varying thickness and density. Its thickness and density depends upon the functional demands for elasticity. Articular *cartilage* is a gristlelike connective tissue that lies in bony cavities and serves as a protective cushion for articulating surfaces. Each of these structures contains different amounts of collagen. It has been suggested that increased rigidity of connective tissues surrounding joints and musculature is due, in part, to greater masses of collagenous substances, particularly among the elderly.[6] Muscular *extensibility* or *amplitude* also determines one's degree of flexibility. Dynamic-type activities that allow joints to proceed through a full range of motion enhance the extensibility of muscular tissue. Heavy resistance-type and isometric exercises tend to shorten fibers and thus restrict flexibility. The contractile qualities of actomyosin within the myofibrils of muscular tissues are continued indefinitely with proper nutrition and physical activity, barring pathological conditions. Morphological changes in muscle with old age do not become noticeable until a very late state, and secondary changes are due primarily to disease and nutritional deficiency.[7] Such activities as swimming and stretching type calisthenics are highly recommended for maintenance of muscular contractility and flexibility.

Functional flexibility performance has been studied by numerous researchers. Early investigators showed that extreme differences existed between right and left body measurements with certain articulations exhibiting as much as 200 percent differentials.[8,9] These data provided initial credence to the premise that flexibility is specific to joints rather than a general functional quality. Other investigators of a more recent vintage reinforce the concept of flexibility specificity to include females and champion athletes.[10,11] General agreement exists that flexibility is a *highly specific factor* rather than a general component, and the measurement of one joint cannot predict the range of motion in other body parts.[12] In addition to supporting the concept of flexibility specificity, the President's Council on Physical Fitness and Sports includes the following points, which have significant implications and relevance for professionals teaching physical education and coaching athletic sports[13]:

Flexibility patterns are different among and between girls and boys; and boys are generally less flexible than girls with flexibility decreasing after adolescence among both sexes.

Different sport activities produce unique patterns of flexibility. Swimmers and baseball players yield greatest flexibility measures, while wrestlers are least flexible.

The concept that weight training causes a muscle-bound condition is a myth.

Hold-stretch method of stretching (static) is an effective technique of improving joint flexibility.

FLEXIBILITY MEASUREMENT

Several techniques and methods have been utilized to measure joint range of motion. Devices such as the *mechanical goniometer* and *Leighton flexometer* are used to determine direct flexion and extension. Indirect methods of determining flexibility are usually integrated in a battery of physical fitness tests. Two simple indirect measures of trunk flexibility are shown in Figures 14.1a and 14.1b. The method utilized depends upon the purpose of gathering mobility data. Employing indirect methods is generally acceptable in determining gross measurement when precision is not necessary. The mechanical goniometer and Leighton flexometer are generally used for therapeutic and coaching purposes when greater precision in degrees of joint angulation is necessary.

Mechanical Goniometer

A popular device for measuring joint flexibility found in educational and clinical settings is the *universal goniometer*. Fundamentally, this tool is a protractor that has a fulcrum or axis with two lever arms attached. One of the arms is movable and is placed in line with the movable part of the body to be measured. Several variations of goniometers are available. Figure 14.2 illustrates three common types currently used by physical educators and allied health professionals.

The mechanical goniometer selected should (1) be durable with solid construction (stainless steel preferred), (2) be easy to read with clear marking with degrees ranging from 0 to 180 or 360 degrees depending on type, (3) have a movable arm with an adjustable pivot to allow for tightening at a fixed position after flexion or extension point is measured, (4) have degree readings numbered in two directions from zero to 180 and/or 360 degrees and from 180 and/or 360 to zero degrees. The lever arms should be approximately 15 inches long for upper and lower limbs. Finger joint goniometers should be three to four inches in length.

Although many variations in goniometer types exist, the authors prefer two basic kinds for general use: (1) 360 degree stainless steel goniometer with 15-inch lever arms, and (2) 180 degree type with four-inch lever arms. These instruments can effectively measure arm, leg, trunk, and finger articulations with reasonable accuracy.

The mechanical goniometer can yield valid information provided the tester uses the instrument correctly and in a consistent fashion. It is particularly important when measuring obese individuals that joint landmarks be carefully identified as reference points. In certain cases, excessive soft tissues may prevent the correct positioning of the instrument; therefore, other devices such as the Leighton flexometer should be employed to insure accurate measurement. Several methods exist to interpret the actual degree range of motion. Scores may be determined by subtracting complete flexion from full extension or expressing flexibility in terms of maximum flexion and extension. The authors recommend the *neutral zero method* offered by the committee for the study of joint motion of the American Academy of Orthopedic Surgeons and the American Orthopaedic Association. The principles indicated are as follows[14]:

1. All motions of a joint are measured from *zero starting positions.* Thus, the degrees of motion of a joint are added in the direction the joint moves from the zero starting position. (See Figures 14.3a through 14.3e).

2. The extended "anatomical position" of an extremity is therefore accepted as zero degrees, rather than 180 degrees.

3. The motion of the extremity being examined should be compared to that of the opposite extremity. The differences may be expressed in degrees of motion as compared to the opposite extremity, or in percentages of loss of motion in comparison with the opposite extremity.

4. A distinction is made between the terms *extension* and *hyperextension.* Extension is used when the position opposite to flexion, at the zero starting position, is a natural motion. This is present in the wrists and shoulder joints. If, however, the motion

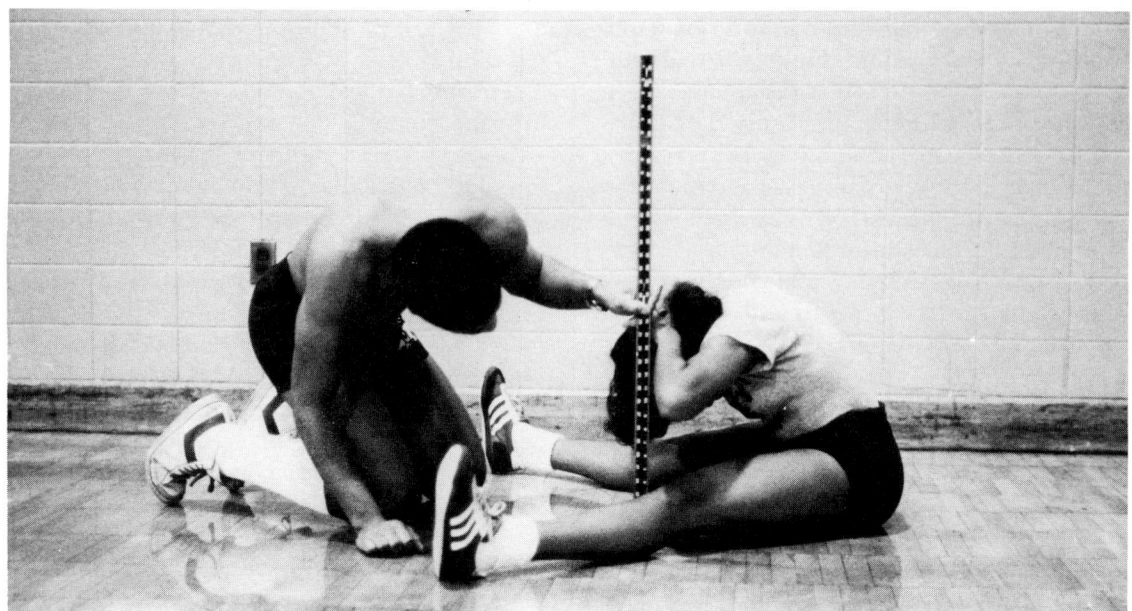

Figure 14.1a Indirect method of measuring trunk flexion (lower back)

Figure 14.1b Indirect method of measuring trunk extension (upper back)

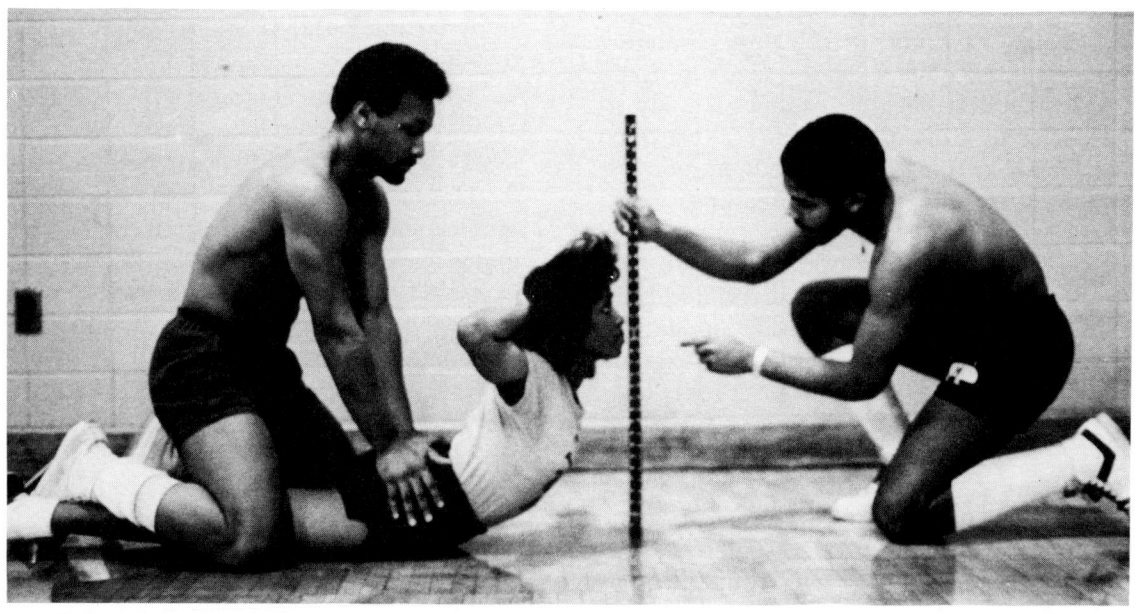

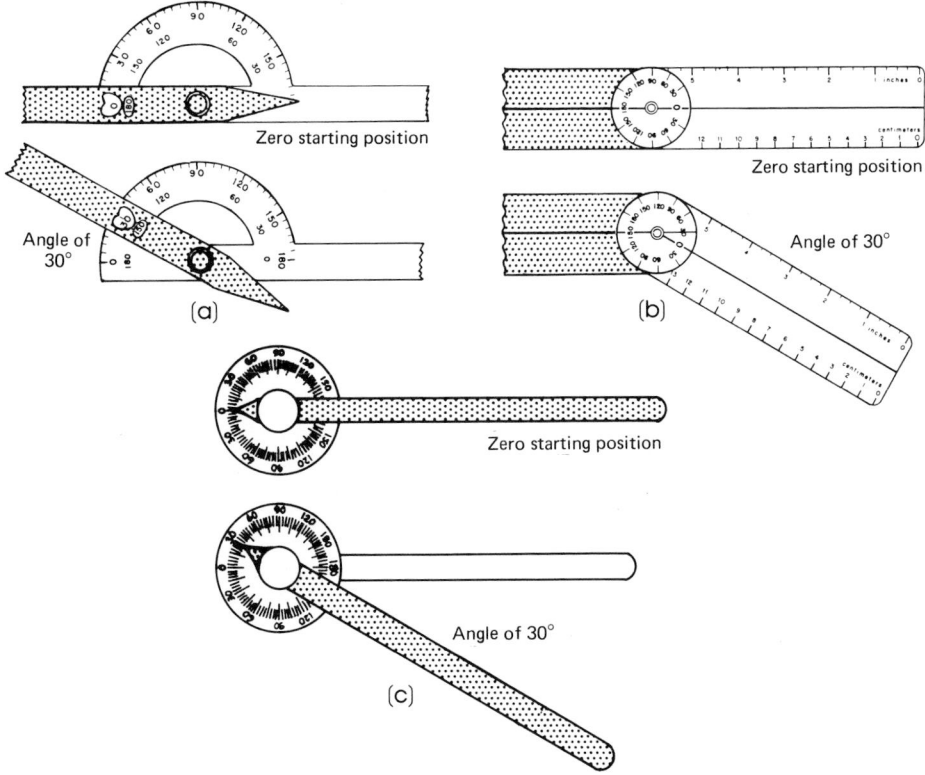

Figure 14.2 Various types of goniometers: **(a)** metal finger type, **(b)** 180 degree type, **(c)** 360 degree type (from C.V. Heck, I.E. Hendryson, and C.R. Rowe, **Joint Motion: Method of Measuring and Recording**, American Academy of Orthopaedic Surgeons, Chicago, Illinois, 1965, p. 9, with permission)

opposite flexion at the zero starting position is an unnatural one, such as that of the elbow or knees, it is referred to as hyperextension.

Figure 14.3, adapted from the manual *Joint Motion: Method of Measuring and Recording*, published by the AAOS, is presented to illustrate typical joints using the zero neutral method.

Studies indicate that a well-informed tester using a reliable and well-constructed tool can measure flexibility with high reliability.[15]

Joint ranges of motion continue to defy definitions of "average." Variations in physique, age and sex, and even temperament appear to affect flexibility among individuals. A recent investigation, prompted by the empirical observation of black superiority in such sports as track and field, basketball, and football, attempted to determine a relationship, if any, between flexibility and ethnic groups. One hundred youngsters ranging in age from 11 to 13 years of black, German, Italian, and Jewish populations were studied. Using a standard universal goniometer, flex-

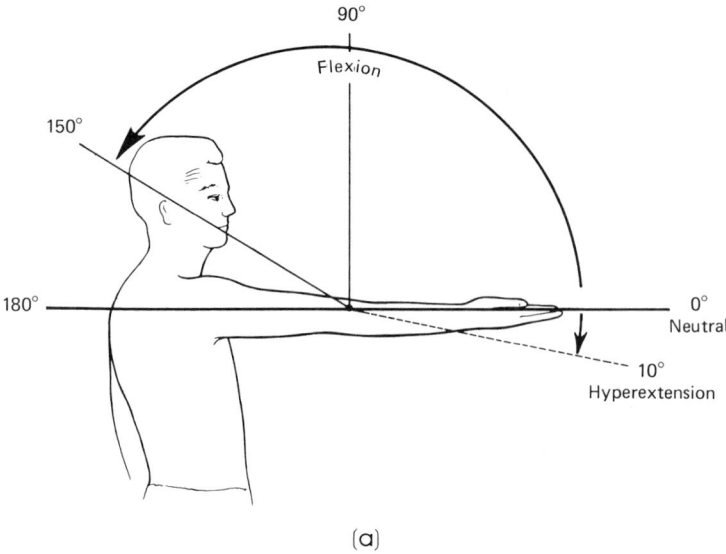

Flexion and hyperextension

90°

Flexion

150°

180°

0°
Neutral

10°
Hyperextension

(a)

Figure 14.3a The elbow (from C.V. Heck, I.E. Hendryson, and C.R. Rowe, **Joint Motion: Method of Measuring and Recording**, American Academy of Orthopaedic Surgeons, Chicago, Illinois, 1965, p. 9, with permission)

ibilities of neck, shoulder, hip, and ankle were determined. The hypothesis—that similar patterns of flexibility exist between members of a similar ethnic background was shown to be invalid; and the study disclosed that the existence of a significant or even casual correlation did not occur between joint ranges and ethnic variables.[16] Considering the findings of this research, we can assume that a great deal of variability is present among individuals of all ages, sexes, and backgrounds; therefore, flexibility norms should be interpreted, at best, as rough guides in assessing flexibility. Table 14.1 presents estimates in average ranges of joint motion. It is emphasized that these data should serve merely as *guides* and not standards.

Leighton Flexometer

The accuracy and reliability of flexibility measurement was improved with the advent of the *Leighton flexometer* developed and refined by its inventor Jack R. Leighton of Eastern Washington College, Washington.[17,18] Leighton pointed out the limitation of linear measurement devices such as the goniometer. He argued that tall persons have longer segments than shorter persons. Therefore, longer segments moving through the same arc (range of motion) would give greater linear measurements (caliper measurements); and the arcs formed (angular measurement) by longer body segments from their starting positions might actually be equal to, greater than, or less than those of shorter segments.

The instrument shown in Figure 14.4 consists of a weighted 360 degree dial and a weighted pointer mounted in a case.[19] These figures illustrate position one and position two following the prescribed procedure established by Leighton.

An instrument called the *electrogoniometer* has been devised to measure continuous

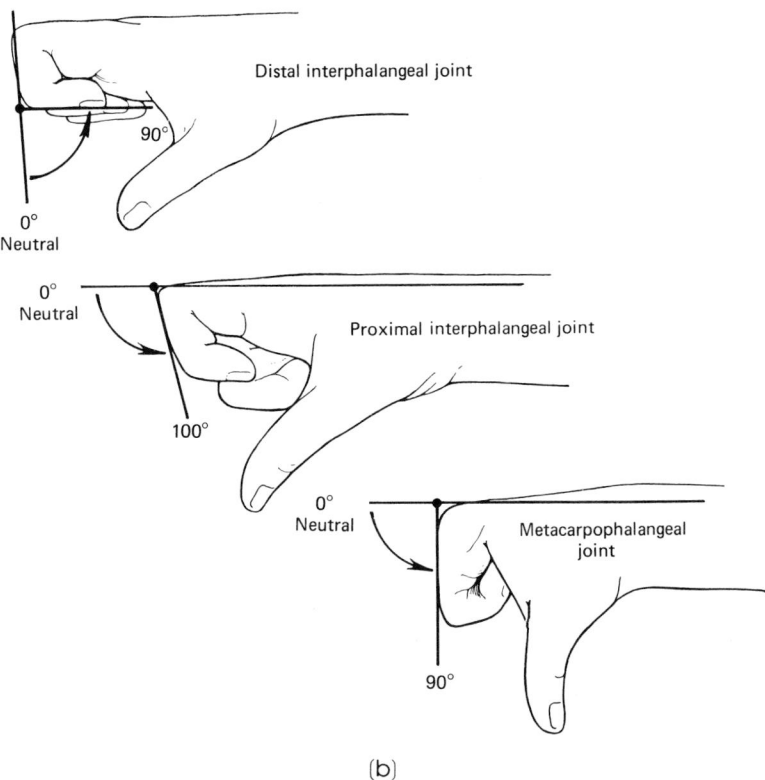

Distal interphalangeal joint

90°

0°
Neutral

0°
Neutral

Proximal interphalangeal joint

100°

0°
Neutral

Metacarpophalangeal joint

90°

(b)

Figure 14.3b *The fingers (flexion) (from C.V. Heck, et al.,* **op. cit.,** *p. 27)*

changes in joint motion. The student is referred to the next chapter, dealing with quantitative assessment instruments, for a detailed discussion of this electronic tool.

PRINCIPLES OF FITNESS AND CONDITIONING

Physical conditioning programs for athletes should develop those qualities of fitness most needed for success in their particular sport. Some sports place a high premium upon aerobic fitness while others demand anaerobic fitness. Different skills require flexibility in different joints and muscular strength in different muscle groups. Certain sports require explosive power whereas others demand muscular endurance. The mentor who wishes

to produce maximal possible success must tailor the conditioning program to the demands of the sport. This almost mandates an *individualized* physical conditioning program since diverse modalities must be used to achieve different objectives.

Whether an activity is classified as aerobic or anaerobic is dependent upon the speed or intensity with which the activity is done. The more the demand for oxygen exceeds the capacity to deliver oxygen to the cells, the greater the anaerobic component and the less the aerobic component. Obviously, some individuals have a greater capacity to deliver oxygen to the cells; therefore, an intensity of activity that is aerobic for one person may be anaerobic for another. Interval training, rope skipping, circuit training, grass drills,

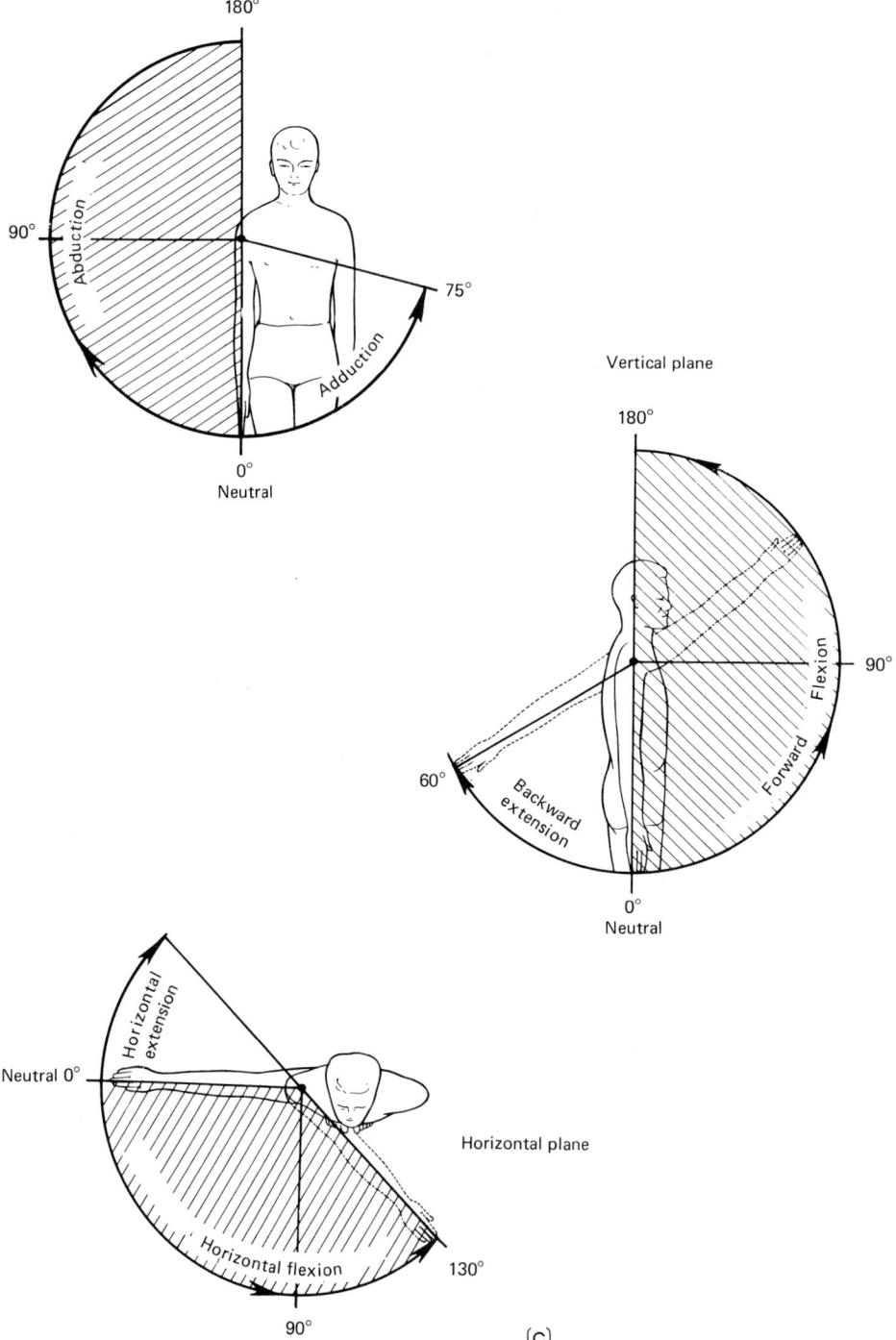

Figure 14.3c Motion of arm at the shoulder (from C.V. Heck, et al., **op. cit.**, p. 33)

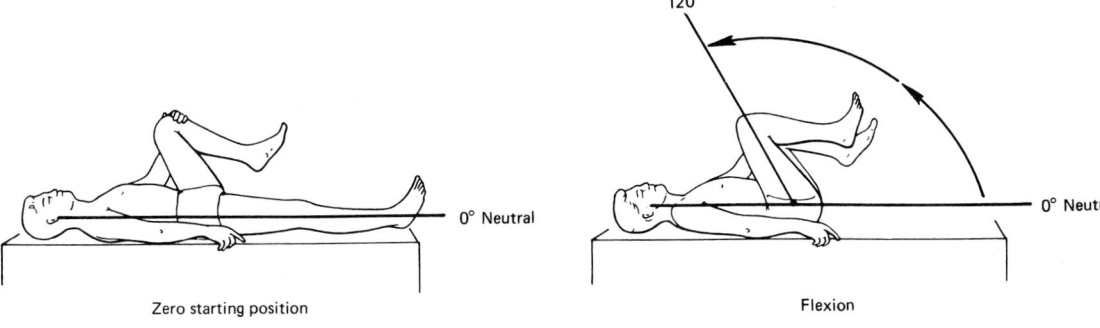

Figure 14.3d The hip (flexion) (from C.V. Heck, et al., **op. cit.**, p. 57)

and wind sprints are activities that improve anaerobic condition. Jogging, distance running, slow cycling, and slow swimming will develop aerobic condition. Intensive bouts of cycling and swimming alternating with rest periods or decelerated speed will develop anaerobic condition by improving the ability of the body to utilize stored adenosine triphosphate (ATP) and creatine phosphate (CP) and to reduce glucose to pyruvic acid

Figure 14.3e The ankle (from C.V. Heck, et al., **op. cit.**, p. 69)

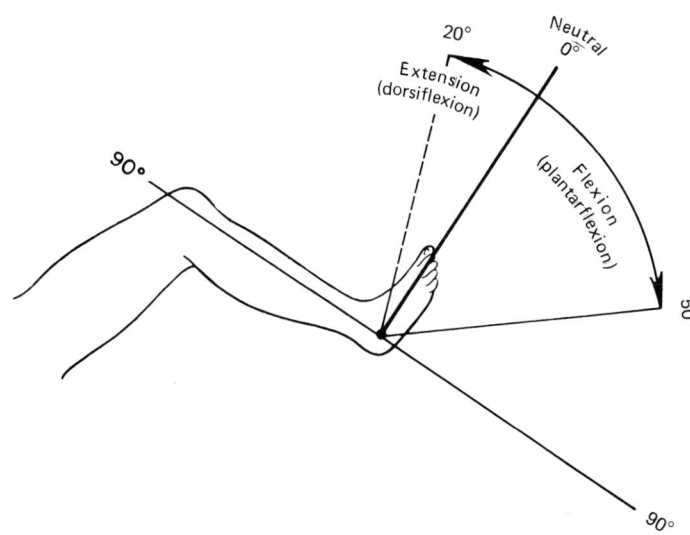

(glycolysis). Recent research also reports that this type of training improves aerobic condition when the exercise bouts are at four-minute intervals.[20]

Different Physical Qualities Needed for Success in Diverse Sports

Every sport requires for success different physical qualities.[21] The long-distance runner needs great aerobic fitness; large muscles would be a handicap. The hammer thrower needs little or no endurance but does need great power and huge muscles. Sprinters and middle-distance runners need great anaerobic endurance; they also need power but must keep bulk as low as possible. The football lineman needs powerful leg and shoulder muscles to execute the explosive block or tackle or to crash through the line. The gymnast needs a strong upper body; it is advantageous if the legs and buttocks are light. Baseball pitchers, javelin and discus throwers, gymnasts, and tennis players need good flexibility in the shoulder girdle. This increased range of motion will increase the length of the backswing and, consequently, the distance through which momentum can be generated while throwing or swinging the racquet.

Different Procedures for Developing Diverse Physical Qualities

Weight training, isometric, and isokinetic exercises can be selected that develop the specific muscle groups upon which the greatest demands are placed in the sport of the athlete's choice. There is a relationship between the amount of resistance that is placed against the muscle and the demands of the sport. For sports in which bulk is an advantage, or at least not a handicap, and where great power is required, fewer repetitions against greater resistance can be done. For sports that place greater demands upon muscular endurance in which greater body weight is a disadvantage, greater numbers of repetitions against less resistance should be practiced.

Some sports are characterized by short intensive bursts of activity followed by a rest or a slower pace. Participants in these sports should develop anaerobic condition and the consequent ability to tolerate an oxygen debt through interval training types of activity.[22] Examples of this type of activity are the all-around in gymnastics, soccer, and football. In other sports the activity is continuous and sustained. Participants in these sports should develop aerobic fitness through jogging, cycling, or other types of sustained activity. They need to develop the ability to take in, distribute, and process enough oxygen to keep up with the cells' demands for oxygen as the activity is continued.[23]

Agility

Agility is the ability to change direction quickly and effectively while moving as nearly as possible at full speed. Agility is primarily a function of strength and power as related to body mass. In all agility tests the performer must establish momentum in one direction as quickly as possible and then decelerate and stop this momentum and explode in a new, slightly altered direction. Starting and stopping quickly is dependent upon power. The muscles decelerate and stop movement or overcome moving inertia by undergoing eccentric contraction. How effectively the muscles do this is dependent upon their power as related to the body mass. Therefore, the way to improve agility (other than through practice on the specific test of agility) is either to increase strength while holding body weight constant or to decrease body weight while holding strength constant.

Table 14.1 Average Ranges of Joint Motion

Joint	Average in Degrees	Joint	Average in Degrees
Elbow		**Shoulder**	
Flexion	150	Forward flexion	180
Hyperextension	0	Horizontal flexion	135
Forearm		Backward extension	60
Pronation	80	Abduction	180
Supination	80	Adduction	75
Wrist		**Hip**	
Extension	70	Flexion	120
Flexion	80	Extension	30
Ulnar deviation	30	Abduction	45
Radial deviation	20	Adduction	30
Thumb		**Knee**	
Abduction	70	Flexion	135
I-P joint	80	Hyperextension	10
M-P	50	**Ankle**	
M-C	15	Plantar flexion (flexion)	50
Extension		Dorsiflexion (extension)	20
Distal joint	20	**Spine**	
M-P	0	Cervical	
M-C	20	Flexion	45
Fingers		Extension	45
Flexion		Lateral bending	45
Distal joint	90	Thoracic and lumbar	
Middle joint	100	Flexion	80
Proximal joint	90	Extension	20–30
Extension		Lateral bending	35
Distal joint	0		
Middle joint	0		
Proximal joint	45		

From C. V. Heck, I. E. Hendryson, and C. E. Rowe, *Joint Motion: Method of Measuring and Recording*, American Academy of Orthopaedic Surgeons, Chicago, Illinois: 1965, pp. 81–86.

Necessity for Kinesiological Analysis When Prescribing Exercises

Analysis of muscle involvement is essential if exercises are to be properly prescribed for development of specific muscle groups. Perhaps the classic example of this concept is provided in the abdominal exercise known as the "leg raiser" when it is used as part of an exercise program to improve posture. Some physical educators have believed that the leg raiser is primarily an abdominal exercise because upon palpation the abdominal muscles are seen to be in hard contraction during the exercise. However, muscular analysis shows that all the abdominal muscles insert on the crest of the ilium and pubis. They cannot flex the hip joint. They do, however, stabilize the pelvis and prevent it from tilting forward (in-

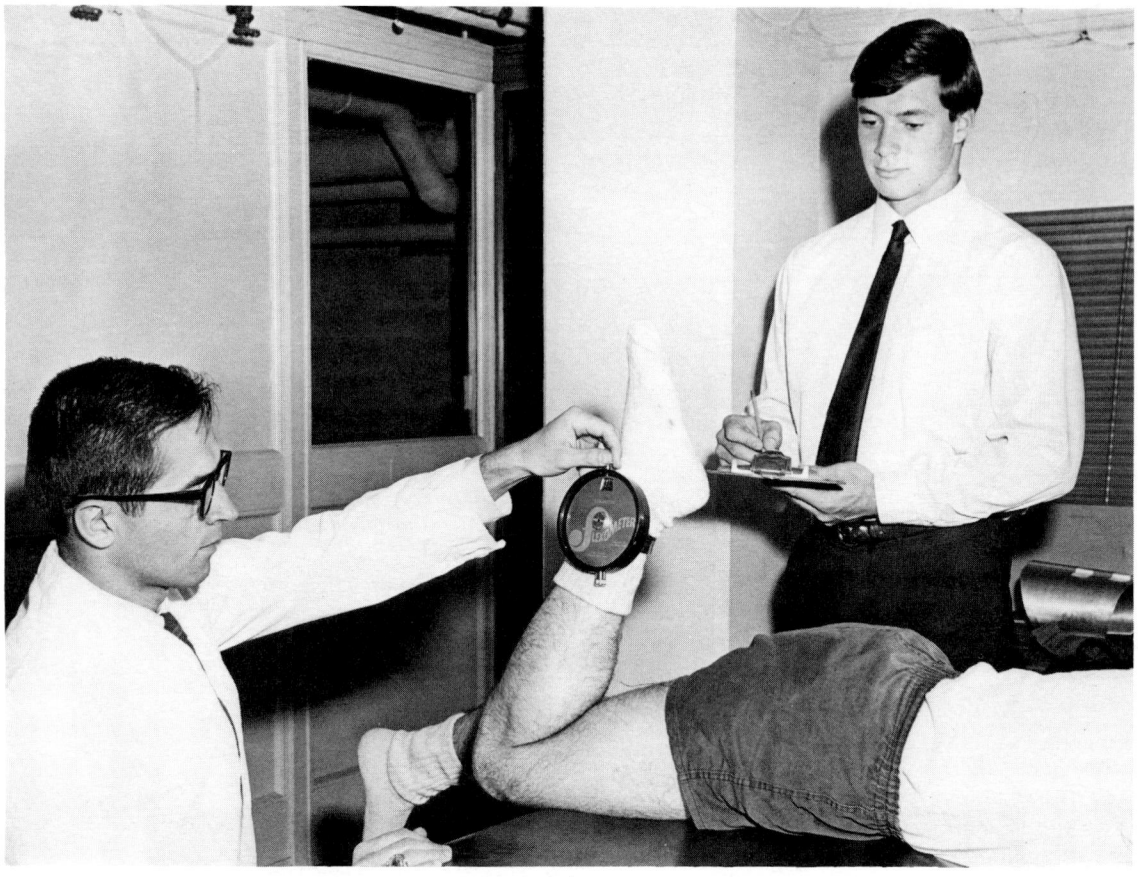

(a)

Figure 14.4 Complete knee extension: **(a)** Position one, flexion **(b)** position two, extension

creased inclination) due to the pull of the iliacus, whose proximal attachment is the anterior surface of the ilium and the base of the sacrum, and the psoas, whose proximal attachment is the sides of the bodies and intervertebral cartilages of the last thoracic and all the lumbar vertebrae and the front and lower borders of the transverse processes of the lumbar vertebrae. Both the iliacus and the psoas have their distal attachment on and below the lesser trochanter of the femur. It can easily be seen that these two muscles are hip flexors and that if the abdominal muscles are insufficiently strong to stabilize the pelvis, the lumbar curve will be exaggerated. That is, the pelvis will be tilted forward and the concavity of the lumbar curve will be increased. The lumbar curve may be sufficiently increased to produce lordosis, a postural deformity, if the difference between the strength of the abdominal muscles and the iliacus and psoas is greatly in favor of the latter two muscles. For this reason, this exercise is contraindicated.

Maximal Resistance, Strength, and Stress

Maximal strength gains can be made only through continuous increments in the resist-

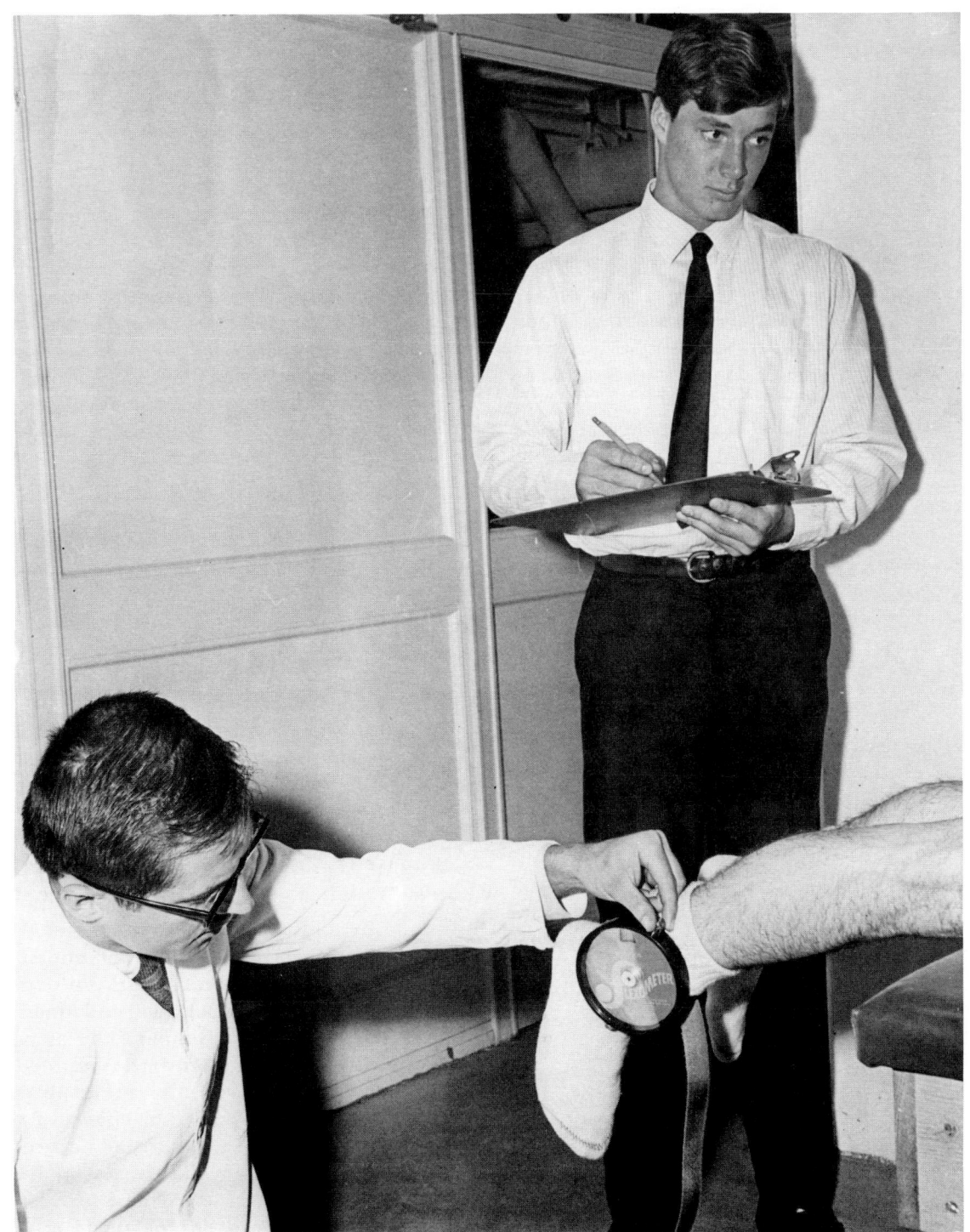

(b)

MOBILITY PATTERNS, FITNESS, AND AGING   **507**

ance provided against muscles whether the contraction is concentric, eccentric, or static (isometric). It is a fundamental law of nature that all living things adapt to stresses to which they are subjected providing the stress is not excessive. Man and other animals have adapted to the stress of extreme cold in Alaska and to the stress of extreme heat in Kenya, to the humidity of the bayous of Louisiana and the aridness of the Mohave Desert, to all sorts of diets, to the altitudes of Salt Lake City and the Andes Mountains. Conditioning for endurance, strength, or flexibility is a manifestation of adaptation to the stress of physical activity.

When muscles are not used they atrophy. When a fractured limb is placed in a cast, the cast fits snugly; however, after a few weeks there is considerable space between the cast and the limb—sometimes enough to insert the hand. The cast did not stretch; the muscles of the limb atrophied. On the other hand, when the muscle is stressed, it hypertrophies.

AGING AND MOVEMENT PATTERNS

Demographic data clearly point to the steadily and continuously increasing number of older persons within our society. The census bureau reported 42 million persons over 55 years of age in 1976, and projections indicate that this group will continue to grow well beyond the year 2000.[24] The consequences of poor health and fitness, particularly among older citizens, are cogently expressed by Dr. Raymond Harris, geriatric physician and cardiologist, in recent testimony to a Senate subcommittee on fitness for older persons[25]:

Impaired mobility in middle-aged and older people, often the result of poor physical fitness, leads to social isolation, personality and emotional deterioration and poor mental health. Physically inactive people past 50 perceive their bodies to be broader and heavier than they really are and they experience bodily activities as increasingly strenuous. Kinesthetic pleasures which young people derive from motor action are steadily reduced in habitually sedentary elderly subjects who eventually become reluctant to move at all. Muscular degeneration, distinct physiological changes and distortion of body image resulting from restriction of physical exercise lead to greater clumsiness, increased fear of physical activity and development of faulty feedback mechanisms between movement and body image. Inactive older people develop increased internal tensions and pent-up aggressions. Physical exercise programs that encourage older Americans to be more active, independent and mobile, provide economic benefits by reducing medical problems and hospital costs. Group exercise programs at all ages assist people to acquire new friends, new interests and lead to better mental and physical health. The rationale of exercise and activity programs in geriatric day care centers is based upon helping older people to rejoin society and thereby feel better mentally and physically. Ludotherapy (treatment by games) is useful to help the aged person who exhibits a tendency to disengage from the world and society.

Although fitness benefits and/or impairments affect the individual holistically, our discussion focuses upon biological and kinesiological changes that accompany the aging process with implications for the improvement of mobility patterns. The authors contend that the need to maintain *physical fitness and mobility* is a basic one for the enhancement of human effectiveness of the individual. Sedation, in its extreme manifestation, ultimately leads to physical, emotional, and, finally, mental degeneration.

FITNESS AND AGING IN HUMANS

Aging is irreversible; it is an inescapable retrogressive process of *structural, functional,* and *chemical* changes in the human organism. Although the process cannot be stopped, we believe that the rate can be slowed down to a significant degree by maintaining sensible standards of physical fitness. This conviction is based upon the overwhelming research evidence supporting the value of exercise and mobility regimens for the improvement of human efficiency, and the profound movement pattern differentials of individuals beyond the age of 55, ranging from the "rocking chair" set to the alert and vigorous life style of "paddle ball" players (see Figure 14.5).

Anthropometrical and Skeletal Changes

It is well known that as individuals age, they become shorter. In fact, decreases in stature of one to three inches, and even more, are reported as occurring over a lifetime.[26] Generally, females lose approximately 4.9 cm (nearly 2 inches). Males lose about 2.9 cm (nearly 1¼ inches) with about half of the decline in sitting height. Most of the stature decrement is due to a "thinning out" or flattening of intervertebral disks. Bones tend to lose their density or mass and become more porous and fragile, particularly among women. Not only does stature decrease, ligaments and tendons lose elasticity with varying degrees of calcification. The results of these changes affect the posture mechanics of older persons. Thoracic kyphosis (round upper back) evolves, further hastened by a pattern of walking and sitting in a "slump" position and characterized by carrying the posture with knees and hips in slight flexion. Habits of walking and sitting in which an erect posture is not assumed contribute to height shrinkage. The appendicular skeleton (long bones) do not shrink as much as the axial skeleton (vertebral column). Therefore, it is not unusual for elderly persons, particularly those individuals beyond 70, to have a stature of long arms and legs with short torsos, the reverse picture of physique in infancy and early childhood.

Another contributing cause of loss in height is a decrease in protein substance called *collagen* from bony tissue. Collagen is a fibrous substance common to bone, cartilage, and intervertebral disks. Coupled with calcium loss, extreme decreases result in *osteoporosis*, which not only produces fragility of bones but causes more loss in height. Studies have shown that aging subjects may lose as much as 5 cm (nearly 2 inches) in total height within relatively short periods of time (1 to 3 years) especially in the case of women at the menopause.[27] Resorption of bone and loss of bone mass occur as a natural change with aging. An interesting study provides some evidence that bone growth can happen when elderly persons participate in regular and systematic exercise programs. Researchers at the University of Wisconsin investigated bone resorption of a group of elderly women aged 69 to 95 before and after an exercise program.[28] These investigators found bone growth following the conditioning program, lending support to the belief that exercise does slow down the rate of bone shrinkage.

A majority of spines, after the fourth decade, show disk degeneration, and the process intensifies sharply after age 50. The cervical vertebrae are frequently involved; it is this segment of the spinal column that requires greater mobility for rotating the head. Because of these bony changes and the stresses of head mobility, it is not uncommon for spinal stiffness and arthritic complaints to prevail among the elderly. Popular exercises such as head-rolling, which moves the head in a continuous circumducting motion, are not recommended for older persons, particularly beyond the age of 60, because of the "grinding" affect that may further aggravate

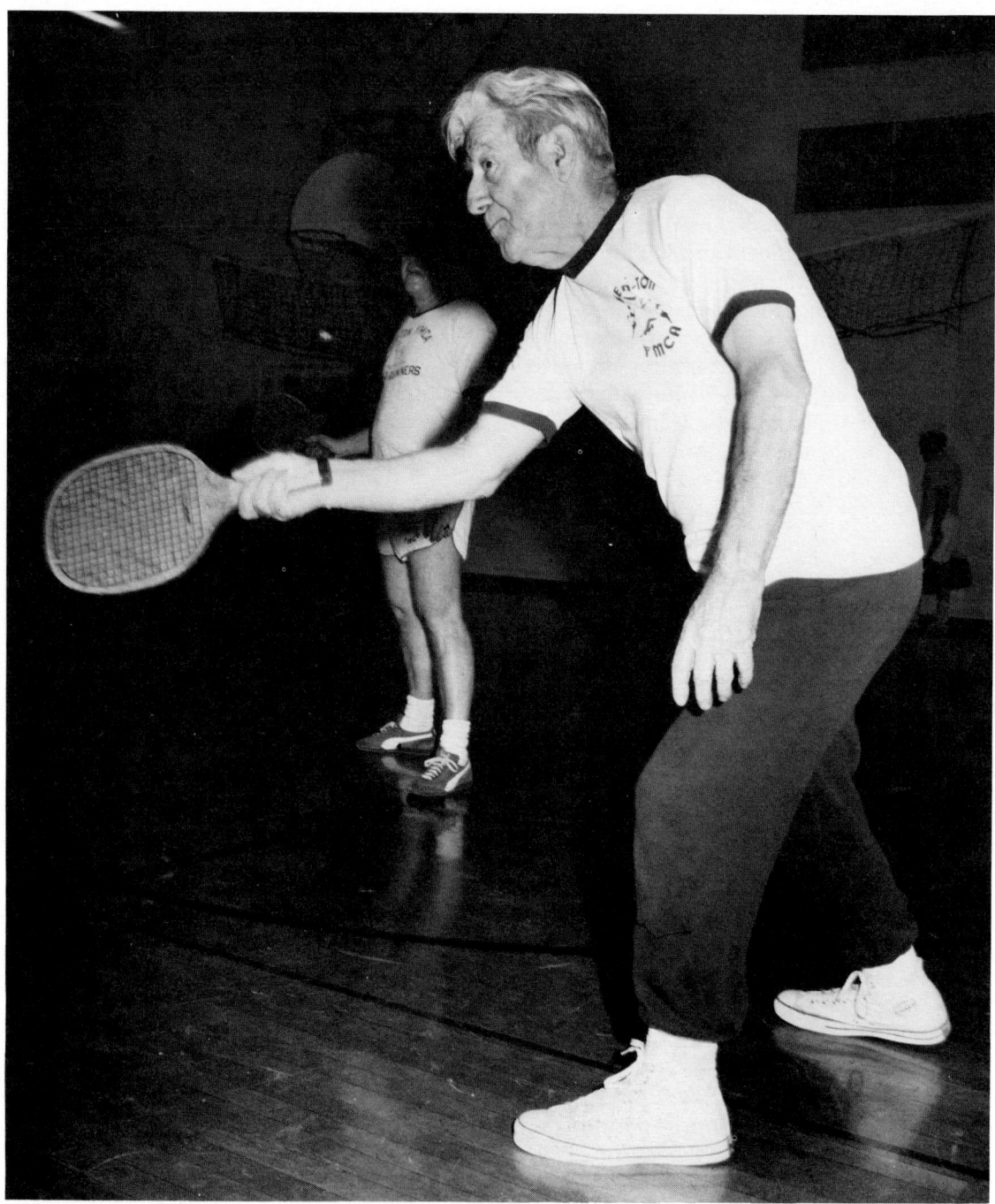

Figure 14.5 Playing paddle ball at 70 (from John Piscopo, "Preparing Geriatric Fitness and Recreation Specialist," **JOPER**, 48:24–29, October, 1977)

the intervertebral disks of the cervical spine. Slow rotation left and right is less traumatic to these joints than continuous head-rolling, which may also disturb the balance mechanism located within the inner ear of the exercising individual. Figure 14.6 illustrates physique and age changes of a male group from ages 20 to 79.

Figure 14.6 shows a change in physical appearance comparing young men with older persons. The young mesomorphic body build with wide shoulders and trim abdominal girth is reversed. Biiliac and abdominal girths gradually increase, thus projecting the pyramid physique with larger buttocks and waist and a narrowing of shoulder width. It should be noted that these changes do not necessarily apply to the well-conditioned older individual. Mesomorphic physique characteristics can be retained indefinitely provided sensible conditioning regimens are maintained.

Body Composition

Body weight typically rises to approximately age 50, then is followed by a gradual decline as shown in Figure 14.6. Women generally hold their weight gain longer than men. Weight in humans is indeed highly variable and subject to continuous change. Lifestyle and nutritional modes have a profound effect on body weight. It is well known that when individuals expend higher levels of energy with restricted food intake, fat gain does not occur. Body weight, especially in the form of

Figure 14.6 Physique and age—selected variables: white veterans, normative aging study (from A. Damon, et al., *Journal of Gerontology*, 27:205, 1972, with permission)

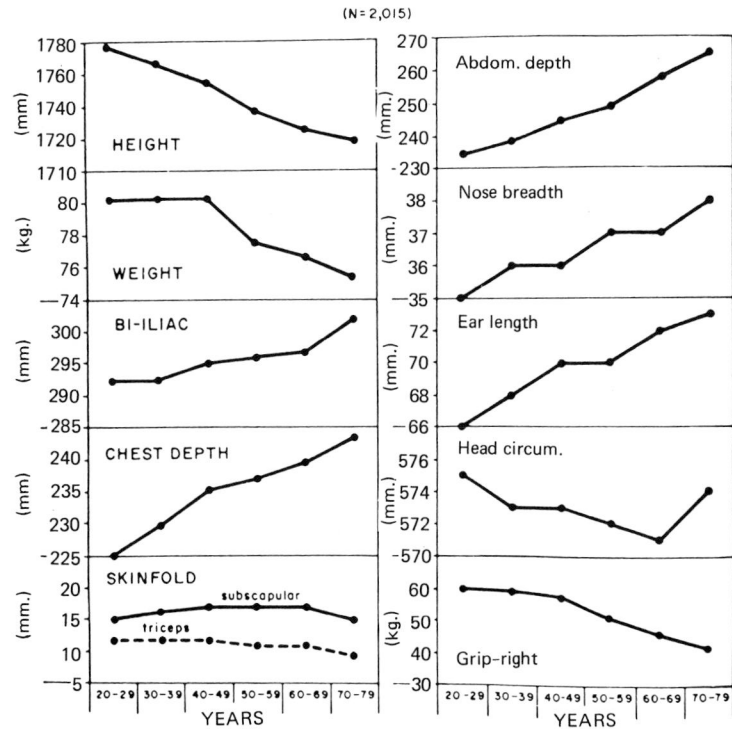

(N = 2,015)

adipose tissue, serves as a morphological restraint to the efficiency of human movement. Fat tissue is inert; it cannot generate muscular contraction, and in some cases, excessive deposits may literally impede motion. For example, an individual with an enormous waistline may not find it possible to perform a sit-up exercise from the supine position. The disadvantage of heavy weight, which is usually due to adipose tissue among middle aged and older persons, is exemplified by applying Newton's first law of motion, which states that the inertia of the body is directly related to its mass, and in order to overcome the body's resting inertia, a force must be exerted on its mass. In this example, body weight is considered mass although technically these properties are different. The heavier an object, the more force is required to move the mass from one point to another. Of course, other facts, such as distance, velocity, density, and gravity, enter in precise quantitative analysis. This discussion points out that greater body weight demands greater energy expenditure and force for generating motion than a lighter one. The source of force emanates from contractile tissue of muscle fibers, which diminish with age unless the individual continues a training program. Increases in body weight coupled with decreases in muscular strength negatively affect the individual's ability to move under his/her own power. It is possible for certain individuals to remain the same weight, yet gain in subcutaneous fatty tissue. Fat increases while muscle decreases, reducing specific gravity. The deterioration in physique is the result of inactivity. Jokl[29] reports the condition of an international wrestler at 28 years of age with his condition at 63 after discontinuance of all training for more than 30 years. Figure 14.7 illustrates the dramatic change in shape without weight change. Specific gravity was down by 5 percent, which implies a reduction in muscle and a deposit of surplus fat.

Practical Adipose Measurement. Body shape and adipose dimensions for young and older persons can be determined by simple girth measurements and skinfold caliper procedures. Calipers are particularly well-suited for older people since this instrument is innocuous and easy to use and to interpret.

Chest, abdominal, arm, and leg circumference provides objective data about size and shape. Caliper techniques furnish evidence about adipose tissue. Although girth measurements yield configurative data, this procedure does not distinguish differences between muscular and fatty tissue. Girth size may be due to adipose deposits or concentrated stores of muscle mass. Since fat is inactive tissue, and muscular fibers provide the energy source for human mobility, it would seem that maintenance of a sensible state of muscular tone and hypertrophy is vital as one advances in chronological years. The skinfold caliper shown in Figure 14.8 is a valid instrument to determine subcutaneous (skinfold) thickness. However, careful attention is needed with the technique. Variability of skinfold scores greatly depends upon the objectivity of the tester's procedure. Careful and consistent bite depths of the subcutaneous folds must be observed using a calibrated caliper with jaw face pressure of 10 gm/mm^2. The skinfold caliper measurement technique provides a quick and accurate estimate of body fat and should be part of the body composition evaluative process of older persons. These data, in conjunction with other anthropometrical measurements such as height, weight, and girth measurements, can be an effective way to appraise the leanness/fatness status of an individual.

The ease and rapidity with which a fold of skin is located and lifted are important factors in site selection of skinfolds. Based on the authors' experience and that of other skinfold caliper researchers, the following body areas are recommended, fulfilling the criteria of

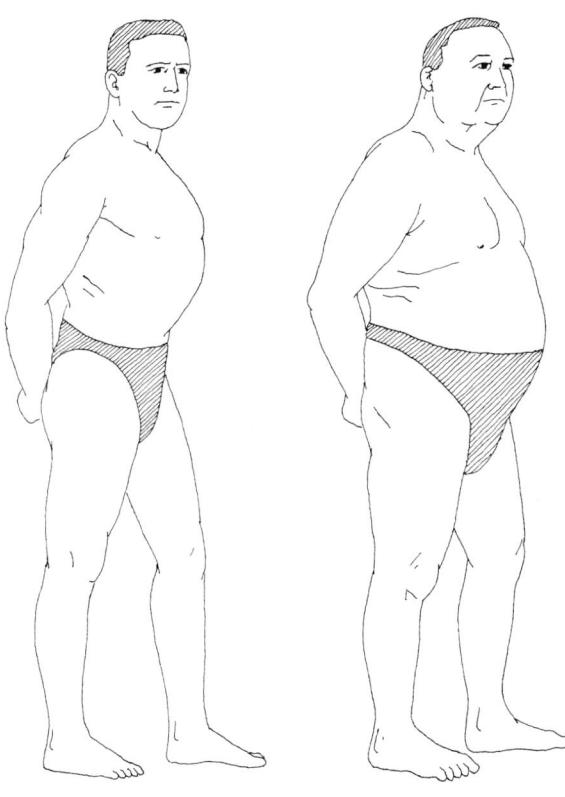

Figure 14.7 Physique at 28 and again at 63 (from Ernest Jokl, M.D., **Physiology of Exercise**, 1964. Courtesy of Charles C. Thomas, Publishers, Springfield, Illinois)

ease, accuracy, and rapidity of measurement[30]:

Posterior Arm. Subject standing, measurement is made at the fold parallel to the long axis of the preferred arm, over the triceps, halfway between the olecranon and acromial processes (Figure 14.9).

Abdomen. Subject standing, measurement is made with skinfold oriented laterally approximately 5 cm to the right of the navel.

Scapula. Subject standing, measurement is made at the fold diagonally from the vertebral column toward the inferior angle and slightly toward the midline of the body.

The upper posterior arm is a popular measurement location and can give reliable estimates when only one site is to be measured. Additionally, this surface area can be measured in men and women without disrobing. Body composition evaluation can be an important motivational tool since many older persons are interested in maintaining their appearance as the inevitable physical changes come about with the aging process. Improvement in body shape can and does occur with regular physical activity.

Fat loss trends with aging tend to be centripetal; that is, fat is lost early and to a greater degree from the extremities and is maintained more consistently and longer on the trunk.[31] Females generally show a greater skinfold thickness pattern throughout the life cycle.

Muscles and Muscular Strength

Empirical observations and scientific investi-

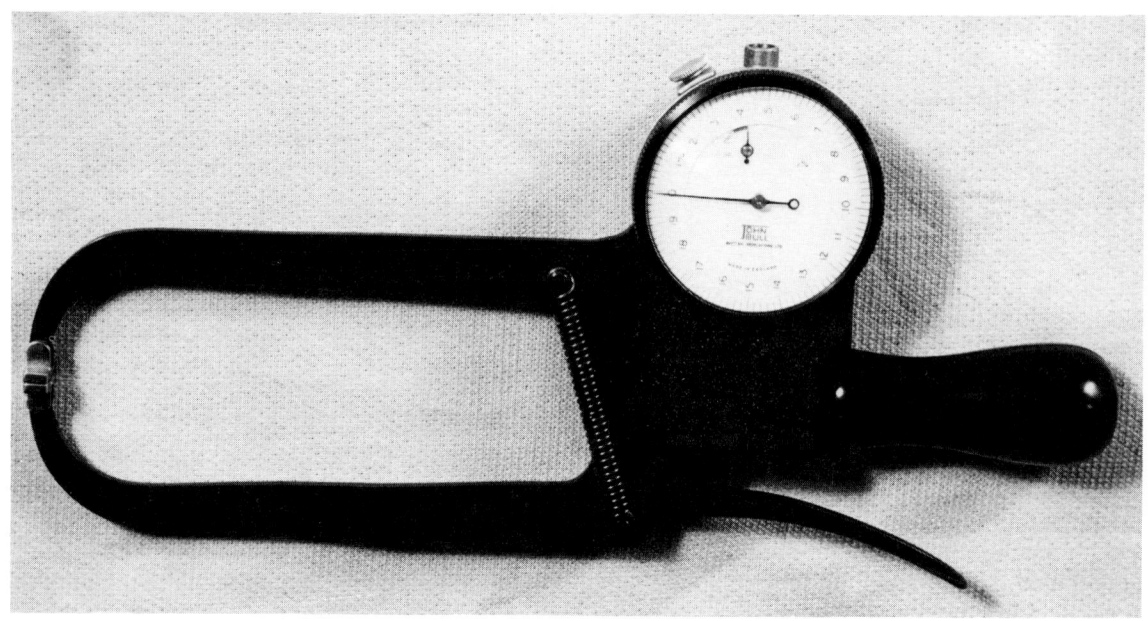

Figure 14.8 The harpenden skinfold caliper (courtesy of British Indicators Ltd., London, England)

gations indicate a gradual decrement in strength with advancing age. However, it should be noted that like adipose tissue, this parameter is variable and subject to extreme differences among individuals. Certainly, morphological and biochemical changes naturally occur such as loss in muscle weight and increase in collagen and fat, but again the degree of change is alterable. As in all biological mechanisms, heredity and nutrition affect muscular performance; however, our discussion centers on the effects of use and disuse of muscles upon the quality of contractile tissue with implications for sustaining mobility and efficient movement well into the mature years. Morphological muscle changes do not become noticeable until a very late date. Disuse is considered one important factor in anatomical and physiological characteristics of declining strength.[32]

Muscles are basically differentiated into two categories: fast and slow types according to the performance demands of speed and/or endurance. Although we know that a gradual loss of cells occurs with a reduction in size and number of muscle fibers, some evidence suggests that a progressive loss of differentiation between fast and slow muscles also takes place in old age.[33,34] Therefore, muscular performance is a multiple process that is affected, not only by the quality of muscle tissue itself, but also by neuronal, hormonal, vasomotor, and other body interactions, which, again, underscore the concept of holistic integrity—all parameters function together as an organic ensemble.

Muscular strength is essential for effective and efficient living of older persons, because of its direct relationship to mobility and volitional movements of the body. Skeletal strength provides the energy and force required by the big muscles used in walking, artwork and typing. Motion cannot evolve unless force is present. That force originates

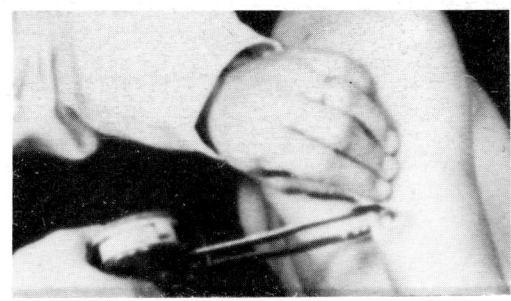

Figure 14.9 Measuring posterior arm skinfold

from the contractile qualities of muscular tissue. Humans may have force without movement (isometric contraction) but never dynamic movement (isotonic contraction) without force.

Muscular development programs have centered around training and conditioning for youth and young adults. Isotonic, isometric, and isokinetic (special machines to control resistance and speed) techniques have been developed. Each type contains training value, depending upon the purpose sought by the participant. Heavy resistive exercises are contraindicated for unconditioned older persons because of their potential danger to the cardiovascular system and probable triggering of the valsalva effect, which increases the intrathoracic pressure surrounding the heart.

Essentially, strength development and maintenance programs for persons over 50 years serve two basic purposes: (1) to provide vital qualitative myogenic tone (muscle firmness through activity) for sustaining good posture, and (2) to provide the energy source of power and force needed for efficient movement in daily work tasks and play.[35, 36] A consequence of poor muscular strength and tone among older persons often reflects itself in defective posture and body mechanics. As muscular strength and endurance decline, posture problems intensify. The characteristics of forward head, trunk, and knees, labeled "posture fatigue," is common among

residents in institutions for the elderly. The extensor or antigravity muscles gradually lose their ability to withstand the constant pull of gravity, and the body is literally weighted into the ground. Kyphosis (round upper back) and ptosis (sagging abdominal wall) are prevalent musculoskeletal dysfunctions of older persons, particularly after a bout with illness. These conditions are described in Chapter 12. Restoration of shoulder girdle, abdominal, and gluteal muscular strength can improve and sustain the efficiency of the structural framework for various stationary and locomotive posture movements.

Kinesiologically, the human musculoskeletal system is not constructed for strength advantages. As indicated in Chapter 7, the anatomical mechanical structure is comprised primarily of third-class levers with long resistance and short force arms, which require considerable muscular strength to produce rotary joint movement. Simple flexion of the elbow joint illustrates a classic internal lever of the third class with the insertion of forearm flexors (force point) located close to the joint (fulcrum) and the resistance applied at the end of the end of the hand (weight). Figure 14.10 demonstrates a short force arm compared to the long resistance arm found in the elbow joint.

In addition to strength loss with age and the problem of overcoming the muscular disadvantage of the third-class lever system, other mechanical factors affect the efficiency of joint movement. For example, flexion of the elbow joint is influenced by the method in which the movement is performed. If the elbow is flexed with the hand in the supine position (palm up) as shown in Figure 14.11a, less muscular force is required than when the same movement is performed with the hand positioned in pronation (palm down). Figure 14.11b illustrates the negative twisting effect of the biceps tendon around the radius as the fibers unwrap with the hand in the pronated position. The biceps brachii is not only a flex-

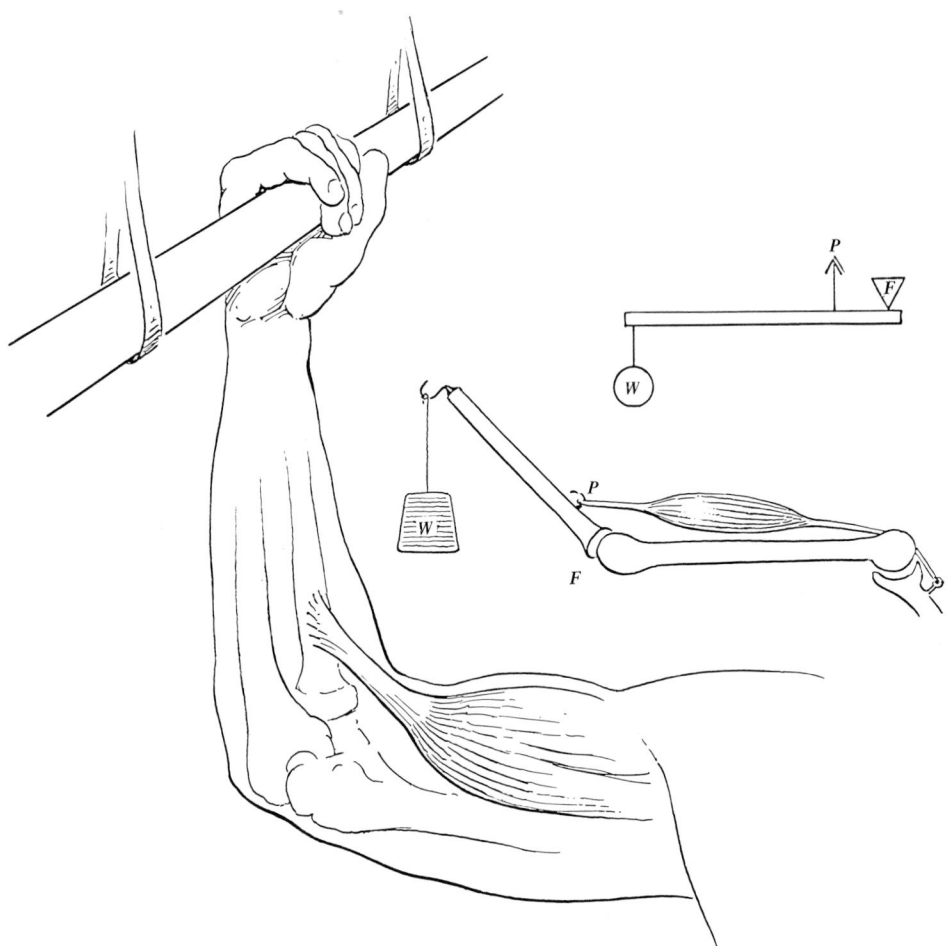

Figure 14.10 W = weight, P = power, F = fulcrum. Muscular disadvantage of the third-class lever. (from John Piscopo, "Assessment of Forearm Positions upon Upperarm and Shoulder Strength Performance," **Kinesiology IV**, AAHPER, 1974, p. 55)

or of the elbow but a prime supinator as well, and this factor affects the pulling efficiency in flexion. The insertion of the biceps on the tuberosity of the radius lies behind the long axis of the latter so that the tendon winds around the ulna border of the radius. It is this supinatory effect that prohibits the full mechanical advantage of the muscle's direct line of pull upon the biceps when the forearm is pronated.[37] The forearm flexors can exert their greatest force with the hand in the supinated position. The correct hand grasp has important implications for physical educators and allied health specialists. Individuals with low strength levels can perform elbow flexion movements with less muscular force and greater efficiency by using the *supinated hand position.* This is especially relevant to older persons who lack strength in the upper arms. Exercise therapists can apply the direct

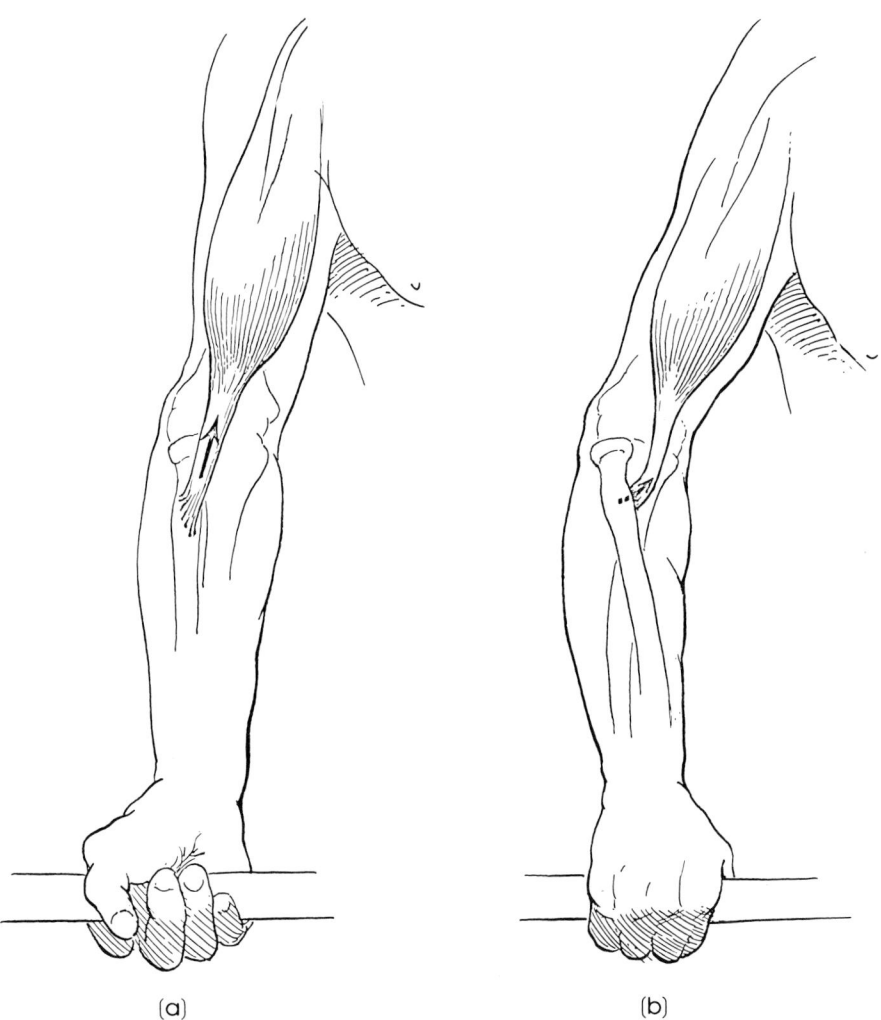

Figure 14.11 **(a)** Supinated forearm (direct line of pull); **(b)** pronated forearm (twisting line of pull) (from J. Piscopo, *Kinesiology IV, op. cit.*, p. 54)

line of pull principle in restoring normal range of motion. The student is referred to reference 37 for further analysis and implications for utilization of correct mechanics entailing flexion and extension of the elbow.

Specific Muscle-Strengthening Plan. Exercise patterns and descriptions are abundant in the literature, ranging from sophisticated textbooks for research scientists to popular magazines for laypersons. Many primers present activities for various regions of the body from shoulder girdle exercises of "push-ups" to full body movements of "jumping jacks." The authors contend that exercises should be carefully prescribed with the following considerations: (1) age and medical/dynamic fitness condition, and (2) prescribed kinesiological movements. The ensuing exercises and activities are recommended specifically for the purpose of strengthening areas of the body that are generally weak among persons over 50.

1. Pectoral Muscles (Anterior Chest Region).

Arm throwing movements, for example, overhead throwing of a ball or other object, or a calisthenic exercise of thrusting arms across the chest (adduction in horizontal plane) will activate the pectoral muscles. These muscles are important for maintaining strength of the upper body and are particularly vulnerable to flaccidity and sagging caused by the constant downward pull of gravity. Disuse further hastens the "posture fatigue" appearance of forward body flexion in advanced age. Crawl stroke swimming, racquet sports utilizing a variety of overhead arm movements, and specific calisthenic exercises—moving arms across the chest toward the body midline—are excellent activities for maintaining sufficient muscle tone and hypertrophy.

2. Abdominal Muscles (Rectus Abdominus, Transversalis, External and Internal Oblique Group).

Ptosis (sagging abdominal wall) is a common condition among adults of all ages. Simply stated, "the waistline is larger than chest girth." The ptosis effect is usually due to an accumulation of subcutaneous tissue (predominantly fat) ranging from two to six inches or more in extreme cases of obesity. The need for maintaining tone and functional strength of the abdominal group probably has as much aesthetic impact as movement efficiency. A protruding waistline affects the anterior-posterior lumbar spinal curvature and presents a striking postural image. Excessive protruberance can cause a forward shift of the body weight, which forces the head and upper trunk backward to maintain standing equilibrium. This compensating backward movement often results in lordosis or swayback.

Improved strength of the abdominals can be developed by assorted sit-up actions from the supine position. In addition to the individual's obesity status, force requirements for this exercise also depend upon weight and length of the trunk (distance from the hip joint to the head). Individuals with heavy and long trunks must exert a greater force than persons with lighter and shorter upper bodies because of the mechanical disadvantage of longer resistance arms inherent in their internal lever structure. Twenty-five sit-ups may be a reasonable sum for a person of short stature, but the same count will require more force and work for an individual over six feet in height. This kinesiological fact should be considered before establishing a target number of sit-ups as a goal for all participants. Certain men and women are unable to perform even one sit-up. These individuals should be taught how to execute this movement by using the arms and legs as auxiliary aids. A downward thrust of the legs with a push from the palm of the hands facing the floor will allow most persons to lift the trunk to an upright sitting position. Number of repetitions and types of sit-up styles should be prescribed according to the individual's somatotype and conditioning objectives.

Participants should be encouraged to perform trunk twisting movements in order to activate the external and internal oblique muscles to supplement the regular sit-up. Exaggerated breath expiration (without strain) is beneficial for toning the transversalis muscle of the abdominal group.

3. Pelvic and Hip Extensor Muscles (Gluteus Medius and Minimus).

These extensor muscles tend to decrease in resiliency and increase in flaccidity with the aging process. Hip girth is usually greater due to excessive adipose tissue and more time spent sitting. This condition, characterized by loss of spring and strength, often results in the body literally sinking within the pelvic ba-sin.[38] This sinking effect, coupled with weakness, impedes the extensor mobility movements of the hip and contributes to the gradual loss of standing height as age advances. Firm gluteal muscles play an important role in preventing sagging of the pelvis in the propulsive phase of walking and running, and these muscles can be strengthened by brisk walking, hopping, and jogging. When certain arthritic and lower joint anomalies are present, however, these exercises may be contradicted. Hip extensor actions (movements in the sagittal plane), either standing or lying prone, are also excellent exercises for the gluteal muscles.

Although exercises and physical activities that activate other body muscle areas are desirable, pectoral, abdominal, and gluteal groups are notably weakened with aging. These muscles significantly affect the posture and appearance, as well as the mobility patterns of older persons. Adequate levels of hypertrophy of these extensors should be maintained throughout life.

Aging and Flexibility

Joint range of motion or flexibility is usually subordinated and often excluded in physical fitness test batteries. Although one may argue the significance of flexibility in the ranking of fitness components among youth, this factor takes precedence over other fitness elements in older persons because it is an indispensable prerequisite of mobility. The anatomical and physiological musculoskeletal conditions of youth and the elderly are different. Several pronounced dissimilarities are (1) greater calcification of cartilage and surrounding tissues among older people, (2) a tendency for muscles to shorten, particularly those groups located on the posterior surfaces and lower regions of the body, including trunk, hamstrings, and leg musculature, (3) increased "stiffness" of males over females with advanc-

ing age, (4) prevalence of arthritic and other orthopedic conditions that intensify the restriction of joint motion, (5) tension and anxiety, which often invade the living environment of older persons and may impede body flexibility, and (6) much lower elasticity and compression tolerance of the spinal column in older persons.

A closer look at human flexibility and aging reveals the influence of genetics and environment. Tissue changes, such as less resiliency and cartilage calcification, are progressive. Sufficient levels of calcium in the diet, in addition to appropriate amounts of protein, iron, and vitamins, in conjunction with regularly performed slow-stretching exercises, can retard the stiffening effect of body joints.

The shortening effect of the muscular system, especially the lower back and hamstrings (see Figure 14.12) can be retarded with regular stretching (nonballistic, slow-stretching type) exercises. Hormonal differences between males and females may reveal clues about the empirical evidence favoring greater flexibility among older women. However, the cause of this phenomenon remains unclear. Exponents of yoga (slow-stretch-hold movements) exalt the beneficial effects of this activity as a superior method of maintaining suppleness. Notwithstanding the merits of low-gear, slow-motion type of stretching exercises, their limited benefits to the cardiorespiratory system should be recognized. Other activities that stimulate the heart/lung mechanisms should also be a part of the exercise regimen.

Arthritic and other orthopedic-type conditions are common ailments of the elderly. Joint mobility can be fostered with activities that relieve the weight-bearing joints of stress and strain and possible further inflammation. Swimming is excellent for orthopedically limited persons who are comfortable in an aquatic environment and possess a minimum level of stroke skills. A bicycle ergometer (stationary bicycle) is another exercise

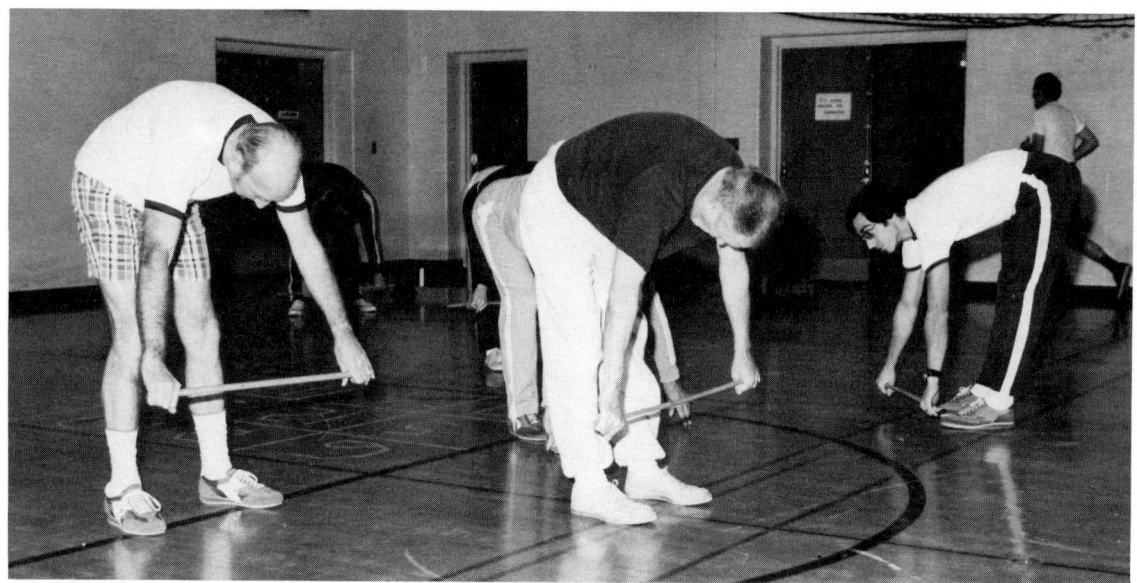

Figure 14.12 Improving hamstring and knee joint flexibility (from J. Piscopo, "Preparing Geriatric Fitness and Recreation Specialists," *JOPER*, 48:24–29, October, 1977)

modality that can be used while relieving body weight stress on the lower limbs.

Mechanical Forces Affecting the Spine

The muscles of the spinal column are involved in most movements of the body either as prime movers or as stabilizing units. For example, the spine is a major mover in sit-ups as the column flexes and extends in the sagittal plane; however, this structure becomes a stabilizing force when the individual is performing push-ups. The extrinsic muscles of the abdomen, thorax, and back stabilize the trunk, thereby allowing the push-up action without hyperextending the spine or sagging in the middle. The spine encounters inevitable structural changes with age. Essentially, as the intervertebral disks thin out, the column loses a significant amount of its shock absorptive qualities. In youth the combined *intrinsic* and *extrinsic* support capabilities of

the spinal column can withstand great forces similar to the function of an elastic rod. As explained in Chapter 4, the critical level of compression stress on the disks is lower in older persons. Strain on the spine, which may be caused by extreme hyperflexion or hyperextension, should be avoided, as well as head-rolling exercises, which grind the cervical segments and hasten the degeneration of the disks.

The mechanical forces that act on the spine arise from the *force of gravity, neurogenic and myogenic muscle tone,* and *assorted body activities.*

Force of Gravity. Since the spine is not a rigid rod, but rather a curved column of concave and convex curves, forces of gravity vary from one segment of the spine to another. Gravity produces rotational stress that must be neutralized by opposing forces. Without these stabilizing forces, the spine would lose its balance and collapse. These rotary forces tend to increase with age since muscles weaken; consequently, posture may assume a kyphotic position. The pull of gravity exerts its greatest force on the lumbar and sacral intervetebral disks. At this level in the erect position, force due to gravity is the result of the weight of the upper part of the body in addition to the weight of the arms. It appears prudent to maintain strength of the low back and abdominal muscles to assist in neutralizing the rotary and unbalancing forces created, in part, by the constant force of gravity acting on the spine.

Body Activities. Movements surrounding the spine are diverse. The forces that affect the spine are also produced by the lever action of the trunk and limbs. These forces on the lower spine can be increased or decreased depending upon the position and lever type involved in a specific movement or series of movements. For example, Figure 14.13 illustrates the third-class lever action and the forces exerted on the spine by forward flexion of the trunk and extension of the arms.

Figure 14.13 Effect of leverage upon the spinal column in ordinary movements (from J.R. Armstrong and W.E. Tucker (Eds.), **Injury in Sport**, Charles C. Thomas Co., Springfield, Illinois, 1964, p. 569, courtesy of Granada Publishing Limited, St. Albans, England)

The reader will note from Figure 14.13 that the anterior lever length leading forward from the fulcrum is much *longer* than the posterior segment leading to the muscular insertions of the back muscles. If a weight of 100 pounds is lifted in this manner, it must be balanced by contraction of the extensor muscles of the spine acting much closer to the fulcrum of joint movement (intervertebral disks). The relationship between the long anterior and short posterior levers has been computed as 15 to 1; and the 100 pounds must, therefore, be balanced by a muscle contraction of 1500 pounds shown by the movement in Figure 14.13. When considering the total *throwing* force, in addition to *counter balancing* contraction as shown in the above example, 3000 pounds of force is exerted on the intervertebral joint.[39] Thus, it can be seen that the forces due to gravity, weight of the body, and bodily activities can exert considerable compression between the intervertebral disks of the spine.

The intrinsic stability of the spine diminishes with age since the thinning process of

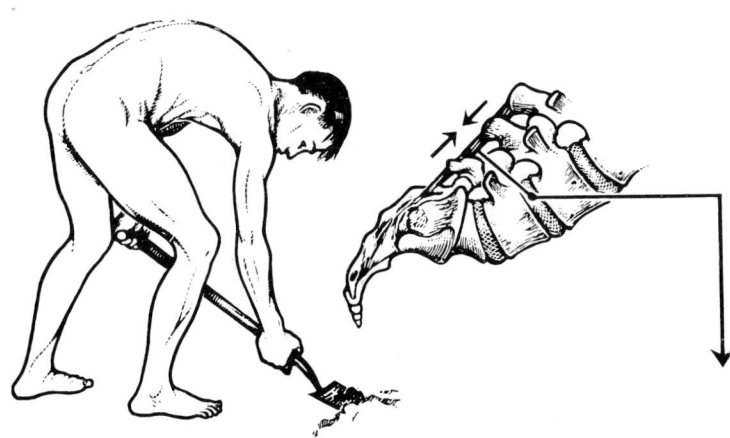

the disks is inevitable; however, the extrinsic support that comes from the quality of external muscles surrounding the spine is alterable and is primarily dependent upon their level of myogenic tone, developed through proper movement and exercise.

AGING AND CIRCULORESPIRATORY FUNCTIONS

Decreased circulorespiratory function occurs with age. Our discussion is limited to consideration of the role of the system with respect to human motor performance.

The ability of the heart and lungs to utilize oxygen decreases with age, and so the resultant complaint of fatigue is frequently heard from the elderly. The thoracic cage and chest wall decrease in *pliability* and *elasticity*, which directly reduces the respiration efficiency of the lungs (inspiration and expiration capacity). The internal structure of the lungs tends to become rigid with cell loss and increases in collagen substances. The net result is manifested in decreased ventilation and muscular force of the chest. Deep breathing and coughing can be a problem among certain older persons. Weakened intercostal muscles, which are used to lift and lower the rib cage for breathing, often fail to maintain an adequate level of vital capacity. It should also be pointed out that the transversus muscle of the abdominal group plays an important part in the expiratory phase of breathing. The diaphragm assumes a prominent role in quiet breathing, particularly during the inspiration phase. Older persons need good breathing and coughing efficiency to rid the respiratory system of congestive mucus, which may serve as a breeding ground for pathological organisms. Activities and exercises of an aerobic nature that stimulate the diaphragm, intercostals, and transversus muscles should be an integral part of a training and conditioning regime for older persons. Brisk walking, jogging, swimming,

and diaphragmatic breathing exercises help to maintain chest wall elasticity.

The cold hands and feet syndrome is also a common disorder of the elderly. This condition is partially explained by the lack of adequate blood circulation to the skin, which is manifested by lower skin temperatures than among younger people. Dynamic exercise improves circulatory efficiency by increasing the pumping action of the heart, which results in delivery of more blood to the extremities. The combined and integrative effect of exercise upon the cardiovascular and respiratory systems helps to bring more blood to the surface and thus serves as a body-temperature regulatory mechanism. Activities that focus upon improving the peripheral vascular circulation by using the big muscles of the legs as in walking, jogging, swimming, and dancing are natural and inexpensive ways to improve blood circulation. Heavy resistive exercises create higher blood pressure and may constrict circulatory flow to the peripherum of the arms and legs. Swimming is especially appropriate for individuals with joint and other orthopedic restrictions since the buoyancy of the water provides a cushion and minimizes load strain upon weakened joints.

Figure 14.14 illustrates an excellent exercise activity for individuals who are affected with vascular problems of the legs.

AGING AND BODY BALANCE

Balance and equilibrium are intricately interwoven with physiological aspects including eyes, ears, and kinesthesia (body position sense). The acuity of these sense mechanisms wanes as we grow older. Maintenance of sufficient balance skills can enhance the personal safety of the elderly. Persons over 65 account for 25 percent of all accidental deaths, and in seven out of ten fatalities from falls, the victim is elderly.[40] This high accident rate is undoubtedly due to reduced dynamic fit-

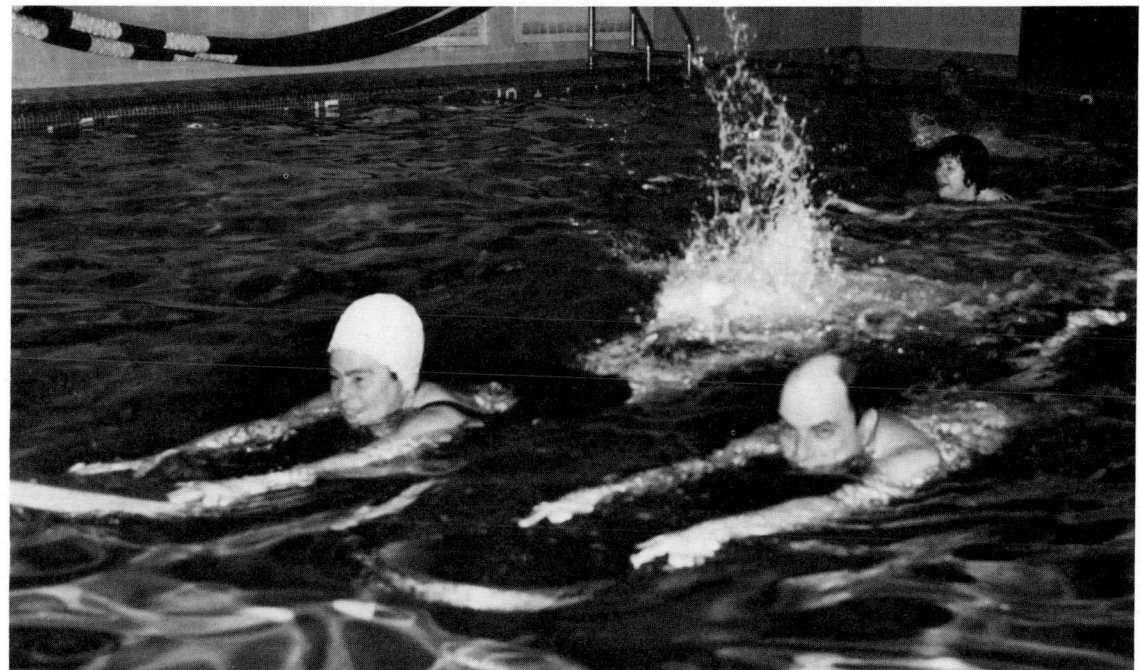

Figure 14.14 Improving peripheral circulation of the legs using a kick-board (from J. Piscopo, "Preparing Geriatric Fitness and Recreation Specialists," op. cit., p. 29)

ness status and, in part, to decreased balance and equilibrium capabilities. Visual impairments are common among older persons. This sensory mechanism is important for maintaining balance because it provides a point of reference for the individual in everyday skills such as walking or standing. The elderly can apply their vision capability for the improvement of balance by the practice of walking on a low balance beam with eyes focused at specific reference points. This exercise enhances better sensorimotor feedback to the cerebellum, which modulates neuromuscular balance control.

Ear impairments are also common among the elderly. Although conductive losses (mechanical defects of ear bones) have little relationship to balance, attention should be directed to those older citizens afflicted with sensorineural defects. Usually these defects affect the internal labyrinth and disturb the vestibular fluid and function of the semicircular canals, which involve the mechanism of equilibrium. Various changes in head movements causing posture adjustments trigger neural signals to the brain, which tend to move the body in the direction initiated by the head. This vestibular mechanism has particular implications for older persons. Sudden and quick head movements can cause the individual to lose balance since the body follows the head. In certain older persons vertigo or dizziness caused by Meniere's disease may be present. In such instances head movements and balance exercises of any kind should be avoided.

Maintaining equilibrium also entails the utilization of neural receptors called proprioceptors, which originate in the muscles, tendons, and joints and are discussed further in

Chapters 4 and 8. These receptors, combined with inner ear vestibular mechanisms, are important components of balance. Muscular contraction stimulates nerve endings in tendons and joints, sending messages to the cerebellum informing it of the actual state of contraction. This information, together with messages from the brain's motor cortex, is integrated by the cerebellum, resulting in an adjustment of the rate and force of muscular contraction necessary for the balancing task at the moment. Information on joint angulation and muscle tension is eventually impressed upon memory. Active body movements contained in dance, bowling, shuffleboard, horseshoes, fitness exercises, and swimming are excellent ways to cultivate proprioceptive impressions and neural efficiency for the improvement of safety balance skills. The development of these sense structures depends significantly upon their stimulation and utilization. Mention should be made about muscular strength and balance efficiency: Strength has little, if any, relationship with the attainment of a balance position. However, this fitness component does have value in correcting balance mechanic errors. The greater force made available by greater strength can alter errors in joint angles, which are important in maintaining the correct alignment of the gravity line within its supporting base. Figure 14.15 illustrates an activity designed to improve upright stationary balance.

AGING AND MOTOR SKILLS

The variability of motor skill performance among persons over 50 is profound. Older people have attained phenomenal performances in athletics. Some notable records indicate that men in their 60s throw a discus over 100 feet; 55-year-old sprinters crack the 24 second mark for 200 meters; and women aged 60 and older set records in swimming, sprinting, and field events. These are the

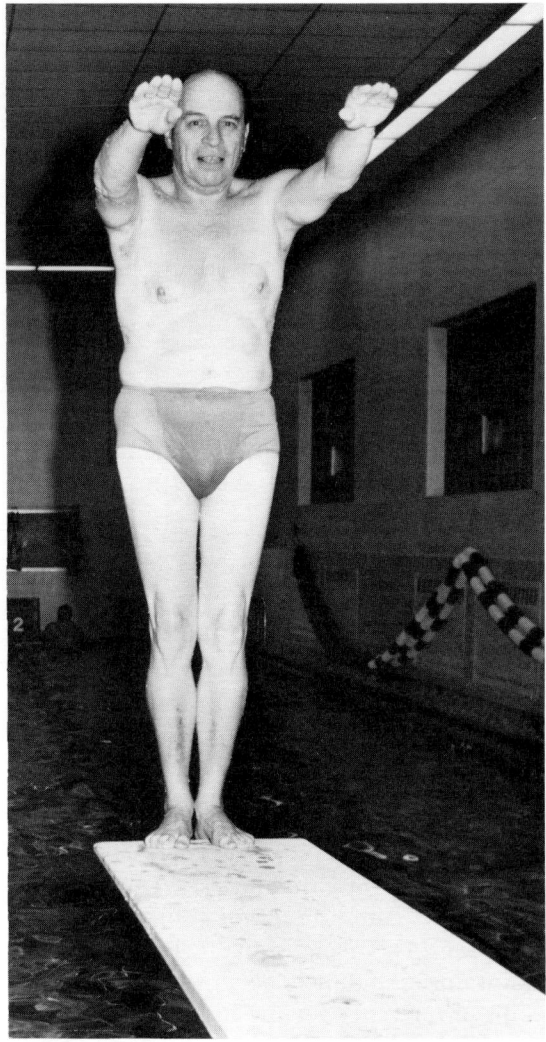

Figure 14.15 Improving upright stationary balance through diving

kinds of athletic performances that reflect superior motor skills demonstrated in the Senior Olympics Program under the auspices of Senior International, which stages yearly games for amateur athletes 25 years old and up.[41]*

*For further information about the Senior Olympics Program, write to *Senior Sports International, Inc.,* 5225 Wilshire Boulevard, Los Angeles, California 90036.

On the other hand, many older persons with one or more chronic incipient conditions possess inadequate locomotion and motor skills required for activities of daily living and personal safety. The level of motor skill and athletic prowess covers a great range and can reach superlative caliber depending upon the *medical* and *dynamic* physical fitness status and motivation of the individual. Although psychodynamics play an important role in the motor skill development of the mature citizen, our discussion is focused upon the biological and kinesiological aspects of motor performance. A direct biological consequence of participating in competitive sport in most instances reflects itself in gaining a high level of dynamic physical fitness. The individual who participates in running, jumping, or cycling activities directly improves his/her physical mobility and efficiency pattern.

Individuals do not lose their ability to learn motor skill after age 50. The central difference is not whether they can learn and perform, but the manner and rate in which skills are presented.[42] Older persons need concrete and clear instructions and an opportunity to learn at their own pace. As noted earlier, most physiological parameters decline at varying rates with the aging process, and, consequently, more time is required for acquisition of motor skills. Although older persons play active recreational games in a slower manner, their performance becomes quite accurate. This characteristic is probably due to their cautious approach in analyzing a task to be learned before accepting the learning challenge.

Certain age constraints should be noted that directly affect physical skill learning and motor performance: (1) limited range of joint motion, (2) limited strength, (3) loss of peak sensory perception, and (4) loss of some neuromuscular coordination. As indicated earlier, motor skill parameters vary greatly among the elderly; however, it should be emphasized that physical performance of older persons should not be expected to exhibit the qualities demonstrated by youth. Rules and regulations for such games as badminton, tennis, volleyball, running, and jumping events may be adjusted whereby high physical demands for successful performance are not a prerequisite. For example, doubles badminton is more appropriate for individuals after age 55 than singles play. Activities that require quick and powerful reactions should be limited. Such activities as trampoline bouncing are contraindicated for older persons simply because of their inherent requirement of fast neuromuscular coordination and the threat to safety. Conversely, an activity such as dancing (square or social) is an excellent aerobic motor skill that presents minimum safety hazards to men and women and enhances coordination without demanding great spurts of speed and muscular power. Heavy isometric-type motor skills such as competitive weight lifting should be avoided in old age. A quick clean and jerk movement is an activity that places sudden and unreasonable physiological demands upon the older organism. This does not preclude weight training provided repetitive light-weight equipment is used.

Losses in special sense response usually begin after age 50. Vision and hearing acuity diminish, with the majority of persons developing presbyopia or farsightedness and loss of sensitivity to sounds in the high-frequency range. Night vision acuity shows a gradual failing with advancing age. Of particular relevance to motor skill performance is the gradual loss of proprioception sensitivity in the feet, which affects one's sense of position and kinesthesia, as described in Chapter 4. Each of these sensory perception losses restricts motor performance. Fortunately, the law of varying rate of individual organ decline prevails, and the senior adult may, and often does, compensate by utilizing remaining well-functioning sensorial mechanisms when one receiver fails. These natural changes provide clues for selection of appropriate and nonappropriate games and activities for the elderly. For example, games that require whisper signals or directions should be avoided. All activities should be conducted in well-lighted rooms and playing areas. Balls and other forms of playing equipment should be large and in bright colors for easy identification. Activities that demand precise dynamic and static balance body movements for success should be avoided.

Loss of brain cells coupled with the hardening of vessels within the brain itself affect the quality of neuromuscular response in voluntary skeletal and motor skill movements. *Reaction time,* which is inherently involved with neuromuscular control, generally slows down. Research studies suggest that participation in vigorous physical activity may retard decrements in neurological efficiency among older persons. Older males actively participating in racket sports and handball were found to have faster reaction time than older inactive men.[43,44] A rationale, which of course needs further supportive evidence but indeed seems plausible, is suggested by Spirduso[45]:

> *When neuronal cells fail to receive and process stimuli, eventually they involute and atrophy. Physical activity, particularly as occurs in competitive sport, generates— both internally and externally—a virtual storm of impinging stimuli. The excitation that occurs during physical activity affects the entire chain of neurons involved, from motor neurons to the higher cortical centers. The continued reaction and speed decision-making in response to the continually changing unpredictable stimuli that is characteristic of men who play racket sports and handball may enhance neuronal longevity and efficiency. According to this rationale, the best protection against senile involution of brain cells in cerebral activity, stimulates metabolism, respiration,*
> *blood circulation, digestion and glands of external secretion.*

Many studies measuring reaction time have been completed in institutional settings involving persons with varying degrees of disabling diseases. These findings investigating neuromuscular efficiency of the aging certainly provide some evidence that reaction time loss may not be due to age alone.

INDICATIONS AND CONTRAINDICATIONS OF ACTIVITIES FOR THE AGING

Throughout our discussion, we have advanced the concept that physical activity is essential for enhancing human efficiency. As research evidence mounts in support of exercise and sports for healthy bodies in the mature years, professionals working with senior citizens, who are well-prepared in social and psychological aspects of gerontology, often embark on activity and exercise programs (although well-meaning) without an understanding of the anatomical, physiological, and kinesological benefits or limitations. Certain types of activities are indicated for some individuals while the same physical movements may be contraindicated for other individuals. The principle of *specificity of conditioning* and *law of individual differences* must be respected. For example, jogging does very little to develop the muscle strength of the shoulder girdle and pectoral muscles, and, therefore, it is erroneous to indicate that one is building strength and power of the deltoids and pectoral muscles by jogging or running activities. Is jogging a suitable exercise modality for everyone? A person in the 250- to 300-pound weight range and/or afflicted with inflammatory arthritis of the knees should not engage in such an activity because insult and further aggravation to body joints may result. Any conditioning program for older persons should begin with an assessment of medical status. Prescribed activities, based upon scientific evidence, relative to *type, frequency,* and *dosage,* should be selected according to individual needs and capabilities. The authors have selected 26 *contraindications* and *indications* with a rationale drawn from kinesiological and physiological foundations. Although research evidence is continually advancing knowledge about the effects of physical activity upon the human organism, we believe that the contraindications and indications given in Tables 14.2 and 14.3 should be taken into account.[46]

PROGRAM IMPLICATIONS

Although our discussion has focused upon the biological perspectives of aging with specific emphasis on human movement, the authors subscribe to the concept that man functions holistically. Each individual is unique, and the human organism behaves and moves as an eclectic whole depending upon his/her own genetic constitution and environment. This assumption places credence upon the importance of developing movement program content and didactics on an *individualized basis* since aging rates occur differentially within and between individuals. The contributions of high levels of mobility and physical fitness toward the enhancement of health can result in the end product of self-fulfillment. No assurance or contention that such programs extend longevity is proclaimed, although medical evidence (not conclusive) supports a positive relationship between high levels of fitness and long life. Notwithstanding the law of individuality, certain commonalities in attitudes and motivation prevail as one grows older.[47] In Baley's[48] research for his doctoral dissertation, he administered a questionnaire to 3000 men between the ages of 20 to 59 covering 67 recreational activities. The three types of activities that showed the greatest decline in interest were (1) those that require quick reaction time, (2) those that require physical stamina

and endurance, and (3) those that satisfy the romantic and erotic impulses. Baley also found that participation in active sports declines with age, and frequency of participation in activities of a sedentary nature increases. These findings substantiate the notion that the drive for physical activity lessens and participation in passive activities increases as one becomes older. A recent sampling of elderly men and women with average age of 65 years also showed that an inactive lifestyle prevailed.[49] These trends are also reported from a national adult physical fitness survey conducted under the auspices of the United States President's Council on Physical Fitness and Sports. Fewer older people were engaged in strenuous forms of activity such as jogging, calisthenics, bicycling, or swimming, with the majority engaging in walking as their favorite exercise modality.[50] Although the physical activity drive decreases, older adults recognize the need for physical exercise for the maintenance of health. The salient issue stems from *motivation.* Motivation is multifaceted and individualized to the point where one's incentive for fitness activity participation may conversely generate negative responses and behavior about the same activity from someone else. For example, physical fitness as a goal may be a powerful stimulus for certain persons. Others may view conditioning and training as a means of attaining the vigor and vitality necessary for enjoying everyday living. Each value judgment is quite different and yet commendable. Respect for these divergent drives should be honored and nurtured. Fitness goals for older adults should be flexible enough to allow for differences in intellectual maturity levels that accent personalization. For example, a person with an arthritic knee can be motivated with exercises and activities designed specifically for the relief of pain and enhancement in joint range of motion through swimming, modified bicycle ergometer, and/or slow-motion yoga-type calisthenics. Certain older

Table 14.2 Contraindications and Indications for Various Exercises, with Kinesiological Rationale

Contraindication	Indication	Rationale
1. Fix or stiffen joints such as trying to touch toes with knees locked.	1. Swing free; bend knees, and move in a comfortable manner.	1. Respects bone, joint, and muscle changes; less danger of joint sprains and muscle strain.
2. Perform trunk twisting in standing position.	2. Perform trunk twister in sitting position on bench or chair.	2. Respects the basic structure and function of the joint, which is essentially a ginglymus or hinge joint. Torque generated by the twisting action of the trunk can be absorbed by the knee when flexed because of its greater capacity for rotation in sitting position.
3. Circumduction of head or head-rolling exercises.	3. Slowly rotate or turn head to left and right; flex and extend head up and down, without jerky movements.	3. Lessen the danger of "grinding" the first two cervical vertebrae (atlas and axis), which may be damaged because of the natural "thinning out" of the intervebral disks.
4. Jog or run when such conditions as arthritis are present.	4. Utilize bicycle ergometer or pool for swimming activities.	4. Weight which creates pressure upon knee and ankle joints is removed; buoyancy of water has hydrotherapeutic effect on muscles and joints.
5. Quick flexion of trunk on thigh in supine position (sit-up) with legs straight.	5. Perform sit-up with legs bent at least 60 degrees.	5. Lessens probability of increasing lordosis angle of spine and allows greater intensity of contraction upon the abdominal muscles, and less on iliopsoas (hip flexors).
6. Double leg raising exercise to angular hold position off the floor.	6. Raise legs to 45 degree angle without hold position, with back flat on floor.	6. Lessens the risk of spinal hyperextension and resultant low back strain.
7. Continuous fast "swirling" and "whirling" movements of the body.	7. Slow rotary and/or circumducting limb movements.	7. Postural changes may induce vertigo or dizziness and loss of balance.
8. Activities that require fast reaction time and explosive power movements, such as trampoline bouncing and vaulting events with springboard.	8. Modify and adapt activities so that success in performance does not require quick or extreme bursts of power, e.g., playing doubles badminton, dancing.	8. Reaction time, perception, and neuromuscular response generally decline; activities that demand high levels of neural acuteness are threats to the mature person's safety.
9. Full flexion of the knee joint from standing position (deep-knee bends).	9. Half-knee bends from stand position.	9. May overstretch and injure supporting structure of knee, including ligaments, cartilages.
10. Stressing static balance hold positions without use of arms or visual clues, such as, standing on one leg with arms along thighs, with eyes closed.	10. Walking wide balance beam (12- to 15-inch width) with arms abducted in frontal plane and eyes focused at end of beam.	10. Improves functional balance in upright position, uses mechanical principle of extending the horizontal distance from the center of gravity with arms, and utilizes vision to establish point of

Table 14.2 Contraindications and Indications for Various Exercises, with Kinesiological Rationale

Contraindication	Indication	Rationale
		reference in maintaining dynamic balance skills.
11. Flexing elbow exercises with hands in pronated position (palms down).	11. Flexing elbow with hands in supinated position (palms up).	11. More strength can be applied in elbow flexion with hand in supination because of favorable mechanical advantage (see Figure 14.11).
12. Present exercises and game instructions quickly without loss of time.	12. Present instruction with slow pace and concrete demonstration; allow for self-pacing of motor skills.	12. Neural information, reception, and capacity for processing decreased; instructional material presented must be reduced accordingly.
13. Execute exercises in a "slump posture" stance.	13. Perform exercises in erect posture (not stiff) with attention to activation of antigravity postural muscles.	13. Lessens tendency toward kyphotic, (hump-back) and postural fatigue in body alignment.

adults may find "shortness of breath" and premature fatigue as impediments to moving efficiently in work and play. Sustained rhythmic aerobic exercise, challenging respiration and lung movements through walking, jogging, or swimming (depending upon medical condition), are meaningful to the chronically fatigued individual seeking relief. This approach gives direct purpose for activity engagement.

Movement is a part of *Homo sapien's* functional living environment; an understanding of biological and kinesiological phenomena affecting mobility patterns of the aging is vital before embarking on a program of exercise and sport for this special population.

SUMMARY

Flexibility is one component of dynamic fitness that is equally important to athletes performing in varsity sports or the atypical individual striving to improve mobility in tasks of everyday living. Joint mobility is affected by such variables as stress, anxiety, body build, tendons, ligaments, fascia and collagen content, and certain pathological conditions like

arthritis. Research studies indicate that flexibility is specific to a particular joint, rather than a general functional quality, and the measurement of one or several body joints cannot be used to predict validly the range of motion in other body parts. Mobility patterns also vary between genders, ages, and types of activities engaged in by the individual. Females tend to be more flexible in various joints, but mobility generally decreases with age.

The mechanical goniometer and Leighton flexometer are tools that can be used by the practitioner in allied health.

The Leighton flexometer can measure flexibility with greater accuracy than the mechanical goniometer, since the former device does not depend upon the careful alignment of the instrument with bony land marks and movable body segments.

Principles of physical and motor fitness require specific exercise modalities for the development of the different qualities needed for success in diverse sports. The relationships, differences, and developmental procedures for improving fitness were examined, compared, and contrasted.

It has been shown that the aging process can be slowed to a significant degree by

Table 14.3 Contraindications and Indications for Various Exercises, with Physiological Rationale

Contraindication	Indication	Rationale
1. Holding breath during exercise.	1. Breathing rhythmically; with expiration at the end of the effort.	1. Holding breath decreases venous return of blood to the heart; may cause dizziness or fainting.
2. Using heavy weights with fast repetitive movements.	2. Use light weights with slow repetitive movements.	2. Heavy weights impede blood circulation to the extremities. [Small size soup cans (8 oz.) excellent for hand weight in shoulder girdle exercises.]
3. Accent overwork and stressful movements of arms in calisthenics.	3. Stress activity of big muscles of trunk and legs.	3. Arm exercises increase blood pressure at higher levels than trunk and leg workouts.
4. Take hot shower after exercise.	4. Take warm shower after exercise, slowly cooling water temperature.	4. Hot shower may elevate blood pressure.
5. Start vigorous movements without warm-up.	5. Always warm up 5 to 7 minutes before jogging, playing sports, etc.	5. Ischemic effect (inadequate blood flow to tissues) may result without warm-up.
6. Immediate rest after exercise.	6. Walk after jogging, or loosen up with calisthenics.	6. Fosters cool-down of the body and allows a natural transition of blood pumping action from muscles to the heart without undue stress.
7. Stress resistive and anaerobic (without O_2) exercises and activities.	7. Accent isotonic and aerobic (with O_2) exercises and activities.	7. Aerobic-type exercises enhance the function of cardiovascular system, whereas resistive work is of little value for heart and lung efficiency.
8. Work out in rubberized clothing in hot weather.	8. Work out in cool perspiration-absorbing type shirt and trunks.	8. Rubberized clothing prevents normal functioning of perspiration mechanism and constricts necessary body cooling process during exercise and after workout.
9. Stretching muscle to extreme range.	9. Stretch to full range without strain or discomfort.	9. Extreme stretching may induce muscle spasm and undue soreness or strain.
10. Short "jerky" or "bouncing" stretching movements.	10. Slow nonballistic, static stretching.	10. Jerky and/or bouncing movement may invoke reverse myotactic reflex in the muscle spindle, which opposes the desired stretching (see Chapter 4).
11. Sit-up exercises on inclined plane or board.	11. Sit-ups parallel with floor, back firmly on the mat.	11. Places undue strain on hip flexors, primarily iliopsoas muscle and resultant soreness to low back.
12. Perform exercises that develop muscle bulk only.	12. Perform exercises that stimulate flexibility, strength, and endurance through stretching, light	12. Exercises that are directed toward increasing muscle bulk do not contribute to cardiovascular fitness.

Table 14.3 Contraindications and Indications for Various Exercises, with Physiological Rationale

Contraindication	Indication	Rationale
	resistance work, and repetitive movements.	
13. Perform daily high-intensity work-outs.	13. Generally, gear exercise intensity to low and moderate levels dependent upon medical and dynamic fitness status.	13. Body needs a minimum of one day's rest for adaptive homeostasis adjustment and avoidance of activity "staleness."

maintaining sensible standards of physical fitness. Anthropometrical and skeletal changes that occur in older persons change height, posture, and bone structure to variable degrees.

Bone growth can occur in older persons when they participate in regular and systematic exercise programs. A majority of spines, after the fourth decade, show disk degeneration, and the process rises sharply after age 50.

Body shape and composition also change with age. Fatty adipose tends to replace muscular tissue, reducing body density and lowering specific gravity. The skinfold caliper technique is a practical and valid manner of assessing body fat when used in a correct and careful way.

Muscular strength decreases with age; however, morphological changes do not become noticeable until a very late stage. Certain types of exercises are contraindicated because of structural and physiological limitations of older persons. Activity and fitness programs should accent exercises that enhance body posture and efficient mobility patterns. Maintaining muscular strength of the *shoulder girdle, abdominals,* and *gluteal* muscles is vital for sustaining various upright stationary and locomotive posture movements. The shortening of muscles due to the aging process, especially of lower back muscles and hamstrings, can be lessened with regular (nonballistic), slow-stretching type exercises. Swimming is an excellent activity for orthopedically limited persons who are comfortable in an aquatic environment. A stationary bicycle is also a recommended activity

that can be used while relieving body-weight stress on lower limb segments.

Extreme hyperflexion and hyperextension of the spinal column are contraindicated for older persons due to changes in spine composition and lower tolerance to disk compression stress.

The *intrinsic* and *extrinsic* stability of the spine can be developed and maintained by applying sound kinesiological principles to regular and systematic exercise regimens.

Activities and exercises of an aerobic nature that stimulate the diaphragm, intercostal, and transversus muscles should be an integral part of a conditioning program for senior citizens.

The elderly can apply their vision capability for the improvement of balance skills by the practice of walking on a low balance beam with eyes focused at specific points. This exercise enhances better sensorimeter feedback to the brain (cerebellum), which modulates neuromuscular control.

New motor skills can be learned by older persons provided they can proceed at their own pace without pressure, when the skill to be learned is presented in a concrete and uncomplicated manner.

Research evidence suggests that regular participation in such sport activity as racquetball and handball can retard decrements in reaction time among older persons and that loss in this neuromuscular parameter may not be due to age alone.

Twenty-six indications and contraindications were advanced with rationales drawn from kinesiological and physiological foundations.

A sound knowledge of biological and kinesiological phenomena affecting mobility patterns of the aging is essential before embarking on a physical program for this special population.

REFERENCES

1. Dickinson, R.V., "The Specificity of Flexibility," *Research Quarterly*, 39:792-794, 1968.

2. Whelan, Christopher D., "An Analysis of Flexibility and Anxiety Levels Among Adolescent High School Boys," unpublished Master's Project, State University of New York at Buffalo, 1975.

3. Rathbone, Josephine, *Relaxation.* New York: Bureau of Publications, 1943, p. 19.

4. Bowman, Kurt, "Effect of Emotional Stress on Spasticity and Rigidity," *Journal of Psychosomatic Research*, 15:107-112, 1971.

5. Vines, Roland H., "The Influences of Race and Anxiety Level Upon Performance of Novel Motor Tasks Under Varying Stressful Conditions," *Dissertations Abstract Internation*, 32, (7-A):3770, January, 1972.

6. Hall, David, *The Ageing of Connective Tissue.* London: Academic Press, 1976, p. 62.

7. Gutman, E., "Muscle," in Calib F. Finch and Leonard Hayflick (Eds.), *The Biology of Aging.* New York: Van Nostrand Reinhold, 1977, pp. 445-469.

8. Cole, H. M., "The Range of Active Motion at the Wrist of White Adults," *Journal of Bone and Joint Surgery*, 10:763, 1928.

9. Hewitt, D. "The Range of Active Motion at the Wrist of Women," *Journal of Bone and Joint Surgery*, 10:775, 1928.

10. Harris, M. L., "A Factor Analytical Study of Flexibility," *Research Quarterly*, 40:62-69, 1969.

11. Hupprich, Florence, and Hupprich, Peter, "Specificity and Reliability of Measures of Flexibility for Girls," *Research Quarterly*, 21:25-33, 1950.

12. Holland, George J., "The Physiology of Flexibility: A Review of the Literature," Council on Kinesiology, *Kinesiology Review.* Washington, D.C.: American Association for Health, Physical Education, and Recreation, 1968, pp. 49-61.

13. Clarke, H. Harrison (Ed.), "Joint and Body Range of Movement," *Physical Fitness Research Digest*, 5:1-22. Washington, D.C.: President's Council on Physical Fitness, October, 1975.

14. American Academy of Orthopaedic Surgeons, *Joint Motion: Method of Measuring and Recording*, Chicago, 1965.

15. Moore, Margaret L., "Clinical Assessment of Joint Motion," in Sidney Licht, *Therapeutic Exercise*, 2nd ed. Baltimore: Waverly Press, 1965, pp. 128-162.

16. Aquilina, Lynore, "A Paradigm for Studying Differential Amounts of Flexibility in Selected Ethnic Groups Predominant in Buffalo, N.Y.," unpublished Master's Degree Project, State University of New York at Buffalo, 1970.

17. Leighton, Jack R., "A Simple Objective and Reliable Measure of Flexibility," *Research Quarterly*, 13:205-216, May, 1942.

18. Leighton, Jack R., "An Instrument and Technic for the Measurement of Range of Joint Motion," *Archives of Physical Medicine and Rehabilitation*, 36:571-86, September, 1955.

19. Leighton, Jack R., "The Leighton Flexometer and Flexibility Test," *Journal of the Association for Physical and Mental Rehabilitation*, 20:86-93, May-June, 1966.

20. Gregory, Larry W., "The Development of Aerobic Capacity: A Comparison of Continuous and Interval Training," *Research Quarterly*, 50:199-206, May, 1979.

21. Baley, James A., *An Illustrated Guide to the Development of Strength, Power, Endurance, Agility, Balance and Flexibility.* Englewood Cliffs, N.J.: Parker Publishing Company, 1976.

22. Costill, David L., Thomason, Harry, and Roberts, Eric, "Fractional Utilization of the Aerobic Capacity During Distance Running," *Medicine and Science in Sports*, 5(4):248-252, 1973.

23. Knuttgen, H. G., Nordesja, L. O., Ollander, B., and Saltin, B., "Physical Conditioning Through Interval Training with Young Male Adults" *Medicine and Science in Sports*, 5:220-226, 1973.

24. U.S. Bureau of the Census, Department of Commerce, *Current Population Reports:* Special Studies, Series P 22, No. 59, "Demographic Aspects of Aging and the Older Population in the United States," May, 1976, p. 1.

25. Testimony on Physical Fitness for Older Persons, from Selected Hearings before the Subcommittee on Aging of the Committee on Labor and

Public Welfare, U.S. Senate, April 23, 1975, Washington, D.C., pp. 713–899.

26. Rossman, Isadore, "Anatomic and Body Composition Changes with Aging," in C.E. Finch and L. Hayflick (Eds.), *The Biology of Aging.* New York: Van Nostrand Rheinhold, 1977, pp. 189–221.

27. Hall, David A., *The Ageing of Connective Tissue.* London: Academic Press, 1976, p. 52.

28. Smith, E. L., and Reddan, W., "Physical Activity—A Modality for Bone Accretion in the Aged," *American Journal of Roentgenology, Radium Therapy and Nuclear Medicine*, 126:1297, June, 1976.

29. Jokl, Ernest, *Physiology of Exercise.* Springfield, Ill.: Charles C Thomas, 1964, pp. 34–35.

30. Piscopo, John, "Obesity: A Noteworthy Method of Assessment," *New York State Journal of Health, Physical Education, and Recreation*, 20:24–27, 1967.

31. Rossman, *op. cit.*, p. 197.

32. Gutmann, E., "Muscle," in C.E. Finch and L. Hayflick (Eds.), *The Biology of Aging.* New York, Van Nostrand Reinhold, 1977, pp. 445–469.

33. Gutman, E., and Hanzlikora, V., *Age Changes in the Neuromuscular System.* Bristol, England: Scientechnica Ltd., 1972, p. 82.

34. McCarter, Roger, "Effects of Age on Contraction of Mammalian Skeletal Muscle," in George Kaldor and William J. DiBattista, (Eds.), *Aging in Muscle.* New York: Raven Press, 1978, pp. 1–21.

35. Piscopo, John, "Fitness After Fifty," *Health Values: Achieving High Level Wellness*, 1:210–217, September/October, 1977.

36. Piscopo, John, "Strength," *The Physical Educator*, 24:66–68, 1967.

37. Piscopo, John, "Assessment of Forearm Positions Upon Upperarm and Shoulder Girdle Strength Performance," in *Kinesiology IV*, Washington, D.C., AAHPER, 1974, pp. 53–57.

38. Thompson, C. W., *A Manual for Structural Kinesiology*, 7th ed. St. Louis: C. V. Mosby, 1977, pp. 59–62.

39. Armstrong, J. R., and Tucker, W. E., *Injury in Sport.* Springfield, Ill.: Charles C Thomas, 1964, pp. 568–569.

40. Accident Mortality at Older Ages, Metropolitan Life Insurance Co., *Statistical Bulletin*, 55:6–8, June, 1974.

41. Yasgur, Stevan L., "The Senior Olympics: Games for Adults Who Won't Quit," *Geriatrics*, 30: 120–125, January, 1975.

42. Piscopo, John, "Aging and Human Performance," in Edmund J. Burke, (Ed.), *Exercise Science and Fitness.* Ithaca, N.Y.: Movement Publications, 1980, pp. 98–126.

43. Spirduso, Waneen Wyrick, "Reaction and Movement Time as a Function of Age and Physical Activity Level," *Journal of Gerontology*, 30:435–440, 1975.

44. Spirduso, Waneen Wyrick, and Clifford, Phillip, "Replication of Age and Physical Activity Effects on Reaction and Movement Time," *Journal of Gerontology*, 33:26–30, 1978.

45. Spirduso, *op. cit.*, 1975, p. 439.

46. Piscopo, John, "Indications and Contraindications of Exercise and Activity for Older Persons," *Journal of Physical Education and Recreation*, 50:31–34, 1979.

47. Baley, James A., "Recreation and the Aging Process," *Research Quarterly*, 26:1–7, March, 1955.

48. *Ibid.*

49. Sidney, Kenneth H., and Shepard, Roy J., "Activity Patterns of Elderly Men and Women," *Journal of Gerontology*, 32:25–32, 1977.

50. Clarke, Harrison H. (Ed.), "Exercise and Aging," *Physical Fitness Research Digest.* President's Council on Physical Fitness and Sports, Washington, D.C., Series 7, No. 2, April 1977.

15

EQUIPMENT AND ASSESSMENT INSTRUMENTS APPLIED TO THE ANALYSIS OF MOVEMENT

CONCEPTS

1. Analysis of motor performance in human movement is particularly well-suited for television because of its distinct action-oriented nature.

2. Television reinforces the learning process through its visual and audio feedback.

3. Television enables observation of detailed close-up motor movements occurring in the gymnasium, field, or laboratory by the student while sitting in the classroom.

4. Video-Tape-Laboratory offers. the unique approach of allowing the student to participate concurrently with television.

5. The electrogoniometer offers a precise means of measuring joint angles and movement patterns; however, body wire attachments may limit motion.

6. The combined utilization of photography, goniometry, and electromyography provides a comprehensive and formidable store of biomechanical information about human movement.

7. Biomechanical quantitative kinematic and kinetic data utilize three general instrumentation systems: (1) mechanical, (2) optical, and (3) electrical.

8. Mechanical instruments such as dynamometers, flexometers, and cable tensiometers have the advantage of ease in usage and durability.

9. Electromyography is the study of muscular activity using the graphic recording of electrical impulses called an electromyogram.

10. Cinematographical data may be collected qualitatively (viewing a videotape) and quantitatively (measuring time and spatial components).

11. Correct application of basic principles of camera, lens, film, and calibration procedures is essential for the accurate collection of photographic data.

12. An ideal camera contains multiple lenses with interchangeble fraction stops.

13. Black and white film is preferred for research purposes. Color film is appropriate for subjective and/or instructional film analysis.

14. The force platform is especially valuable for quantifying data about the magnitude and direction of force generated by the subject against the ground during a skill in a limited area.

TELEVISION AND VIDEOTAPE APPLIED TO THE ANALYSIS OF MOVEMENT

Characteristics of the Medium

While investigating the uses of television as an instructional tool, it is important to consider the characteristics inherent in the medium and particularly the characteristics that enable television to lend itself most effectively to the instruction of kinesiology.

Television offers the following instructional benefits by reinforcing visual and auditory perceptions:

1. Television can transmit sound and picture, in black and white or color, still or moving pictures.

2. Through closed-circuit and broadcast networks, television may be viewed by an unlimited number of persons in an unlimited number of locations.

3. Television enables the recording (videotaping) of special programs.

4. Videotaping permits the immediate playback of a recording or the repeating of a program at a future date.

5. A television program may include the use of any other type of medium as well as live action. For example, a program could combine live action, narration, a film, a lecture with illustrations as slides, charts, or drawings, an explanation of some apparatus that is viewed at close range, and numerous other media.

6. Portable equipment allows videotaping at nearly any location.

7. Television can be used for close-up demonstration and is readily adaptable to magnification and the display of highly detailed objects.

8. Videotaping equipment with slow-motion record and playback capability enables motion study of movement as well as time-lapse programing.

9. An editing machine may be used to edit and correct a videotape.

Characteristics 2, 4, 5, 6, 7, and 8 are of particular value to educators in kinesiology. A class studying the body movement during a diving motion can watch the movement close up from a better than poolside position while sitting in a classroom. Recordings may be made at a convenient time and played back for many classes simultaneously or whenever doing so meets the objectives of the course. Videotaping also permits review of a program for further study. Slow-motion playback of a program recorded in real time allows detailed study of human body movement.

Television Equipment with Special Features for Kinesiology

Television equipment is available in a vast array of models with features useful in the instruction of human biokinetics. The continual updating of television products makes it impossible to guarantee current information in a text discussion. The most up-to-date "state of the art" information on television and videotape systems should be obtained from qualified engineers, television specialists, and audiovisual equipment distributors.

The student may be particularly interested in equipment that features portability, slow motion, editing, freeze frame or stop motion, and ease of use. Several manufacturers of television equipment exhibit one or more of the above features.*

Portability is featured by the Porta-Pac video system (see Figure 15.1) developed and manufactured by the Sony Corporation.† The Sony Porta-Pac is light-weight and easy to operate with a carrying case for the videotape recorder and a mono pod for the camera. The camera is equiped with a zoom lens and is available with either a fixed or roving microphone. Sony also manufactures another tape recorder that permits voice dubbing and editing of programs. Stop motion may be done during the playback of a videotape on

*Note: The discussion that follows is offered to represent the variety of products available. Since the design of TV equipment changes so rapidly, the most current information should always be explored.
†The Sony Corporation of America, 47-47 Van Dam Street, Long Island City, New York 11101.

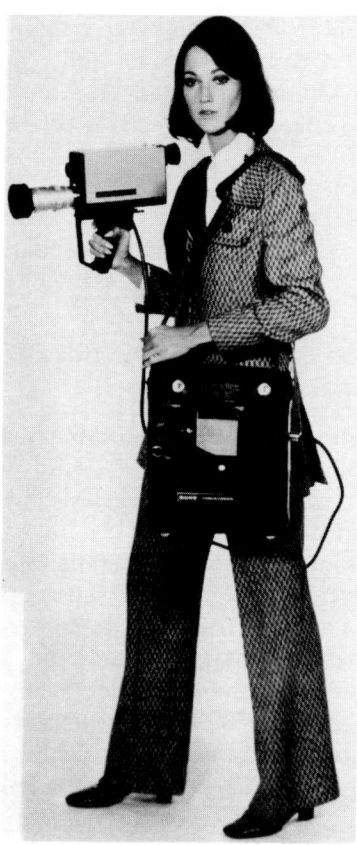

Figure 15.1 Porta-Pac video system (courtesy of Sony Video Products Co.)

models featuring freeze frame capability. The handling of videotape and machine threading has become increasingly easy with the marketing of the new video cassette recorder. A video cassette is inserted into the slot provided and the recorder is ready to record or play back a program.

The capability of presenting action in slow motion is a particular feature of the videotape recorder system designed and manufactured by Javelin Electronics Company.* The Javelin videotape recorder contains two recording and playback speeds. One one-hour program may be played back at the normal

*Javelin Electronics Company, 5556 W. Washington Boulevard, Los Angeles, California 90016.

speed of 7½ intervals per seccond (IPS) or at 1 1/16 IPS to show motion at one-seventh the original speed (seven hours). Program playback may also be accelerated by recording at the slower speed (1 1/16 IPS) and playing back at the faster speed (7 1/2 IPS). The Javelin recorder also features still frame stop action, insertion editing, and independent audio erasure rerecording.

Sony and Javelin videotape recorders typify television equipment that can be used for kinesiological instruction. Black and white as well as color systems are available in most models. Videotape recorders are manufactured in 1/2-inch, 3/4-inch, 1-inch and 2-inch models. Most 1/2-inch systems have been standardized to permit interchangeability of videotapes and the equipment. The video cassette systems, which are developed by many manufacturers, utilize 3/4-inch videotape.

When the decision is made to invest in television, the selection of equipment should be based upon local user needs. Although the videotape industry is constantly developing new products and more sophisticated equipment, the reader should bear in mind that a well-engineered piece of equipment will produce an excellent program, despite the fact that a new model may be easier to operate or offer a new feature. The audiotape industry is undergoing a similar evolution of design (reel to reel, cassette, cartridge, stereo, 2-track, 8-track, etc.). Television has many advantages of particular use in the instruction of kinesiology. Equipment is on the market today that can serve analysts well for many years.

Development of Instructional Television

Television, as a significant instructional medium in physical education, began with sporadic exposures in elementary schools, secondary schools, and colleges during the early Fifties. Instructional programs were generally demonstrations of exercises, sport skills, and physical fitness activities whereby the viewer watched the action projected on the screen. The method of presenting "live" or "taped" telecasts to audiences large or small scattered throughout various geographic locations appeared to many educational theorists as an eminent discovery of allowing the best teachers to bring their expertise of instruction to large groups of people.

Television programs at the elementary school level have been used to demonstrate assorted motor skills, conditioning concepts stunts, games, and posture exercises. This electronic medium at the elementary grade level has established a solid foundation as a teaching supplement. Television and videotape systems at the secondary level have been used principally for the improvement of sport skills in gymnastics, baseball, and basketball. An interesting system called the "isolated camera" technique was devised by Robinson[1] whereby a closed-circuit replay enabled the coach to rerun a football play immediately during a game, pin-pointing errors to players. This equipment also made it possible for the coach to show tape replay in the dressing room at halftime. Coaches have taken greater advantage of television procedures as a means of self-instruction and analysis of team play than physical education teachers in regular class settings. This situation may be due to pressure exerted for excellence in performance and winning, impelling the coach to seek out every available teaching aid for the improvement of his players.

Videotape procedures have been successfully utilized in examining the skeletal system, where knowledge of minute landmarks and articulations are important aspects of study. Floyd and Willson[2] developed television tapes on 12 segments of the skeleton system including such structures as the skull, vertebral column, shoulder girdle, and upper and lower extremities. Close-up views via television were shown accompanied by verbal explanation by the instructor and manipulation of the reference bone by the student, as shown in Figure 15.2a and b.

Reid[3] devised a technique that entailed synchronous videotaping of a subject during a movement and recording of electrical potentials produced by the muscles involved. Simultaneous filming of the electromyograms and actions of a subject is shown in Figure 15.3.

Reid's technique allows the student to compare visually the amount of stress placed on each muscle for each exercise performed and provides an opportunity for the teacher and student to record and examine electrical potentials produced during the performance of various motor skills. These techniques allow the student to study intricate skeletal and muscular characteristics in detail.

Television techniques in kinesiology are extremely limited. This electronic instrument can be an effective tool for the enrichment of learning through its exciting and stimulating effect on the senses, primarily seeing and hearing, when employed in an appropriate manner.

Television and videotape in physical education have largely centered around a "one-way" communication system; that is, motor activity is shown without immediate viewer response. The predominant method of program projection places the subject in a passive role as an observer. The medium continues to lean heavily on the one-way communication system with sophisticated techniques designed to hold attention and interest of the viewer in an inactive fashion. The authors are convinced that mere television observation of motor activities, regardless of its content, with passive attention to its view is of limited instructional value in the teaching/learning process.

A new approach to utilizing television is presented, advancing the concept of allowing the viewer to share in the action shown on the television screen. A prototype instructional

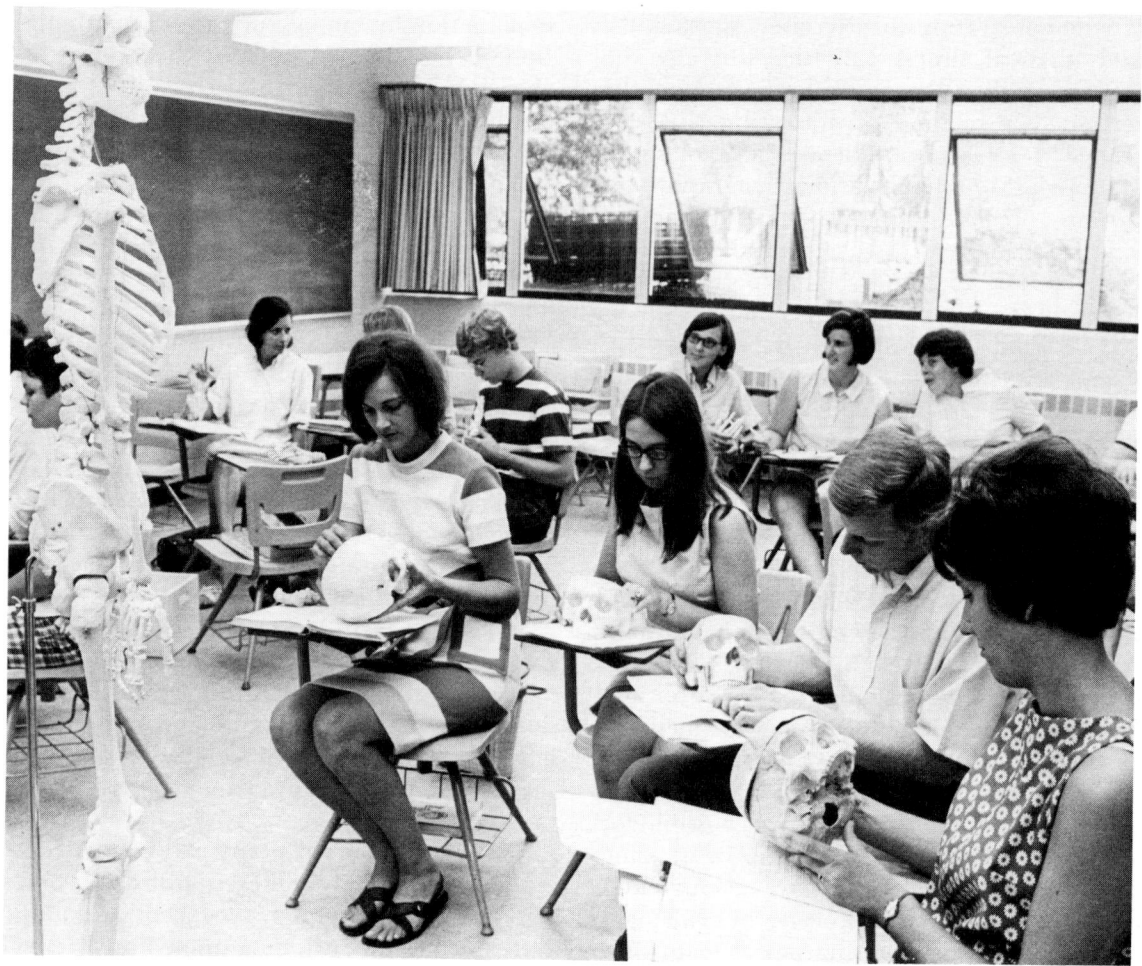

Figure 15.2a Studying the skeleton through videotapes and manipulation of the reference bones
(from William A. Floyd and Philip K. Willson, "Videotape in Skeleton System Study," **JOPER,** 41:81–82,
April, 1970, with permission)

program (V.T.L.) developed by Piscopo[4] and
captioned *Video-Tape-Laboratory* puts forth
the notion of permitting the student to participate concurrently with the television program through a laboratory booklet attuned
to the visual and audio elements. The program entitled "Selected Motor Performance
in Human Movement: A Kinesiological Analysis" is described in a subsequent section.

SELECTED MOTOR PERFORMANCE IN HUMAN MOVEMENT: A KINESIOLOGICAL ANALYSIS

Video-Tape-Laboratory

To counteract the restricted nature of traditional television programing, a program was
designed to activate the viewer for immediate
response with the action projected on the

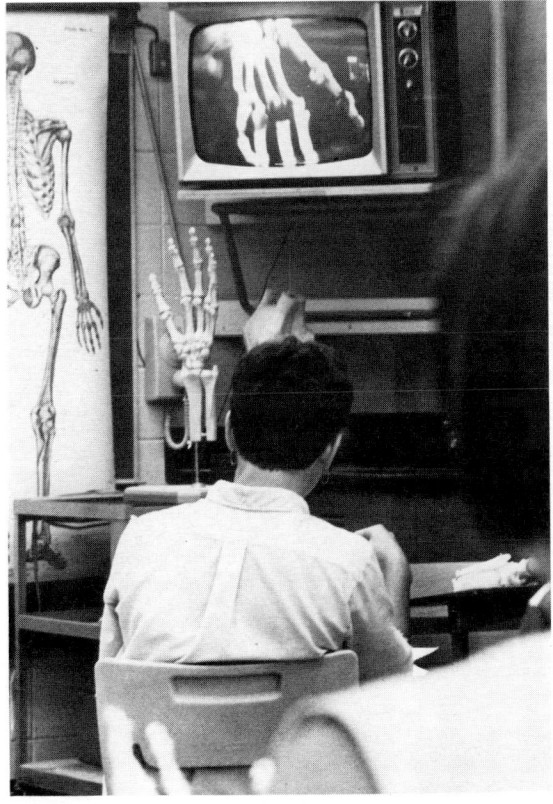

(b)

Figure 15.2b Close-up view of the skeleton using videotapes (from Floyd and Willson, **op. cit.**, p. 82, with permission)

screen; it contained a videotape and parallel kinesiology laboratory booklet.*

Principles and concepts underlying human motion including (1) *balance and leverage,* (2) *transfer of momentum,* (3) *rotation and velocity,* and (4) *direction and magnitude of forces* were illustrated through selected tumbling and gymnastic motor skills. A classroom laboratory booklet was written in such a fashion that it permitted students to participate with the viewing screen. Immediate response

*John Piscopo, *Selected Motor Performance in Human Movement: A Kinesiological Analysis;* Video-Tape and Laboratory booklet, State University of New York at Buffalo, 1973. (Funded through a Biomedical Science Support Grant made to the Research Foundation of the State University of New York ay Buffalo, by the Nation-

questions and relevant study/analysis problems were arranged in a two-part series. Part I contains questions sequenced to allow the learner to respond immediately to actions on the screen. Part II entails in-depth explanatory analysis queries supplementing the immediate-response questions in Part I.

Subject Matter

The first precept, *balance and leverage,* is illustrated by a variety of handstands, couples balancing, still ring movements, and balance beam exercises. The second area, *transfer of momentum,* is shown through demonstrations of forward somersaults utilizing two different arm-lift techniques, mat kip-ups, backward handsprings, and vaulting activities. *Rotation and velocity* fundamentals are demonstrated and analyzed by backward roll variations, twisting movements on the floor, trampoline, and a free turntable apparatus. *Direction and magnitude of forces* are explored through basic jumping movements at specific points on the trampoline. Figures 15.4 through 15.7 present illustrative motor skills of the four concepts contained in this program.

Procedures for Developing the Videotape

After each kinesiological concept was identified and appropriate skills selected, a plan of filming the sequence in a logical pattern was determined. Motor movements were filmed and subsequently edited according to the following design: (1) *lead action* showing a variety of skills containing several illustrations of a kinesiological concept under study, (2) *specific motor skill* exhibiting a concise example of the concept selected for analysis.

The specific skill requiring analysis was

al Institutes of Health, U.S. Department of Health, Education, and Welfare. Appreciation is extended to the staff of the Instructional Communications Center of the State University of New York at Buffalo for the technical assistance in the completion of this project.)

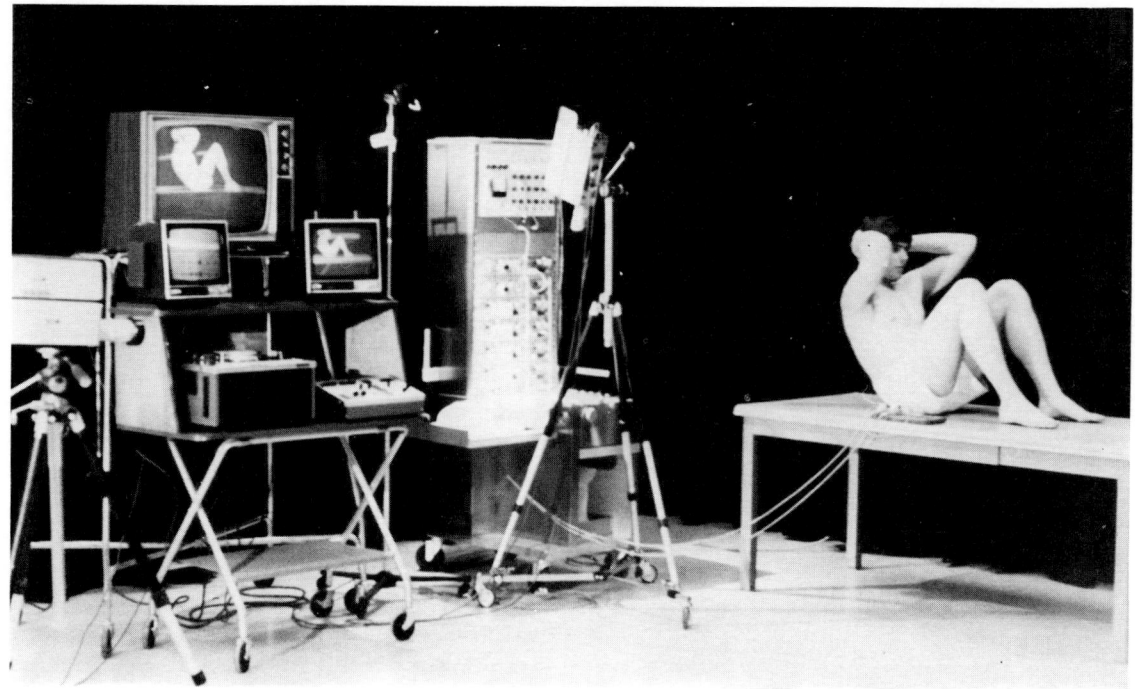

Figure 15.3 Electromyographic recording and videotape in action (from Gavin J. Reid, "Muscles in Action: Use of Videotape and Electromyography," *JOHPER*, 42:61–62, September, 1971, with permission)

shown in slow motion at established points and interlocked with the narration of the television instructor posing pertinent questions at appropriate intervals in the sequence. It is at this moment that the student becomes involved in the program by answering an immediate-response question in the booklet.

Figure 15.8 represents the program flow sequence and its integration with the participant utilizing the laboratory booklet format.

The flow sequence schematically exhibits the specific motor skill twice with the answer box flashed on the screen between the appropriate specific skill. The answer box is repeated to terminate each immediate-response question. The pattern of repeating motor skills and answer boxes allows students neces-

sary time to check the appropriate response in the laboratory booklet. From the student's viewpoint, repetition permits learning reinforcement with the sequence cues on the television screen. A basic principle of "frequent repetition," a characteristic of programmed learning techniques, prevades the entire program. See Figure 15.15a in the appendix for a script segment exhibiting the blend of visual, audio, and laboratory booklet elements.)

Sound Aspects

The sound portion of the videotape was inserted after the film segment was completed. Two narrators were employed. One described the kinesiological subject matter germane to demonstrated actions and the second posed

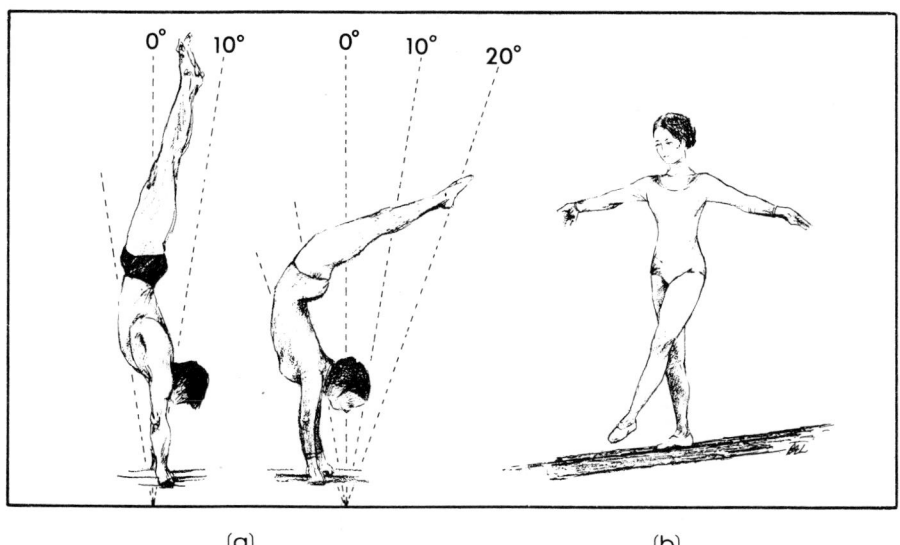

(a)

(b)

Figure 15.4 (a) Maintaining balance with variations in arch magnitudes. (b) first-class lever (arms serve as balance pole) keeps line of gravity within supporting base (feet). (from John Piscopo, "Video-Tape-Laboratory: A Programmed Instructional Sequence," **JOPER**, 44:32–35, March 1973)

Figure 15.5 (a) Floor kip-up: hip and leg extension (body part) transfers momentum to whole torso raising gravity center from floor to hip area over feet in standing posture. (b) Front salto: reverse or backward arm thrust transferred to hips creating upward and rotary motion of the body (from John Piscopo, **op. cit.**, p. 33)

(a)

(b)

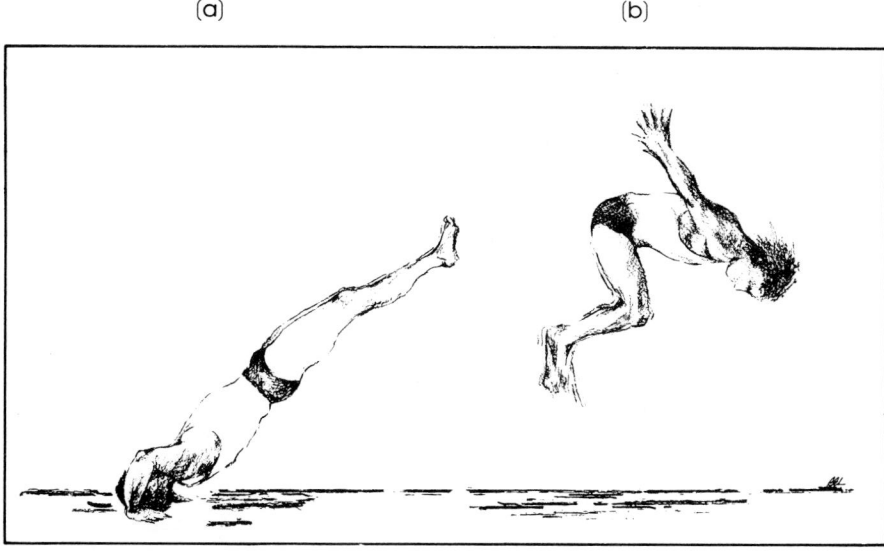

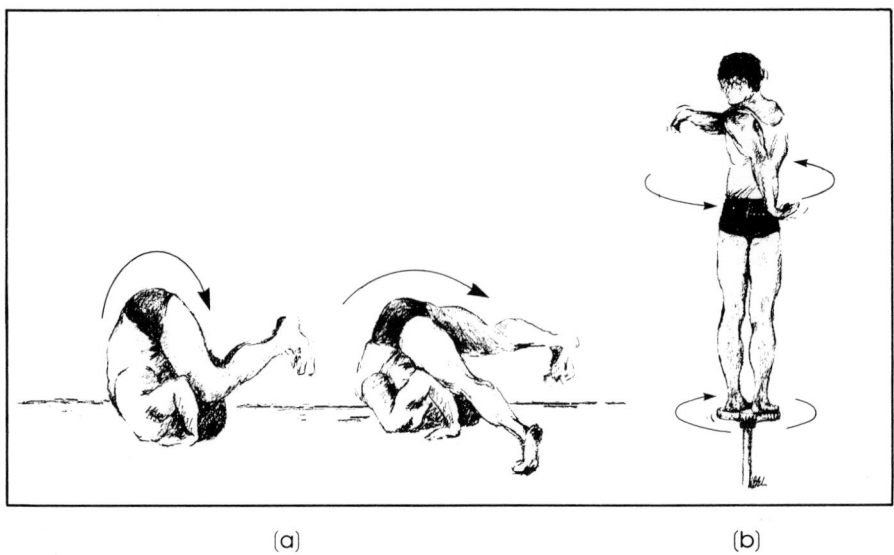

(a)   (b)

Figure 15.6 (a) Backward rolls: speed of rotation (turning phase) is governed by the length of the radius about its center of gravity. (b) Turntable movement: counterclockwise thrust of the arms producing a clockwise movement of the body (law of action and reaction) (from John Piscopo, **op. cit.,** p. 33)

Figure 15.7 Direction and magnitude of forces (jumping at the end of the trampoline)—line of force angular (upward/forward) as performer rebounds on the lift (from John Piscopo, **op. cit.,** p. 33)

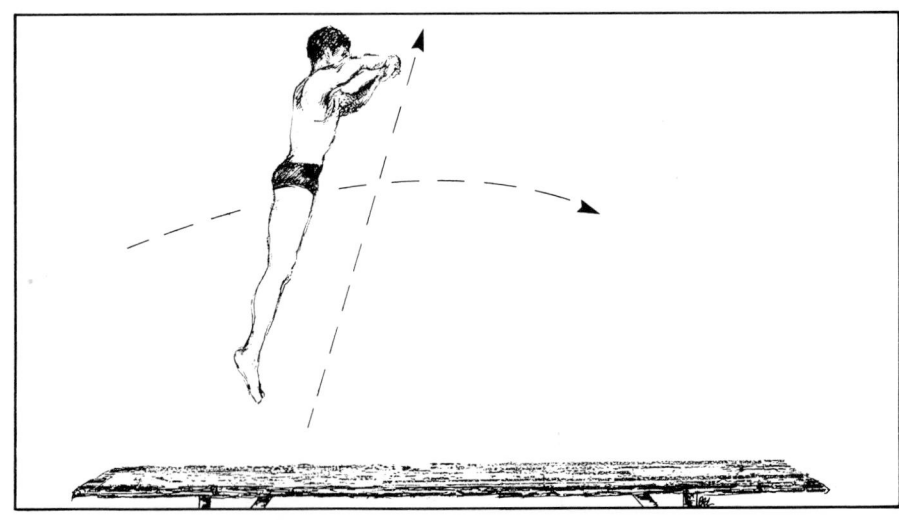

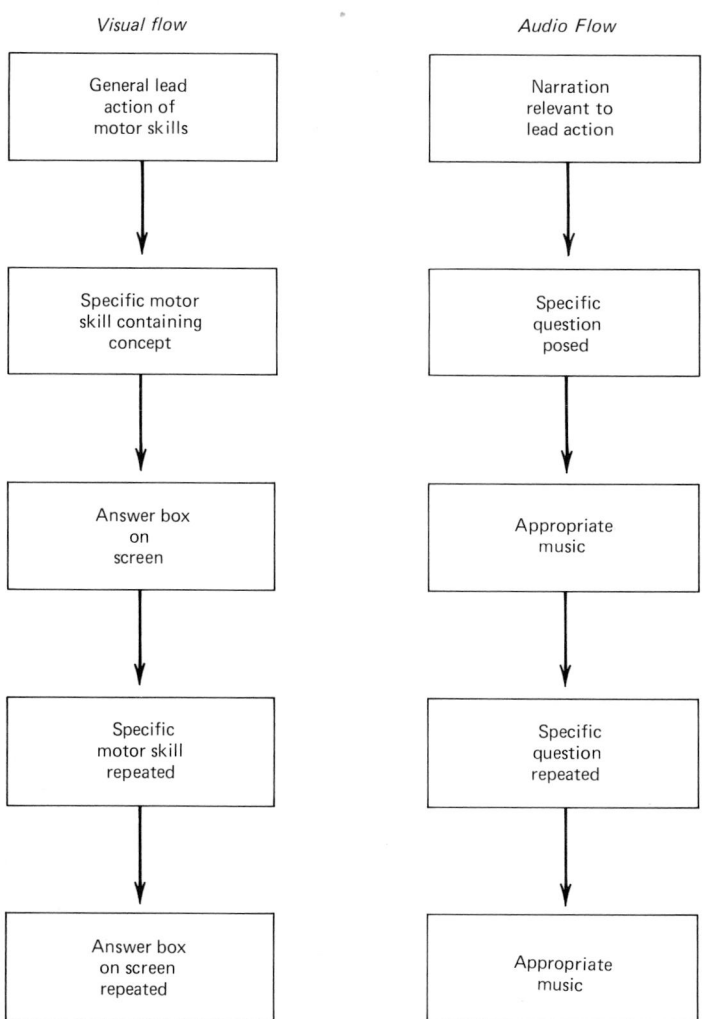

Visual flow

| General lead action of motor skills |
| Specific motor skill containing concept |
| Answer box on screen |
| Specific motor skill repeated |
| Answer box on screen repeated |

Audio Flow

| Narration relevant to lead action |
| Specific question posed |
| Appropriate music |
| Specific question repeated |
| Appropriate music |

Figure 15.8 Program flow chart (from J. Piscopo, **op. cit.**, p. 34)

each immediate-response question. The application of two different voices provided a distinct cue for the learner to respond and mark the appropriate answer in the booklet. Suitable music was utilized to complement screen actions. Careful attention was accorded to the softness and loudness of the background music to enhance visual actions without distracting from the instructional narration.

Visual Aspects

The entire visual aspect of the motor skills was filmed with a 16-mm Arriflex camera. Narrative portions and questions were recorded on a separate magnetic tape. Accompanying music was also recorded on magnetic tape and subsequently both tapes were interlocked on the 16-mm film. The final procedure entailed the development of a one-inch video recording (VTR), copied from the completed sound film.

Laboratory Booklet

A unique feature of the program is reflected by a parallel laboratory booklet format. The booklet is conceived as an integral part of the program and is divided into two sections. Part I contains 17 immediate-response questions. Part II comprises corresponding explanatory analysis queries designed for completion as "homework" utilizing collateral readings. Instructions included in the booklet are presented in the appendix at the end of the chapter.

Careful attention to the preparation of the sequential pattern of screen actions and student participation with the laboratory booklet is vital for the success of this instructional sequence. Student response at appropriate points must be cued in an orderly fashion in the program without viewing distraction. The placement of answer boxes at certain points, shown in Figure 15.15a, is critical for a natural blending of screen actions and response to questions posed by the narrator.

Figures 15.15a, b, and c show the integration of the audiovisual, immediate-response, and explanatory elements pertaining to the "transfer of momentum" concept through the kip-up.

OTHER AREAS FOR V.T.L.

Piscopo and Bennett[5] experimented with the application of V.T.L. in selected diving rotary movements. The analysis of the front dive in pike position was filmed and subsequently videotaped utilizing the basic labora-tory format of allowing the student to follow the television program with immediate-response questions. Relevant follow-up explanatory analysis queries were also included in the laboratory form.

The format (see Figure 15.16 in the appendix) from Laboratory XIV B, currently in use, illustrates how V.T.L. can be applied to diving skill analysis. Although more than one question can be presented on a single page with satisfactory results, it is recommended that the booklet format described in the chapter appendix be utilized. Similar V.T.L. programs have been developed in sports skills of paddle ball and basketball by Albaneze[6] and Hill.[7]

The models described may well expand beyond gymnastic and diving analyses. V.T.L. formats afford distinctive opportunities for augmenting knowledge in dance, aquatics, posture education, and many other forms of motor skills in human movement.

Learner participation is a vital element of the instructional sequence presented in this text. With the rapid advance of technology, V.T.L. can assist the learner to better understand and appreciate human motor performance.

The technique of combining video projection and instant participation laboratory exercises in human performance is unexplored, and this design represents a unique approach to studying kinesiology.

QUANTITATIVE ASSESSMENT INSTRUMENTS FOR THE ANALYSIS OF MOVEMENT

Quantitative analysis implies a precise method of measuring human movement. The sub-area of kinesiology termed *biomechanics*, which studies the motion of living organisms, is particularly well-suited for quantitative analysis whereby an exact and accurate record of performance is desired. *Quantitative kinematic* methods entail the measurement of geometric parameters such as velocity, acceleration, and linear and angular displacement. *Quantitative kinetic* methods involve the measurement of forces that affect motion such as mass, force, power, momentum, and inertia. Kinematic and kinetic methods of assessment require the numerical calculations of a measurable quantity and are typically utilized in the domain of research laboratories. Such external mechanics as Newton's laws of motion are kinetic parameters; linear velocity such as covering a distance per unit of time, $V = D/T$, is considered a kinematic variable. The concepts of kinematics and kinetics are further considered and described in Chapter 5.

Biomechanics specialists generally use three basic instrumentation systems to collect kinematic and/or kinetic data about human movement. These instruments may be categorized as *mechanical, electrical,* and *optical.* The mechanical types involve such appliances as dynamometers (springs, levers, etc.); electrical instruments include electromyography and electrogoniometry to record data about muscular contraction and joint range of motion; optical systems utilize assorted cameras and film types whereby the investigator analyzes motion through photography.

Another electronic device that has been used to measure the magnitude and direction of forces of an individual in sport and therapeutic activities is a *force platform.* This appliance can measure forces exerted on it in three perpendicular directions as well as the center of pressure of the resultant force in such movements of jumping, running, and standing posture.

Mechanical systems such as hand dynamometers, flexometers, and cable dynamometers are standard tools that have the advantage of ease in usage and durability and are particularly well-suited for undergraduate student class use. However, such tools as hand grip dynamometers, tensiometers, and goniometers are gradually being replaced by sophisticated electronic systems that offer greater accuracy and precision in data determination and recording.

Our discussion will focus on *electromyography, cinematography,* and *force platforms.* Each of these systems range from homemade types to sophisticated automated commercial instruments. The basic constituent parts, principles, and applications are considered in the subsequent paragraphs.

Electrogoniometer (Elgon)

An *electrogoniometer* is a sophisticated version of a goniometer and/or protractor. Essentially, the instrument is electrified to measure output signal proportional to an angular change between two pivot arms, and it is used to record joint angle variations. The "elgon," as it is commonly called, was developed in the late Fifties at Springfield College by Karpovich (father) and Karpovich (son).[8] A basic advantage of this device over the mechanical goniometer and flexometer is that it has the capability of measuring continuous changes in degrees of joint angles during motion. However, this device is not considered a practical tool for gymnasium or field activities in everyday teaching and coaching duties. The elgon is a research instrument that provides valid and reliable information of body joints *in vivo* and *in motion.* Basically, the elgon is a goniometer in which a small potentiometer (electrical control device used in hearing aids), has been substituted for a protractor. The electrogoniometer is connected to a control panel used to balance the electrical circuit, and the panel is connected to a recording device where degrees of motion are read from a recording paper called a *goniogram.* Figure 15.9 illustrates an electrogoniometer utilizing the basic equipment recommended by Karpovich.

Such variables as range, amplitude, angular velocity and sequence of movement, and

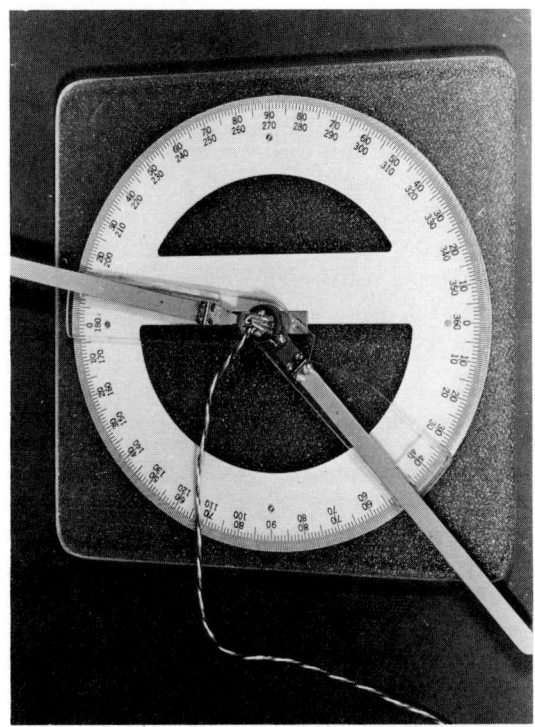

Figure 15.9 Electrogoniometer and calibration board (courtesy of Dr. Thomas J. Sheeran)

It should be noted that the elgon described measures the action in one plane. The above illustrations are examples of joint ranges of movement of the knee and ankle moving in the sagittal plane around a frontal-horizontal axis.

Figure 15.10 Goniogram of the knee and ankle movement during the performance of the front crawl. Point A = maximum knee extension; point B = maximum knee flexion; point C = maximum ankle extension; point D = maximum ankle flexion. (from Dr. Thomas J. Sheeran, "An Electrogoniometric Analysis of the Knee and Ankle in Competitive and Noncompetitive Swimmers," unpublished Doctoral Dissertation, State University of New York at Buffalo, 1976, p. 59)

angle of a joint at specific points can be calculated from goniograms.[9] Figure 15.10 illustrates knee and ankle goniograms of a swimmer performing the front crawl.

The elgon is attached by tape or elastic wrap bandages to the body parts forming a joint. In a recent study at the State University of New York at Buffalo, investigating the design of motion in competitive and noncompetitive leg kicks, waterproof elgons were used to gather flexibility data about the knee and ankle. Waterproofing involved a covered potentiometer and adjacent connections with a rubber balloon. Balloon ends were closed with a silicon rubber adhesive sealant. Figures 15.11 and 15.12 illustrate two elgons fastened to a subject (Figure 15.11) and a swimmer (Figure 15.12) performing the Dolphin stroke with attached electrogoniometers transmitting signals to a recording panel.

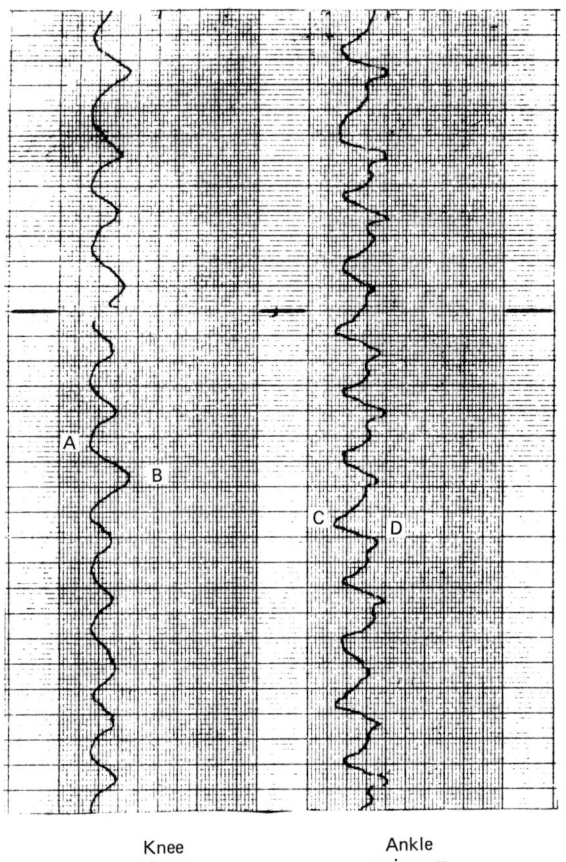

Knee
goniogram

Ankle
goniogram

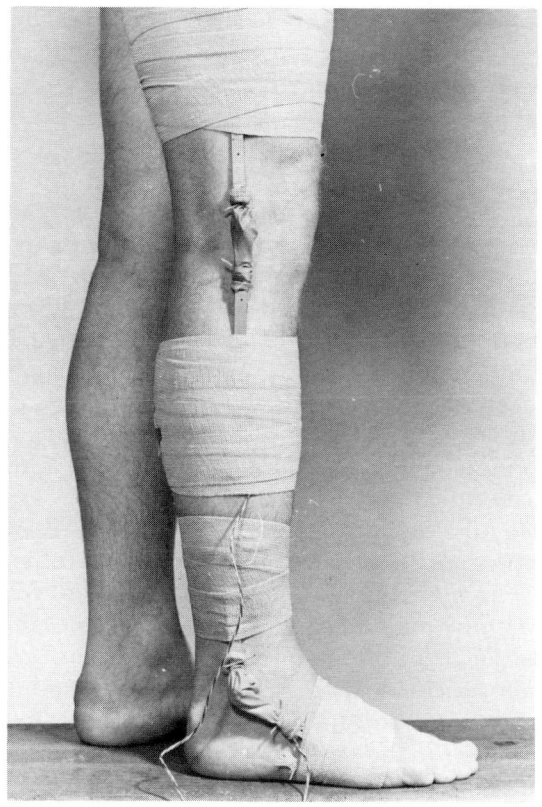

Figure 15.11 Electrogoniometers fastened to a subject: knee and ankle (courtesy of Dr. Thomas J. Sheeran)

Elgons have been used to study walking on high heels, normal and pathological gaits;[10-12] tumbling, sprint starts, baseball throw, shot put, swimming, jumping events;[13-16] weight lifting and other types of movements including gait analysis of hemiplegic patients.[17,18] A simplified elgon was devised by Peat and Fulford for the purpose of studying movements of shoulder muscles following hemiplegia.[19] The unit operates on a gravity reference principle that eliminates the need for accurate alignment of the elgon with the center of joint rotation. Detailed description and procedural technique are found in reference 19. The validity, and reliability of the elgon has been established using comparisons with manual measurements and photometric procedures.[20] Although the elgon offers a precise means of measuring angles and movement patterns while the individual is in dynamic motion, certain limitations are associated with this device; namely, that the instrument, by its wire attachment to the limbs of the subject, may alter the normal movement patterns and, further, analysis is restricted to a limited number of joints whose motion is in a single plane. These problems are continually being studied, and it is the authors' conviction that such limitations will eventually be overcome by applying telemetry to triaxial-type electrogoniometers.

In summary, the elgon offers valuable and precise data about dynamic movement patterns in the following ways:

1. Provides information about angular movement during motor performance.

Figure 15.12 Electrogoniometric attachments to the knee and ankle while swimming the dolphin stroke (courtesy of Dr. Thomas J. Sheeran)

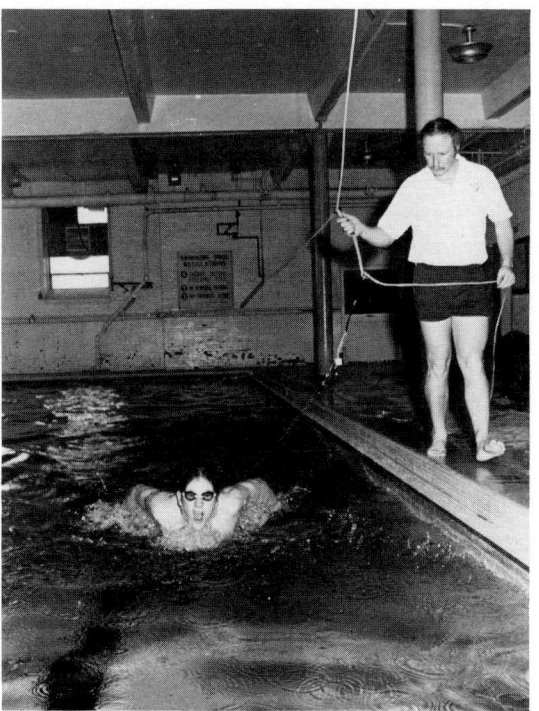

2. Provides an effective method of evaluating sport technique.

3. Provides information about the rhythm, coordination of movements, and form.

4. Provides precise information about the joint range of motion and its relationship to basic motor patterns such as walking, running, and jumping.

5. Provides information in the time sequences of angular changes of movements.

6. Provides information about joint range of motion in pathological and/or therapeutic situations.

Electrogoniometric procedures may also be combined with cinematographic and electromyographic techniques. The triad of photography, goniometry, and electromyography employed in concert provides a formidable gathering of scientific information that can be used for a better understanding of human movement.

Electromyography

Electromyography (EMG) is the study of muscular activity through the graphic recording of electrical impulses called an *electromyogram*. EMG instrumentation systems give quantitative information about the *electrical potential* of muscle contraction. Physiatrists (M.D.s specializing in physical medicine) apply EMG to analyze defects in normal functional tasks such as grasping, walking, and turning and investigate the characteristics of nerve conduction velocity from motor nerves to muscle spindles, which governs the quality of muscular contraction. Various neuropathies affecting the speed of nerve conduction and their influence on muscular movement is of chief interest to the physiatrist. Problems of alcoholism, diabetes, drug abuse, and tumors may inhibit or slow the transmittal of motor nerve conduction to the muscle. Thus, physicians use EMG as a method of diagnosing and correcting atypical and abnormal deviations of human movement. Kinesiologists and physical educators are interested in whether or not a muscle or group of muscles is active during a given normal movement or sequence of movements.

The physical educator, kinesiologist, and corrective therapist are concerned with the question: "Which muscle(s) does 'what' at a particular point or series of points in a given motor or athletic skill?" EMG provides this kind of information through electrical signals recorded on an oscilloscope or graphic recorder. Signals can also be amplified in sound; such acoustical magnification, popularly called *biofeedback*, allows the subject to hear the action potential or the intensity of muscular contraction. Biofeedback is often used for testing and recording activity of the frontalis muscle (front of the skull) relevant to the relief of emotional stress and, in certain types of stroke patients, to determine whether or not motor nerves are conducting impulses to the atrophied muscles. EMG electrodes are so sensitive that they can pick up action potentials of muscular activity whether or not external movement results.

Although EMG is a valuable tool for the evaluation of muscle action, it is not without limitations. Allied health professionals should possess a sound background in anatomy and physiology before embarking upon electromyographical experimentation. Some knowledge in electrical engineering is desirable as well. This does not imply that detailed and sophisticated preparation is a prerequisite in these areas, but a student who possesses a base in each of the above scientific disciplines can develop expertise in electromyography.

Electromyography is an indispensable tool for scientists that has practical implications for the practitioner conducting exercise and activity programs. Researchers throughout the world continue to use this modality to study human and animal movement. Recent studies have been reported analyzing such biomechanical phenomena as motor nerve/muscle characteristics; action potentials and firing patterns of lower limb muscles; analysis of breaststroke swimming; spinal muscle characteristics and postural tone; EMG and isometric endurance; and other topics entailing static and dynamic muscular movements.[21-23]

Basmajian,[24] one of the world's foremost electromyographical kinesiologists, has investigated most aspects of EMG, including such topics as muscle tone and fatigue, coordination of muscle function, effects on handedness, gait, relaxation, and specific actions of other muscles of the body. The student is referred to references 23 and 24 for a comprehensive review of electromyography and a sampling of topics that have been analyzed by EMG methods and procedures.

Cinematography

Cinematography is an optical tool whereby the action information is recorded on photographic movie film using such devices as lights, tripods, and assorted cameras. Two subareas of cinematography are classified as *qualitative* and *quantitative* analysis. Qualitative analysis refers to non-numerical observation that uses movie film as a primary ingredient. An example of qualitative analysis combining film with electronic videotape was described earlier. Quantitative analysis implies numerical calculations of temporal and spatial components of movement from film in a prescribed and objectifying manner.

Several advantages are found with film-analysis techniques. First, wires are not necessary for recording the visual image of the performer. Therefore, the subject is not restricted by gear that may impede his/her performance. Movie film also lends itself well to competitive sport situations where the performer's actions can be divorced from shooting the film. Another advantage of film anal-

ysis rests with degree of permanency. For example, direct visual observation can be recaptured only by memory, which invites gross error in assessment. Films provide a resource whereby images can be reviewed at any time, without pressure, and this advantage allows greater accuracy in analyzing the motor performance of the participant.

Perhaps two of the primary limitations of cinematography are the inability of film to assess muscle functions and the problem of analyzing a three-dimensional action from a two-dimensional film. Errors in recording spatial (displacement of points) and temporal (time) pattern relationships can occur. However, the problem of these numeral quantities has been greatly reduced by using biaxial (two-cameras) and triaxial (three-cameras) setups. Early film analyses were also limited by the extensive amount of time involved in obtaining, recording, and analyzing the data; however, modern motion analyzers, automated data-gathering systems, and high-speed computers have overcome this obstacle. Notwithstanding the limits of precision in interpreting recorded data and lack of information about muscle function, cinematography can give meaningful quantitative knowledge provided fundamental principles are observed. These principles incorporate a functional working knowledge of *cameras, lenses, film types,* and *calibration basics.* A detailed and comprehensive treatment of the elements is not within the scope of this text; however, a general description of these vital components follows in the subsequent paragraphs.

Camera and Lens. Cinematography is the most common optical technique used to record human movement. Cameras range from speeds of 32 frames per second to 500 frames per second.

Sixteen-millimeter movie cameras provide a workable balance between exposure and picture image and are especially popular for high-speed photography. Fast ballistic-type actions require shorter exposure time, which can usually be accommodated with a 16-mm motor-driven camera. It should be noted that, as exposure time is reduced, more light is necessary for clear pictures. Table 15.1 presents important factors for consideration in selecting a camera for movement analysis.

Cameras should have interchangeable lens systems to accommodate various film shooting requirements. High-quality lenses are essential to reduce film distortion. A telephoto lens with zoom provisions is desirable since this feature reduces the *parallax error*, which is the displacement of the object or action caused by a change in the position of the filmmaker. The telephoto feature allows the photographer to be farther away from the object to be filmed, thereby minimizing the error. An ideal camera with a multiple lens apparatus should have the following f (fraction) stops: (1) the standard lens should have an f stop range from 1.9 to 22; (2) wide-angle lens should have f stop settings from 1.8 to 16;

and (3) telephoto lens should provide an f stop setting from 2.5 to 3.2.[25]

Film and Calibration. Films are rated according to their ASA index (American Standard Association). Films that exhibit high numbers are fast films and are more sensitive to light. Therefore, the choice of film depends upon lighting conditions, type of action to be filmed, and purpose of utilization. Black and white film is usually the choice of researchers because of its clarity of images as compared with color. However, if film is to be used for qualitative, subjective evaluation of a motor skill, color film may be preferred.

Temporal (time) data extraction is an important part of film analysis. Therefore, time, which is derived from the frame rate, and must be considered, especially if exact and accurate information is desired. Motor-driven cameras operate at a constant speed and are preferred over the spring-wound type, which may be affected by humidity and other climatic conditions. It is also desirable

Table 15.1 General Specifications of 16-mm Cameras

Camera drive	Spring or motor (AC-DC) driven?
Type	Intermittent film transport or rotating prism?
Pin registration	Prevents image drifting when film is projected.
Sampling rate	Minimum and maximum frame rates possible? Fixed or continuously variable?
Speed regulation	Time to reach designated frame rate? Consistency of frame rates?
Image quality	Resolution and steadiness of image?
Lens mount	Types of lenses accepted? Single lens or revolving turret?
Shutter	Fixed, variable, or interchangeable?
Focusing and viewing	Through-the-lens reflex viewing?
Ease of loading	Film magazines? Self-threading?
Footage indicator	Self-setting?
Internal timing or event marker lights	Availability? Number? Location with respect to the gate?
Operational environment	Effect of temperature and humidity variation?
Film capacity	100, 200, or 400 feet? Can smaller reels also be used?
Weight and dimensions	Influence portability.
Construction	Sturdy or easily damaged?
Warranty and repair	Availability of parts and repair facilities?
Cost	Can optimal features be added later?

From D. I. Miller and R. C. Nelson, *Biomechanics of Sport: A Research Approach*, Lea and Febiger, Philadelphia, 1973, p. 125.

to have an indication of the frame rate while filming the actual performance, in addition to a stopwatch before or after the action. The student is referred to reference 26 for several sophisticated methods of calibrating camera speed to ensure accuracy of film interpretation.

Cinema Basics. Certain basic plans and procedures should be followed by the investigator conducting ciné analysis. The points indicated include some important requirements for successful production and analysis[27]:

1. Secure appropriate facilities when filming under *laboratory conditions*, such as blackcloth, scales for distance measurements, horizontal and vertical lines to determine x and y coordinates, timing device to check framing rate.

2. Subject should move at right angles to the camera.

3. Use telephoto to increase the size of picture.

4. Reduce perspective error by avoiding close-up shots when possible without affecting the purpose of the film.

5. Use a fixed or stationary camera to permit distance computation.

6. Set distance limit marks of the line of action before filming the action.

7. Action field should contain points of reference such as a pole, part of building.

8. The operating speed at which the camera should be set depends upon the movement to be filmed, number of movement segments needed for analysis, and camera type.

9. Segmental end-points to be used for analysis should be clearly marked on the subject.

10. Use appropriate film for specific lighting conditions—faster film necessary for low-lighting situations.

Film Analysis. Sophisticated techniques involve triaxial cinematographical analysis of velocity, acceleration, space displacement, changing centers of gravity, and angular and linear patterns. Although these methods and parameters serve as valuable facilitators for augmenting new knowledge about the biomechanics of motion, coverage of such analytical quantities would require a comprehensive textbook on cinematography given the advanced technical software and hardware now available. Our discussion focuses on the practical use of cinematography equipment available to the student seeking a better understanding of human movement through film analysis.

Basic film analysis does not necessarily have to utilize complicated mathematical calculations. Films can provide objective answers to such questions as: What is the angle of trunk flexion in a tuck somersault? Where is the position of the lead foot in relation to the hips as the hurdler passes over the hurdle? What is the angle at the knee in sprint running? What is the typical arm-swing pattern in normal walking? Does the ankle dorsiflex or plantar flex in the breaststroke leg thrust? Where is the center of gravity in the sprint start? What is the takeoff angulation of the body in a highly skilled swimming racing start? What is the difference in the motion pattern of a hitter or pitcher when performing "well" or when in a "slump"? How does a superior performer get height in doing a back somersault on the parallel bars? Does the reverse arm-lift (Russian front) create greater height and faster rotation in the execution of a forward somersault?

With reference to the last query, Cianfrini[28] completed a cinematographical study showing that the conventional forward two-arm-lift achieved a two-inch greater height advantage over the reverse arm-lift technique. A simple system of using a 16-mm camera (speed of 64 frames per second), grid screen, marking tapes, stopwatch, and still photos made from a movie film negative was employed. Such analysis proved to be of practical value to the investigator, who was coaching the performer at the time. These questions and problems about motor and athletic skills can be answered, at least in part, through film analysis.

Data analysis can be made from basic methods of observing film from frame to frame in a film reader to precise measurement of velocity, acceleration, spatial displacement, moments of force, and angular body changes using triaxial photography. The complexity of the data derived from triaxial cinematography requires a sophisticated knowledge of mathematics, physics, and computer programming beyond the scope of this text.

Logan and McKinney suggest a useful and practical procedure for analyzing film as follows:[29] (1) review film several times, making notes regarding the various joint or body-segment motions during the performance phases (such review should include form of total performance and violation of motion principles); (2) analyze film frame by frame with a record made of each joint motion during each phase of the performance (ranges of motion should be noted as well as whether motion was against resistance or with gravty); (3) observe implications of the extraneous motion and evaluate in terms of the performance objectives; and (4) rank faults and list teaching suggestions to eliminate each fault.

If the student is seeking specific joint angulation data, tracings of the contour or body outline called a *contourogram* can be made. Drawings should be accurate enough to determine joint angles. It should be remembered that *absolute joint angles* cannot be determined with photographic techniques because of the perspective error described earlier. However, usable information can be gained from contourogram drawings (batting) shown in Figures 7.18a through 7.18e.

Another basic analysis procedure is called the *point-and-line* technique.[30] This procedure is as follows: a point is used to indicate the estimated joint or anatomic landmark, and the lines that connect these points indicate body segments as shown in Figure 15.13.

Each point indicates the center of the pelvic segment used to estimate the line of movement. The student may elect to use the contourogram or the point-and-line drawing. Drawing of every frame is not essential. In a series of 30 or 40 frames, every fourth frame could be drawn, reflecting a consistency of time interval between drawings. Another method of selecting frames would be to determine the critical phases of a performance after the film has been observed several times. This mode emphasizes the crucial points of a skill where the performer's faults may occur. The preceding steps pertain to a basic level of analysis. The student is referred to reference 31 for a comprehensive approach to calculating various angles, accelerations, velocities, moments of force, moments of inertia of individual segments, and kinetic energy of the body. An excellent review of cinematographic analysis of such movements as walking, running, throwing, striking, pushing, pulling, locomotion on and from land, locomotion in water, and other sports activities are described by Anne E. Atwater[32] with an extensive bibliography on all phases of film analysis. Each activity is analyzed in synoptic form. The student seeking a general overview of motor skills and patterns will find this review a valuable resource for further study.

Force Platform

The amount and direction of forces that a performer applies to an implement, apparatus, or environment determines, to a significant degree, success or failure in performance of a motor or athletic skill. The *force*

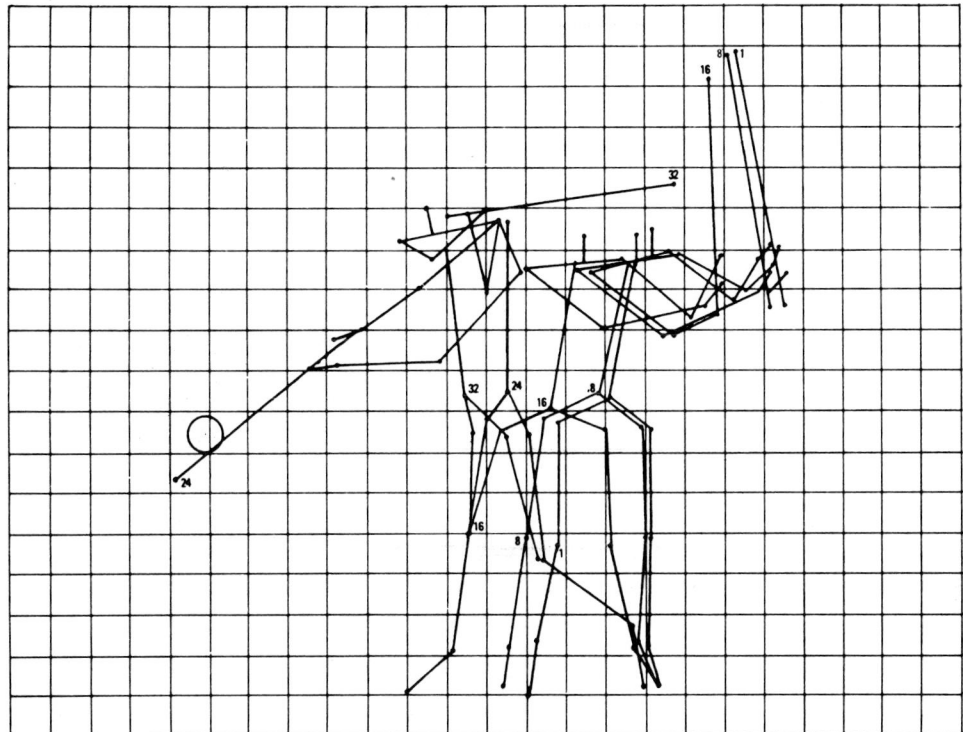

Figure 15.13 Point-and-line technique (male performer numbers indicate film frames. Film was taken at 32 frames/second. Left-handed hitter.) (from Gene A. Logan and Wayne C. Mc-Kinney, **Kinesiology,** 2nd ed., Wm. C. Brown Co., Dubuque, Iowa, 1977, with permission)

platform is an instrument designed to measure direct force exerted against the ground through the feet. This platform is generally about 3 feet by 3 feet by 5 inches and, with such sensing instruments as variable transformers, strain gauges, and other electronic devices for amplification and recording, can measure forces in the sagittal, frontal, and horizontal planes. The ideal platform should be rigid, light, and very stiff so that its displacement is imperceptible to the person performing an activity on it.[33] Force platforms have been used for gait analysis in orthopedics, posture control, and athletic sports of broad jumping, sprint starting, shot put, and weight lifting. The instrument can be utilized to quantify forces that a performer exerts on the ground during running, jumping, walking, balancing, or any activity in which ground reaction forces are important for efficient performance. A properly equipped platform generates electrical signals proportional to the magnitude and direction of forces exerted on the surface. These signals are transmitted to such recording devices as a tape recorder, chart recorder, or light oscillograph for analysis. A. H. Payne[34] of the University of Birmingham, England, conducted a number of sport studies on weight lifting, tennis, and shot putting and emphasizes the important requirement that analysis should be carried out, as much as possible, under natural conditions for a particular movement under investigation. Since the measuring area of the platform is rather small, activities that require large surface space may necessitate the use of two platforms. Certain activities are better suited than others, simply because of varying playing dimension needs. For example, the study of upright static balance mechanics shown in Figure 15.14 has excellent possibilities for determining force variations as well as center of gravity shifts in different directions. Such quantitative information can pinpoint mechanical deficiencies in standing and walking movements. These data can provide valuable information on rehabilitation and the design of prosthetic devices.

The Kistler Instrument Corporation of Switzerland* has developed a quartz multicomponent measuring platform, a measuring system that determines three components: force, location of point of force application, and moment about a vertical axis.

An interesting study was done to compare the accuracy of the force platform method of determining the center of gravity applied to the standing vertical jump with that of the classical cinematographic analysis.[35] Twenty-five college students performed vertical jumps on the force platform and were also filmed simultaneously at 100 frames per second. The results showed a high positive relationship between the two methods, with the conclusion that the platform method is an accurate technique for measuring the vertical component of takeoff velocity. Commercial-type platforms are available that satisfy the requirements of sensitivity, sturdiness, and electronic reliability; however, the cost of

*Kistler Instruments AG, CH-8408 Winterthur, Switzerland.

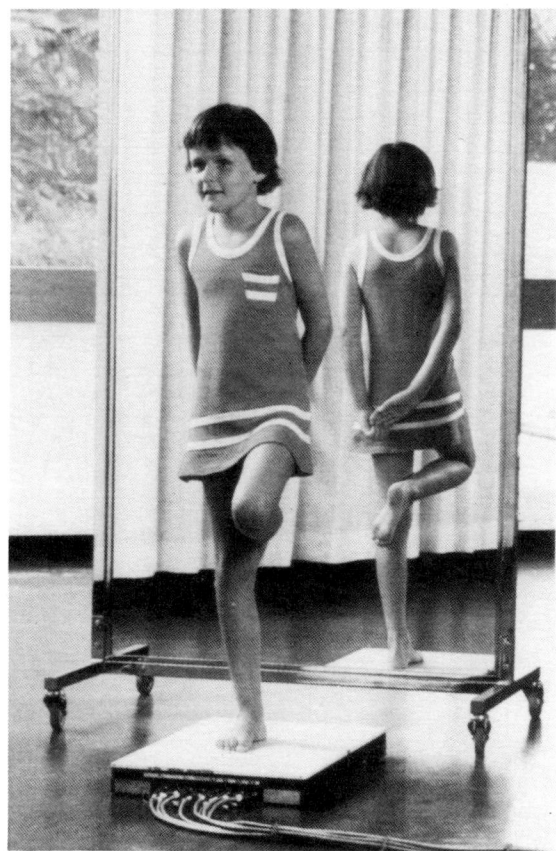

Figure 15.14 Measuring forces during an upright standing position (courtesy of Kistler Instrument Corporation, Switzerland)

these units is high, and they are generally found in colleges and universities where research in motor performance is pursued.

SUMMARY

Use of television in physical education emerged during the early Fifties with various one-way communication systems primarily directed toward skill demonstration types of programs.

Characteristics of the television medium delineated are particularly valuable in the instruction of kinesiology. Several models of equipment that feature slow motion, portability, and ease of utilization were described.

Kinesiologists have used closed-circuit systems studying landmarks and articulations of the human skeleton. Other investigators have used television with electromyography.

The application of television as a teaching medium predominantly focuses upon one-way systems of communication. Video-Tape-Laboratory offers a new instructional design allowing the viewer to participate actively with the passive projection shown on the television screen.

Quantitative data about human movement can be collected with *mechanical, optical,* and *electrical* instrumentation systems. Mechanical tools have the advantage of durability and ease of use; however, in certain instances they lack precision and accuracy. Cinematography is the most common optical technique used to record human movement and can be adapted for practitioner and researcher use.

The electrogoniometer (elgon) is an electronic instrument with the capability of measuring continuous changes in degrees of joint angles. Such variables as range, amplitude, angular velocity, sequence of movements, and angle of joints at specific points can be calculated from goniograms.

Electromyography (EMG) is the study of muscular activity through the graphic recording of electrical impulses called an electromyogram. Physical educators and other allied health professionals interested in motor skills and sport can use this electronic tool to study muscle activity during a given movement or sequence of movements.

Cinematographical data can be collected qualitatively and quantitatively. Qualitative analysis refers to non-numerical observations, such as viewing movie film reproduced on videotape and subjectively analyzing the action. Quantitative analysis implies numerical calculation of temporal and spatial components of movement from film in a prescribed and objectifying manner. Meaningful quantitative data can be secured by movie film techniques provided the filmmaker follows basic principles pertaining to (1) camera, (2) lenses, (3) film types, and (4) calibration. Sixteen-millimeter movie cameras provide a workable balance between exposure and picture image and are especially popular for high-speed photography. Telephoto lenses are a desirable feature since their use reduces the parallax error. An ideal camera should contain multiple lenses with interchangeable f stops. The choice of film depends upon lighting conditions, type of action to be filmed, and purpose or use. Generally, black and white film is the choice of researchers because of its clarity; however, color film is appropriate for qualitative and instructional purposes.

Certain cinema basics pertaining to facilities and laboratory conditions, camera angulation, lens type, photographic technique, fixed-camera devices, line of action markings, background reference points, camera speed, marked reference points on the subject, and correct film type are essential factors to consider in the preplanning phase of filming motor activity.

A practical method of analyzing film includes reviewing film and analyzing motion and positions frame by frame at selected intervals. Joint angulation data can be secured by developing tracings of body drawings called a contourogram. Another basic method known as the point-and-line technique may be used for data analysis.

A force platform is an instrument designed to give quantitative information about direct forces exerted against the ground through the feet. This device is an excellent apparatus to measure the vertical component of takeoff velocity when movement is confined to a restricted action area.

APPENDIX: V.T.L. BOOKLET*

Instructions

This booklet is designed to be used in conjunction with the film/videotape entitled, "Selected Motor Performance in Human Movement: A Kinesiological Analysis."

Part I contains seventeen questions which will be asked during the program. Complete each question by selecting one answer from among the choices given. Place a check mark in the box next to your answer; then turn the page for the next question.

Part II requires you to analyze the kinesiological concepts presented in Part I of the program. The references given in Part II list sources of additional information which should be consulted to assist you with each explanatory analysis.

Figure 15.15 (a) V.T.L. Transfer of Momentum script segment; (b) immediate response segment (booklet question #9); (c) explanatory analysis segment (booklet question #9)

Video	Audio
Concept: Transfer of Momentum	
A. *General lead action*	A. *Kinesiological Narration* (Dr. Piscopo) *Music* (under)
1. Variations of kip-ups on *parallel bars*.	Transferring momentum from one part of the body to the whole torso is exemplified by the kip-up.
a. Single kip-up	The kip-up entails raising the center of gravity from below the parallel bars to a point of support above the apparatus.
b. Alternate kip-ups (two persons)	
c. Simultaneous kip-ups (one person at each end)	The gravity center must also be raised when the movement is performed on the mat. Raising the center of gravity depends largely upon the force and angle of leg thrust.
2. Series of floor mat kip-ups	Observe the kip-up with particular attention to the leg thrust. 21 sec.
	Music (full) completes lead action 19 sec.
Total lead time: 40 sec.	total: 40 sec.
B. *Specific Motor Skill*	B. *Alternate Announcer* (Mrs. Bennett) *Music* (under)
Kip-up from floor mat:	At what angle is the body fully extended? 07 sec.
(Freeze frame to show angulation) 09 sec.	*Music* (full) completes specific motor skill 02 sec.
	total: 09 sec.

*From J. Piscopo, "Video Tape Laboratory: A Programmed Instructional Sequence," *Joper*, 44:34, March, 1973.

Video		Audio	
☐ 10°			
☐ 20°			
☐ 30°			
C. Answer box:	*10 sec.*	*C. Music* (full)	*10 sec.*
D. Specific Motor Skill (repeated)		*D. Alternate Announcer* (repeat question) *Music* (under)	
Kip-up from floor mat (Freeze frame repeated)		At what angle is the body fully extended?	*07 sec.*
		Music (full) completes specific motor skill	*02 sec.*
	09 sec.	total:	*09 sec.*
☐ 10°			
☐ 20°			
☐ 30°			
E. Answer box (repeated)	*10 sec.*	*E. Music* (full)	*10 sec.*

QUESTION 9

At what angle is the body fully extended?

☐ 10°

☐ 20°

☐ 30°

ANALYSIS 9

Explain the effect of the angle of leg thrust upon projection of the performer to a standing position.

_____

_____

_____

_____

_____

_____

_____

Figure 15.16 V.T.L. analysis of the front dive in the pike position.

Name: _____

Date: _____

I. *PURPOSE:*   To identify and examine basic mechanical and kinesiological principles affecting a running front dive.

II. *EQUIPMENT:*   Protractor or goniometer (optional).

III. *REFERENCES:*   Bunn, John W., *Scientific Principles of Coaching*, Englewood Cliffs, New Jersey: Prentice-Hall, Inc., 1972.

                    Councilman, Roger L., "The Dynamics of Entries in Diving," *Athletic Journal*, XLV (May 1965):14–63.

                    Groves, William H., "Mechanical Analysis of Diving," *Research Quarterly*, 21:2 (May 1950):132–144.

IV. *DIRECTIONS:*   Study *individually*. Answer each question designated 1a, 2a, 3a, etc. immediately as directed by the video announcer. Complete questions designated 1b, 2b, 3b, etc. *after* the screen projection is concluded. Refer to references above for study and analysis.

A. *RUN*

1a. HOW MANY STEPS DOES THE DIVER COMPLETE INCLUDING THE HURDLE STEP?

          (a) 3 steps   _____

          (b) 4 steps   _____

          (c) 5 steps   _____

1b. Explain the effects of forward momentum and body angulation of the run upon the performance of the dive.

_____

_____

_____

_____

2a. CHECK THE APPROXIMATE LOCATION OF THE CENTER OF GRAVITY DURING THE RUN.

          (a) over feet   _____

          (b) slightly in front of feet   _____

          (c) slightly behind the feet   _____

2b. Explain the effect of the center of gravity upon the dive as checked in question 2a.

_____

_____

3a. CHECK THE APPROXIMATE DEGREE OF BODY LEAN
ON THE RUN.

(a) 40° _____
(b) 60° _____
(c) 90° _____
(d) other _____

3b. Explain how body lean affects dive height.

_____

_____

_____

B. *HURDLE*

4a. INDICATE THE HURDLE LEG SELECTED BY
THE DIVER.

(a) left leg _____
(b) right leg _____

4b. What initial move or action in the run determines which leg is raised in the hurdle?

_____

_____

5a. APPROXIMATE THE HEIGHT OF THE DIVER'S
HURDLE LEG FROM THE BOARD.

(a) 10 inches _____
(b) 20 inches _____
(c) 30 inches _____
(d) other _____

5b. Explain the effect of hurdle height upon dive height in terms as governed by Newton's Law of Motion.

_____

_____

_____

6a. INDICATE THE LANDING DISTANCE OF BOTH FEET
FROM THE END OF THE BOARD (WATER EDGE END)
ON THE HURDLE.

(a) 3 inches _____
(b) 6 inches _____
(c) 12 inches _____

6b. Explain the mechanical advantages or disadvantages of the diver's hurdle landing position as indicated in 6a.

_____

_____

C. *TAKEOFF*

7a. INDICATE THE DIVER'S APPROXIMATE
ANGULATION OR BODY LEAN ON THE TAKEOFF.

    (a) 45° _____
    (b) 60° _____
    (c) 80° _____
    (d) other _____

7b. Explain how the degree of lean affects the following:

(1) height of dive — _____

_____

(2) rotatory velocity — _____

_____

_____

(3) execution phase of the dive — _____

_____

8a. MARK THE APPROXIMATE LOCATION OF THE
CENTER OF GRAVITY DURING THE INITIAL
TAKEOFF.

    (a) in front of
        the body _____
    (b) directly over feet _____
    (c) slightly behind
        the body _____

8b. How does the initial position of the center of gravity affect the execution of dive? What implication does your answer have for all diving categories?

_____

_____

9a. INDICATE THE APPROPRIATE LOCATION OF THE
ARMS EXHIBITED BY THE DIVER ON THE TAKEOFF.

    (a) parallel to
        humeroscapula
        joint _____
    (b) below humero-
        scapula joint _____
    (c) above humero-
        scapula joint _____

9b. How is the arm lift related to body inertia on the takeoff? (Explain)

_____

_____

D. *EXECUTION*

10a. OBSERVE THE MOVEMENT OF THE LEGS AS THE
DIVER EXECUTES THE PIKE POSITION. SELECT ONE
OF THE FOLLOWING:

(a) feet move
toward hands   _____

(b) feet move away
from hands   _____

(c) feet remain
stationary   _____

10b. Explain your answer in terms of Newton's Law of Motion.

_____

_____

11a. INDICATE THE POSITION OF THE HIPS DURING THE
"HOLD" ACTION OF THE PIKE.

(a) above shoulder
height   _____

(b) parallel to
shoulders   _____

(c) below shoulders _____

11b. Draw a parabolic curve or flight path from takeoff to the point of entry indicating the gravity
center at the following points: (1) beginning of the flight, (2) point of greatest flight, (3) point of
entry. Explain the mechanical phenomenon affecting the center of gravity in the flight path of
the demonstrated dive.

_____

_____

_____

12a. INDICATE THE APPROXIMATE ANGULATION OR
MAGNITUDE OF "PIKE TIGHTNESS" DURING THE
EXECUTION PHASE OF THE DEMONSTRATED DIVE.

(a) 40°   _____
(b) 90°   _____
(c) 10°   _____

12b. Explain how the angulation of the pike dive position affects the following:

(1) rotatory velocity — _____

_____

(2) dive height — _____

_____

(3) magnitude of rotation — _____

_____

E. *ENTRY*

13a. APPROXIMATE THE ANGLE OF ENTRY ATTAINED
 BY THE DIVER.

          (a) over 180°   _____

          (b) under 180°   _____

          (c) 180°   _____

13b. Explain the effect of the entry as indicated by your answer in 13a. If the entry is unsatisfactory, explain the mechanical principle causing the error.

_____

_____

_____

_____

14a. INDICATE THE APPROPRIATE ANSWER RELEVANT
 TO THE "ENTRY" PHASE OF THE DEMONSTRATED
 DIVE.

          (a) splash toward
 board   _____

          (b) splash away
 from board   _____

          (c) no splash   _____

14b. Explain the mechanical principle governing the speed of rotation applicable to the Jackknife Dive entry.

_____

_____

_____

15a. INDICATE THE APPROXIMATE DISTANCE OF THE
 DIVE FROM THE BOARD ON THE ENTRY.

          (a) 1 foot   _____

          (b) 2 feet   _____

          (c) 3 feet   _____

          (d) over 3 feet _____

15b. Explain the cause of excessive distance, if any, by the demonstrated dive.

_____

_____

_____

REFERENCES

1. Robinson, Frank, "Coaching with Video Tape," *Scholastic Coach*, 35:36-56, January, 1966.
2. Floyd, William A., and Willson, Philip K., "Using Videotape in Skeletal System Study," *Journal of Health, Physical Education and Recreation*, 41:81-82, April, 1970.
3. Reid, Gavin J., "Muscles in Action: Use of Videotape and Electromyography," *Journal of Health, Physical Education and Recreation*, 42:61-62, September, 1971.
4. Piscopo, John, "Video-Tape-Laboratory: A Programmed Instructional Sequence," *Journal of Health, Physical Education and Recreation*, 43:32-35, March, 1973.
5. Piscopo, John, and Bennett, Stephanie, "Television Applied to Human Motor Performance," *The Physical Educator*, 30:35-37, March, 1973.
6. Albaneze, Dennis, "Paddleball: An Analysis of Selected Skills and Kinesiological Concepts," unpublished Master's Project, State University of New York at Buffalo, 1973.
7. Hill, John D., "A Mechanical and Videotape Analysis of the Jump Shot in Basketball," unpublished Master's Project, State University of New York at Buffalo, 1974.
8. Karpovich, Peter V., and Karpovich, George P., "Electrogoniometer: A New Device for Study of Joints in Action," *Federation Proceedings*, 18:79, 1959.
9. Adrian, Marlene J., "An Introduction to Electrogoniometry," *Kinesiology Review*. Washington, D.C.: American Association for Health, Physical Education, and Recreation, 1968, pp. 12-18.
10. Gollnick, Philip D., Tipton, Charles M., and Karpovich, Peter V., "Electrogoniometric Study of Walking on High Heels," *Research Quarterly*, 35, pt. 2:370-378, October, 1964.
11. Adrian, Marlene J., and Karpovich, Peter V., "Foot Instability During Walking in Shoes with High Heels," *Research Quarterly*, 37:168-175, May, 1966.
12. Finley, Ray F., and Karpovich, Peter V., "Electrogoniometric Analysis of Normal and Pathological Gaits," *Research Quarterly*, 35, pt. 2:379-384, October, 1964.
13. Gollnick, Philip D., and Karpovich, Peter V., "Electrogoniometric Study of Locomotion and of Some Athletic Movements," *Research Quarterly*, 35 pt. 2:357-369, October, 1964.
14. Ringer, Lewis B., and Adrian, Marlene J., "An Electrogoniometric Study of the Wrist and Elbow in the Crawl Arm Stroke," *Research Quarterly*, 40:353-363, 1969.
15. Sheeran, Thomas J., "An Electrogoniometric Analysis of the Knee and Ankle in Competitive and Noncompetitive Swimmers," unpublished Doctoral Dissertation, State University of New York at Buffalo, 1976.
16. Klissouras, Vassilis, and Karpovich, Peter V., "Electrogoniometric Study of Jumping Events," *Research Quarterly*, 38:41-48, March, 1967.
17. Singh, Mohan, and Buck, T.M., "Leg-Lift Strength Test with Electrogoniometric Analysis of Knee Angle," *Archives of Physical Medicine and Rehabilitation*, 56:261-264, June, 1975.
18. Bajd, T., Stanic, U., Kljajic, M., and Trnkoczy, A., "On-Line Electrogoniometric Gait Analysis," *Computers and Biomedical Research*, 9:439-444, 1976.
19. Peat, Malcolm, and Fulford, Raymond, "An Electrogoniometer for the Measurement of Single Plane Movements," *Journal of Biomechanics*, 9:423-424, 1976.
20. Kettlekamp, Donald B., et al., "An Electrogoniometric Study of Knee Motion in Normal Gait," *Journal of Bone and Joint Surgery*, 52A:775-790, June, 1970.
21. Asmussen, Erling, and Jorgensen, Kurt (Eds.), *Biomechanics VI-A*, Baltimore: University Park Press, 1978, pp. 135, 183-265.
22. Asmussen, Erling, and Jorgensen, Kurt (Eds.), *Biomechanics VI-B*, Baltimore: University Park Press, 1978, pp. 126, 167, 195, 319, 325, 332.
23. O'Connell, A. L., and Gardner, E. B., "The Use of Electromyography in Kinesiological Research," *Research Quarterly*, 30:166-183, May, 1963.
24. Basmajian, John V., "Electromyographic Analysis of Basic Movement Patterns," in Jack H. Wilmore (Ed.), *Exercise and Sport Science Re-*

views, Vol. I. New York: Academic Press, 1973, pp. 259-284.

25. Logan, Gene A., and McKinney, Wayne C., *Kinesiology*. Dubuque, Iowa: Wm. C. Brown, 1970, p. 197.

26. Miller, Doris I., and Nelson, Richard C., *Biomechanics of Sport: A Research Approach*. Philadelphia: Lea & Febiger, 1973, pp. 173, 135.

27. Smith, A. J., "Photographic Analysis of Movement," in D. W. Grieve, D. I. Miller, D. Mitchelson, J. P. Paul, and A. J. Smith (Eds.), *Techniques for the Analysis of Human Movement*. Princeton, N.J.: Princeton Book Co., 1976, pp. 3-10.

28. Cianfrini, Dennis M., "A Comparative Cinematographic Study of Two Forward Somersault Techniques," unpublished Master's Project, State University of New York at Buffalo, 1974.

29. Logan, Gene A., and McKinney, Wayne C., *Anatomic Kinesiology*, 2nd ed. Dubuque, Iowa: Wm. C. Brown, 1977, pp. 230-231.

30. *Ibid.*, p. 230.

31. Plagenhoef, Stanley, *Patterns of Human Motion*. Englewood Cliffs, N.J.: Prentice-Hall, 1971.

32. Atwater, Anne E., "Cinematographic Analyses of Human Movement," in Jack H. Wilmore (Eds.), *Exercise and Sport Sciences Reviews*, Vol. I. New York: Academic Press, 1973, pp. 217-258.

33. Payne, A. H., "The Use of Force Platforms for the Study of Physical Activity," in J. Wartenweiler, E. Jokl, and M. Hebbelinck (Eds.), *Biomechanics I*. Basel: Karger, 1968, pp. 83-86.

34. Payne, A. H., "A Force Platform System for Biomechanics Research in Sport," in R. C. Nelson and C. A. Morehouse (Eds.), *Biomechanics IV*, Baltimore: University Park Press, 1974, pp. 502-509.

35. Lamb, W. H. and Stothart, P., "A Comparison of Cinematographic and Force Platform Techniques for Determining Take-Off Velocity in the Vertical Jump," in Erling Asmussen and Kurt Jorgensen (Eds.), *Biomechanics VI-A*, Baltimore: University Park Press, 1978, pp. 387-391.

16

KINESIOLOGIC CONCEPTS APPLIED TO TEACHING MOTOR SKILLS: A SUMMARY

CONCEPTS

1. Internal mechanics refers to mechanics within the body such as angle of insertion of muscles, relative lengths of force and resistance arms, stress resistances of body tissues, internal friction, and other aspects.

2. External mechanics refers to forces, leverage, and visible movements outside the body.

3. When making a kinesiologic analysis of a motor skill, it is necessary to describe the starting position, execution of the movement, and the final position.

4. When determining the starting position, consideration must be given to (a) the objective of the movement to follow, (b) external forces that might be brought to bear upon the body, (c) the need for stability, and (d) the need to move in one of several possible directions.

5. A prime consideration when making a kinesiologic analysis of the execution of a motor skill is the objective of the movement, although there may be a number of other factors to be considered.

6. All people involved in teaching motor skills, including those who administer motor programs, should understand and be familiar with not only those kinesiologic principles of import to the learning of motor skills but also those having to do with body type, evalua-

tion, racial characteristics, growth, physical conditioning, neural functions, learning, resolution of vectors, influences of orthopedic deviations upon balance and movement patterns, posture, and injury.

7. The efficiency of a motor performance is evaluated on the basis of the ratio of the mechanical work accomplished in a period of time to the total energy expended.

8. The effectiveness of a movement is determined by the degree to which the goal has been accomplished.

9. The effectiveness with which a movement is achieved is determined by many factors including the difficulty of the goal, genetic characteristics, and qualities of physical fitness.

10. A **kinetic analysis** is one in which the various movement variables such as interacting forces that produce other movements and changes in movement are studied.

11. A **kinematic analysis** is one in which the movement variables are observed and described.

12. Learning of all new motor skills occurs in the cerebral cortex; however, the cerebral cortex gradually relinquishes its control to the lower brain levels as the skill is mastered.

13. The cerebral cortex continues to monitor skills after they are mastered.

14. The learning of many motor skills is quite complex and, for this reason, learning should

565

progress from the simple to the increasingly complex.

15. New motor skills should not be presented to children until their state of physiological maturation has progressed to a level at which they are ready to learn the skill.

GENERAL CONSIDERATIONS

In this, the summarizing and closing chapter of this textbook, the objective is to suggest approaches to application and utilization of all the information previously presented to the solution of problems that occur in learning and teaching motor skills. Although this has been done to some degree throughout the text, the primary objective has been to illustrate the concept and *secondarily* to illustrate how the concept can be used in teaching and learning motor skills. In this chapter, these priorities are reversed.

What are the procedures for analyzing the reasons for failure to execute a skill with efficiency? Why did the diver overspin his forward one-and-a-half somersault? How could the kicker have gained more distance on his kick? How can the sprinter decrease his time out of the blocks? What body types are most likely to succeed in marathon runs? Gymnastics? Football? Swimming? Basketball? How can the probability of injury in skiing be minimized? Kinesiology can provide a large part of the answer to these practical questions to help the practitioner become more effective.

Procedures have been developed that have proven successful for making kinesiologic analyses of motor skills. The instructor needs to know the factors in determining the most effective starting position as well as those for determining the best method of execution.

It is important for the instructor to know all the kinesiologic concepts. Furthermore, the learner should also know and understand certain of these concepts. In this chapter we will list those concepts that we believe learners should know and apply in their efforts. These learnings constitute a portion of the cognitive precepts that should occur in physical education classes. Other concepts are of prime, and in some cases, exclusive, interest to the teacher or coach. These concepts have implications for evaluative procedures, administrative decisions, selection of players for teams, selection of activities for students and classes, conditioning procedures, teaching methods, adaptations of activities for the handicapped, postural standards, exercises selected for students with postural deviations, and prevention of injuries. Concepts having to do with execution of movement skills, on the other hand, are of interest to student participants as well as to teachers and coaches.

The efficiency and effectiveness of movement patterns must be evaluated. Kinetic and kinematic analyses of a nominal or quantitative type may be made either deductively or inductively.

INTERNAL MECHANICS APPLIED TO MOTOR PERFORMANCE

Internal mechanics refers to mechanics within the body such as angles of insertion of involved muscles, relative lengths of force and resistance arms, stress-resistances of body tissues, range of motion, internal friction, and other aspects. While internal mechanics contribute to skillful performance as much as do external mechanics, adjustments of internal mechanics are made on a subconscious level through the proprioceptive and kinesthetic mechanisms and are also primarily the result of genetically determined structure and function. Consequently, little can be done by the coach or physical educator to improve internal mechanics, and as a result attention is generally focused on *external mechanics* when teaching motor skills.

EXTERNAL MECHANICS APPLIED TO MOTOR PERFORMANCE

External mechanics refers to forces, leverage, and movement outside the body. External mechanics are easier to observe, measure, and study than are internal mechanics. Consequently, those who teach and study movement skills give more attention to external mechanics. There have been hundreds of books and thousands of articles written describing the external mechanics of sports and other movement skills. These have included descriptions of the dolphin kick in the butterfly, angle of the legs with respect to the floor at the moment of lift-off in a front somersault, procedures for use of crutches or a cane, relations of the several body segments on a downfield tackle, and many others. Coaches and teachers of all sorts of movement skills must continually analyze movements and positions of their students in light of the biomechanical and anatomical principles discussed throughout this text.

An illustration of the above point can be provided in the teaching of a running forward somerault. The instructor might note that the student experiences difficulty in completing the somersault in spite of correct "blocking" action, good height, and a tightly tucked position. He also notes that the student rotates slowly and that his arms do not extend above the head prior to initiation of rotation but are thrown downward from shoulder level. Because he knows that the center of rotation during the forward somersault is the frontal-horizontal or lateral axis and that it is forward of the hips, and also because he knows that *the further a force is applied from the center of rotation, the greater the speed of rotation,* he will recognize that the student must extend his arms above his head before whipping them downward. This will lengthen the moment arm to increase the moment of inertia to produce more kinetic energy or force to apply for rotation.

Another example of the aid knowledge of principles of external mechanics can provide for the performer or coach comes from the area of track and field. Most people believe that the best angle of projection is 45 degrees where maximum distance is the objective as in the shot put, javelin throw, or hammer throw. However, those who have studied external mechanics dealing with projection will know that *when throwing downhill* (when the landing point of the projectile is at a lower elevation than the starting point) *at low projection velocities, the optimum angle of projection may be as low as 37 degrees.* An understanding of the principles of projection (Chapter 5) will enable the athlete to add distance to the throw.

KINESIOLOGIC ANALYSES OF MOTOR SKILLS

When describing or teaching movement skills, it is necessary to describe the starting position, execution of the movement, and the final position. These descriptions must take into consideration all relevant principles of external mechanics. They will be more complete and, consequently, more helpful if all relevant kinesiologic principles are included.

Starting Positions

When determining the starting position, consideration must be given to the objective of the movement to follow, external forces that may be brought to bear upon the body, the need for stability, and the need to move in one of several possible directions. The objective of the racing start in swimming is to project the body in a horizontal direction as far as possible over the surface of the water as quickly as possible and to enter the water with the body in a streamlined position. In the 100-yard dash, the objective is likewise to project the body as rapidly as possible in a horizontal direction; however, the body itself must be nearly vertical. In both starts, *the line of gravity must be at the forward edge of the base of support to facilitate a quick start at the sound of the gun.* In the swimming start, the body rotates 90 degrees at the feet and the thrust is directly backward in a horizontal direction since maintenance of vertical balance is unnecessary. Consequently, the feet are in line laterally and the toes project beyond the forward edge of the starting block. In the start for the 100-yard dash, one foot is placed forward of the other and the thrust of the feet against the starting blocks must have a downward (vertical) component of force because of the necessity for maintaining the vertical position of the body. The objectives of these two racing starts are similar in that in both the body must be accelerated quickly in a horizontal direction; however, the body position after the start is horizontal in one and nearly vertical in the other.

The starting position of the "clean," in the clean and jerk in weight lifting, is different from that in racing starts because the objective is to move a weight upward to the shoulders in the most efficient and explosive manner while maintaining balance. The feet are in line laterally and about two feet apart to permit full knee and hip flexion as well as to facilitate maintenance of balance in a lateral direction. Since the barbell must be pulled directly upward in a vertical line to culminate in a resting position across the chest and directly above the center of the base of support, it is inadvisable to place one foot in front of the other in the starting position. Downward thrust resulting from extension of the knees and hips is greater when the feet are parallel than when one is forward of the other because all the force is directed downward and none forward and backward as when the feet are separated in an anterior-posterior direction. Also, an anterior-posterior separation of the feet will make a vertical pull of the barbell less likely since the shoulders may be positioned behind the barbell.

Like the racing start in swimming and the 100-yard dash, the clean requires an explosive extension of the knee and hip joints. However, unlike these movements, in the clean, the line of gravity must be centered over the base of support.

The differences between the starting position or stance of the defensive and the offensive lineman are due as much to the differences in the external forces that will be brought to bear against their bodies as they are to their differing objectives. It is of greater importance for the offensive lineman to maintain a low center of gravity than it is for the defensive lineman because the defensive lineman is permitted to use his hands and can apply lateral forces upon the offensive lineman. Also, the offensive lineman must move his opponent out of the line of play. This can be accomplished more effectively when contact is made below the opponent's center of gravity. The defensive lineman must maintain a higher center of gravity in order to possess greater maneuverability; however, if his stance is too erect, he can be more easily knocked over. Consequently, the stance is a compromise between that required for maneuverability and maintenance of stability when subjected to an external force.

The offensive lineman maintains his line of gravity near the forward edge of his base of support because he must react quickly with a forward lunge on the signal to make contact with his opponent. However, since his opponent may grasp and pull him forward onto his face easily when his weight is forward, he may not place his weight too far forward unless he is confident his reaction will be faster than that of his opponent. Again, an intelligent compromise is required.

In some skills the most desirable starting position is one that facilitates a quick response and movement in any one of several directions. This is the case when in the "ready" position waiting to receive the service in tennis, badminton, handball, squash, paddleball, or racquet ball. The player does not know until the last moment whether it will be necessary to move forward, backward, right, left, or somewhere in between. When quick movement in any of several unknown directions is necessary, *the center of gravity should be located above the center of the base of support. The area of the base of support is reduced so that a small displacement of the center of gravity results in an unbalanced position.* This narrowed stance facilitates a faster movement of the center of gravity and the feet in the desired direction. For the same reason, an excessively low center of gravity should be avoided. The weight should be on the balls of the feet; the ankles should be slightly dorsi flexed, the knees and hips should be slightly flexed, and the muscles should be in mild static contraction. When the decision is made to move in a certain direction, the muscles that will move the body go from static to concentric contraction while their antagonists relax. Reaction time is decreased as a result of this procedure because the muscles responsible for moving the body have been preshortened.

The squat balance or "frog stand" taught in beginning tumbling classes provides an example of a skill requiring delicate balance and great stability. The center of gravity is lowered by beginning from a full squat position. The arms are placed between the knees and the hands are placed on the floor at shoulder width with the fingers well spread. The medial aspects of the thighs are placed on the upper arms while the elbows are flexed to 130 degrees. The feet are then elevated off the mat. The forearms are maintained in a vertical position so that the body weight passes down the bones of the forearms. The center of gravity is directly over the hands with the head elevated to compensate for the weight of the legs on the opposite side of the fulcrum. It should be noted that the starting position is a highly stable one with a very low center of gravity and with four points of sup-

port—the two hands and the two feet. The weight is very carefully shifted forward from the feet entirely onto the hands to complete the skill, as shown in Chapter 8.

In many movements in sports, a prime objective is maximal production of force. Examples are throwing a cross or straight right in boxing, putting the shot, pitching in baseball, or throwing a javelin. *Production of force by the body must always conform to Newton's third law, i.e., for every action there is always an equal and opposite reaction.* If a boxer's right cross is to have maximal force on impact, it is essential that none of the impact be absorbed by partially flexed joints or by insecure footing. Therefore, at the moment of impact, the rear or driving leg must be extended so that the reaction is through the bones and to the floor. As has been stated many times in earlier chapters, each successive force (plantar flexion, knee extension, hip extension, hip rotation, shoulder flexion, and elbow extension) should be initiated at the point of greatest speed and least acceleration of the preceding movement (*summation of forces*). The starting position must be such that it is possible that the several involved body segments are in as nearly as possible a straight line relationship at the conclusion of the movement. It is not possible that the arm be in line with the trunk at the conclusion of a right cross (unless a four-foot boxer is striking a seven-foot boxer). Consequently, the scapula and the shoulder must be stabilized by static contraction of the muscles of this area. Obviously, these muscles must be sufficiently strong to stabilize these joints completely. However, the lower leg, upper leg, and trunk can be in a straight-line relationship and must be if the punch is to be delivered with maximum impact.

Other factors that determine whether the punch will produce a knock-out are amounts of momentum, mass, force, velocity, and acceleration. *The amount of momentum generated determines how damaging the blow will be. Momentum equals mass times velocity.* Although the boxer cannot change his own mass, he can increase the amount of the mass available that he gets into the punch. He can "get his body into the punch" by following through to the extent possible without losing balance or moving beyond the opponent. Terminal velocity is determined by the rate of acceleration, in turn determined by the amount of force generated by the muscles and the time over which this force acts. *The stronger the muscles, the more force they can generate.* If the boxer attempts to increase the time (length of the backswing) of the punch, he will "telegraph" his punch; therefore, strength is a major factor in determining terminal velocity of the punch.

Execution

When analyzing the kinesiological requirements for execution of motor skills, the first consideration is to determine the objective of the movement. In the case of a projectile, the objective may be to hurl it as far as possible, to throw it from point A to point B as quickly as possible, to pitch it with precise accuracy and great speed, or to deceive an opponent by causing the ball to follow other than a straight path. There are thousands of motor skills, each with different objectives. Invariably, there are considerations such as actions of opponents (rushing the passer, man on first, etc.), wind, weight, size and shape of various projectiles, size of throwing area, etc., which dictate variations in the mechanics used. However, these variations and adaptations of style are not illustrations of exceptions to kinesiologic principles. Kinesiologic principles are derived from the laws of nature and are irrevocable. If they are amended, it is because the principle was incompletely or incorrectly stated.

We will now provide illustrations of kinesiological analyses of several motor skills.

Volleyball Spike

The objective of this skill is to strike a volleyball that has been set up by teammates so that it is driven over the net and into the opponent's court in such a manner that the opponents are unable to return the ball into the spiker's court. Opposing players endeavor to block the ball just after it passes over the net. Occasionally, the ball may be set up too close to or too far from the net.

Physical prerequisites for most effective spiking require good jumping ability, shoulder flexibility, and height. Jumping ability can be enhanced by increasing the strength of the knee and hip extensors, plantar flexors, and shoulder flexors through progressive resistance exercises (with heavy resistance) such as the rise on toes, half squat, dead lift, and dumbell lifts forward with the arms extended. Shoulder flexibility can be increased through static stretching exercises of the shoulder joint. Taller players should be selected as spikers.

The spiker starts from a position eight or nine feet from the net in order that the ball may be set up in front of him. To be certain that he/she moves in the correct direction, the spiker waits until the ball has been set up. Then, from a position facing the net, the spiker takes two steps toward the net to generate forward momentum. The horizontal momentum generated in these two steps is converted into vertical momentum by landing after the second step with the legs angled backward. Upon landing, the knees and hips are flexed and the extended arms are swung backward while continuing to watch the ball (Figure 16.1*a*). The extended arms are then swung forcefully upward, the hips, followed by the knees, are extended and the feet are plantar flexed (Figure 16.1*b*)—each segmental action being initiated at the point of greatest speed and least acceleration of the preceding segment and culminating in the thrust of the feet against the floor (summa-

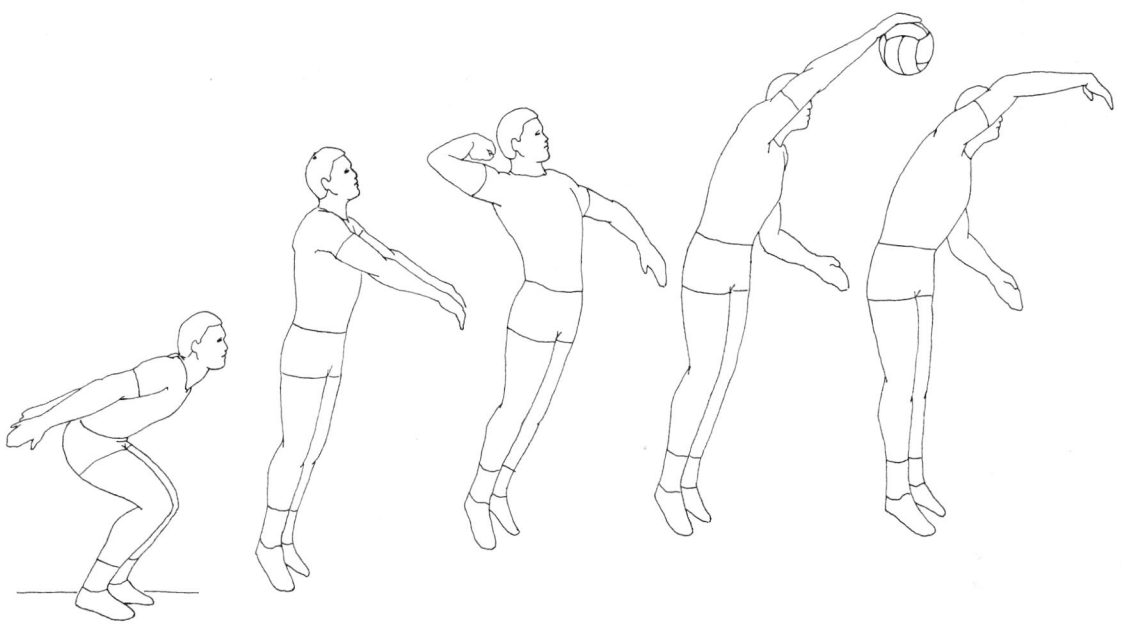

Figure 16.1 Volleyball spike

tion of forces). The more forceful this thrust, the higher the jump, as expressed by Newton's third law: *For every action, there is an equal and opposite reaction.*

The jump must be timed or synchronized with the flight of the ball during the set up in such a manner that the ball is just forward and above the spiker's head when the highest point of the jump is reached. At this point, *the spiker's back is arched to increase the distance through which the force acts and to thereby increase the amount of acceleration of the hand and consequently, its final velocity* (Figure 16.1c). As contact with the ball is made, the spine moves from an arched or hyperextended to a flexed position (Figure 16.1a). This action increases the amount of mass involved. The action increases both mass and velocity and, consequently, there is a substantial increase in the amount of momentum transferred to the ball. (The student will recall that *momentum equals mass times velocity*.) The distance through which the

hand may accelerate is further increased through clockwise rotation of the thoracic spine, drawing the shoulder of the striking arm farther backward prior to the forward swing of the arm. During the striking action, the thoracic spine is rotated counterclockwise. Rotation of the trunk and shoulder girdle will produce a *reactive twist in the lower part of the body in the opposite direction as per Newton's third law.* However, after the first reactive twist of the lower body, it will be brought back into its original position by the reactive twist produced as a result of the counterclockwise rotation of the thoracic spine and the shoulder girdle as the arm and hand swing forward toward the ball.

Additionally, at the height of the jump, the elbow is flexed to bring the hand behind the head, the wrist is hyperextended, and the humerus is outward rotated, abducted, and sideward elevated. Elbow flexion, as in pitching a ball, decreases the length of the resistance arm as the hand is brought forward during the first portion of the movement. The speed of rotation of the hand is more easily accelerated with the elbow flexed. As the hand is brought forward with the elbow flexed, the humerus moves from an outward-rotated to an inward-rotated position producing great speed in the hand. Before the hand meets the ball, the elbow is extended. While this action will not increase the speed of rotation of the hand around the shoulder joint, it will increase the linear velocity of the hand.

The heel of the hand hits up into the back of the ball and the wrist is flexed to snap down and forward onto the ball, the hand wrapping around the ball (Figure 16.1e). This action drives the ball downward and produces a topspin on the ball. The wrist snap is the final and culminating lever action brought into the total striking action. *The principle of summation of force is operative throughout the sequential actions* of inward rotation of the humerus, sideward elevation of the humerus, spinal rotation, elbow extension, and wrist flexion. Since *action and reaction are always in opposite directions*, the direction of the final force against the ball determines its direction. Top spin on the ball will increase air resistance on the top of the ball and decrease it on the underside of the ball. This will cause it to drop downward more rapidly.

After the spiker has struck the ball, he/she will drop to the floor. He must return to the floor on his feet, in good balance, and ready to continue play. The hips need to be flexed slightly to bring the feet under the body as it drops downward. The landing should be on the balls of the feet with the feet spread shoulder width apart to improve stability. *Impact should be absorbed over a greater period of time through eccentric contraction of the extensor muscles of the feet, ankles, knees, hips, and spine.*

The preceding discussion explains the procedures and applicable kinesiologic princi-

ples for execution of the basic spike. Back court spikes, dumping, and placement require slight adaptations of these basic techniques.

Track and Field—Running Broad Jump

Maximum distance in the running broad or long jump is achieved by coordinating horizontal and vertical acceleration at the moment of leaving the takeoff board. The primary requisite is the development of power achieved through velocity during the run and powerful contraction of the extensor muscles of the hip, knee, and ankle joints. The jumper should accelerate at such a rate that maximum speed is attained, at least three or four strides before reaching the takeoff board. Since full speed is attained within 45 feet by even the slowest runners, the run need not exceed 60 feet.[1]

Weingartner[2] found that use of the sprint start produced fewer fouls than the stand-up start more commonly practiced. During the last three strides, the jumper lowers the center of gravity slightly by increasing the amount of flexion of the hips and knees. This action decreases velocity slightly but is necessary in order to prepare to give the body a vertical component of force upon leaving the takeoff board. The jumper should strive to achieve a *takeoff angle of 45 degrees since it has been shown that the optimal angle for achievement of distance of projectiles is usually 45 degrees.* Few jumpers obtain a takeoff angle of 45 degrees; however, they should strive to accomplish this without excessive loss of horizontal velocity.

The jumper should avoid looking down at the board since this will impart an undesirable forward rotational force to the body, which will decrease the distance of the jump. To convert horizontal momentum to an upward thrust, the takeoff board is hit with the heel of the takeoff foot with the leg angled backward in the manner used by tumblers and high jumpers to convert horizontal into vertical momentum (Figure 16.2a). Use of plastic heel cups will help to absorb this impact and to prevent damage to the calcaneal bone. On the takeoff, the arms and the striding leg should be swung upward as high as possible (Figure 16.2b). *The momentum generated by these parts will be transferred to the entire body to impart a vertical component of force to the body.* As the striding leg is swung upward, the head and chest should be lifted. The knee of the takeoff leg is bent after the foot leaves the board to *shorten the radius of this leg and thereby increase its angular velocity,* which will bring it in front of the body more quickly.

Cinematographic analyses of the movement of the center of gravity of the body during the long jump show that it is lowered slightly during the last three or four strides as the body is gathered for the leap and that the trajectory on the takeoff is seldom as high as 45 degrees. The trajectory and distance of travel of the body's center of gravity is determined at the moment of takeoff and, consequently, movements during the flight will add nothing to distance. The objectives during flight are to maintain balance and to so position the body that the feet will land as far forward of the center of gravity as possible without falling backward. A natural running action is continued in the air. This "hitch kick" technique enables the jumper to reach further forward with the feet. The feet should be held above the ground as long as possible (Figure 16.2c).

As the feet approach the ground, the arms are brought forward and the hands reach toward the feet (Figure 16.2d). These actions will place the locus of the center of gravity forward of the hips. When the feet strike the ground, the arms are swung forcefully to the rear and the knees are flexed to absorb the impact of the landing. *The rearward swing of the arms produces a reaction in the opposite direction in the trunk causing it to move forward over the feet.* The angle of the legs to the ground before the feet strike the ground should be approximately 30 degrees. If the jumper falls forward onto the hands after the landing, the feet have not been held off the ground long enough.[3] After the feet have hit the ground, the arms are swung forward and the body bends forward to insure that

Figure 16.2 Sequence drawings of long jump

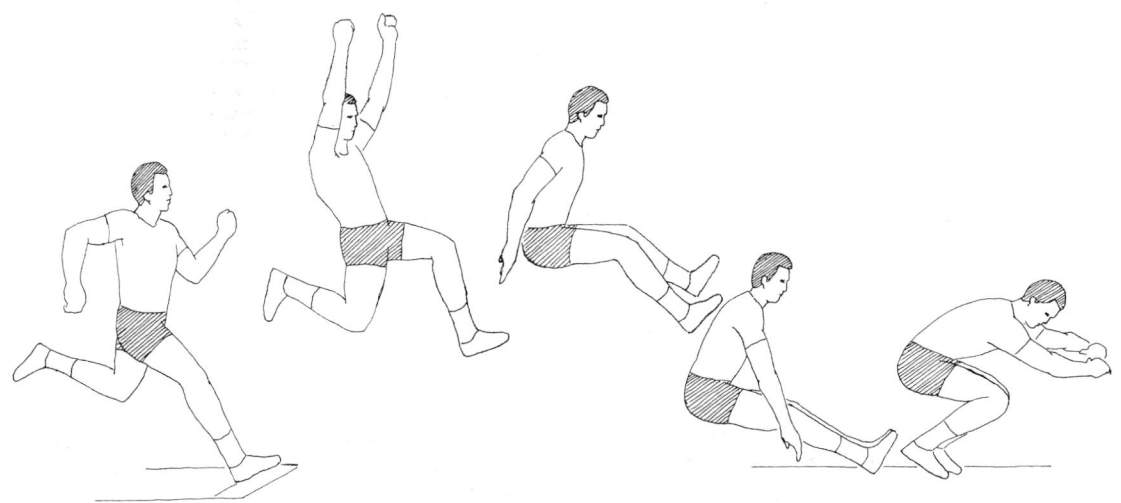

the jumper does not fall backward (Figure 16.2*e*).

Football—Tackling

The objective in tackling is to bring down the ball carrier as quickly as possible and to prevent him from progressing forward after contact has been made. As they approach one another, both the ball carrier and the tackler possess momentum. *The amount of momentum each possess is the product of mass times velocity.* A light tackler can stop a heavier ball carrier if the tackler has sufficient velocity that the product of his mass times his velocity will be greater than the product of the ball carrier's mass times his velocity. If the tackler's momentum is equal to or greater than the ball carrier's momentum, he should make his tackle at the ball carrier's center of gravity and from directly in front. If the tackler's momentum is less than that of the ball carrier, the tackle should be made below the ball carrier's center of gravity and at an angle to his line of motion. This move will permit the ball carrier to advance after contact has been made but he will be brought down.

If it is apparent that the ball carrier is in a position to dodge, the tackler must enhance his equilibrium by lowering his center of gravity, widening his base of support, and taking short steps. These measures will enable him to adjust more quickly to the evasive movements of the ball carrier.

Just before making contact, the tackler should dip under the ball carrier's arm. He should move in close and low to direct maximal force more vertically by maintaining a straight-line relationship between his feet, legs, center of gravity, and point of contact with the ball carrier. This will direct all the muscular force generated along a straight line and in the same direction (summation of forces) and enable the tackler to lift the ball carrier off the ground so that he will be unable to continue securing drive from his legs.

The neck should be stabilized via isometric contraction of the muscles of the neck. The arms pull inward from behind the ball carrier and below his center of gravity. At the moment of contact, the knees and hips are extended in an explosive movement. The feet are separated laterally about one or two feet, and the legs continue to drive with short steps throughout the tackle.

PRECEPTS APPLIED TO THE LEARNER

With knowledge of kinesiologic principles, the participant will understand not only the *how* but also the *why* of prescriptions by the teacher or coach concerning techniques and procedures. Explanations of the precepts by the teacher or coach should be terse and brief since the purpose of physical education classes is to motivate students to move their bodies. However, if students experience success, they are more likely to continue participation in the activity. The authors believe that understanding of these precepts will enhance the probability of success.

The authors further believe the precepts should be presented along with explanations of the techniques. The applicability of each precept to similar skills should be briefly explained as the precept is presented. For example, hip flexion to shorten the radius of rotation occurs at the same point during rotation in both the giant swing on the horizontal bar and the shoulder roll on the parallel bars. The mechanical principles involved in the sidearm throw and the forehand and backhand drives in tennis are basically identical.

On the following pages we have listed a number of precepts we believe can be taught during regular physical education activity classes. Selection of these precepts for inclusion has been necessarily arbitrary. Certain concepts might be taught during the upper elementary years, others during the junior high school years; presentation of still others might best be delayed until senior high school or college years. The precepts or instructions will not be discussed here since each has been thoroughly discussed earlier in the text.

Somatotype and Leanness

1. Body type is an important determinant of success in sports. It is fortunate, since people do vary in body type, that different body-type characteristics are required for a high level of success in different sports. This gives a greater proportion of people an opportunity to become truly outstanding performers. The small and lean are favored in cross-country and marathon running, the tall and thin in basketball and jumping, the big and heavy in football, the short, strong, and lean in gymnastics, etc. It would be well that students who wish to achieve excellence in sports select sports for which they are best adapted.

2. Since the number of fat cells can be delimited through exercise during the growing years and since the number of fat cells determine propensity toward obesity throughout the life span, an exercise regimen is of particular importance during the growing years.

3. The probability of success in athletics is enhanced through increasing body density or decreasing fat.

Structural and Physical Fitness Considerations

1. Good flexibility or range of motion in body joints is an asset in performance of most sports skills.

2. When a muscle is first placed on a stretch, it can contract with greater force.

3. The quality of coordination and timing is decreased as a result of localized and general fatigue. This increases the probability of error in the performance of mo-

tor skills and, consequently, the probability of injury.

4. Performance capacities of females as well as of males in sports can be enhanced as a result of participation in progressive-resistance exercises.

Neural and Physiological Elements

1. When learning skills that require both speed and accuracy, both should be stressed concurrently.

2. Mental rehearsal of motor skills is more effective when the learner has previously physically experienced the motor skill.

Mechanical Elements

1. To initiate rotary motion, as in a somersault or twist, a force must be applied off-center and at an angle to the radius of rotation. The greater the distance from the point of application of force on the radius to the axis of rotation, the more rotational force results per unit of force applied.

2. To initiate translatory motion as in running or jumping, a force of sufficient magnitude to overcome the pull of gravity must be applied at the object's center of gravity.

3. The best angle of projection, as when throwing a ball, varies according to whether the objective is distance, speed, or maximal time in flight.

4. The best angle of projection when distance is the sole objective may range between 37 and 45 degrees depending upon the initial velocity of the projectile and the difference in elevation between the projection and landing points. The higher the landing point with reference to the projection point, the nearer the projection angle should approach 45 degrees.

5. The amount of force that can be generated by muscles and their speed of contraction determines how fast and how far a projectile such as a ball, discus, or javelin can be thrown.

6. A force must be applied to an object to initiate, accelerate, decelerate, stop, or change its direction of motion. The amount of force necessary is dependent upon the momentum of the object and the distance or time over which the force can be applied.

7. Momentum is equal to mass times velocity. It may be transferred from one part of the body to the entire body and may also be transferred from one object to another. Specific applications of this principle to tumbling, gymnastics, striking, kicking, pushing, and other motor skills should be learned by students at the time the skill is presented.

8. Sequential joint actions require that the joints below be stabilized to avoid dissipation of force.

9. Maximum acceleration is achieved most effectively when all available forces are applied sequentially at the proper time and in the desired line of motion with all unnecessary body actions reduced to a minimum.

10. Speed of rotation is accelerated by shortening the radius of rotation and decelerated by lengthening the radius of rotation.

11. The flight path of the center of gravity of the body is determined at the moment of lift-off by the relationship of the center of gravity to the point of application of force and the direction of thrust of the feet.

12. When a circling object is released, it will follow a path at a right angle to the radius of rotation at the moment it was released.

13. Impulse is the product of force and the time over which the force acts. This precept can be taught in connection with braking falls and catching balls.

14. An increase in the time over which kinetic energy is absorbed can help in the prevention of injury.

15. Air resistance increases when footballs or javelins wobble or arrows quiver, decreasing their velocity rapidly and, consequently, the distance they cover.

16. Muscles and their tendons are the first line of defense against trauma to bones and joints.

17. The stronger the muscles whose tendons pass over joints, the less the probability of a sprain or dislocation of these joints.

Actions of Levers

1. External levers can be shortened or lengthened according to the demands of the situation. Where speed of rotation is desired or when a resistance must be overcome (as in lifting a weight), levers should be shortened to decrease the length of the resistance arm. When linear speed is desired as in throwing or kicking, levers should be lengthened.

2. When pushing against or lifting a heavy resistance, all levers utilized should be brought into action simultaneously.

3. The pelvic lever contributes more force than any other lever in all four throwing and striking patterns described in the text.

4. To achieve maximal possible force when throwing or striking, it is necessary to maintain contact with the supporting surface.

Strength, Power, Flexibility, and Agility

1. The greater the range of motion in the shoulders, trunk, hips, and ankles, the more forward propulsion that can be provided when swimming.

2. Competitive swimmers should know that the grab start technique is faster than the conventional arm swing method in the racing start; the experimental standing screw start is faster than the in-water start in the backstroke event, and the one-arm glide technique is faster than the two-arm glide method in both the forward and backward crawl strokes.

3. The abdominal muscles are the most important muscles involved in the maintenance of posture, while those next in importance are the muscles that lift the thoracic cage.

4. When an object is being lifted, it should be kept as close as possible to the body's line of gravity throughout the lift.

5. When lifting, the trunk should be held as nearly vertical as possible.

6. The spine should not be rotated while lifting.

7. Strength resides in muscle fibers while flexibility resides in tendons and ligaments. Consequently, a person can possess great strength and great flexibility at the same time.

8. Development of strength through progressive-resistance exercises by female athletes will not cause them to appear less feminine.

9. Improvement of strength and flexibility will decrease the probability of spraining a joint.

10. Continuous increase in strength can be accomplished only through continuous increase in the amount of resistance provided against muscular contraction.

11. Participation in sports alone will not develop maximal possible levels of physical fitness.

12. There is little difference in the results derived in increased strength and power between isometric and isotonic exercises.

13. Large muscles are detrimental to performance in endurance events.

14. During a maximal muscular effort,

the glottis should be kept open in order to maintain uniform intrathoracic pressure.

15. In conditioning for athletic events that require utilization of explosive power, exercises should be done that exert a sharp pull on the muscles and tendons. The intensity of these exercises should be increased progressively.

16. Agility and quickness can be improved by improving strength when body mass is not excessively increased.

17. Increased range of motion in joints will enable the athlete to exert force against an implement over a greater distance and consequently improve performance.

18. Flexibility is specific to a body joint and in only one direction; that is, a person may have good flexibility in the hip joints and poor flexibility in the shoulder joints and a good range of flexion in the hip joint but poor range of motion in the direction of hyperextension of the hip joint.

Injury Prevention

1. Injury can be prevented by increasing the distance over which force can be brought to bear upon an object to absorb its kinetic energy.

2. Injury can sometimes be prevented by decreasing the length of a lever arm through which an injury-producing force acts.

3. Soft tissues of the human body, such as muscle or fat, possess greater elasticity than bone and, for this reason, injury can sometimes be prevented by turning or twisting to receive an impact upon the buttocks, thighs, or shoulder rather than an area where bone is near the surface.

4. Injury can be prevented by distributing an impact over a greater surface area since there will then be less force per square inch.

5. The incidence of injuries in skiing is greater on wet heavy snow than under ice or powder conditions.

6. Spotters in gymnastics and tumbling should stand as close as possible to the performer whom they are spotting.

Stability

1. Lowering the center of gravity increases stability and thereby may prevent a fall.

2. Stability is increased when the base of support is increased in the direction of an impending force.

3. In vertically segmented bodies, stability is enhanced when the center of gravity of each segment lies in the line of gravity of the entire body or when deviations in one direction are exactly balanced by deviations in the opposite direction. This precept has particular application to posture and to sports acrobatics stunts.

4. The relationship of the line of gravity to the base of support should be such as to facilitate the desired movement—forward, backward, or sideward.

5. Friction between the base of support and the feet will decrease probability of loss of balance.

6. Injury resulting from landing on water can be minimized by entering the water with the body vertical or as nearly vertical as possible, streamlined, and stabilized.

PRECEPTS APPLIED TO THE TEACHER

The precepts that follow are those that teachers of various forms of human movement—physical education teachers, teachers of dance, physical therapists, and coaches—should know, fully understand, and apply daily during their work to become maximally effective. A few of these precepts are specifically directed at teachers or coaches of certain activities. Most, however, are of general applicability. All of the precepts contain implications for the conduct, administration, provision of facilities and equipment, and/or teaching techniques utilized.

Somatotype and Leanness

1. Students low in mesomorphy should not be encouraged to set unrealistic goals in athletic achievement. However, all students, including potentially outstanding athletes, should be encouraged to utilize sports and other physical activities for their recreational benefits.

2. Students who are low in mesomorphy and high in endomorphy or ectomorphy cannot be expected to perform well on tests of motor fitness regardless of their efforts.

3. Body density can be measured through indirect methods such as hydrostatic weighing or measurement of girth of various body segments and skinfold measurement.

4. Persons of the black race have a higher crural index, which presents an advantage in jumping and running, while their higher body density presents a disadvantage in floating and beginning swimming skills.

5. Although various bones of the body ossify at different rates, ossification of all bones is not fully completed until about age 20. This has implications for the selection and conduct of athletic activities for young people, particularly those in their teens.

Neural and Physiologic Considerations

1. The structural integrity and the functional capacity of the central and peripheral nervous system is one determinant of the quality of motor performance.

2. Motor skills are modulated and coordinated by the cerebellum.

3. The all-or-none law acting through the motor unit explains why it is necessary to make muscular contractions of maximal force in order to increase strength and power so important to success in athletic endeavors.

4. Children learn motor skills most effectively when consideration is given to the level of maturation of the child with respect to the specific skill or skills to be taught. These considerations include (*a*) biological elements such as skeletal maturation, neural development, strength and endurance, (*b*) psychological elements, and (*c*) social maturation.

5. The decision whether to utilize the whole or part method of teaching should be based on the maturity of the learner and the complexity of the task.

6. Proficiency in one motor task does not necessarily transfer to a similar skill unless the neuromuscular requirements are directly related.

7. Practice does not inevitably lead to perfection unless the conditions of motivation, use of correct mechanics, and teacher effectiveness are present.

8. The decision whether to utilize massed or distributed practice should be based on the purpose and characteristics of the motor skills to be learned.

9. Motor learning can be facilitated through "feedback" or frequent and accurate knowledge of results.

10. Manual guidance may accelerate learning of motor skills and is most helpful in learning of closed skills, particularly with young learners and older individuals whose reaction time has increased.

11. Continuous-type skills such as cycling, skating, and swimming are easily recalled after long periods of abstinence, whereas discrete skills such as kicking or throwing are not remembered well after long periods of abstinence.

Forces Affecting Motion

1. In skills that involve the action of several body joints, each joint action should be initiated at the point of greatest speed and least acceleration of the preceding joint action. When this is accomplished, physical educators, coaches, and athletes usually say "The athlete's timing or coordination is good."

2. In sports like football, the coach should understand utilization of a parallelogram to compute the resultant direction and velocity of an object acted on by two or more forces.

3. The energy cost of muscular contraction varies with the cube of the speed of contraction.

4. Physical education classes present many opportunities to illustrate Newton's three laws of motion. The implications of these laws for execution of motor skills should be pointed out.

Human Levers

1. The longer the lever, the greater the force required to move the lever.

2. Somatotype has an influence on the effective use of internal levers because of the relative length of limbs and the distribution of weight over the limbs influencing the amount of angular momentum.

Equilibrium

1. Stationary and dynamic balance are uniquely different and each requires specific skills.

2. Upright and inverted balance skills are not necessarily related.

3. Individuals of short stature generally are able to maintain balance more easily than tall persons.

4. Muscular strength aids in balance control.

5. Stability and balance are primarily a matter of aligning the center of gravity over the center of the base of support.

6. Some people with middle ear impairment display superior balance ability.

7. Balance and buoyancy in water are dependent upon the relationship between the locus of the center of gravity and the center of buoyancy.

8. Orthopedic aberrations usually change the locus of the center of gravity and make control of balance more difficult.

9. The greater the body density, the less the buoyancy.

10. Body drag in water is less in females than in males.

11. Hydroplaning is the result of velocity and buoyancy.

Postural Considerations

1. One postural standard should not be applied to all people because of individual variations due to differences in body type, weight distribution, structural anomalies, disease, congenital defects, and injury.

2. Psychological and emotional states influence posture.

3. During the sprint, the feet strike the ground under the center of gravity and the horizontal component of force is as great as possible as a result of the forward inclination of the body.

4. Round shoulders may develop as a result of weak or stretched scapular adductors.

5. Long continued participation in certain sports or occupations may cause postural deviations.

6. Certain sports activities and exercises may be used to correct postural deviations before they become structural.

7. Scoliosis begins as a C curve that usually develops into an S curve.

8. In the fatigue slouch, in which muscles used in maintenance of posture are relaxed and in poor tone, excessive stress is placed upon ligaments, which may become stretched.

9. Lordosis is often associated with kyphosis or round upper back.

10. Students in classes for postural correction need to be highly motivated.

11. Exercise programs for postural correction should progressively increase in intensity and duration.

12. It is possible for students to pass the plumb line test and yet exhibit poor posture.

Physical Fitness

1. When prescribing exercises for physical fitness maintenance and improvement, exercises that may damage the stability and integrity of joints or be harmful to efficient posture should be avoided.

2. Deep breathing exercises are of little value for healthy young people. However, they are advisable for the elderly.

3. When designing physical fitness programs for athletes, development of the specific physical fitness qualities required for success in the athlete's sport should receive primary attention.

4. Static stretching exercises are preferable to ballistic stretching exercises from the standpoint of both effectiveness and avoidance of small muscle tears.

5. Use of videotape can facilitate the teaching/learning process of motor skills by making possible leisurely analysis of performance, self-assessment, and increased motivation.

Prevention of Injury

1. Spearing and use of helmets with nose guards greatly increase the probability of

cervical fracture, severing of the spinal cord, and paralysis.

2. Coaches of ice hockey can contribute substantially to reduction in the incidence of injuries through purchase of the most effective protective equipment and by insisting that players play in a sportsmanlike manner.

3. Physical educators can minimize the incidence of injuries in gymnastics and trampolining by insisting that students learn moves in their progressive order of difficulty and practice proper spotting procedures.

IMPROVING EFFICIENCY AND STYLE OF MOVEMENT THROUGH APPLICATION OF MECHANICAL PRINCIPLES

Force is necessary to cause an object to move, to change the direction of motion of an object, to stop a moving object, and to hold an object in position against the pull of gravity or some other force. In the human body, force is created by the contraction of muscles. The amount of force that can be created via muscular contraction and the speed of muscular contraction, which together make up power, are determined prior to the performance of a neuromuscular skill. The available strength and power cannot be increased during execution of a skill although psychic factors can cause variations in the percentage of the total available strength and power utilized.

The human body in motion, like all other objects, must conform to the laws of gravity and all other laws of nature. Unlike inanimate objects, the human body can change its shape, the length of its external levers, the sequence in which various levers are used, the location of the line of gravity relative to the base of support, the location of the center of gravity relative to various body segments, the velocity of various movements, and the point of application of force against supporting surfaces as well as objects against which force is being applied. Levers can be lengthened and then shortened or vice versa according to the objectives of the movement. When these adjustments and movements are executed in conformity with physical laws, the most efficient movement results. *Efficiency* of a performance is evaluated on the basis of the ratio of the mechanical work accomplished in a period of time to the total energy expended. Since all motor skills are goal oriented, the *effectiveness* of a movement is determined by the degree to which the goal has been achieved. The difficulty of the goal may range from the first efforts of a baby to walk to a world record in the pole vault. The effectiveness of a movement, or whether the goal is achieved, is dependent not only on the efficiency of movement but also upon the difficulty of the goal, length of body levers, body type, speed of neural transmissions, quality of the central nervous system, viscosity of muscle, appropriateness of body mass and height to the task, and other genetically determined variables.

Achievement of the goal is also dependent upon such qualities of motor fitness as strength, power, range of motion (flexibility), endurance, static and/or dynamic balance, and agility. Development of these qualities and their relationship to level of performance in sports has been thoroughly discussed throughout the text.

A substantial proportion of the research completed in physical education and movement-related fields has investigated the relative efficiency of different procedures for execution of various skills. Such questions as the following have been researched: Is the grab start faster than the standard start in swimming? Is more height secured with a backward or with a forward throw of the arms in the running front somersault? Can greater distances be achieved in the shot put by executing a half turn during movement across the circle? All of these are studies of the efficiency of movement.

Athletes, physical educators, coaches, and others in allied movement fields continuously analyze the efficiency of movement. In analyzing a skill, the total movement may be broken down into its parts to determine the nature of the total movement and to determine the proportions, functions, and relationships of the several parts. An analysis may be made of the various movement variables as interacting factors that produce movements and changes in movement. This type of analysis is known as *kinetic* analysis. An analysis in which the movement variables are observed and described is called a *kinematic* analysis. Kinematic or descriptive analysis may be of two types: (1) *qualitative*, in which the components are identified and named and in which the relative excellence of the movement is evaluated, and (2) *quantitative*, which deals with the determination of the amount of the various components of a thing. A qualitative analysis can be further divided into nominal and evaluative types.

In a nominal analysis the movements of the several body parts are identified and named. In an evaluative analysis, on the other hand, the objective is to rank or order the several components. In the judging of diving, synchronized swimming, and figure skating, evaluative comparisons are made. Quantitative analyses can also be made as in determining the time on a 100-yard dash, the distance on a running broad jump, or the height on a pole vault. In these events performance is counted or measured.

A mechanical analysis may be made either *deductively* or *inductively*. A deductive analysis proceeds from the known to the unknown, from the general to the specific, or from known laws of motion to a logical conclusion. For example, we know that shortening the radius of rotation will accelerate the speed of rotation; therefore, we know that a diver who tucks tightly is more likely to complete an inward two-and-one-half somersault than one who does not tuck tightly.

Inductive analysis proceeds from individual cases to general conclusions. It could be noted that all champion shot putters have certain common movement patterns. The conclusion could be reached that these movement patterns are essential to success. Further analysis could show that these patterns are in conformity with physical laws. After they are verified through research procedures as being essential for maximal performance, they will be accepted as valid kinesiological principles and can then be used for deductive analysis of shot putting mechanics.

We will now proceed to illustrate how efficiency and style of movement can be improved through the application of mechanical principles.

Back Handspring from a Stand

The immediate objective of a back handspring is to move backward from a standing position through a handstand and back to the standing position with a minimal expenditure of energy and in good form. The ultimate objective is to be able to do a series of back handsprings with increasing velocity and, consequently, sufficient momentum to enable the gymnast to execute a backward somersault, somersaults with multiple twists, or double somersaults.

Gravity is utilized to initiate the backward movement of the body by sitting backward with the lower legs and trunk held in a vertical position. This will place the center of gravity behind the feet. During the sit back, the arms are swung backward in an extended position as far backward as shoulder flexibility will allow. This action increases the distance through which the arms can accelerate as they next swing forward to generate greater momentum. During this action, the head should be held erect. *The momentum generated by the arms during their forward* swing is transferred to the trunk when they reach the end of their range of motion to cause it to rotate around its center of gravity at the hips. As the arms pass the head in their forward-upward-backward swing, the head is thrown backward to add its momentum to that of the arms. If the lower legs and trunk have been held in a vertical position during the sit-back, the thrust of the hips during their hyperextension will be directly upward. The upward-backward moving body will pull the feet off the mat. (The gymnast should not spring from the feet.) As the body passes through the handstand position, at which time the shoulders should be directly over the hands with the arms vertical, the hips should be vigorously flexed and the shoulders extended to bring the feet forcefully to the mat with sufficient momentum to move the body easily into the succeeding back handspring or back somersault.

If the succeeding move is to be another back handspring, the center of gravity must be moved backward in a horizontal direction and rebound from the feet must be minimized. To accomplish this, the knees are flexed somewhat when the feet contact the mat to absorb impact and the feet are brought closer to the hands to facilitate rearward movement of the center of gravity. Additionally, the feet remain in contact with the mat for a longer period, that is, until after the sit-back.

If the succeeding move is to be a back somersault, somersault with one or more twists, or a double back somersault, the feet must strike the mat with greater force and further from the hands to facilitate "blocking action." In the "blocking action," the legs form a more acute angle with the floor after the feet contact the mat; that is, the hips are forward of the feet at this moment. The lift-off is in a vertical direction and with maximal force in order to secure maximal height, which will permit more time for rotation. With the hips forward of the feet and the legs

angled forward, it may appear that the lift-off will be forward of the vertical. It must be remembered, however, that the body still possesses backward momentum and its center of gravity is moving backward as the feet are leaving the mat.

In the following paragraphs we will explain what will happen if the principles explained are not observed to illustrate detrimental effects upon the efficiency and style of the execution. If, in the back handspring, either the lower legs or trunk, or both, are angled forward during the sit-back, the center of gravity will not be moved backward an adequate amount to establish backward movement, and when the hips are hyperextended, the thrust will be forward-upward rather than directly upward.

If the arms are not swung sufficiently far rearward during the sit-back, the distance through which they can accelerate to develop speed and momentum will be decreased and the handspring will not be as fast. *If the elbows are flexed as the arms are swung forward-upward, the linear speed of the hands and forearms will be decreased, decreasing the momentum generated through the arm swing so that less rotational force is imparted to the trunk.* If the head is thrown backward too soon, its momentum, which is considerable due to its weight and the fact that it is on the end of the lever (the trunk) giving a long moment arm, will not be added to that of the arms. Additionally, a too early backward movement of the head will cause the hands to land too close to the feet. Failure to move the head backward may result in insufficient momentum being transferred to the trunk.

If the backward swing of the arms beyond the head is checked too soon before the shoulders have reached the limits of their range of motion or before the arms are in line with the trunk, the gymnast will land on the hands in the handstand with shoulders forward of the hands and the arms angled forward rather than in a vertical position. This will result in inadequate rebound from the hands, an unbalanced position through the handstand, and decreased effectiveness in the snap-down. See page 328 for illustrations of back handspring sequences.

The preceding description of the mechanics of a back handspring illustrates application of mechanical principles to improve efficiency and style of movement. Instructors involved in teaching movement skills should utilize analyses such as the preceding to improve teaching effectiveness. In the following paragraphs we will follow the same procedures in analyzing the sprint start.

Sprint Start

The objective in the sprint start is to overcome standing inertia and to achieve maximal forward speed as quickly as possible. All three of Newton's laws are easily demonstrable in this skill. The first law states that *every body continues in a state of rest or uniform motion in a straight line unless external forces are applied.* The second law states that *the acceleration of a body is proportional to the force causing it.* The third law states that *for every action or force there is an equal and opposite reaction.*

On the signal "Get on your mark," the runner comes to position on the track with the feet in the starting blocks, one knee on the track and both hands just behind the starting line and parallel to one another. Starting blocks are made advisable by Newton's third law. The feet must have a firm surface against which to act. If some of the force generated by the extensor muscles of the runner's legs is absorbed because the starting blocks are not firmly planted and slide, the start will not be as explosive as it would otherwise be. The action is the thrust of the runner's legs backward while the reaction is the forward push of the blocks against the runner's feet. If the blocks are solidly implanted, action and reaction are equal and in opposite directions.

Starting blocks determine the width of the stance; however, when they are not used, the feet should be placed at such a width that the thrust is directly forward and not such that the lines of force from each leg intersect so that some of the force is dissipated. This implies that the feet be placed no more than shoulder width apart.

The distance between the hands and feet should be such that in the "Get set" position. there is the smallest possible angle between the horizontal and a line connecting the center of gravity of the body with a point on the ground midway between the feet without minimizing the thrust possible from the legs.

In the "Get set" position, the angles at the knee and hip joints should be such that the greatest possible force is exerted over the longest possible distance in the shortest time in the forward direction. There is general agreement that the angle at the forward knee should be about 90 degrees. The greater the strength of the legs, the smaller these angles may be. A smaller angle will make possible thrust through a greater distance. However, many other variables such as experience of the athlete, type of starting block, track surface, and body structure will influence both the optimal distance between the hands and feet and the angles at the hip and knee joints.

On the "Get set" signal, the knee is raised off the ground, the hips are elevated above the shoulders to a point where the line from the hips to the shoulders forms an angle of 25 to 30 degrees with the horizontal, and the center of gravity is shifted forward toward the hands. This position will *place the line of gravity near the forward edge of the base of support so that when the starting gun is fired, the force of gravity is utilized to get the runner underway.* This position will also permit maximum thrust in a horizontal direction since the body, after extension of the hip and knee joints, will be at a fairly acute angle to the ground. The eyes should be focused about three feet in advance of the starting line. This will maintain the head in line with the spinal column so that all body segments are in the line of thrust from the legs and hips. If the runner looks down the track toward the finish line, the head will not be in this line.

The runner should concentrate on reacting to the gun. When the gun is fired, the hands are lifted from the track and the rear foot and then the forward foot explode against the starting blocks. The arm opposite the rear foot is swung forward with great force with the elbow flexed while the other arm, also with the elbow flexed, is swung rearward with equal force. The action of the arms counters the action of the legs in causing the body to rotate around its vertical axis and insures that the frontal plane of the body is perpendicular to the direction of movement. This is an illustration of the principle that *the momentum of a part* (the arms) *is transferred to the whole* (the body).

Since *acceleration is proportional to the force producing it and can only occur when force is being applied, the runner should take relatively short strides and gradually increase the stride* until top speed is attained. The knees should be lifted high and the feet should be pulled backward rather than pounded into the ground. As the runner gains speed, a more erect position can be assumed and the length of the stride can be increased. A high knee lift and knee flexion *shortens the radius of rotation of the leg and thereby accelerates the speed of rotation of the leg* to hasten its return to the forward position and delivery of a new thrust. Even at top speed, the sprinter's body should be angled 20 degrees forward of the vertical to overcome air resistance and to keep the center of gravity forward of the base of support. If the center of gravity is behind the foot as it contacts the ground, there is a braking action imparted to the body. Full speed is reached in 30 to 45 feet. As speed increases, the stride lengthens. Speed is increased by lengthening

the stride through application of greater force against the ground rather than by taking more steps in a unit of time. The runner must eliminate any weaving of the body down the track to insure that all the force is directed in a straight line down the track. See page 432 for illustration of sprint start.

In the preceding paragraphs, we have illustrated application of mechanical principles to improvement of efficiency in the sprint start. People involved in executing and teaching human movement skills of all types could and should utilize this method for all skills.

PROGRESSIVE SKILL LEARNING THROUGH THE APPLICATION OF SCIENTIFIC CONCEPTS

It has long been an accepted practice in all areas of education to present information in its progressive order of difficulty. This axiom is no less applicable to that area of education concerned with the teaching of motor skills. A commonly used expression of this axiom is: "One should learn to walk before he runs." In this section we will review the scientific concepts presented earlier, principally in Chapter 4, which have implications for progressive skill learning.

Learning of all new motor skills occurs in the cerebral cortex. However, as the skill is mastered as a result of correct practice, the cerebral cortex gradually relinquishes control to lower brain levels. Nevertheless, it continues to monitor the total response and imposes modifications in force, direction, and time of movement as dictated by varying external circumstances. For example, when catching a ball, vision provides clues regarding the direction and velocity of the ball that the catcher's cerebral cortex processes to provide instructions to muscles as to where to position the various body segments as well as the entire body. Sometimes, due to the sun, background, or lack of adequate reference points as the ball approaches, visual clues are inadequate or distorted, resulting in the player completely missing the ball or, at best, only getting his gloved hand in front of the ball. As the ball impacts the gloved hand, the Pacinian corpuscles in the hand inform the cerebral cortex of the amount of pressure. The cerebral cortex interprets this as force and computes the amount of counterforce the muscles involved in this act must generate during their eccentric contraction as they absorb the impact. The Ruffini's corpuscles in the joints inform of the movements around the joints and of the joint positions. The cerebral cortex then provides instructions to the muscles as to where to position the various body segments to absorb the momentum of the ball most effectively.

Inner ear receptors in the labyrinth, the vestibular receptors, and the righting reflexes all provide clues as well as reflex corrections to help the player maintain balance as the catch is made. Golgi tendon organs inform of the tension within the tendon and muscle so that corrections can be made if the tension is excessive and thereby prevent injury produced by excessive strains on the tendons or muscles. In some sports activities, the athlete must learn to inhibit or to ignore, to a degree, the stimuli emanating from the Golgi tendon organs in order to make a greater effort. This probably occurs in such activities as shot putting, some instances in wrestling, the crucifix on the rings, weight lifting, and wrist or arm wrestling. It is commonly observed in arm wrestling that the arm suddenly gives way to the opposing force. It is likely that this is due to the inhibitory action upon the force of muscular contraction of the Golgi tendon organs.

The cerebral cortex stores memories of successful and unsuccessful motor skill efforts and selects from these memories patterns of force, direction, velocity, balance, pressure, tension, and joint position and movement that are most likely to lead to success. The cortex receives a large number of messages, which it interprets and transmits to the cerebellum and the brain stem. The learning of complex motor skills is little different from any other kind of learning.

The learning of many motor skills is complex. For this reason and in order that the learner experience as great a frequency of successful efforts as possible, *the presentation of motor skills in teaching-learning situations should proceed progressively from the simple toward the more complex.* Further, *motor skills should not be presented until the learner's state of physiological maturation has progressed to a level at which he is ready to learn the skill.* An example of this precept is provided in catching balls. The development of neuromuscular control does not, on the average, progress sufficiently rapidly in the area of hand–eye coordination to make it advisable to introduce catching balls and other objects prior to age five. Therefore, in kindergarten and first and second grade, students should be taught to catch large, brightly colored fleece balls. The size of the ball can be progressively decreased through grade four. After age ten, the velocity of the ball can be progressively increased and a greater variation in direction can be introduced.

Throughout this process, the cerebral cortex will accumulate a greater store of memories of correct and incorrect adjustments. Information from the Pacinian and Ruffini corpuscles, the labyrinth, and Golgi tendon organs will become interpreted and integrated with increasing accuracy. With each experience in catching a ball, the student's neuromuscular system will become increasingly prepared to meet the challenge of a more difficult catch and to improve the odds of executing the skill successfully. Obviously, we always work with the whole child and must be concerned with self-image and social relationships as well as with physiological and anatomical considerations and skill learning. Skill learnings are really only means to an end and not ends in themselves in an educational setting. For this reason, physical educators and others involved in teaching children motor skills have a moral obligation to study the scientific concepts concerned with progressive skill learning.

SUMMARY

Internal mechanics refers to the study of mechanics within the body such as the angle of pull of muscles, relative lengths of internal force and resistance arms, stress resistances of body tissues, range of motion of joints, and internal friction. These are all legitimate areas of study in kinesiology since they provide answers to such questions as why some people perform certain movement skills better than others, how much force is required to fracture bones, and what the factors are that limit performance. A study of internal mechanics also provides a rationale for improvement of qualities of motor fitness such as flexibility, strength, power, speed, and agility.

External mechanics refers to forces, leverage, and positions outside the body. A great number of articles, textbooks, and research studies have been published that explain the external mechanics of execution of a large variety of athletic skills.

When constructing a kinesiologic analysis of motor skills, it is necessary to describe the starting position, execution of the movement, and the final position. All relevant principles of external mechanics must be taken into consideration. An analysis of the starting position must take into consideration the objective of the movement to follow, external forces that might bear upon the body, stability, and the need to move in any one of several directions. Illustrations of application of these principles from racing starts in track and swimming, offensive and defensive lineman positions in football, tumbling, tennis,

boxing, pitching, and weight lifting were presented.

In making a kinesiologic analysis of the execution of motor skills, a determination of the objective of the movement is the first consideration. Kinesiologic principles are then used to help accomplish the objective. Secondary influences upon the performance such as wind, actions of opponents, etc., should next be considered. Detailed kinesiologic analyses of the volleyball spike, long jump, and football tackle were developed to provide illustrations of the process.

Teachers of movement skills can improve their effectiveness by incorporating brief explanations of kinesiologic principles relevant to the particular skills they are teaching. Additionally, teachers are urged to explain briefly the applicability of specific kinesiologic principles to skills related to the one being taught. Kinesiologic precepts, an understanding of which will facilitate the learning of a variety of motor skills, were presented. These precepts can be taught at various times throughout the 12 years of public school education and in college physical education classes at the time motor skills are being presented in which these precepts are utilized.

A number of kinesiologic precepts of concern to teachers of various forms of human movement were presented. Knowledge, understanding, and application of these precepts will enable teachers and administrators of various kinds of movement programs to serve their clientele more effectively. Athletes can be given advice that will improve their performance; the incidence of injuries can be decreased; students can be guided into activities in which they are most likely to experience success; the learning process can be accelerated; the implications of structural differences for performance levels in various activities will be better understood, thereby facilitating establishment of more realistic goals for individual students. A knowledge of kinesiologic principles will also enable the teacher to detect postural deviations and to present exercises and activities that can alleviate these conditions.

Techniques for improving the efficiency and style of movement were next discussed. Efficiency was defined as the ratio of the mechanical work accomplished in a period of time to the total energy expended. Effectiveness was defined as the degree to which the goal has been achieved. Mechanical analyses may also be either deductive or inductive. Examples of mechanical analysis of the back handspring from a stand and of the sprint start were provided.

In the closing pages of this summarizing chapter, we have presented the case for progressive skill learning. Justification was presented primarily from a neural stand-point, in view of the fact that all feedback information provided by Ruffini's and Pacinian corpuscles, Golgi tendon organs, visual clues, the labyrinth, game situations, memories of past experiences, and game rules must be processed by the cerebral cortex.

The more one studies the moving human body, the more one is fascinated by the miracle of human movement.

REFERENCES

1. Bunn, John W., *Scientific Principles of Coaching*, 2nd ed. Englewood Cliffs, N.J.: Prentice-Hall, 1972, p. 132.

2. Weingartner, Jay E., "A Comparison of the Sprint Start and a Stand-up Start in Broad Jumping," Masters thesis, Springfield College, 1965.

3. Parker, Virginia, and Kennedy, Robert, *Track and Field for Girls and Women*, Saunders Physical Activities Series. Philadelphia: W. B. Saunders, 1969, p. 104.

GLOSSARY

Acceleration. The time rate of change in velocity.

Action Potential. The electrical changes that occur in a muscle as determined by electromyography.

Actin. A protein of the muscle's myofibril, localized in the I band and acting with myosin particles; responsible for contraction and relaxation of muscle.

Aerobic. Muscular work that requires the presence of oxygen such as running a two-mile event.

Agility. A component of neuromuscular control that refers to the ability of the individual to change body direction and position efficiently.

Agonist. A muscle(s) primarily responsible for a movement.

All-or-None-Law. A single nerve fiber or a motor unit responds maximally to a stimulus if it is of sufficient intensity, or not at all if it is of insufficient intensity.

Amphiarthrosis. A slightly movable joint.

Anaerobic. Muscular work that does not require the presence of oxygen such as running the 50-yard dash.

Anatomical Position. Standing position in an erect posture with feet together, arms at the side, and the thumbs pointing away from the body.

Angle of Incidence. The angle of approach before a ball strikes a surface.

Angle of Pull. The angle formed between the muscle's line of pull and the long axis of the bone being moved.

Angle of Reflection. The line of flight of an object after rebounding from a surface.

Angular Motion. Movement around an axis; also called rotary motion.

Anthroposcopy. The description of physical variations in the human body by inspection as opposed to exact measurements.

Appendicular Skeleton. That part of the skeleton composed of the upper and lower limbs.

Applied Anatomy. A part of kinesiology that deals with locomotion, primarily from the point of view of the human organism's musculoskeletal system.

Archimedes' Principle. The principle that states that a body immersed in a fluid is buoyed up by a force (buoyant force) equal to the weight of the fluid displaced by the body.

Arthrodia. A form of a joint permitting a gliding movement.

Articulation. The junction of two or more bones.

Axial Skeleton. That part of the skeleton composed of the vertebral column, skull, hyoid bone, ribs, and sternum.

Ballistic Movement. A movement initiated by muscular contraction and then continued as a result of momentum or the pull of gravity.

Bernoulli's Principle. The pressure of a fluid is decreased when the velocity is increased; and inversely the pressure is increased when a lower velocity is created.

Biarticular. Muscles that cross two joints.

Biokinetics. The study and analysis of loco-motion applied to living organisms.

Biomechanics. The science dealing with the mechanics of living organisms.

Body Density. Quality of compactness; mass per unit volume.

Buoyancy. Degree of power to float or rise in a liquid.

Center of Buoyancy. A point in the body about which the buoyant forces acting on an object in water are balanced.

Center of Gravity. A point in an object about which it balances, or a location at which the weight of the body is concentrated.

Centrifugal Force. The force moving or directed outward from the center (opposed to centripetal). A "pulling out" force.

Centripetal Force. The force acting upon a body moving along a curved path that is directed toward the center of the path. A "pulling in" force.

Cervical Vertebrae. The first seven vertebrae of the spinal column.

Circular Motion. A type of angular motion in which a part or whole object moves in an arc or curvilinear path around an axis of rotation.

Closed Motor Skill. A motor task in which the environment of the activity does not change, such as bowling.

Concentric Contraction. A force generated by muscles resulting in a shortening contraction.

Concurrent Force. Sum of forces that act or meet at a point.

Conditioned Reflex. A learned form of response to a stimulus.

Conservation of Angular Momentum. The total angular momentum of a system remains constant unless an external torque acts upon it; also known as Newton's First Law.

Conservation of Energy. The principle that in a system that does not undergo any force from outside the system, the amount of energy is constant, irrespective of its changes in form.

Conservation of Linear Momentum. The principle that the linear momentum of a system has a constant magnitude and direction, if the system is not subjected to an external force.

Continuous Motor Skill. A motor skill without a specific beginning or end, such as running.

Contourogram. A drawing or outline of a series of figures in action.

Contralateral Muscle. Muscle acting in unison with a similar part on the opposite side of the body.

Curvilinear Motion. The movement of an object moving in a curved path.

Cyclo-cross Racing. A type of bicycle road race in which the course is routed through woods, streams, and remote paths that force the riders to carry their bicycles on their backs at certain junctions.

Deceleration. A decrease in velocity.

Deductive Analysis. A logical process in which a conclusion drawn from a set of premises contains no more information than the premises taken collectively.

Diarthrosis. A freely movable joint articulation.

Discrete Motor Skill. A motor task that has a specific beginning and end, such as a softball throw.

Displacement. The distance and direction of movement.

Dorsal Flexion. Moving the top of the foot toward the anterior portion of the lower leg.

Dynamometer. A mechanical instrument used to measure muscular strength.

Eccentric Contraction. A type of muscular contraction that occurs in controlled lengthening tension such as the action of the biceps brachii in the lowering phase of a pull-up exercise.

Ectomorphy. A component of physique denoting linearity, fragility, and delicacy of structure; a third component of a somato-type number.

Elasticity. The property of a substance that enables its length, volume, or shape to change in response to a force effecting such a change, and then to recover its original form upon removal of the force.

Electrogoniometer. An electronic instrument for measuring angular positions of body joints such as arms, legs, and trunk while in motion.

Electromyography. A procedure for the study of muscular contraction utilizing measurement of the electrical discharges of muscles when contracting to identify the muscles used in execution of a movement.

Enarthrosis. A ball-and-socket joint, such as the hip joint.

Endomorphy. A component of physique denoting the presence of excessive fatness, softness, and roundness of the body; the first component of somatotype.

Energy. The capacity to do work.

Equilibrium. A state of balance due to the equal action of opposing forces.

External Mechanical Analysis. A term used to examine and analyze the appropriate kinematics and kinetics, laws, and motion principles outside the body.

External Work. The product of a force and the distance through which the force is applied, expressed by the formula $f \times d$ (force times distance).

Fine Motor Skill. A term used to describe delicate or precise movements of the body requiring sensitive neuromuscular coordination such as handwriting or dart throwing.

Flexibility. The range of motion in a single joint or a series of joints.

Flexometer. A circular mechanical instrument that operates on the gravity principle to measure flexibility.

Force. Energy or power that originates, accelerates, or arrests motion.

Force Arm. Part of a lever that represents the perpendicular distance between the line of force application and the axis of the lever.

Force Platform. An electronic instrument designed to measure the magnitude and direction of force patterns generated by a performer from the ground.

Friction. The resistance of a surface to relative motion, such as sliding or rolling of a surface of one body against that of another.

Frontal Plane. A line passing through the body vertically from side to side dividing it into two equal but not symmetrical halves, anterior and posterior.

Ginglymus. A hinged body joint.

Glycogen. A carbohydrate stored in the liver where it is converted as the system requires into sugar (glucose).

Goniometer. A mechanical instrument for measuring the range of joint motion.

Gravity. The force of attraction by which bodies tend to fall toward the center of the earth.

Gross Motor Skill. A term used to describe big muscle activity that requires full body motion, such as jumping, running, and throwing skills.

Homeostasis. The maintenance of equilibrium, or constant conditions in the internal environment of the body.

Horizontal Axis. A lateral axis passing horizontally from one side to the other side of the body at right angles to the sagittal plane (sagittal-horizontal), or at right angles to the frontal plane (frontal-horizontal).

Hydroplaning. A body position in swimming that permits skimming over the water with head and shoulders in an elevated position.

Hyperextension. Extension of a body limb or part beyond the straight position.

Hypertonic. Exceeding the normal muscular tone.

Hypertrophy. An increase in muscle

strength that may be due to greater amounts of protein concentration as well as increased packing density of contractile elements within the muscle cell.

Impulse. The product of the force acting upon a body and the time during which it acts, equivalent to the changes in the momentum of the body produced by such a force.

In vivo. Occurring in the body.

In vitro. Occurring outside the body.

Inductive Analysis. A logical process in which a conclusion is proposed that contains more information than the observations or experience on which it is based.

Inertia. The property of matter by which it retains its state of rest or its velocity so long as it is not acted upon by an external force.

Internal Mechanical Analysis. A term used to indicate the application of mechanics to internal body actions with a primary focus on the musculoskeletal system.

Internal Work. Contraction of muscle(s) without producing motion but consuming energy.

Interneuron. A neuron in a chain of neurons, situated between the primary sensory neuron and the motor neuron.

Ipsilateral Muscle. Muscle situated on, pertaining to, or affecting the same side, as opposed to contralateral muscle.

Isometric Contraction. The development of muscular force without a change in length of muscles and no skeletal movement.

Isotonic Contraction. A dynamic form of concentric or eccentric contractile muscle movement.

Joule. A meter-kilogram-second unit of work or energy equal to the work done by a force of one newton when its point of application moves through a distance of one meter in the direction of the force. Also called a Newton-meter.

Kinesiology. The science of movement composed of applied anatomy, neuromuscular physiology, and mechanics.

Kinesthesia. A position sense; an awareness of position and movements of body segments or the whole body as a unit.

Kinematics. A branch of mechanics that deals with the description of bodies in motion without concern to the causes of an object in motion.

Kinetics. The study of forces that analyzes the causes and production of motion.

Kinetic Chain. A sequential combination of several successively moving joints, such as in throwing a ball, in which the action of the shoulder joint, elbow joint, wrist joint, and, finally, joints of the fingers act in series.

Kinetic Energy. The energy of a body or a system with respect to motion of the body or of the particles in the system.

Lever. A simple machine consisting of a straight or curved bar that rotates around a pivot or fixed axis.

Ligaments. A band of fibrous tissue that connects bones or cartilage serving to support and strengthen joints.

Line of Gravity. An imaginary vertical line that passes through the center of gravity.

Linear Acceleration. The time rate of change in linear velocity.

Linear Force. A force that pulls or pushes along a straight line.

Linear Motion. Motion in a straight line.

Linkage System. Body joint linkage from large joints found in the trunk continued to the small articulations of the fingers or toes.

Lordosis. An exaggerated inward or concave curvature of the lumbar spine.

Ludotheraphy. Therapeutic modality of treatment by games.

Lumbar Vertebrae. The five vertebrae of the spinal column between the thoracic and sacral segments.

Manual Guidance. Leading or directing the learner by assisting and guiding the whole body or limbs in a motor skill.

Mass. The amount of a body's matter expressed as weight divided by the acceleration of gravity.

Mechanical Advantage. The ratio of the output force doing the work of a mechanism to the input force of the machine.

Mechanics. The study that deals with the actions of forces on bodies and with motion, comprised of kinetics, statics, and kinematics.

Mesomorphy. A component of physique denoting prominent musculature with broad shoulders and narrow hips; the second component of somatotype.

Mitochondria. Cellular structure found in the cytoplasm of cells; in muscle, mitochondria are associated with myofibrils and serve as principal sites in the generation of energy.

Moment Arm. The distance from the point of application of force to the axis of rotation.

Moment of Inertia. The sum of the products of the mass and the square of the perpendicular distance from the line of force to the axis of rotation of each particle in a body rotating about an axis.

Momentum. The mass of a body multiplied by its linear velocity.

Morphological Change. Changes that occur in the form and structure of organisms, as distinguished from consideration of function.

Motor Ability. The ability to perform motor skills.

Motor End-plate. Myoneural junction where the motor nerve fiber makes functional contact with the muscle cell.

Motor Neuron. Neurons that conduct impulses from the central nervous system to the muscles and other effectors.

Motor Unit. A group of muscle fibers and the single motor nerve that innervates these muscle fibers.

Movement Time. Refers to the period from the beginning of the response to the completion of a specified movement.

Multijoint Muscle. Muscles that pass over or affect movement at more than one joint.

Muscle Amplitude. The total range or extent of a muscle's change in length from a fully stretched to a maximally contracted state.

Muscle Fiber. A threadlike structure that contains the contractile elements called actin and myosin.

Muscular Atrophy. Diminution or wasting away of size and function of muscular tissue.

Myosin. A protein substance (68 percent in muscle) occurring in the A band for the contraction and relaxation of muscle.

Myotatic Reflex. A muscle spindle reflex, also called a stretch reflex, that by its stretching effect, excites a muscle spindle to contract automatically.

Negative Work. Work done by a muscle that is eccentrically contracting while lengthening.

Neuron. A complete nerve cell including the cell body, axon, and dendrites; specializes as a conductor of impulses.

Newton's Laws. Classic laws in mechanics, which include the law of inertia, law of acceleration, and law of action and reaction.

Oblique Axis. A diagonal line passing at right angles to the oblique plane of motion.

Ontogenetic Activities. Motor skills such as manipulating objects, swimming, bicycling, and skating that rely upon training and practice.

Open Skill. A motor skill in which the environment of the activity is constantly changing, such as badminton.

Opposition. A unique characteristic of the thumb (carpometacarpal) joint, which allows the tip of the thumb to be brought forward to the tip of each finger.

Osteoporosis. A bone disorder characterized by the loss of total bone mass.

Oxygen Debt. A physiologic condition that arises when the intensity of the exercise is such that the need for oxygen exceeds the supply.

Parabolic Flight Path. Motion that follows a curved path that is an equal distance from a given point and a given line.

Parallel Forces. Forces that lie parallel and in the same plane to each other but do not act on the same action line.

Parallelogram of Forces. A vector analysis in which two sides and a diagonal represent two forces acting on a body and their resultant force.

Pendulum. A body suspended from a fixed point so as to move to and fro by the action of gravity and acquired momentum.

Peripheral Nervous System. That part of the nervous system that consists of (1) the cranial nerves, (2) the spinal nerves, and (3) the sympathetic nervous system.

Phylogenetic Activities. Motor skills, such as grasping, reaching, turning, crawling, that appear to proceed according to maturation.

Plantar Flexion. Movement of the sole of the foot toward the ground.

Point-and-Line Technique. A film analysis procedure using line drawings to identify anatomic landmarks and body segments.

Poppelreuter's Law. The hypothesis that advocates that accuracy is gained more effectively at a low rate of speed and that accuracy obtained at low rates is sustained when speed is increased.

Positive Work. Work accomplished by muscles used concentrically against gravity, such as walking uphill.

Potential Energy. The power possessed by a body at rest by virtue of its position, such as the potential energy of a suspended weight.

Power. Work done or energy transferred per unit of time; the time rate of doing work.

Pronation. The turning of the palm of the hand inward.

Proprioception. A sensory feedback mechanism that provides information about the relative activity of muscles, joints and tendons; frequently used as a synonym for kinesthesis.

Ptosis. Sagging abdominal wall resulting in protrusion of the abdomen.

Qualitative Analysis. The analysis and evaluation of a movement or motor skill by identifying the components as a whole, such as viewing film or television action.

Quantitative Analysis. The examination and study of movement by determining precise and exact numerical motion components.

Reaction Time. The period from stimulus to the beginning of the response.

Reciprocal Innervation. A reflex mechanism that provides the neuromuscular coordination between the agonistic and antagonistic muscles. The antagonistic muscles relax while the agonists contract.

Rectilinear Motion. A form of translatory motion whereby an object moves linearly as a whole.

Red Fibers. Slow-twitch muscle fibers capable of sustaining long-term endurance-type activity.

Reflex Movement. The sum total of any particular involuntary activity.

Resistance Arm. The perpendicular distance between the fulcrum and the line of resistance force.

Resolution of Forces. The process of separating one force of a given magnitude and direction into two elements.

Resultant of Forces. Determining the resultant forces of two or more forces (vectors) acting at one point.

Sagittal Plane. A line passing through the body from front to back dividing it vertically into two symmetrical halves, right and left.

Salto. Forward or backward somersault; a turning movement in the air from feet to feet in the sagittal plane around a horizontal axis.

Scalar Quantity. A quantity possessing only magnitude.

Scoliosis. An excessive lateral deviation of the spinal column.

Sensory Neuron. Neurons that conduct impulses from the periphery to the central nervous system.

Sine. The ratio of the side of the triangle opposite a given angle to the hypotenuse.

Somatic. Pertaining to the body.

Somatotype. A particular category of body build, determined on the basis of certain physical characteristics.

Specific Gravity. The ratio of density of a substance to the density of some other substance taken as a standard, water being the standard for liquids and solids.

Stance. The posture or initial position at the beginning of a movement pattern in a motor or sport skill.

Static Stretching Exercise. A method of holding a stretch position without movement; also known as a nonballistic exercise.

Statics. The analysis of forces acting on bodies at rest or at equilibrium, relative to some given state of reference.

Supination. The opposite of pronation, turning the palm of the hand outward.

Synapse. The point at which an impulse passes from an axon of one neuron to the dendrites or to the body of another.

Synarthrosis. A joint articulation in which the bones are immovable, such as the sutures of the skull.

Temporal Data. Deals with timing or rhythm of human performance.

Tendon. A band of dense fibrous tissue forming the termination of a muscle and attaching the latter to a bone.

Tensiometer. A mechanical apparatus used to measure the tensile strength of a muscle.

Tetanus. A fusion of rapid successive stimuli to a muscle.

Tuberosity. An elevation or protuberance on a bone.

Thoracic Vertebrae. Twelve vertebrae between the cervical and lumbar segments.

Tonus. A quality of muscle firmness at rest.

Torque. The tendency of a force to rotate a body or segment around its axis; the force multiplied by the perpendicular distance from the center of rotation to the line of force application.

Transverse Plane. A line passing through the body horizontally from front to back dividing it into equal but not symmetrical upper and lower halves.

Valsalva Maneuver. Breath holding during the expiratory effort of exercise with the glottis closed, creating increased intrathoracic pressure.

Vector Quantity. A quantity possessing magnitude and direction.

Velocity. The time rate of change in position of a body with reference to a specific direction; the rate of speed.

Vertical Axis. The axis at right angles to the horizontal plane, which passes through the body vertically.

V.T.L. Video-Tape-Laboratory; a programmed instructional sequence designed to initiate immediate viewer response with actions projected on a television screen.

White Fibers. Fast-twitch muscle fibers that are capable of high-speed activity of short duration.

Work. Transference of energy through the performance of external or internal processes.

NAME INDEX

SUBJECT

Acceleration, 188
  angular, defined, 189
    formula for, 189
  efficient sports performance and, 180
  energy costs of, 180
  force and, 179
  formula for, 188
  in gymnastics, 345
  law of, 179
  linear, 188
  measurement of, 179
  muscle contraction and, 180
  velocity and, 179–180
  see also Deceleration
Accuracy:
  motor skill learning and, 156–157
  projectiles and, 258–259
  sport skill and, 398
ACH index, 117
Actin, 29–31
Adipose tissue:
  aging and, 123
  athletes, values of, 119
  cellular characteristics of, 126
  essential, 124
  girth measurements and, 119
  loss of, 125
  measurement of, 113–115, 117, 512–513
    specific gravity and, 115
  storage, 129
  types of, 124, 129
  see also Fat cells
Aerobic conditioning, 501
Age, physique compared to, 511 (fig.)
Aged:
  activities for, 525, 527
    contraindications of, 526–527, 528–529 (tab.), 530–531 (tab.)
    indications of, 526–527, 528–529 (tab.), 530–531 (tab.)
  circulorespiratory functions of, 522

conditioning program assessment for, 527
  ear impairments, 523
  fitness goals for, 527
  lifestyle and, 527
  musculoskeletal conditions of, 519
  neuromuscular response and, 526
  poor health and fitness in, 508
  reaction time and, 526
  visual impairments and, 523
  see also Aging
Agility:
  defined, 504
  sport skill and, 398
Aging:
  anthropometrical changes and, 509, 511
  balance and, 522–524
  body composition and, 511–513
  bone growth and, 509
  circulorespiratory functions and, 522
  collagen and, 509
  disk degeneration and, 509
  equilibrium and, 522–524
  exercise and, 123
  fat loss and, 513
  fitness and, 509–522
  flexibility and, 519–520
  lifestyle and, 527
  motor skills, 524–526
  movement patterns and, 508
  movement program implications for, 527, 529
  muscles and, 513–519
  muscular strength and, 513–519
  Newton's first law of motion and, 512
  physiologic changes in, 123
  posture and, 509
  sensory perception losses and, 525
  skeletal changes and, 509, 511
  spine and, 520–522
  decrease in stature and, 509
  strength loss and, 514
  see also Aged

Agonist muscles, 24, 25, 145
Alertness, sport skill and, 398
All-or-none law:
    motor neurons and, 148
    muscle contraction and, 148
    neural conduction and, 140
Alpha motor units, of nervous system, 147
American crawl, *see* Front crawl
Anaerobic conditioning, 501
Angle of incidence, 236, 238 (fig.)
Angle of obliquity, 46, 56
Angle of projection, *see* Projection angle
Angle of rebound, *see* Rebound, angle of
Ankle, 60-65
    muscles of, 63-65
Antagonist muscles, 24, 25, 145
Anthropometrical measurements, ethnic comparisons
    of, 121-122
Anthropometry, defined, 94
Anxiety:
    flexibility and, 495
    motor skills and, 495
Appendicular skeleton, parts of, 9, 18
Arachnoid mater, of spinal cord, 134
Archimedes' principle, 365
Articulations, *see* Joints
Athletic ability, performance components of, 397-399
Athletics, *see* Sports
Autonomic nervous system, 133, 137
Axes of body, definition of, 22
Axial skeleton, parts of, 9, 18
Axons, of neuron, 139

Back crawl:
    arm action in, 373-374
    arm/leg coordination of, 374 (fig.)
    breathing and, 374
    compared with front crawl, 373
    components of, 373
    conventional start, 380 (fig.)
    experimental start, 380 (fig.)
    leg action in, 374
    mechanics of, 373-374
    start, mechanics of, 379
    turn, 382
Back salto, *see* Somersault, back salto
Back stroke, *see* Back crawl
Backward somersault, *see* Somersault, back salto
Badminton:
    arm movements in, 402
    backhand stroke, 404 (fig.)
    descriptive analysis of, 401
    forehand stroke, 405 (fig.)
    kinesiological principles of, 401-405
    external mechanical analysis of, 404-405
    general motor classification of, 401-402
    internal mechanical analysis of, 403-404
    mechanical precepts of, 404-405
    muscles of lower extremity in, 403
    muscles of upper extremity in, 403
    muscular analysis of, 402

    overhead smash, 402 (fig.)
    sidearm flat drive, 402 (fig.)
    underhand service, 402 (fig.)
    see also Racquetball; Racquet sports
Balance:
    activities requiring, 292-293
    aging and, 522-524
    attaining, 291-293
    base of support and, 291-292
    center of gravity and, 291-292
    center nervous system impairments and, 295-296
    cerebral palsy and, 306-307
    control of, 294
        levers and, 294-296
        muscular strength and, 307-309
        physical activities for, 307-309
    deafness and, 297
    dynamics, defined, 287
    ears and, 296-297
    eyes and, 296-297
    injury prevention and, 488-489
    kinesthesia and, 298
    line of gravity and, 291-292
    maintenance factors of, 291
    motor dysfunctions and, 306-309
    Newton's laws of motion and, 304
    orthopedic aberrations and, 306
    sense factors and, 296-298
    sensorineural nerve loss and, 297
    somatotypes and, 293-294
    special problems of, 304-306
    sport skill and, 398
    stationary, defined, 287
    strength development and, 294
    tests of, 300-304
    vision and, 296
    in water, 304-305
    see also Equilibrium
Balance beam-walking test, 302
Balance board machine, 303-304
Balancing skills, 317
Balls, *see* Projectiles
Base of support:
    balance and, 291-292
    center of gravity and, 318
    enlargement of, gymnastics and, 350
    equilibrium and, 288-289
    in gymnastics, 345, 350
Baseball:
    base running, 415
    batting, 276 (fig.)
        mechanics of, 273-274
    catching, 585-586
    injury prevention in, 483-484
    types of injuries in, 483-484
    "Little League elbow," 484
    pitching, 260 (fig.)
    pitching injuries in, 483-484
    running between bases, mechanical elements of,
        416
    running to first base, mechanical elements of, 415

muscular analysis of, 412, 414
popularity of, 411
posture and, 415
road races in, 411
sprint racing, 413 (fig.)
track races in, 411

Deceleration, in gymnastics, 345. *See also* Acceleration
Descriptive analysis, of movement, 582
Diagonal planes, 23
Discus throwing, *see* Throwing, discus throw
Disk, intervertebrate, *see* Intervertebral disk
Displacement, equation for, 189
Distance, projectiles and, 258-259
Diving:
    absorption of momentum in, 490
    angular velocity and, 390
    backward, mechanics of, 392
    backward vs. inward, 392
    body position and, 490
    categories in competition, 383
    competition, 383
    flight arc in, 386-387
    forward running approach, 384-387
    inward, mechanics of, 392
    mechanics of, 384-392
    Newton's first law of motion and, 392
    Newton's third law of motion and, 385, 387, 390, 392
    parabolic trajectory in, 387
    performance components in, guidelines for, 383-384
    physical characteristics of divers, 383
    principles and procedures in, 489-491
    rules in competition, 383
    "saving" of dive, 390-391
    scoring in competition, 383
    somersault, mechanics of, 387
    springboard, 382-383
    standing backward takeoff, mechanics of, 391-392
    twisting, mechanics of, 387-389
    water entry in, mechanics of, 389-391
    water entry and takeoff, 490
Dura mater, of spinal cord, 134
Dynamic balance test, 302
Dynamics, defined, 175
Dyne (force), definition of, 179

Eating, physical activity and, 124-126
Ectomorphs, levers and, 257
Ectomorphy, 96-97
    athletic performance and, 121
    characteristics of, 96-97
Elbow, 77-84
    ligaments of, 78-79
    movements of, 79-80
    muscles of, 80-84
Elderly, *see* Aged
Electrogoniometer, 500-501, 545-549
    limitations of, 547

movement data provided by, 547-548
other analysis instruments and, 548
use of, 547
validity of, 547
Electromyography (EMG), 548
    application of, 548-549
    as diagnostic instrument, 548
    evaluation of muscle action by, 548
    limitations of, 548
    movement analysis and, 548-549
    use of, 548
"Elgon," *see* Electrogoniometer
EMG, *see* Electromyography
Endomorphs, levers and, 256-257
Endomorphy, 94
    athletic performance and, 120-121
    characteristics of, 94
Endurance:
    motor skill learning and, 152
    sport skill and, 398
Energy, 226
    conservation of, 227-228
    kinetic, 227
    potential, 226
Equilibrium, 286-287
    aging and, 522-524
    base of support and, 288-289
    center of gravity and, 289-290
    cerebral palsy and, 306-307
    elements of, 287-288
    injury prevention and, 488-489
    internal ear (labyrinth) and, 297
    levers and, 294-296
    line of gravity and, 290-291
    mass and, 288
    motor dysfunctions and, 306-309
    orthopedic aberrations and, 306
    proprioception and, 297-298
    in water, 304
    weight and, 288
    see also Balance
Exercise:
    aging and, 123
    effects on fat cells, 126-127
    food intake and, 124-126
    for older persons, 518-519
    for postural deviation, 453-469
    prescribing of, kinesiological analysis and, 505-506
External mechanics, 567
Exteroceptors, 141

Falling (free in air):
    distance of, formula for, 193
    force of impact and, 193
    injury factors and, 192
    kinetic energy and, 193
    time of, formula for, 193
Fast-twitch neurons, 147
    exercise performance and, 147-148
Fat (body), *see* Adipose tissue
Fat cells, size and number of, 126

summation of forces in, 339
swinging moves in, 353
swinging on parallel bars, 323–326
teaching of, 317
thigh stand, 321 (fig.)
trajectory in, 340
transfer of momentum in, 341, 343
twisting movements, 354–356
uneven parallel bars, 343
velocity in, 339–340, 345
Veronin, 356 (fig.)
visual clues in, 318
V-sit, 359 (fig.)
walkover, 327 (fig.)
Gymnastics Safety Manual, 484

Hand, 84–89
    ligaments of, 85–86
    movements of, 86
    muscles of, 88–89
Handball, 266–268
Handspring, *see* Gymnastics, handspring
Haversian system, 12
Health, inadequate, consequences of, 508
Heath-Carter somatotype rating form, 107, 109, 110,
        113, 114 (fig.)
Height and weight measurements, body composition
        and, 117–119
Height-weight charts, inadequacies of, 123–124
Higher brain (cerebral cortex), nervous system func-
        tion of, 136–137
High jumping, *see* Jumping, high jump
Hip, 45–51
    ligaments of, 46–47
    movements of, 47–48
    muscles of, 48–51
Hydroplaning, in swimming, 366–368
Hydrostatic weighing, 114–115, 117
Hypertonicity, 149
Hypertrophy, muscular, 150–151
    weight training and, 151

Ice hockey, 483
Impact, absorption of, 185
Impulse, 190
    force and, 234
Inertia, 177
    in gymnastics, 345
    law of, 177
    moment of, 191–192
Injury:
    prevention of:
        balance/equilibrium precepts and, 488–489
        base of support and, 488
        baseball, 483–484
        basketball, 479
        "crash pads" and, 475
        equipment and, 475–476
        football, 477–479
        distribution of force and, 475–476
        friction and, 489

gymnastics, 484–488
    kinesiology and, 473
    line of gravity and, 488, 489
    skiing, 479–483
    soccer, 484
    soft tissue and, 474–475
    stability and, 488
rebound precepts and, 474–476
in sports, 473
Instructional television, 536–538
Internal mechanics, 566
Interoceptors, 141
Intervertebral disk:
    anatomy of, 35
    compression ranges of, 135
    stress and bending effects on, 252
"Isolated camera" technique, described, 537

Jabbing, body levers in, 279–282
Javelin throwing, *see* Throwing, javelin throw
Javelin videotape recorder, 536
Joint Motion: Method of Measuring and Recording,
        499
Joint movements, *see* Movements
Joint receptors, 142–143
Joints:
    acromioclavicular, 67
    amphiarthrodial, 14, 16
    ankle, 60–65
    carpometacarpal, 85–86
    classification of, 13–14
    diarthrodial, 14–16
    elbow, 77–84
    foot, 60–65
    function of, 16
    hand, 84–89
    hip, 45–51
    improving mobility of, 519–520
    intercarpal, 85
    intermetacarpal, 86
    intermetatarsal, 61
    interphalangeal, 63, 86
    knee, 55–60
    linkage of, dynamic body motion and, 401
    metacarpophalangeal, 86–88
    metatarsophalangeal, 62
    movement of, factors affecting, 515
    pelvis, 32–33
    radiocarpal, 85
    radioulnar, 77–80
    range of motion in, 16, 499, 505 (tab.)
        ethnicity and, 499–500
    sequential actions of, 178–179
    shoulder, 65–77
    stability of, 16
    sternoclavicular, 66
    structure and functions of, 13–18
    synarthrodial, 14, 16
    talonavicular, 61
    thorax, 51–55
    vertebral column, 33–45

wrist, 84–89
Jumping:
  high jump:
    application of force and, 233
    predicting height achieved in, 121
  running broad jump:
    kinesiological analysis of, 572–574
    landing in, 573–574
    principles and procedures of, 572–574
    takeoff in, 572, 573
    trajectory in, 572, 573

Kill spring, 185
Kinematic analysis, 582
Kinematic movement data, instrumentation systems
    for, 545
Kinematics, 175, 217
Kinesiologic precepts:
  action of levers, 576
  agility and, 576–577
  equilibrium, 579–580
  flexibility and, 576–577
  forces affecting motion, 579
  human levers, 579
  implementation of, 578–581
  injury prevention, 577–578
  and learner, 574–578
  mechanical elements, 575–576
  neural elements, 575, 578–579
  physical fitness, 580
  physiologic elements, 575, 578–579
  postural considerations, 580
  power and, 576–577
  prevention of injury, 580–581
  somatotype and leanness, 575, 578
  stability, 578
  strength and, 576–577
  structural and physical fitness, 575
  and teacher, 578–581
  teaching of, 574–578
Kinesiology, 1, 175
  competency levels in, 4–5
  history of, 1–3
  instruction of, television and videotape for, 535
  programmed instruction and, 538–539
  study of, 4
  television equipment and, 535–536
  television techniques and, 537
Kinesiology Academy, educational guidelines and
    standards of, 5
Kinesthesia, balance and, 298
Kinesthesis, 157–158
Kinesthetic learning points, motor skill learning and,
    159–160
Kinesthetic perception, tests of, 158–159
Kinesthetic receptors, response of, 158
Kinetic analysis, of movement, 582
Kinetic energy:
  absorption of, 473–474
  formula for, 473

Kinetic movement data, instrumentation systems for,
    545
Kinetics, 175, 217
Kistler Instrument Corporation, force platform, 554
Knee, 55–60
  bursae of, 57
  injuries to, 57
  ligaments of, 57–58
  movements of, 59
  muscles of, 59–60
Knock knee, 56
Knowledge of results, 160–161
Kyphosis, described, 450

Law of acceleration, *see* Newton's second law of
    motion
Law of inertia, *see* Newton's first law of motion
"Leg raiser" (leg raises), 505–506
Leighton flexometer, 500
Leverage:
  projectiles and, 257–282
  rotary motion and, 253–256
Lever length:
  momentum and, 178
  rotary force and, 351
Levers, 244
  actions of:
    in baseball throwing, 259–261
    in batting, 274
    in discus throwing, 272–273
    in golf stroke, 268–271
    in handball underhand stroke, 267–268
    in javelin throwing, 261–264
    in one-handed push shot, 280–281
    in overarm patterns, 259
    in shot put, 281–282
    in sidearm patterns, 272
    in tennis drive, 274–275, 277–279
    in tennis serve, 264–265
    in underarm patterns, 265
    in underarm throw, 266
  anatomic:
    lengthening of, 253–254
    shortening of, 253–254
    sports success and, 253
  balance and, 294–296
  external, 245–247, 249–250
  first class, 245–247, 249
  in human body, 249–250
  internal, 245–247, 249–250
  in jabbing, 279–282
  principle of, 250–253
  projectiles and, 258–259
  second class, 245, 247
    wheel and axle, 256
  somatotypes and, 256–257
  speed and, 255–256
  sports implements as, 246
  third class, 245–247, 249–250
    muscular disadvantage of, 516 (fig.)
    wheel and axle, 256

length of, 222
resistance, 251
torque and, 222–224
Momentum, 190
  angular, 191
    conservation of, 191–192
    sports and, 192
  body mass and, 190
  conservation of, 190–191
  distance and, 356–357
  in gymnastics, 339–340, 351, 356–357
  impulse and, 190
  lever length and, 178, 343, 345
  mass and, 177–178
  rotary, 178
  in sports skills, 178
  techniques for increasing, 178
  transfer of, 193–194, 341, 343
Motion:
  angular vs. linear, 176
  circular, 228
    control of, 230
  curvilinear, 176
  description of, 175
  human, Newton's laws applied to, 177–185
  linear, 176
  negatively accelerated, 188
  Newton's first law of, 177
  Newton's second law of, 179
  Newton's third law of, 182, 184
  principles and concepts of, programmed instruction
    for, 538–540, 543–544
  rotary, 176
    leverage and, 253–256
  translatory, 176
  twisting, principles and procedures of, 197–210,
    254–356
  types of, 175
  uniform, 186
  uniformly accelerated, 188
  variable, 186
  variable accelerated, 188
  see also Movement
Motor activity, levels of, 135
Motor dysfunctions:
  balance and, 306–309
  cerebral palsy and, 306–307
Motor endplate, of neuron, 139
Motor learning, *see* Motor skills, learning of
Motor performance:
  anatomical aspects of, 399
  kinesiological construct of, categories of, 399–400
  measurement of, 225–228
  mechanical aspects of, 399–400
  mechanical laws and principles of, 399–400
  reflexes and, 143–146
"Motor sense," 158
Motor skill learning, *see* Motor skills, learning of
Motor skills:
  ability to learn, 525
  analysis of, 399–400

anxiety and, 495
cerebral cortex and, 585–586
classification of, 163–166
closed, 163–165
continuous, 165–166
discrete, 165–166
execution of, 570
fine, 166
gross, 166
growth and changes in, 153
kinesiologic analyses of, 566, 567–574
learning of, 151–163, 566, 585–586
  age constraints and, 525
  defined, 151
  development of, 152
  effects of distributive practice on, 155–156
  effects of mass practice on, 155–156
  effect of speed and accuracy on, 156–157
  facilitators for, 153–157
  feedback and, 157–162
  generality and, 154
  kinesthetic learning points and, 159–160
  knowledge of mechanical principles and,
    161–162
  knowledge of results and, 160–161
  manual guidance and, 162
  maturation and, 152–153
  mechanical guidance and, 162–163
  mechanoreceptors and, 585–586
  mental practice and, 157
  open, 163–165
  part method, 154
  progression and, 153
  progressive nature of, 586
  reaction time and, 163
  specificity and, 154
  whole method, 154
outline of, 400–401
performance of, age constraints and, 525
starting positions of, 567–570
teaching of, 566, 585
  mechanical principles and, 161–162
Motor unit, 146–148
Movement:
  effectiveness of, 581
  efficiency of, 581–585
  electrical analysis of, 545
  force and, 581
  human, rhythmic patterns of, 213
  human performance and, 5
  kinesiological analysis of motor performance in,
    538–540, 543–544
  mechanical analysis of, 545
  mechanical principles and, 581–585
  optical analysis of, 545
  quantitative analysis of, 544–554
    kinematic methods, 544–545
    kinetic methods, 545
  see also Motion
Movement analysis:
  cinematography and, 549–552

efficiency of, 582
electrogoniometer and, 545–549
electromyography and, 548–549
film analysis and, 551–552
force platform and, 552–554
instruments for, 544–554
kinematic, 582
kinetic, 582
mechanical, 582
television and, 534–538
videotape and, 534–538
Movements:
abduction, 17, 47, 69, 86
adduction, 17, 47, 69, 86
backward tilt, 32, 69
circumduction, 18, 40, 47–48, 69, 86, 87
decreased inclination, 32
depression, 18, 69
dorsiflexion, 17, 63
downward rotation, 18, 69
elbow, 79–80
elevation, 18, 69
eversion, 18, 52, 63
extension, 17, 38, 47, 59, 69, 79, 86, 87
fingers, 86
flexion, 17, 47, 59, 63, 69, 79, 86, 87
foot, 63
forward tilt, 32, 69
hand, 86
hip, 47–48
horizontal extension, 17, 69
horizontal flexion, 17, 69
horizontal hyperextension, 17
hyperabduction, 17
hyperadduction, 17, 86
hyperextension, 17, 38, 47, 69, 79, 86, 87
hyperflexion, 69, 86
increased inclination, 32
interphalangeal joints, 87–88
inversion, 18, 63
inward rotation, 18, 69
knee, 59
lateral flexion, 17, 38–39
lateral rotation, 18
lateral tilt, 32
lateral twist, 32
medial rotation, 18
metacarpophalangeal joints, 86–88
opposition, 86
outward rotation, 18, 69
pelvic, 32–33
pronation, 18, 63, 79
protraction, 18, 69
radial flexion, 17, 86
radioulnar, 79–80
reduction, 18
repetitive angular, 175
retraction, 18, 69
rotation, 17, 32, 39–40, 48, 59
scapula, 69
shoulder-arm mechanism, 69

supination, 18, 63, 79–80
thorax, 52
thumb, 86–88
ulnar flexion, 17, 86, 87
upward rotation, 18, 69
vertebral column, 38–40
wrist, 86
Movement time, 163
Muscle contraction, 24, 25–27
all-or-none law and, 148
angle of pull and, 150
concentric, 26
eccentric, 26
force-length relationship in, 149–150
force-velocity relationship of, 150
gradation of, 148
isometric, 26
isotonic, 26
maximum force, 25
microscopic muscle structure and, 31–32
rapid tension, 26
slow tension, 26
static, 26
types of, 25
Muscle fibers:
hypertrophy and, 150–151
microscopic structure of, 27–32
pale, 27
red, 27
Muscle receptors, 141–142
Muscles:
action of, 25
aging and, 513–519
agonist, 24, 25, 145
amplitude of, 149
angle of pull of, 150
ankle, 63–65
antagonist, 24, 25, 145
arrangement of, 24
attachments of, 24
contractility of, 149
contraction of, see Muscle contraction
described:
abductor digiti minimi, 65, 89
abductor hallucis, 65
abductor pollicis brevis, 89
abductor pollicis longus, 88
adductor brevis, 51
adductor hallucis, 65
adductor longus, 51
adductor magnus, 51
adductor pollicis, 89
biceps branchii, 76
biceps femoris, 49
brachialis, 80
brachioradialis, 80–81
coracobrachialis, 76
deltoid, 69–71
diaphragm, 52–53
dorsal interossei, 65, 89
erector spinae, 43–44, 54

Reaction board method, center of gravity and, 298-299
Reaction time, 163
    motor skill learning and, 163
    sport skill and, 398-399
Rebound:
    angle of, 236, 238 (fig.)
    back spin, 239
    clockwise spin, 239
    coefficient of restitution and, 235-236, 237 (tab.)
    counterclockwise spin, 239
    forces of, 234-236
    left spin, 239
    momentum and, 235
    right spin, 239
    spin and, 238-239
    surface resistance and, 235
    top spin, 239
Receptors:
    balance, 143
    cutaneous, 143
    inner ear, 143
    joint, 142-143
    kinesthetic, 158
    muscle, 141-142
    for muscle sense, 141
    for muscle tension, 141
    neck, 143
    for pressure, 143
    sensory, 140-143
        head movements and, 143
    skin, 142-143
Reciprocal inhibition, 25
    as reflex mechanism, 145
Reciprocal innervation, as reflex mechanism, 145
Reciprocal ponderal index, 113, 116 (tab.)
Rectilinear motion, see Motion, translatory
Red muscle fibers, 27
Reflex:
    conditioned, 144-145
    crossed extensor, 24
    extensor thrust, 144
    innate, 143-144
    knee jerk, 136
    motor performance and, 143-146
    myotatic, 143
    postural, 145-146
        effect of aging on, 146
    spinal cord level, 135-136
    stretch, 143
    types of, 143
    upright posture, 136
    withdrawal, 136, 144
Repetitive angular movements, 175
Resistance moment arm, 251
Resolution of forces, 220
Reuther board, use of, 339-340
Rhythm pattern, sport skill and, 398
Ribs, 51-52
Rising on toes, mechanics of, 247-249
Rotary force, balancing lifts and, 319

Rotation:
    axes of, 19
    radius of, 180-182, 228-229
    speed of, 180-181, 353-354
Rotator cuff, 76
Rotatory force, lever length and, 351
Round shoulders, 451
    exercises for, 458-459, 460 (fig.)
    muscular aspects of posture and, 444
Round upper back, 451-452
    exercises for, 461, 463, 464 (fig.), 465 (fig.)
Ruffini's corpuscles, 142
Running:
    compared to walking, 432
    mechanics of, 432-433
    one hundred yard dash, 567, 568
    spring, mechanics of, 433
    sprint start, 584-585
Running broad jump, see Jumping, running broad jump

Sagittal-horizontal axis, 22
Sagittal plane, 19
Salto, see Somersault
Scalar quantities, 217-218
Scapula, 65
    movements of, 69
Scoliosis, 444-445, 446 (fig.)
    C curve, 452
        exercises for, 463, 465, 466 (fig.), 467 (fig.)
    described, 452-453
    muscular aspects of posture and, 444-445
    S curve, 452-453
        exercises for, 466-469
Selected Motor Performance in Human Movement:
    A Kinesiological Analysis, 538, 539 (n.), 556
Senior Olympics Program, 524
Sense organs, 141. See also Receptors, sensory
Sensory attention, sport skill and, 398
Sheldon somatotype, 105, 107
Shot put, see Throwing, shot put
Shoulder, 65-77
    muscles of, 69-77
Shoulder-arm mechanism, 65-77
    ligaments of, 67-69
    movements of, 69
Shoulder blades, protruding, 451
    exercises for, 459, 460 (fig.), 461, 462 (fig.), 463 (fig.)
Shoulder girdle, see Shoulder-arm mechanism
Sideward leap test, 303
Sit-ups:
    force aspects and performance of, 223-224
    mechanics of, 518
Sitting, as postural variation, 428
Skeleton:
    motor skill learning and maturation of, 152
    structural aspects of, 9-13
Skiing injuries, 479-480
    mechanics of, 480-481
    prevention in, 479-483

Skill learning, *see* Motor skills, learning of
Skill outline, analysis of motor skills and, 400–401
Skin receptors, *see* Receptors, skin
Skinfold thickness,
    body composition and, 117–119
    ethnic comparisons of, 121–122
    measurement of, 512–513
        recommended body areas for, 513
Slow-truth neurons, 147
    exercise performance and, 147–148
Slug (force), definition of, 179
Soccer, injury prevention in, 484
Somatic nervous system, 133, 137
Somatotypes, 94–98
    athletic performance and, 119–121
    of champion athletes, 101, 104 (tab.), 106 (fig.),
        107 (fig.), 108 (fig.), 109 (fig.), 110 (fig.),
        111 (fig.), 112 (fig.), 113 (fig.)
    comparative studies of, 101–103
    crural index and, 99–100
    determination of, 105, 107, 109, 110, 113
        Cureton, 113, 115 (tab.)
        Heath-Carter, 107, 109, 110, 113, 114 (fig.)
        Sheldon, 105, 107
        skinfold measurements and, 107, 109
    effect of age on, 122–123
    effect of exercise on, 122
    endurance and, 98
    ethnic considerations, 121–122
    of female athletes, 101, 104 (tab.), 112 (fig.)
    football and, 100–101
    gymnastics and, 320
    levers and, 256–257
    of male athletes, 101, 104 (tab.), 106 (fig.), 107
        (fig.), 108 (fig.), 109 (fig.), 110 (fig.), 111
        (fig.), 113 (fig.)
    mixed, 97–98
    of nonathletes, 111 (fig.)
    obese classifications of, 123–127
    of Olympic athletes, 120
    racial considerations, 121–122
    skill performance and, 98–105
    somatochart of, 101, 105 (fig.)
    somatoplots of, 101, 106 (fig.), 107 (fig.), 108
        (fig.), 109 (fig.), 110 (fig.), 111 (fig.), 112
        (fig.), 113 (fig.)
    sport counseling and, 103, 105
    strength and, 98–99, 120
    weight lifting and, 98–99
    see also Ectomorphy; Endomorphy; Mesomorphy
Somersault:
    back salto:
        back handspring into, 328–334 (fig.)
        principles and procedures of, 212–213
        spotting for, 337–339
    back salto with twist:
        action-reaction method, 201
        direct method, 197–199, 199–206 (fig.)
    front salto, 348–350 (fig.)
        principles and procedures of, 211–212

    direct method, 207–211 (fig.)
    injuries in, 487
    landing and, 212
    lift-off and, 212
    principles and procedures of, 210–213
    rotation and, 212
    thrust in, 184
    torque and, 210–211
    with twist, action-reaction method, 199–201
Somersault dismounts, time of release in, 340–341
Sony Porta-Pac video system, 535, 536 (fig.)
Spasticity, *see* Motor dysfunctions
"Spearing," 478–479
Specific gravity:
    body fat and, 115
    formula for, 115
    hydrostatic weighing and, 115
Speed, 186
    motor skill learning and, 156–157
    sport skill and, 398
Spiking, *see* Volleyball spike
Spin:
    back, 237–238
    clockwise, 238
    counterclockwise, 238
    forces of, 236–238
        functions of, 236
    left, 238, 239 (fig.)
    rebound and, 238–239
    right, 238–239 (fig.)
    top, 237–238
Spinal column, *see* Spine
Spinal cord, 134
    extrinsic support factors of, 135
    intrinsic support factors of, 135
    membranes of, 134
    nervous system function of, 135–136
    reflex activity of, 135–136
Spine, 33–45
    aging effects on, 520–522
    aging and stability of, 521–522
    body activities and, 521–522
    bones of, 34
    curves of, 34
    effect of leverage on, 521 (fig.)
    effect of standing erect on, 423–425
    force of gravity and, 520–521
    injuries to, 135
    ligaments of, 36–38
    mechanical forces affecting, 520–522
    movements of, 38–40
    muscles of, 40–45
Spinning, *see* Motion, rotary
Sports:
    analysis of skills in, 401–419
    characteristics of activity in, 397
    efficient performance in acceleration and, 180
    performance:
        analysis of, 399–400
        body density and, 119–121

internal mechanical analysis of, 407
kinesiological principles of, 405–411
leverage in, 410–411
motion in, 407–408
motor classification of, 405
muscular analysis of, 405
stability and, 408–410

strength and, 405–406
Wrist, 84–89
  carpal bones of, 84
  ligaments of, 85–86
  movements of, 86
  muscles of, 88–89